Children with Down syndrome

Children with Down syndrome

A developmental perspective

Edited by

DANTE CICCHETTI
University of Rochester

MARJORIE BEEGHLY
Harvard Medical School and
The Children's Hospital, Boston

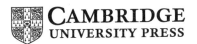

CAMBRIDGE
UNIVERSITY PRESS

Published by the Press Syndicate of the University of Cambridge
The Pitt Building, Trumpington Street, Cambridge CB2 1RP
40 West 20th Street, New York, NY 10011-4211, USA
10 Stamford Road, Oakleigh, Melbourne 3166, Australia

© Cambridge University Press 1990

First published 1990
Reprinted 1993, 1995

Printed in the United States of America

Library of Congress Cataloging-in-Publication Data is available

British Library Cataloging in Publication applied for

ISBN 0-521-37458-8 hardback
ISBN 0-521-38667-5 paperback

Contents

v

Contributors

Marjorie Beeghly, Ph.D.
Harvard Medical School and Scientific
  Director
Child Development Unit
The Children's Hospital
Boston, MA

Jiri Berger, Ph.D.
Helgamagrastraeti 13
600 Akureyri
Iceland

Dante Cicchetti, Ph.D.
Professor
Departments of Psychology and
  Psychiatry
University of Rochester
Director, Mt. Hope Family Center
Rochester, NY

Keith A. Crnic, Ph.D.
Department of Psychology
The Pennsylvania State University
State College, PA

Carl J. Dunst, Ph.D.
Human Development Research and
  Training Institute
West Carolina Center
Morganton, NC

Anne E. Fowler, Ph.D.
Haskins Laboratories
New Haven, CT

Jody Ganiban
Department of Psychology
University of Rochester
Mt. Hope Family Center
Rochester, NY

Robert M. Hodapp, Ph.D.
Department of Psychology
Yale University
New Haven, CT

Claire Kopp, Ph.D.
Department of Psychology
University of California at Los Angeles
Los Angeles, CA

Carolyn B. Mervis, Ph.D.
Department of Psychology
Emory University
Atlanta, GA

Bedonna Weiss-Perry, Ph.D.
Children's Memorial Hospital
Chicago, IL

Felicisima C. Serafica, Ph.D.
Department of Psychology
The Ohio State University
Columbus, OH

Donna Spiker, Ph.D.
Infant Health and Development
  Program
Stanford University
Palo Alto, CA

Sheldon Wagner, Ph.D.
Department of Psychology
University of Rochester
Rochester, NY

Edward Zigler, Ph.D.
Sterling Professor of Psychology
Yale University
New Haven, CT

Preface

Beginning with the writings of Esquirol (1838), who provided the first description of a child with Down syndrome, and John Langdon Down, whose article "Observations on an Ethnic Classification of Idiots" (1866) describes some of the characteristics of the children who are his namesakes, theorizing and research about Down syndrome have proliferated in the scientific literature (see Booth, 1985; Gibson, 1978; and Rynders & Pueschel, 1982, for historical reviews). Although earlier explorations into unraveling the complexities of this condition were conducted primarily by researchers interested in its biomedical aspects, increasingly the study of Down syndrome has become a multidisciplinary endeavor. As the most common organic form of mental retardation, it is not surprising that Down syndrome has captured the attention of so many talented research investigators, educators, and clinicians.

Down syndrome occurs in approximately 1 out of every 600 live births (Hook, 1982), resulting in nearly 7,000 infants in the United States and 1,000 in the United Kingdom born with Down syndrome each year (Wishart, 1988). Down syndrome arises from an abnormality on chromosome 21 (Thuline & Pueschel, 1982). Chromosome pair 21 is the smallest of the 23 human chromosome pairs, possessing only about 1.5% of the total genetic material. Moreover, gene-mapping studies have revealed that only 10% to 20% of chromosome 21, the 21q 22 band on the long arm, is involved in Down syndrome (Patterson, 1987a, 1987b; Patterson et al., 1985; Smith, 1985). Nonetheless, the presence of an additional copy of this small chromosome exerts a profound impact on the developmental biology and psychology of Down syndrome (Benda, 1960, 1969; Breg, 1977; Cicchetti & Ganiban, in press; Cicchetti & Pogge-Hesse, 1982; Coyle, Oster-Granite, & Gearhart, 1986; Epstein, 1986; Lane & Stratford, 1985; Nadel, 1988; Penrose & Smith, 1966; Pueschel & Rynders, 1982; Smith & Berg, 1976).

Most cases of Down syndrome are caused by a meiotic non-disjunction of autosomal chromosome pair 21, resulting in the triplication of the entire 21st chromosome (Lejeune, Grautier, & Turpin, 1959). Approximately 95% of all cases of Down syndrome are characterized by this autosomal trisomy of the 21st chromosome; hence, in the literature Down syndrome has been referred to as "trisomy 21." In addition to the trisomy 21 type, there are two other cytogenetic subtypes of Down syndrome. Of these cases, 4% to 6% manifest translocation of a portion of chromosome 21 to another chromosome. Furthermore, 1% to 4% are a mosaic of normal and trisomic cells as an outcome of a non-disjunction that occurs during early embryogenesis (Thuline & Pueschel, 1982).

Major congenital anomalies, involving virtually all senses and each organ system, are present in one-half of infants born with Down syndrome (see Cicchetti & Beeghly, Chapter 2, this volume; Coyle et al., 1986; Lane & Stratford, 1985; Pueschel & Rynders, 1982; Smith & Berg, 1976). Of all individuals with Down syndrome, 1% develop leukemia, a rate between 20 and 50 times greater than that found in the normal population (Coyle et al., 1986). While 30 to 40 years ago only 50% of all infants with Down syndrome survived infancy, recent medical advances (particularly in cardiology and immunology) have resulted in a significant increase in the life expectancy of persons with this condition. Because many individuals with Down syndrome now survive into their 50s and 60s, the prevalence of Down syndrome has increased fourfold during the course of the 1980s (Coyle et al., 1986; Hook, 1982; Wishart, 1988). In concert with these biomedical breakthroughs, the findings of recent psychological and educational investigations have led to increased expectations for persons with Down syndrome (Lane & Stratford, 1985; Pueschel, Tingey, Rynders, Crocker, & Crutcher, 1987; Rynders, Spiker, & Horrobin, 1978).

Important discoveries in neurobiology likewise have occurred within the past several decades (Coyle et al., 1986). Among the most notable is the finding that the majority of adults with Down syndrome develop pervasive Alzheimer-like brain pathology by their mid-30s. Importantly, only about one-third of all individuals with Down syndrome manifest symptoms of a clinically diagnosed dementia (Thase, 1988). Thus, future investigations of the mechanisms that underlie the uncoupling of the Alzheimer-like neuropathology and dementia in Down syndrome could contribute greatly to the understanding of the ontogenesis and pathogenesis of Alzheimer's syndrome.

As a direct consequence of these advances and changes, it has become increasingly critical to bring a life-span developmental perspective to bear in planning medical, educational, and psychological interventions for children with Down syndrome and their families. During the course of the past several decades, investigators have begun to employ a developmental perspective in their studies of infants and children with Down syndrome. Especially throughout the 1970s and 1980s, major advances have been achieved in several areas of the developmental psychology of Down syndrome, most prominently in the perceptual, social, emotional, cognitive, and representational domains. Contemporaneously, developmental neuroscientists have made significant progress in unraveling many of the genetic, biochemical, and neurophysiological mysteries of Down syndrome. As a consequence, we are approaching the point where a comprehensive developmental theory of Down syndrome may be formulated.

A unifying theme of this volume involves the premise that an organismic–organizational developmental approach can be applied to the study of any discipline (e.g., education, neuroscience, pediatrics, psychiatry, and psychology) and to any population, normal or otherwise atypical. Specifically, the contributors to this book believe that despite the constitutional and biomedical problems described earlier, children with Down syndrome can be studied through this developmental framework. The particular thesis espoused is that the study of children with Down syndrome from such a developmental perspective will increase our knowledge of this condition, thereby minimizing the generation of stereotypes about it and maximizing our understanding of Down syndrome from a lawfully organized viewpoint. Conversely, through the study of Down syndrome from a developmental perspective, advances can occur in the formulation of a truly integrative theory of human development. Such a study also highlights the respective roles of biological, perceptual–cognitive, linguistic, social, emotional, and representational factors in the developmental process. Furthermore, the study of Down syndrome permits us to identify alternative pathways or processes to adaptive and maladaptive outcomes. Finally, to the extent that we now possess a great deal of information on the genetic, biochemical, physiological, and psychological aspects of infants and children with Down syndrome, the developmentalist interested in this condition is in the unique and enviable position of examining the interaction between heredity and environment on the developing organism.

Advances such as these also can be instrumental in informing and guiding methods of intervention. Efforts influenced by developmental principles in psychology, education, and biology are more likely to result in informed knowledge about how best to help children with Down syndrome and their families. Too often parents of these children are presented with inaccurate information that builds false hopes and ultimately causes grave disappointment. Adherence to the developmental perspective should lead to the implementation of timed, guided, and appropriate forms of intervention.

In this volume, authors have contributed theoretically informed chapters on the state of current knowledge of the various domains of psychological development in infants and children with Down syndrome. Where the data base permits, the biological systems that play important roles in the ontogenesis of these psychological domains are discussed. Additionally, a comprehensive treatment of temperament in Down syndrome and its relation to biological and psychological processes, is provided. Furthermore, interventions for children with Down syndrome are reviewed from a developmental perspective. Finally, throughout the volume, suggestions for future research are suggested. We believe that many exciting ideas have been generated by the contributors to this volume and eagerly anticipate the new wave of multidisciplinary developmentally guided research on Down syndrome across the life-span.

We would like to explain our decision to employ ''Down'' rather than ''Down's'' throughout this volume. For several decades, parents of children having this condition have advocated that the term *Down syndrome* be utilized because of their concern that their children were being viewed as simple extensions of the syndrome they possessed. By adopting the terminology of the parents, we are expressing our support for the individuality of the children, despite their shared syndrome. We believe that agreeing with the philosophy of these parents, as well as that of the many scientists in the area who also have begun to use this term, is essential.

On a more personal note, we would like to thank all of the children with Down syndrome and their parents who have participated in our research in Pittsburgh, Minneapolis–St. Paul, and Boston over the years. We feel privileged to have gotten to know them (some extremely well), and feel that our lives are richer as a result. We wish them continuing happiness in their lives together. To them, as well as to all children with Down syndrome and their families, we dedicate this book.

We would like to acknowledge the grants that we received from the John D. and Catherine T. MacArthur Foundation Network on Early Childhood, the March of Dimes Birth Foundation, the Milton Fund of the Harvard University Medical School, and the Spencer Foundation. Special thanks are due to Greg Bialecki, Judy Bigelow, Mary Breitenbucher, Fran Bridges, Cindy Carter, Jody Ganiban, Michelle Gersten, Linda Mans-Wagener, Dan Nichols, Bedonna Weiss-Perry, and Mark Shinagel for their assistance with data collection and coding over the years of our longitudinal studies. In addition, we would like to thank Victoria Gill for her superb secretarial assistance throughout the preparation of this volume.

Dante Cicchetti would like to acknowledge the support he received from the Norman Tishman Associate Professorship that he held at Harvard University. Dante would also like to thank his mentors and friends Drs. William Charlesworth, Alan Crocker, Christine Cronk, Norman Garmezy, Paul Meehl, John Rynders, Sigfried Pueschel, Felicisima Serafica, Alexander Siegel, George Smith, Donna Spiker, Alan Sroufe, and Edward Zigler for their guidance, support, and inspiration over the years – and to single out Linda Mans-Wagener for her superlative efforts, input, support, encouragement, and assistance on many of these projects. Without her brains, energy, and dedication, we would be much further behind in our knowledge of Down syndrome. Finally, Dante would like to extend his heartfelt thanks to his mother, Dolores, his grandmother, Josephine, and his colleagues and friends, Dorothy Dittman, Heidi Mitke, Sheree Toth, and Jennifer White, for their concern, wise counsel, and support.

Marjorie Beeghly would like to thank her mentors and friends, Drs. Elizabeth Bates and Inge Bretherton, for their support and guidance. In addition, Marjorie wishes to acknowledge her husband, Glenn K. Wasek, for his love, patience, and support.

Dante Cicchetti
Marjorie Beeghly

References

Benda, C. (1960). *The child with mongolism*. New York: Grune & Stratton.
Benda, C. (1969). *Down's syndrome: Mongolism and its management*. New York: Grune & Stratton.

Booth, T. (1985). Labels and their consequences. In D. Lane & B. Stratford (Eds.), *Current approaches to Down's syndrome*. New York: Praeger.

Breg, W. (1977). A review of recent progress in research. *Pathobiological Annuals, 7,* 257–303.

Cicchetti, D., & Ganiban, J. (in press). The organization and coherence of developmental processes in infants and children with Down syndrome. In R. M. Hodapp, J. A. Burack, & E. Zigler (Eds.), *Issues in the developmental approach to mental retardation*. New York: Cambridge University Press.

Cicchetti, D., & Pogge-Hesse, P. (1982). Possible contributions of the study of organically retarded persons to developmental theory. In E. Zigler & D. Balla (Eds.), *Mental retardation: The developmental–difference controversy*. Hillsdale, NJ: Erlbaum.

Coyle, J., Oster-Granite, M., & Gearhart, J. (1986). The neurobiologic consequences of Down syndrome. *Brain Research Bulletin, 16,* 773–787.

Down, J. L. (1866). Observations on an ethnic classification of idiots. *London Hospital, Clinical Lecture and Report, 3,* 259–262.

Epstein, C. J. (Ed.) (1986). *The neurobiology of Down syndrome*. New York: Raven.

Esquirol, J. (1838). *Des maladies mentales considérées sous les rapports médical, hygienique et médico-legal*. 2 vols. Paris: Bailliere.

Gibson, D. (Ed.) (1978). *Down's Syndrome: the psychology of mongolism*. Cambridge: Cambridge University Press.

Hook, E. (1982). The epidemiology of Down syndrome. In S. Pueschel & J. Rynders (Eds.), *Down syndrome: advances in biomedicine and the behavioral sciences*. Cambridge, MA: Ware Press.

Lane, D., & Stratford, B. (Eds.) (1985). *Current approaches to Down's syndrome*. New York: Praeger.

Lejeune, J., Gautier, M., & Turpin, R. (1959). Etudes des chromosomes somatiques de neuf enfants mongoliens. *C.R. Acad. Sci., 248,* 1721.

Nadel, L. (Ed.) (1988). *The psychobiology of Down syndrome*. Cambridge, MA: MIT Press.

Patterson, D. (1987a). Genetic mapping in chromosome 21 and its implications for Down's syndrome and other diseases. *Somatic Cell and Molecular Genetics, 13,* 365–371.

Patterson, D. (1987b). The causes of Down syndrome. *Scientific American, 257,* 42–48.

Patterson, D., et al. (1985). Molecular analysis of chromosome 21 using somatic cell hybrids. *Annals of the New York Academy of Sciences, 450,* 109–120.

Penrose, L., & Smith, G. (1966). *Down's anomaly*. Boston: Little, Brown.

Pueschel, S., & Rynders, J. (Eds.) (1982). *Down syndrome: Advances in biomedicine and the behavioral sciences*. Cambridge, MA: Ware Press.

Pueschel, S., Tingey, C., Rynders, J., Crocker, A., & Crutcher, D. (Eds.) (1987). *New perspectives on Down syndrome*. Baltimore: Brookes.

Rynders, J., & Pueschel, S. (1982). History of Down syndrome. In S. Pueschel & J. Rynders (Eds.), *Down syndrome: Advances in biomedicine and the behavioral sciences*. Cambridge, MA: Ware Press.

Rynders, J., Spiker, D., & Horrobin, J. (1978). Underestimating the educability of Down's syndrome children: Examination of methodological problems in recent literature. *American Journal of Mental Deficiency, 82,* 440–448.

Smith, G. (Ed.) (1985). *Molecular structure of the number 21 chromosome and Down syndrome* [Special issue of the *Annals of the New York Academy of Science, 450*].

Smith, G., & Berg, J. (1976). *Down's anomaly*. New York: Churchill Livingstone.

Thase, M. (1988). The relationship between Down syndrome and Alzheimer's disease. In L. Nadel (Ed.), *The psychobiology of Down syndrome*. Cambridge, MA: MIT Press.

Thuline, H., & Pueschel, S. (1982). Cytogenetics in Down syndrome. In S. Pueschel & J. Rynders (Eds.), *Down syndrome: Advances in biomedicine and the behavioral sciences*. Cambridge, MA: Ware Press.

Wishart, J. (1988). Early learning in infants and young children with Down syndrome. In L. Nadel (Ed.), *The psychobiology of Down syndrome*. Cambridge, MA: MIT Press.

1 Applying the developmental perspective to individuals with Down syndrome

Robert M. Hodapp and Edward Zigler

The application of the developmental perspective to atypical populations is characterized by two historical trends. First, the developmental perspective has itself evolved, expanding from its original focus on cognitive and linguistic development to the recent focus on the whole child (Zigler & Hodapp, in press) and the environment in which that child develops (Bronfenbrenner, 1979; Sameroff, 1975). Second, workers have gradually applied the developmental perspective to a wider array of clinical populations (Cicchetti, 1984a). The result is that neither theory nor application has remained static: an expanding theory has increasingly been applied to more varied populations.

In this brief historical review, we attempt to chart trends both in developmental theory and in its application to retarded individuals. After describing the shift from "classical" to "expanded" developmental perspectives, we attempt to show the progression in the application of developmental theory, first to retarded persons not demonstrating organic symptomology (the so-called familial or cultural–familial retarded), later to individuals with Down syndrome and other organic etiologies. Throughout these discussions, we emphasize the strengths and weaknesses of the developmental approach to an understanding of Down syndrome and other retarded individuals.

Classical and expanded developmental perspectives

Classical developmental theory

Any list of developmental theorists must begin with Jean Piaget and Heinz Werner. Even though Piaget is currently undergoing a series of criticisms (e.g., Fischer, 1980; Flavell, 1982), while Werner has experienced a rediscovery by the field (e.g., Wapner & Kaplan, 1983; White, 1984), both are undeniably the developmental

The preparation of this chapter was supported by grant HD 03008 from the National Institute of Child Health and Human Development. We would like to thank Dante Cicchetti for his comments on an earlier draft of this chapter. The assistance of David Evans and Nancy Hall is also gratefully acknowledged.

theorists *par excellence*. A brief overview of the basic principles of both men is therefore in order, if only to delimit the proper domain of "developmental psychology" when we later discuss its expanded version.

According to Piaget and Werner, development involves two processes: differentiation and hierarchic integration. Differentiation is the process by which an organism evolves various parts that are functionally or structurally distinct. As opposed to the undifferentiated mass of cells present in the first few days after conception, for example, the human neonate is characterized by many different organs, each with its own structure and function. The second, and complementary, process is hierarchic integration, or the organization of these separate parts within the structure of the overall organism. In our embryological metaphor, each organ comes increasingly under the control of the brain. Thus, while differentiation leads to the emergence of parts that are distinct and separate, hierarchic integration ensures the organization of such disparate parts in the (now more complex) organism.

Examples of differentiation and hierarchic integration are ubiquitous as the child matures. In early language development, infants first communicate their needs via "holophrases" in which one word, or a word plus a gesture, connotes the child's entire meaning (Greenfield & Smith, 1976). Over time, children develop in their communicative abilities, as an increasing vocabulary of individual words (differentiation) becomes organized into sentences (hierarchic integration) (Brown, 1973; Werner & Kaplan, 1963). Through the use of sentences, children are able to speak of objects and events not in the "here and now," greatly expanding their communicative capabilities. In cognitive development, too, we see instances of differentiation and hierarchic integration. Piaget (1952) has delineated the ways in which neonatal reflexes eventually become the differentiated sensorimotor skills characteristic of later infancy; such skills are then used by the child in combination in order to operate on the external world. Other examples could also be mentioned; the point is simply that increasing differentiation and hierarchic integration can be seen in various domains as the child matures.

Three additional ideas are central to both Piagetian and Wernerian (i.e., classical) views of development. First, classical developmental theory postulates an active organism. According to this view, "the organism is inherently and spontaneously active; the organism is the source of acts, rather than being activated by external or peripheral forces" (Overton & Reese, 1973, 70). This view contrasts sharply with behaviorist and other mechanistic views, which conceptualize the child as the passive recipient of, or respondent to, external stimuli. As summarized by Overton and Reese (1973). "In its ideal form the reactive organism model characterizes the organism as inherently at rest, and active only as a result of external forces" (p. 69). Such views are incompatible with developmental theories, in either their classical or expanded versions.

Second, development is thought to be characterized by regular and invariant sequences, all leading toward a clear endpoint. Zigler (1963) speaks of "the orderliness, sequentiality, and apparent lawfulness of the transition taking place from [birth] to the attainment of maturity" (p. 344), and it is this regular acquisition of progressively more adaptive skills that allows developmental theorists to guide practitioners and researchers. Thus, in Piagetian theory, the child traverses a series of stages in invariant order, beginning with sensorimotor modes of thinking, ending with the acquisition of formal operational thought. In Werner and Kaplan's (1963) analysis of symbol formation, the sequence of development is less well-articulated, but a clear endpoint (the "contemplation of objects") is still present. In short, although different developmental theorists speak of different sequences and endpoints (depending on the domain of interest), each postulates the orderly acquisition of progressively more difficult skills, leading to an endpoint considered to be most adaptive.

Third, development consists of change in internal mental structures, not in behaviors alone. Indeed, behavioral change is thought to reflect changes in underlying mental structures. Thus, the language-using child is thought to be demonstrating an understanding of semantic and grammatical rules when uttering complex sentences. Similarly, the infant who uncovers a ball in an object permanence test, laughs when the mother hides herself in peek-a-boo, or cries when mother leaves the room in Ainsworth's "strange situation" is in each instance considered to be demonstrating an understanding of "object permanence"; that is, the child realizes that objects continue to exist even though out of sight. Again, such a view contrasts sharply with the behaviorist emphasis on the performance of behavior in the absence, or at least without specification, of the nature of the child's internal mental structures. In developmental theory, behavior reflects underlying mental structures.

These three major tenets – active organism, invariant acquisition of progressively more adaptive skills, and changes in internal mental structures – could be considered the strengths of classical developmental theory. These are features that characterize all developmental theories, both "classical" and "expanded" versions. However, classical developmental theory is also characterized by several omissions. We now turn to these inadequately specified areas and to their elaborations in expanded developmental theory.

Expanded developmental theory

The two major contributions of expanded developmental theory involve its emphasis on the "whole child" and its elaboration of both the temporal and ecological aspects of the child's environment. These two contributions help to round out classical developmental theory, but they do not replace it. As we hope to demonstrate below, the issues of development in noncognitive areas and the nature of the environment were at times addressed by Piaget and Werner. The contribution of recent developmentalists has primarily consisted of more comprehensive treatments of both topics.

The first contribution of expanded developmental theory involves the examination of development in areas other than cognition or language. Classical developmental theory, although amply detailing achievements in the cognitive and linguistic domains, has generally neglected the areas of social, emotional, motivational, and personality development. For Piaget, this lack of attention to noncognitive areas is partly due to his overriding interest in cognitive development (Kessen, 1971; Youniss, 1978; although see Cicchetti & Hesse, 1983; Piaget, 1981), partly to his interest in epistemology (''he is a student of the development of thinking more than he is a student of children''; Kessen, 1962, 77). Werner also wrote little on the areas of social, motivational and personality development, although Werner and Kaplan (1963) did briefly address the issues of psychopathology and dream states from a developmental perspective. The result of the omission of non-cognitive domains in developmental theory is a psychology which does not look at the individual ''whole child'' (Zigler, 1971) in all of his or her many aspects. In particular, developmentalists have only recently explored the development of self-image, mastery motivation, learned helplessness, and wariness. We address this issue further when discussing the application of developmental theory to retarded individuals, but we should mention here that these areas of the child's development must be included in any expanded version of the developmental perspective.

The second issue involves the nature and effects of the environment. Piaget always considered himself an ''interactionist'' and Werner spoke of the organism's *Umwelt* (i.e., the environment in the organism's terms), but neither adequately specified what the environment consists of or how it affects development. In fact, it is surprising that two theorists so interested in the development of an active child would view the environment as static. For example, Piaget (1977) spoke of the environment as ''aliment'' to the developing child, and continually emphasized the child's, rather than the environment's, role in promoting development (c.f., Hodapp & Goldfield, 1985). Werner (1948) also conceptualized the *Umwelt* as changing only in response to changes in the developing organism. Thus, although each theorist realized the importance of the environment, neither elaborated on its nature or role in development.

This need for a ''developmental perspective'' on the environment has in recent years been partially met by Sameroff's (1975) ''transactional model of development''. In the transactional model, the environment itself is conceptualized as changing due to its interactions (''transactions'') with the developing child. The changing environment in turn serves as an important factor affecting the child's developmental change. According to Sameroff ''if developmental processes are to be understood it will not be through continuous assessment of the child alone, but through continuous assessment of the transactions between the child and his environment to determine how these transactions facilitate or hinder adaptive integration as both the child and his surroundings change and evolve (p. 283).''

Although many examples could be given to demonstrate research employing the transactional model, a study by Clarke-Stewart (1978) clearly demonstrates the dynamic nature of the child's environment. Examining the relationships among the behaviors of mothers, fathers, and children in the period from 15 to 30 months, Clarke-Stewart found that the amount of maternal stimulation and play with the baby at 15 months was closely related to the child's intellectual performance at 18 months. For fathers the opposite was true, as children's intellectual performance at

15 months correlated with paternal talk and play at 30 months. Furthermore, the amount the father talked and played with the child at one age was associated with mother's talking and playing at later ages. As summarized by Clarke-Stewart, these findings suggest that "the most plausible causal direction . . . is mother influencing child, child influencing father, and father influencing mother" (p. 476). This type of research, examining the changing nature and effects of the environment over time, is clearly consonant with the transactional model, a view of the environment that complements the developmentalist's traditional view of an active and developing child. The areas of input language (e.g., Furrow, Nelson, & Benedict, 1979) and of mother–infant interaction (see Hodapp & Mueller, 1982, for a review) have particularly benefited from research employing the transactional model.

In another elaboration of the nature of the environment, psychologists are now beginning to investigate the entire ecological context in which children develop. Family, school, friends and neighborhood are all considered open to study. Most research on the ecology of childhood is just beginning, however, and the amount of research into such phenomena as the role of the father in the child's development (c.f., Lamb, 1981; Parke, 1979), the newborn's effect on siblings (Dunn & Kendrick, 1981), or the effects of the birth of a baby on family functioning (Lamb, 1978) remains limited. Even the current "family focus" in developmental research (Bronfenbrenner, 1979; Crnic, Chapter 12, this volume; Crnic, Friedrich, & Greenberg, 1983; Kaye & Furstenberg, 1985) dates only to the late 1970s. But given the developmentalist's interest in the organism's *Umwelt* and in the transactional model, such ecological research is rapidly becoming common in developmental psychology.

The resultant, expanded developmental perspective is one that retains the classic view of the child's development while further elucidating unexamined and underemphasized areas. This expanded developmental theory is characterized by a focus on the "whole child" and on the effects of a changing and multifaceted environment, previously neglected areas that add to and strengthen developmental work. It is this expanded, filled-in version of the developmental perspective which is currently being applied to the Down syndrome population.

Applying the developmental perspective to retarded individuals

The two-group approach to mental retardation

Before examining the application of the developmental perspective to Down syndrome individuals, we should discuss the two-group approach to mental retardation. From the beginning of this century, mental retardation has typically been separated into two diagnostic categories: retardation with a known organic etiology, and cases of unknown or uncertain etiology. In the first type, a circumscribed cause of the individual's retardation is indicated.

For example, mental retardation may be due to a dominant gene, as in epiloia; to a single recessive gene, as in phenylketonuria and amaurotic idiocy; to infections, such as congenital syphilis, encephalitis, or rubella in the mother; to chromosomal defects, as in [Down's Syndrome]; to toxic agents, as in retardation caused by radiation in utero, lead poisoning, or Rh incompatibility; and to cerebral trauma. (Zigler, 1967, 292)

Thus, damage may occur, pre-, peri-, or postnatally, but an organic etiological factor is present. The group of organically retarded individuals is thought to constitute less than half of the retarded population.

In the second type of retardation, no organic determinants can be identified. Because retarded individuals of this subtype are typically offspring of low-IQ parents and often are raised in poor environments, both polygenic and environmental etiologic factors are possible. Such labels as "sociocultural retardation," "familial retardation," and "retardation due to sensory deprivation" have been used to describe this type of retardation. This group of individuals is thought to constitute the large majority of the retarded population (see Zigler & Hodapp, 1986, for a review of the two-group approach).

This nomenclature, although it provides order to the mental retardation field, may itself be open to further specification, as organically retarded individuals do not constitute a homogeneous group (Lubs & Maes, 1977, have identified more than 200 types of organic retardation). Differences in degree and type of brain pathology may in turn affect overall intellectual functioning (i.e., levels of retardation) and the specific areas of greatest deficit (see Gardner, 1982 for a discussion of how specific brain lesions may cause behavioral deficits). For example, as we discuss later in the chapter, individuals with Down syndrome seem to have particular difficulties with language functioning; this deficit, which is greater than their overall level of abilities (mental age, or MA), may not be present in individuals whose retardation is caused by other organic etiologies.

It is also noteworthy that, even within a single etiological group, individual characteristics vary widely. Among individuals with Down syndrome, for example, there are several types of chromosomal abnormalities (e.g., trisomy of the 21st chromosome; mosaicism, etc.), a wide range of intellectual levels (from profound to mild retardation, with an occasional reported case of a Down syndrome individual of average intelligence; Fishler, 1975), and many other individual variations (see Gibson, 1978). It is with this caveat in mind that we discuss in the next section the developmental approach to mental retardation in general and, later, to Down syndrome in particular.

Developmental versus difference approaches to mental retardation

Early theorists in the retardation field envisioned all retarded children as being "defective" in their functioning as compared to normally intelligent children. Although different theorists emphasized different defects, each defect theorist hypothesized that one or a small set of circumscribed defects was the cause of mental retardation in all retarded individuals. Some theorists (Kounin, 1948; Lewin, 1935) saw retarded children as being more "rigid" in their cognitive systems; others hypothesized that retardation was caused by a defect in selective attention (Zeaman & House,

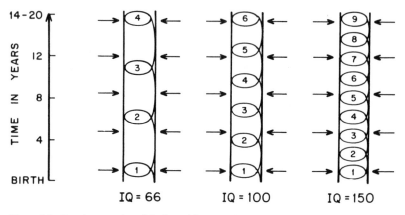

Figure 1.1. Developmental model of cognitive growth. The single vertical arrow represents the passage of time. The horizontal arrows represent environmental events impinging on the individual, who is represented as a pair of vertical lines. The individual's cognitive development appears as an internal ascending spiral, in which the numbered loops represent successive stages of cognitive growth.

1963; 1979), verbal mediation (Luria, 1982), or the prolongation of stimulus traces (Ellis, 1963). In every instance, one or another specific defect was thought to be responsible for the lower level of cognitive functioning in all retarded individuals.

Zigler's developmental formulation of retardation (Zigler, 1969) arose as a direct reaction (c.f., Zigler, 1984) to one of these defect views, the Lewin–Kounin rigidity formulation. In contrast to the idea that all retarded individuals were more inherently rigid than normal children, and that this rigidity was the ultimate cause of their retardation, Zigler stated that retarded children do not suffer from cognitive rigidity but are, rather, globally delayed in the same way that a child with an IQ of 100 is delayed in development compared to a child with an IQ of 130. The only differences between retarded and normally intelligent children are that the retarded child will proceed through the stages of normal development at a slower rate and will stop developing at a lower level. As such, retarded individuals are not different in kind from individuals of normal intelligence; they do not suffer from rigidity or any single defect that causes their retardation.

As originally stated, Zigler's developmental formulation applied only to those retarded children who demonstrate no organic etiology for their retardation. The application to only the group showing no obvious organic etiology is due to the belief that the "nonorganically" retarded population, although composed of several subgroups (Zigler & Hodapp, 1986), essentially comprises the lower end of the Gaussian distribution of intelligence. As Zigler noted, "I have asserted that the same principles of cognitive development apply throughout the normal range of intelligence with the familial retarded representing the lowest end of this distribution" (p. 553).

This model is shown in Figure 1.1. Children of three IQ levels (IQ = 66; 100; and 150) are shown developing across Piagetian, or some other, sequence of developmental stages. Children of higher intellect proceed at a faster pace and asymptote at a higher level, but the successive stages are identical.

A final feature of the original developmental formulation is that cognitive factors alone do not adequately account for the functioning of retarded children (or of normally intelligent children). One of Zigler's earliest criticisms of much of the defect research was the comparison of institutionalized retarded children to home-reared normal children. The effects of institutionalization, of repeated failure, and of a strong desire for interaction (and a simultaneous wariness to interact) with supportive adults were all shown to differ in the two groups even when retarded and normal children were equated on mental age.

This is not to say that the cause of retardation is motivational: the cognitive functioning of the retarded unquestionably has a profound and pervasive influence on their behavior. The crucial questions are: just how great is this influence and how does it vary across tasks with which the retarded are confronted? What often is not realized is that the behavior of the retarded, as for all human beings, reflects more than formal cognitive processes. (Zigler & Balla, 1977, 20)

Thus, there was a concern for the whole child in even the earliest formulations of the developmental approach to mental retardation.

Three major hypotheses derive from the developmental perspective as it applies to familial retarded children. First, it is predicted that familial retarded children progress through the same universal stages of development that normally intelligent children traverse. This prediction, called the *similar sequence* hypothesis, applies to Piagetian cognitive, to linguistic, and to other universal stages of development. Second, the developmental perspective predicts that familial retarded children and nonretarded children have a *similar structure* to their intelligence. Thus, across all areas of cognitive functioning, the familial retarded group should perform about equally well from task to task (i.e., at their level of MA), just as normal children do. Third, the developmental perspective predicts that familial retarded children respond to institutions and external factors in ways similar to the responses of normal children (the *similar responses* hypothesis). Retarded children may, because of their retardation, be more likely to experience "non-normal" life experiences (e.g., more failure, more institutionalization, etc.), but their responses should approximate those of normal children who also undergo such experiences.

Although a detailed review of data on each of these hypotheses is beyond the scope of this chapter, all three have generally been supported for familial retarded children. Summarizing across 28 cross-sectional and 3 longitudinal studies on the similar sequence hypothesis, Weisz and Zigler (1979) concluded that "the great preponderence of the evidence is consistent with the hypothesis that retarded and nonretarded persons traverse the same stages of development in the same order, differing only in the rate at which they progress and in the ultimate ceiling they attain" (Weisz & Zigler, 1979, 846). In 30 of 33 studies employing only familial retarded children, the similar structure hypothesis was also supported; that is, familial retarded children matched on MA to nonretarded children performed equally well on a variety of experimental tasks (Weisz & Yeates, 1981). Finally, in a long line of work (c.f., Zigler & Balla, 1977), Zigler and his colleagues have shown that retarded children respond similarly to normal children when experiencing failure and institutionalization.

It must be noted that each of these studies tests developmental hypotheses only as they relate to familial retarded children. How to conceptualize retarded individuals who show clear organic etiologies is a more difficult matter. These individuals may not be a part of the normal distribution of intelligence because of their organic insults. Furthermore, Zigler (1969) believes it is "illogical to extend those principles to individuals with organic defects (whatever their IQs may be). . . . If the etiology of the phenotypic intelligence (as measured by an IQ) of two groups differ, it is far from logical to assert that the course of development is the same, or that even similar contents in the behaviors of two such differing individuals are mediated by exactly the same cognitive process" (p. 533).

In contrast, other developmentally oriented workers are of the opinion that the developmental perspective is applicable to organically retarded individuals. Conceptualizing development as "organized" or "coherent" across domains, Cicchetti and Pogge-Hesse (1982) advocate the application of the developmental perspective to Down syndrome and other organically retarded individuals. Having shown that Down syndrome children follow the same sequence of development as do nonretarded children in the domains of early affect (Cicchetti & Sroufe, 1976), sensorimotor skills (Cicchetti & Mans-Wagener, 1987), and symbolic play (Motti, Cicchetti, & Sroufe, 1983), they propose that Down syndrome children do indeed traverse a "similar sequence" to that of nonretarded children. In addition, Cicchetti and his colleagues have attempted to examine similar structures of abilities in Down syndrome children across several domains. These workers have shown that the sensorimotor abilities of Down syndrome children correlate to their levels of positive Cicchetti & Sroufe, 1976) and negative (Cicchetti & Sroufe, 1978) affective responses, and that levels of symbolic play and intellectual level are related in 3-, 4-, and 5-year-old Down syndrome children (Motti, Cicchetti, & Sroufe, 1983). Although we will have more to say on this matter later in the chapter, the overall thrust of this work is to apply the similar sequence *and* similar structure hypotheses to the Down syndrome population.

Again, we offer only a brief review of the evidence. As concerns the similar sequence hypothesis, it seems that retarded and nonretarded children do progress along the same sequence of stages "regardless of etiology" (Weisz & Zigler, 1979, 846). With the possible exception of children with electroencephalogram (EEG) abnormalities, all retarded children seem to follow the invariant sequences proposed by Piaget and other developmentalists. This finding, examined more fully in a later section, amply justifies at least a partial "developmental approach" to intervention with Down syndrome and other organically retarded children.

As Table 1.1 demonstrates, however, etiology does seem to matter in relation to the similar structure prediction. Organically retarded children are much more likely to perform worse on a variety of tasks than are MA-matched nonretarded children, whereas familial retarded children performed equally well to the nonretarded group

Table 1.1. *Directional comparisons of MA-matched retarded and*
nonretarded persons summed across various Piagetian tasks

	Direction of difference		
Group	MR > NMR	MR ≅ NMR	MR < NMR
Etiology controlled	0	30	3
Etiology uncontrolled	4	45	22

Note: The abbreviation MR stands for mentally retarded subjects; NMR stands for nonretarded subjects; the symbol = indicates that there was no reliable group difference. Adapted
from Weisz, Yeates, & Zigler (1982).

in 30 of 33 studies. (We elaborate the exact nature of the intellectual structure of
Down syndrome intelligence in the next section.) There are not enough studies
employing etiology of retardation as an independent variable to test differentially
the "similar reaction" hypothesis for organically retarded versus familial retarded
children.

Applying the developmental perspective to Down
syndrome individuals

First described in 1867, Down syndrome may be the most investigated of all types
of mental retardation. Because of its early identification and relatively high incidence, it has been the subject of much research employing the Down syndrome
population. This situation has not necessarily led to a clearer understanding of the
behaviors of Down syndrome individuals, however, as a whole range of myths and
stereotypes have been advanced (with little empirical support) over the past 100
years. Some of these stereotypes – that Down syndrome individuals are especially
musical, good-natured, imitative, and sociable – have begun to receive research
attention (c.f., Belmont, 1971; Gibson, 1978), but the "typical" behavior of Down
syndrome persons remains far from clear.

Spurred by the developmental perspective and the recent explosion in research
knowledge about children, many researchers have examined the performance of
Down syndrome children on a number of tasks. As above, we begin our review of
this work by examining the similar sequence and similar structure hypotheses, after
which we address two developmental issues particular to the Down syndrome population. We end our review with a brief discussion of specific implications of the
expanded developmental perspective as it applies to research and intervention with
Down syndrome individuals.

Similar sequence hypothesis

Like all organically retarded children, Down syndrome individuals seem to progress
in the same sequence as that followed by normal children. Weisz and Zigler (1979)

reviewed studies on the development of retarded children in the domains of senso-rimotor functioning, conservation, and space, time, and moral judgment concepts. In the majority of these studies, Down syndrome children were not distinguished from other retarded children, but each study supported the similar sequence hypoth-esis. With the possible exception of children with severe EEG abnormalities, all retarded children – regardless of level of functioning, etiology, or living environ-ment – demonstrated the usual ordering of achievements in each area of Piagetian functioning.

More recently, Kopp (1983) has reviewed a number of studies on the early de-velopment of Down syndrome and premature children. Compared to nonretarded groups, Down syndrome infants appear to develop along similar paths in sensori-motor cognitive domains (Cicchetti & Mans-Wagener, 1987; Kahn, 1977); in social smiling and laughter (Cicchetti & Sroufe, 1976); in play (Hill & McCune-Nicholich,1981; Motti, Cicchetti & Sroufe, 1983); and in numerous other early skills. Kopp concludes that ''these sensorimotor behaviors have a firm biological basis that reflects strong evolutionary pressures and are distorted only in the wake of profound organic damage'' (Kopp, 1983, 1119). Beeghly, Weiss-Perry, and Cic-chetti, (Chapter 10, this volume; for communicative development) and Fowler, (Chapter 9, this volume; for syntax) have found that stages of later language devel-opment are also traversed in the normal sequence by Down syndrome children (see also Rosenberg, 1984). Across a wide range of developments, then, Down syn-drome children seem to progress through the same sequence of stages as do nonre-tarded children.

Similar structure hypothesis

The bulk of the evidence seems to suggest that Down syndrome children, like other organically retarded groups, do not possess a similar structure to their intelligence as that found in nonretarded children of the same cognitive level (i.e., MA). When matched on mental age to normally intelligent (or to familial retarded) children, Down syndrome children perform worse on certain skills, better on others.

The deficit most often cited in the Down syndrome population involves language functioning. Mahoney, Glover, and Finger (1981) matched 18 Down syndrome and 18 nonretarded children on the Bayley Scales of Infant Development (Bayley, 1969; Developmental Ages for each group equaled 17 months). They then examined scores of the two groups on the Receptive and Expressive Language (REEL) Scales (Bzoch & League, 1970) and on the Piagetian-based Ordinal Scales of Infant Development (Uzgiris & Hunt, 1975). On both the expressive language and receptive language portions of the REEL, Down syndrome children were behind the normal children of equivalent mental age. This deficit in language seemed to be related to the lower levels of Vocal Imitation skills displayed by the Down syndrome children. Other studies have also found that Down syndrome children are lower in vocal (and ver-bal) abilities when compared to normal children of similar developmental levels (e.g., Cardoso-Martins & Mervis, 1985; Greenwald & Leonard, 1979). Even when institutionalized Down syndrome children are compared with non-Down syndrome retarded children in institutions (Johnson & Abelard, 1969), or when the language scores of Down syndrome children are compared to their own scores on other portions of intelligence tests (e.g., Share, 1975), Down syndrome children demonstrate particular difficulties in their performance on language tasks. It may be, as Gibson (1978) suggests, that "the manipulation of symbols and images [i.e., language] provides something of a developmental wall for the syndrome" (p. 33).

In addition to deficits due to the nature of the disorder, it also may be the case that Down syndrome children often receive a less adequate linguistic environment than do nonretarded children, especially in the months just before their beginning productive speech. Comparing Down syndrome children to three nonretarded control groups, one matched on chronological age, one on mental age, and one on linguistic age (i.e., prelinguistic children who, based on chronological age, appeared ready to enter language), Cardoso-Martins and Mervis (1985) have recently found that mothers of prelinguistic Down syndrome children provide lesser amounts of labeling and deictic information than do mothers of nonretarded children. The authors explained their findings in terms of maternal expectations of their Down syndrome children. They noted that the "infrequent use of lexical deixis and nouns by mothers of children with Down syndrome may result from reduced maternal expectations concerning their children's ability to learn language. Some of the mothers who participated in the present study spontaneously stated that they were afraid that their children would never learn to talk" (Cardoso-Martins & Mervis, 1985, 456; also, Jones, 1980, 219–222). Although such differences in linguistic input do not totally account for the difficulties experienced by Down syndrome children in acquiring language, they may exacerbate their problems.

Recent work has also pointed to the possibility that not all aspects of language are particularly deficient in the Down syndrome population. In a study attempting to determine *which* particular aspects of language are or are not differentially impaired in Down syndrome children, Leifer and Lewis (1984) matched Down syndrome children (aged 3.5 to 4.5 years) to normal children (aged 18 to 23 months) on mean length of utterance (MLU, a rough measure of the child's level of grammar; Brown, 1973). They then examined the conversational skills of both groups in 30-minute mother–child interactions. These skills included the ability to uphold one's conversational turn and the ability to give a relevant answer to the mother's question. The Down syndrome children demonstrated better conversational skills than the normal children of the same MLU. Even within language, then, some areas (e.g., social aspects) seem relatively less impaired in Down syndrome children, while other areas (grammatical and "relational" aspects) seem especially deficient (see also Beeghly & Cicchetti, 1987; Rosenberg, 1984).

The relative strength of Down syndrome children in the social aspects of language functioning is consistent with the general finding that Down syndrome children show a relatively better performance (than their mental ages) on tasks of social maturity. In a study by Centerwell and Centerwell (1960), for example, the performances on tests of intelligence (Stanford–Binet) and social adaptation (Vineland) were compared in two groups of institutionalized Down syndrome children. The first group (Group P) had been placed in institutions very soon after birth. The second group (Group H) was institutionalized after two and a half years in their homes. While Group H outperformed Group P on both tests, a wide divergence between IQ and SQ (Social Quotient) scores emerged: at 7 years, Group P had an average IQ of 16 and SQ of 24, Group H had an IQ of 23 and an SQ of 32. Other studies have shown a similar discrepancy in home-reared retarded children (Cornwell & Birch, 1969) and in institutionalized Down syndrome children compared to institutionalized non-Down syndrome children (Johnson & Abelard, 1969). Just as the literature strongly suggests that Down syndrome children have a relative weakness in linguistic functioning, they seem to have a relative strength in social adaptation skills.

Kopp (1983) has further elaborated on the differences in the structure of intelligence between Down syndrome children and nonretarded children of the same mental age, stating that early visual perceptual abilities and reduplicated babbling are relatively immune to delay in Down syndrome infants. "Both of these may be so basic to human existence and so tied to biological underpinnings and maturational factors that [Down syndrome] conditions are not severe enough to disrupt the timing of their emergence" (Kopp, 1983, 1119). Kopp also identified later perceptual–cognitive tasks (e.g., visual scanning of the environment in order to encode information) as more deficient in Down syndrome children than in MA-matched nonretarded children (Jones, 1980; Krakow & Kopp, 1982; MacTurk, Vietze, McCarthy, McQuiston, & Yarrow, 1985). Other researchers note the difficulties Down syndrome children have in attending to, discriminating, and encoding complex stimuli (e.g., Cornwell, 1974).

This is not to say that the pattern of intellectual development is totally "disorganized" in Down syndrome children, however. Cicchetti and his colleagues, in a number of studies, have pointed to the "coherence" of development in Down syndrome infants and preschoolers. They have found, for example, that different affective responses of Down syndrome children are intercorrelated (Cicchetti & Serafica, 1981); that the levels of sensorimotor cognitive abilities closely correspond to levels of laughter (Cicchetti & Sroufe, 1976) and fear (Cicchetti & Sroufe, 1978); and that the symbolic play behaviors of Down syndrome children 3-, 4-, and 5-year-olds are related to the child's mental age (Motti, Cicchetti, & Sroufe, 1983), just as in nonhandicapped children. Thus, Cicchetti and his colleagues have demonstrated a certain degree of "structure" in the development of Down syndrome children, and the nature of this structuralization is similar to that found in nonretarded children.

A possible solution to this problem of whether or not Down syndrome children do indeed possess a "similar structure" of development (and in which areas) is provided by Mundy, Seibert, and Hogan (1984). In a study of developmentally delayed children of 2 to 7, 8 to 13, and 14 to 21 months of mental age, these workers found that retarded children possessed a pattern of correlations among individual sensorimotor abilities that was similar to the one previously demonstrated with nonretarded children (Bates, Benigni, Bretherton, Camaioni, & Volterra, 1979).

Particularly in the mental age range of 8 to 13 months, children's levels of means–ends abilities (i.e., use of one object as a means to retrieve another) and of schemes for relating to objects (e.g., child drinking from a cup; putting on toy sunglasses) were highly correlated with several domains of early social communication (child responding to adult's attempts to direct visual attention; child responding to, or initiating, behavior regulation of the interactive partner). In contrast, children's levels of skills in object permanence, spatial, and causality subscales of the Uzgiris–Hunt test (Uzgiris & Hunt, 1975) were *not* highly correlated with abilities in social communication. Mundy, Seibert, and Hogan (1984) therefore concluded that, as in Bates et al.'s (1979) nonretarded sample, there are "local homologies" in development, or relationships among tasks that require common underlying capacities. These homologies involve subsets of skills that appear together; other skills of the same sensorimotor stage may appear separately.

The position that there are local homologies in development may reconcile the findings of Cicchetti and his colleagues (supporting a certain degree of similar structure in the developments of Down syndrome children) and the findings of Weisz and Yeates (1981) that organically retarded children do not possess a "similar structure" of intellectual skills to that shown by nonretarded children of the same mental age. The idea of local homologies is shown, for both nonretarded and Down syndrome children, in Figure 1.2. The solid line between skills 1 and 2, for example, denotes a local homology (Homology A); these skills are analogous to those found to intercorrelate in Cicchetti's work. Similarly, skills 3, 4, and 5, and skills 6, 7 and 8, also form local homologies (Homology B and Homology C, respectively). All the skills involved in local homologies are to a large extent "in sync"; individual (nonretarded or Down syndrome) children demonstrate similar levels of development on diverse skills within a single homology. Comparison of the two figures for nonretarded and Down syndrome children shows, however, that overall there is not a similar structure to the intellectual abilities of Down syndrome children to that shown by nonretarded children. Thus, although skills 1 and 2 are at similar levels in both Down syndrome and nonretarded children, the levels of development on the three homologies differ. Whereas, on average, Homologies A, B, and C are at the same level as the child's MA in nonretarded children, they differ widely in Down syndrome children. The best example of this sort of dissynchrony would be the linguistic developments of Down syndrome children. As mentioned in a preceding section, language skills are especially deficient in the Down syndrome population. However, various "linguistic like" abilities, for example, various pretend play measures (Motti, Cicchetti, & Sroufe, 1983), may still intercorrelate, in both Down syndrome and nonretarded samples. The concept of local homologies explains how Down syndrome children may indeed not possess a similar structure to nonretarded children across all intellectual domains, even as they still demonstrate some degree of coherence to their development.

Overall, then, Down syndrome children do not seem to possess the same structure to their intelligence as that demonstrated by normal children of the same cog-

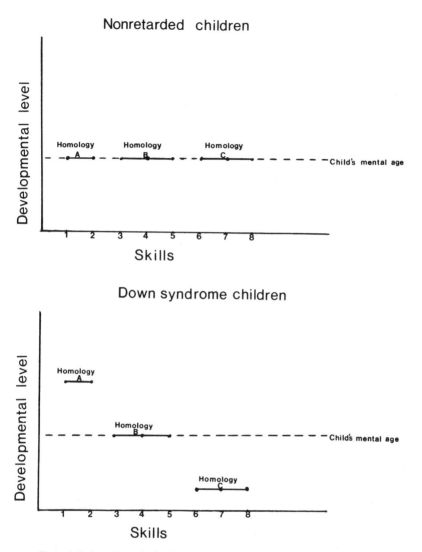

Figure 1.2. Local homologies for nonretarded and Down syndrome children.

nitive level, although they nevertheless show organized patterns of development. Their abilities in several areas (e.g., social adaptation, simple visual perceptual skills, babbling) seem less delayed than their overall level of mental abilities. At the same time, these children have particular difficulty in expressive language, abstract thinking, and dealing with complex stimuli. Further research is necessary to replicate this list of intellectual strengths and weaknesses in the Down syndrome population.

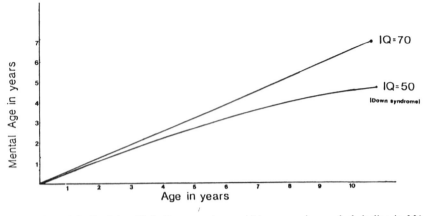

Figure 1.3. Declining IQ in Down syndrome children assuming gradual decline in MA relative to CA over time.

Trajectory of development

Unlike normally developing children, Down syndrome children do not seem to have a constant, or near constant, trajectory of development. The rate of development of Down syndrome children, as measured by the IQ, seems to become progressively slower over time. In a study by Dicks-Mireaux (1972), for example, Down syndrome infants progressed approximately 12 weeks in the first 16 weeks of life (Developmental Quotient = 12/16 = 75), 20 weeks in the first 28 (DQ = 71), 30 in the first 40 (DQ = 75), 36 in the first 52 (DQ = 69) and 45 in the first 78 (DQ = 58). Other studies in the infancy period (e.g., Dameron, 1963; Dicks-Mireaux, 1972) also indicate a deceleration in the rate of intellectual growth over time in Down syndrome infants. In each study, although the Down syndrome children continued to develop in the first year and a half, the rate of development slowed noticeably after the first year. It is unclear at the present time exactly when this decelerated rate of development ends. An illustration of declining IQ in Down syndrome children is shown in Figure 1.3.

From a developmental point of view, a decelerated rate of development implies another difference between Down syndrome children and normal children (or familial retarded children). Data from the Berkeley and Fels growth studies (Honzik & MacFarlane, 1973; McCall, Appelbaum, & Hogarty, 1973), although showing some individuals with large IQ changes over time, do not indicate any consistent, progressive decline in the rate of development over the early years for normally developing individuals. Similarly, the evidence for familial retarded children, although less abundant, indicates some small IQ changes in both directions and a possibility that there is slightly more variation in this group but, again, no progressive deceleration (Silverstein, 1982).

The reason for deceleration in the IQs of Down syndrome children is not known,

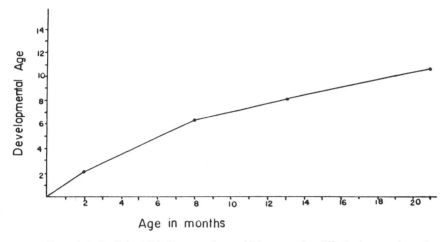

Figure 1.4. Declining IQ in Down syndrome children assuming difficulty in mastering tasks at each transition point in development.

but several theories have been advanced. McCall, Eichorn, and Hogarty (1977) have identified 2 months, 8 months, 13 months, and 21 months as "transition points" in development; it was at these times that a different factor structure of intelligence emerged among children in the Berkeley Growth Studies (i.e., new tasks characterized "intelligent behavior" at each of these points). Kopp and McCall (1982) hypothesize that Down syndrome and other handicapped children fall farther behind at each transition point. To quote them:

We speculate that these transitions may mark the time when infants with known central nervous system impairment begin to separate from their peers, not just in rate of developmental change but also in respect to density, richness, and adaptability of sensorimotor repertoire. Specifically, we suggest that organic impairment distorts or limits this qualitative shift. Thus, earlier, more immature forms of behavior are consistently used, rather than more mature patterns. (p. 55)

Figure 1.4 demonstrates the decline in the rate of development in Down syndrome children as hypothesized by Kopp and McCall. In contrast to Figure 1.3, the rate changes at each transition point. Thus, a child with a Developmental Quotient (the infancy equivalent of the IQ) of 75 at 8 months has a DQ of 52 at 21 months. The decelerated rate of development is clearly linked to the "transition points" identified by McCall, Eichorn, and Hogarty (1977). It remains to be seen if the decelerated rate of development of Down syndrome children is a general phenomenon (as shown in Figure 1.3) or if it is indeed specifically related to a "separation from their peers" that occurs at each successive transition point, as in Figure 1.4. (For discussion of this issue, see Dunst, 1988, and Dunst, Chapter 6, this volume.)

Following the Kopp and McCall hypothesis, language development may still be implicated in the declines at several of the later transition points. It may also be the case that social skills decelerate less than IQ and that linguistic deficits affect functioning in other areas. Cornwell and Birch (1969), studying home-reared 4- to 17-year-old Down syndrome children, found an increasing divergence between measures of intelligence and social skills. At the 4 to 6 year period, Social Quotients exceeded IQs by an average of 4.1 points, whereas at 7 to 9 years and at 10 to 17 years the discrepancies were 15 and 14 points, respectively (our calculations, from Cornwell & Birch, 1969, table 1). Gradually, however, declines in the rates of the children's Social Quotients were also observed, a phenomenon Cornwell and Birch relate to the effect of linguistic deficits on social functioning. These authors conclude that "as these children grew and SA [Social Age] became increasingly dependent upon concepts of language and of symbolic numerical units, the discrepancies between SA and CA came to correspond to the discrepancies between MA and CA" (Cornwell & Birch, 1969, 347–348). Thus, the linguistic deficits of Down syndrome children may increasingly come to affect other areas of development as Down syndrome children get older.

Familial resemblance in IQ

A final issue of interest to developmentalists is the possibility that the intelligence level of 2 children may be influenced by the level of parental intelligence. Correlations in IQ between parents and their nonretarded children suggests a heritability of intelligence of from .45 to .80 (Plomin & DeFries, 1980; Scarr & Carter-Saltzman, 1982; Vernon, 1979), the remainder of the variance being accounted for by environmental influences and gene-environment interactions. If Down syndrome children start with a "projected" level of intelligence before trisomy occurs (and if trisomy damages all children to a similar degree), then some correlation between the levels of intelligence in parents and their Down syndrome children might also be expected. Such a correlation is predicted from polygenic theory and the two-group approach to retardation (Zigler, 1967; Zigler & Hodapp, 1986), which states that the intellectual functioning of Down syndrome children is primarily a function of polygenic inheritance and organic damage caused by trisomy (with a smaller influence due to environmental factors). A correlation between the intelligence of parents and their Down syndrome children would in turn be helpful in identifying which children are in particular need of intensive intervention efforts.

   To date, the question of a familial resemblance between parents and their Down syndrome children is suggested but not clearly demonstrated. Fraser and Sadovnick (1976) examined the IQ scores of 25 institutionalized Down syndrome children, 23 home-reared subjects, and their respective parents and siblings. All correlations involving home-reared Down syndrome children (father–Down syndrome child; mother–Down syndrome child; sibling–Down syndrome child) approached .50, the parent–child and sibling correlations expected under polygenic theory (and generally found between parents and their nonretarded children). For institutionalized Down syndrome children, however, only the IQs of mothers and Down syndrome offspring were significantly correlated ($r = .69$); neither the father–Down syndrome child ($r = .29$) nor the sibling–Down syndrome child ($r = .20$) correlations were significant. Fraser and Sadovnick (1976) conclude:

The data for the children with Down syndrome raised at home suggest that in the presence of an extra chromosome 21 the IQ is reduced by roughly two standard deviations from the population average, that the distribution of scores is similar in form to that of the unaffected parents and siblings, and that the correlation of IQ scores between affected children and their parents or sibs is about where it would be in the absence of trisomy. How much of the correlation results from the genes determining intellectual functions that these children share with their parents and sibs, and how much from familial environmental factors influencing these functions, cannot be determined from the data. (p. 181)

Two other studies have shown similar results when highest level of parental education is used in place of parental IQ scores (c.f. Harrell & Harrell, 1945). Golden and Pashayan (1976) found that the Down syndrome offspring of parents with postgraduate, college, and high school educations were almost identical (IQ = 50), whereas the Down syndrome children of parents with grammar school educations scored much lower (IQ = 35). Similarly, Gibson (1967) found that in two of three institutional samples, Down syndrome children reared at home for a long period and those examined five years after institutionalization, the expected correlations between parental educational level and the IQ scores of Down syndrome offspring were observed. In a third sample (children tested at institutionalization in the 0 to 2 year period), no such correlation was found. Although this lack of correlation in the third sample may have been due to the instability of infant IQ scores (even for handicapped children; Kopp & McCall, 1982), Gibson (1967) concluded from these findings that the familial resemblance between parents and their Down syndrome offspring may be due mainly to environmental factors.

In contrast to the studies just cited, Bennett, Sells and Brandt (1979) have challenged both the polygenic and the environmental explanations for the observation of familial resemblance. These authors claim that the decline in intellectual levels of Down syndrome children over time may be spuriously producing the correlation between parents and their Down syndrome children. In their study, Bennett et al. first adjusted for the chronological age (CA) of the Down syndrome child by comparing the degree to which the child's IQ differed from the averaged IQ of Down syndrome children of the same chronological age (from Melyn & White, 1973). The resultant "deviation score," or the deviation of the child's IQ from the average for Down syndrome children of the same CA, was then used in all analyses. They found no evidence of different "deviation scores" for the Down syndrome offspring of parents with 12 or less years of education, of 13 to 16 years, and of more than 16 years of schooling.

Although the Bennett et al. study did account for the effects of declining Down syndrome IQ with increasing chronological age, other studies have not found this lack of parent–child correlation. For example, Libb, Myers, Graham, and Bell (1983), using similar methods to those of Bennett and his co-workers, found that the Down syndrome offspring of non–high school graduates scored lower than the offspring of parents at other educational levels. The Bennett et al. study, which did not separate parents who were high school graduates and those who were not, may have masked this correlation. In addition, perusal of the ages of the subjects in Fraser and Sadovnick (1976) (all subjects above 5 years of age) and in Gibson (1967) (subjects of different ages were in three different samples) suggests that none of the studies obtained spurious correlations – for this to have been the case, the majority of the younger Down syndrome subjects would have had to be the off-spring of high IQ parents, older subjects the children of low IQ parents.

In spite of the Bennett et al. findings, then, it seems likely that there is a familial resemblance between the intelligence levels of Down syndrome children and their parents. Clearly, however, more research is needed in this area.

Implications of the developmental perspective for intervention with Down syndrome individuals

Until now, we have reviewed research employing Down syndrome individuals in order to determine the extent to which this population conforms to several hypotheses generated by developmental theory. Our conclusions have been that Down syndrome individuals go through a sequence similar to that traversed by nonretarded children and the Down syndrome children may share a "familial resemblance" in intellectual level with their parents when compared to other Down syndrome children. However, in contrast to nonretarded persons, Down syndrome individuals do not seem to possess a similar structure to their intelligence (although they do show evidence of local homologies), and they seem to progress at a decelerating rate over time. Down syndrome children therefore share certain development similarities with nonretarded children, but there are also important differences in development in the two groups. We conclude with a few brief remarks concerning the implications of each finding for intervention work with individuals with Down syndrome.

Similar sequence of development

The most important finding from all of the developmental research on children with Down syndrome is that they do indeed traverse the various stages of development in the same order as that followed by nonretarded children. Thus, in sensorimotor development, these children develop in order through Piaget's six sensorimotor stages (Cicchetti & Mans-Wagener, 1987; Kahn, 1975), in language development they proceed from prelinguistic communication, to holophrases, to complex grammatical speech (Beeghly, Weiss-Perry, & Cicchetti, Chapter 10, this volume; Fowler, Chapter 9, this volume).

The implications of this straightforward finding are important to any intervention effort. Once one knows that Down syndrome children develop along the normal sequence in a particular domain, all of the accumulated knowledge about normal development in that domain can be applied in an intervention program. One can provide training in each of the six sensorimotor domains of infancy, conservation training, language training, even training in the stages of moral reasoning (Kohlberg, 1976). Research into and knowledge about normal development becomes the bedrock upon which to base intervention efforts for Down syndrome children (see Spiker, Chapter 13, this volume).

Examples of such "developmentally based" programs of intervention are best shown in the domain of language. In accordance with recent emphases in developmental psycholinguistics on semantics and pragmatics, various developmentally based early intervention curricula have been suggested (e.g., Bricker & Bricker, 1974; MacDonald & Blott, 1974; McLean & Snyder-McLean, 1978; Miller & Yoder, 1974). Proposed at various times in the past two decades, each program incorporates to a different degree the current knowledge about grammatical, semantic, and pragmatic aspects of language. More importantly, each adheres to the sequence of development followed by nonretarded children in their acquisition of language. Due to the similar sequence shown by Down syndrome children in *their* development of language, these developmentally based programs are thought to incorporate the optimal sequence in which to introduce the various elements of language to Down syndrome children.

Similarly, the assessment of Down syndrome children can now be performed using "developmentally based" testing instruments. Dunst (1980), for example, has taken the Piagetian-based Ordinal Scales of Infant Development (Uzgiris & Hunt, 1975) and modified this test to allow for the assessment of infant behavior in retarded and in physically handicapped children. Items of equivalent cognitive difficulty – but which are easier motorically – have been added where necessary, and the scoring has been simplified. The early intervention worker is left with a useful clinical instrument. In addition, due to the Piagetian base of the Scales, those intervening with retarded children can also teach the skills measured by the test, secure in the knowledge that skills in object permanence, means–ends, causality, and imitation are necessary for later developments (Bates, Benigni, Bretherton, Camaioni, & Volterra, 1977; Brown, 1973; Curcio, 1978).

The structure of intelligence and local homologies

The finding that Down syndrome children have particular difficulties in certain areas (i.e., that they have a different structure to their intelligence than MA-matched nonretarded children) can also be used in intervention efforts. Language skills may need to be taught more intensively, social skills less so. If Mahoney, Glover, and Finger (1981) are correct, it may be that vocal imitation skills demand particular attention in early intervention efforts. As these workers state, the finding that the receptive language difference [between MA-matched nonretarded and Down syndrome children] was related to their relative verbal-imitation proficiency might be interpreted as indicating that training children to imitate verbally . . . will increase their rate of acquiring language'' (p. 26). Other weak areas of functioning in Down syndrome children (e.g., visual scanning of the environment) may also be amenable to more intensive intervention efforts.

The finding that there are local homologies in the development of children with Down syndrome can also inform intervention efforts. If indeed certain skills cluster together in development, whereas others are independent, interventionists can help foster several at one time, as each is indicative of a single underlying skill. For example, object permanence tasks, person permanence tasks (Paradise & Curcio, 1974), and attachment behaviors (Decarie, 1978) might all be taught concurrently, as each seems indicative of the concept of the permanent object. Similarly, work by Bates et al. (1979), Mundy, Seibert, and Hogan (1984), Curcio (1978), and Snyder (1978) seems to point to the importance of some (e.g., means–ends skills) but not all (object permanence and spatial skills) sensorimotor developments for the acquisition of early communicative competence. Although the exact nature of these proposed homologies needs to be clarified, such knowledge is invaluable to the developmentally oriented intervention worker.

Rate of development and familial resemblance

The findings that Down syndrome children demonstrate decelerated rates of development and that there are familial resemblances between Down syndrome children and their parents might also be beneficially employed. The decelerated rate of development in Down syndrome children over the first several years of life may indicate a need for more intensive intervention programs in the earliest years. Indeed, if the IQ were to stop decreasing after the early years (which is not yet known), a strategy of ''the earlier the better'' might be called for. Finally, the probable presence of a familial resemblance between the intelligence levels of Down syndrome children and their parents may indicate a need to intervene more intensively with children whose parents are less intelligent, even in cases in which these children appear to be progressing well at early ages.

The intervention process

A final contribution of the expanded version of the developmental perspective is that it provides clues to the processes by which one can best intervene with Down syndrome children. Work on mother–infant interactions and Sameroff's transactional model seem to indicate that mothers ''match'' their behaviors to the level and needs of their infants (Cairns, 1979; Hodapp & Mueller, 1982; Kaye, 1976), but also that mothers structure the environment for their infants, thereby helping them to develop (Hodapp, Goldfield, & Boyatzis, 1984; Kaye, 1982). Such techniques as teaching mothers to position infants physically, to get their infants' attention, and then to provide appropriate contextual support may all be essential in early intervention efforts (Hodapp & Goldfield, 1983). Work with mothers of Down syndrome infants suggests that these mothers may need to allow the child more chances to initiate interaction (Jones, 1977; 1980), although it is also the case that mothers of Down syndrome children are generally responsive to their child's level of development (Rondal, 1977). In short, the many findings relating to how mothers of nonretarded children help their children to develop can be used to instruct mothers of Down syndrome children.

Maternal expectations of their Down syndrome infants may also be important in early intervention work. Studies by Jones (1980) and Cardoso-Martins and Mervis (1984) have both indicated that the ways in which mothers behave toward their Down syndrome children is at least partially dependent on what their expectations are for their children. As Jones (1980) notes,

> . . . the mothers of the Down's syndrome children expressed some clearly different viewpoints from those of the mothers of the normal children. . . . One mother reported being "afraid to expect any words from her child," explaining that in that way she would not risk disappointment. Although this is a very understandable approach, the difficulty with such an interaction system is that it risks further delaying the development of language as the mother may be reluctant to interpret, expand, and extend her child's vocalizations. (Jones, 1980, 220–221)

Such vignettes point out the importance of both maternal behavior *and* maternal perception to the success of intervention efforts.

Conclusion

It is clear from the many diverse findings reviewed in this chapter that the developmental perspective has an important place in work with Down syndrome individuals. In spite of the relatively high prevalence and many years of research on Down syndrome, there is still much to be known about the development of children with the disorder. For example, although there is a general finding that organically retarded individuals traverse the same sequences of development as those of nonretarded children (Weisz & Zigler, 1979), few studies have examined the Down syndrome population per se. Similarly, the specific reasons for the slowing trajectory of IQ in Down syndrome children, the exact nature of their linguistic deficit, and the nature and effects of the environment in promoting linguistic and other developments are all unknown at this time. Indeed, it appears that the practice of examining Down syndrome children through the lens of normal development has just started to pay dividends.

Although this chapter has focused on the ways in which the developmental perspective aids work with the Down syndrome population, it is also true that findings from research employing Down syndrome individuals tell us much about development in nonretarded children. For example, the use of Down syndrome infants has helped clarify the entire issue of local homologies (Mundy, Seibert & Hogan, 1984), while the many findings that Down syndrome children are relatively advanced in social skills but behind in language (especially syntax) demonstrate the extent to which these two domains can remain independent. Only by examining populations traversing developmental stages at a slower rate (and which have certain asynchronies across domains) can one see which developments "must go together" as opposed to which developments usually, but not necessarily, do so. It is in this sense that we "can learn more about the normal functioning of an organism by studying its pathology, more about its pathology by studying its normal condition" (Cicchetti, 1984b, p. 1). The resultant cross-fertilization should be beneficial to both Down syndrome and nonretarded children.

References

Bates, E., Benigni, L., Bretherton, I., Camaioni, L., & Volterra, V. (1977). From gesture to the first word: On cognitive and social prerequisites. In M. Lewis & L. A. Rosenblum (Eds.), *Interaction, conversation and the development of language*. New York: Wiley.

Bates, E., Benigni, L., Bretherton, I., Camaioni, I., & Volterra, V. (1979). *The emergence of symbols: Cognition and communication in infancy*. New York: Academic Press.

Bayley, N. (1969). *Bayley scales of infant development*. New York: Psychological Corporation.

Beeghly, M., & Cicchetti, D. (1987). An organizational approach to symbolic development in children with Down syndrome. *New Directions for Child Development, 36*, 5–29.

Belmont, J. (1971). Medical-behavioral research in retardation. In N. R. Ellis (Ed.), *International Review of Research in Mental Retardation* (Vol. 5). New York: Academic Press.

Bennett, F., Sells, C., & Brandt, C. (1979). Influences on measured intelligence in Down's Syndrome. *American Journal of Disabilities in Childhood, 133*, 700–703.

Bricker, W., & Bricker, D. (1974). An early language training strategy. In R. L. Schiefelbusch & L. Lloyd (Eds.), *Language perspectives: Acquisition, retardation, and intervention*. Baltimore: University Park Press.

Bronfenbrenner, U. (1979). *The ecology of human development: Experiments by nature and design*. Cambridge, MA: Harvard University Press.

Brown, R. (1973). *A first language*. Cambridge, MA: Harvard University Press.

Bzoch, K., & League, R. (1970). *The receptive-expressive emergent language scale for the measurement of language skills in infancy*. Gainesvile, FL: Tree of Life Press.

Cairns, R. (1979). *Social development: The origins and plasticity of interchange*. San Francisco: Freeman.

Cardoso-Martins, C., & Mervis, C. (1985). Maternal speech to prelinguistic children with Down Syndrome. *American Journal of Mental Deficiency, 89*, 451–458.

Centerwell, S., & Centerwell, W. (1960). A study of children with mongol reared in the home compared to those reared away from home. *Pediatrics, 25*, 678–685.

Cicchetti, D. (Ed.) (1984a). Special issue: Developmental psychopathology. *Child Development, 55* (whole no. 1).

Cicchetti, D. (1984b). The emergence of Developmental Psychopathology. *Child Development, 55*, 1–7.

Cicchetti, D., & Hesse, P. (1983). Affect and intellect: Piaget's contributions to the study of infant emotional development. In R. Plutchik & H. Kellerman (Eds.), *Emotion: Theory, research and experience* (Vol. 2.). New York: Academic Press.

Cicchetti, D. & Mans-Wagener, L. (1987). Stages, sequences, and structures in the organization of cognitive development in Down Syndrome infants. In I. Uzgiris & J. McV. Hunt (Eds.), *Research with scales of psychological development in infancy*. Urbana: University of Illinois Press

Cicchetti, D., & Pogge-Hesse, P. (1982). Possible contributions of the study of organically retarded persons to developmental theory. In E. Zigler & D. Balla (Eds.), *The delay-difference controversy*. Hillsdale, NJ: Erlbaum.

Cicchetti, D., & Serafica, F. (1981). Interplay among behavioral systems: Illustrations from the study of attachment, affiliation, and wariness in young children with Down's Syndrome. *Developmental Psychology, 17*, 36–49.

Cicchetti, D., & Sroufe, L. A. (1976). The relationship between affective and cognitive development in Down syndrome infants. *Child Development, 47,* 920–929.

Cicchetti, D., & Sroufe, L. A. (1978). An organizational view of affect: Illustration from the study of Down syndrome infants. In M. Lewis & L. A. Rosenblum (Eds.), *The development of affect.* New York: Plenum.

Clarke-Stewart, A. (1978). And Daddy makes three: The father's impact on mother and young child. *Child Development, 49,* 466–478.

Cornwell, A. (1974). Development of language, abstraction, and numerical concept formation in Down's Syndrome children. *American Journal of Mental Deficiency, 79,* 179–190.

Cornwell, A., & Birch, H. (1969). Psychological and social development in home-reared children with Down's Syndrome (mongolism). *American Journal of Mental Deficiency, 74,* 341–350.

Crnic, K., Friedrich, W., & Greenberg, M. (1983). Adaptation of families with mentally retarded children: A model of stress, coping, and family ecology. *American Journal of Mental Deficiency, 88,* 125–138.

Curcio, F. (1978). Sensorimotor functioning and communication in mute autistic children. *Journal of Autism and Childhood Schizophrenia, 8,* 282–292.

Dameron, L. (1963). Development of intelligence in infants with mongolism. *Child Development, 34,* 733–738.

Decarie, T. G. (1978). Affect development and cognition in a Piagetian context. In M. Lewis & L. A. Rosenblum (Eds.), *The development of affect.* New York: Plenum.

Dicks-Mireaux, M. (1972). Mental development of infants with Down's syndrome. *American Journal of Mental Deficiency, 77,* 26–32.

Dunn, J., & Kendrick, C. (1981). Interaction between young siblings: Association with the interaction between mother and first-born child. *Developmental Psychology, 17,* 336–343.

Dunst, C. (1980). *A clinical and educational manual for use with the Uzgiris and Hunt Scales of Infant Psychological Development.* Baltimore: University Park Press.

Dunst, C. J. (1988). Stage transitioning in the sensorimotor development of Down's syndrome infants. *Journal of Mental Deficiency Research, 32,* 405–410.

Ellis, N. (1963). The stimulus trace and behavioral inadequacy. In N. Ellis (Ed.), *Handbook of mental deficiency.* New York: McGraw-Hill.

Fischer, K. (1980). A theory of cognitive development: The control and construction of a hierarchy of skills. *Psychological Review, 87,* 477–531.

Fishler, K. (1975). Mental development in Mosaic Down syndrome as compared with Trisomy 21. In R. Koch & F. de la Cruz (Eds.), *Down's Syndrome (mongolism): Research, prevention and management.* New York: Brunner/Mazel.

Flavell, J. (1982). Structures, stages, and sequences in cognitive development. In W. A. Collins (Ed.), *The concept of development: The Minnesota symposia on child psychology* (Vol. 15). Hillsdale, NJ: Erlbaum.

Fraser, F., & Sadovnick, A. (1976). Correlations of IQ in subjects with Down syndrome and their parents and sibs. *Journal of Mental Deficiency Research, 20,* 179–182.

Furrow, D., Nelson, K., & Benedict, H. (1979). Mothers' speech to children and syntactic development: Some simple relationships. *Journal of Child Language, 6,* 423–442.

Gardner, H. (1982). *Frames of mind.* New York: Basic Books.

Gibson, D. (1967). Intelligence in the mongoloid and his parent. *American Journal of Mental Deficiency, 71,* 1014–1016.

Gibson, D. (1978). *Down's Syndrome: The psychology of mongolism.* Cambridge: Cambridge University Press.

Golden, W., & Pashayan, H. (1976). The effect of parental education on the eventual mental development of noninstitutionalized children with Down Syndrome. *Journal of Pediatrics, 89,* 603–605.

Greenfield, P., & Smith, J. (1976). *The structure of communication in early language development.* New York: Academic Press.

Greenwald, C., & Leonard, L. (1979). Communicative and sensorimotor development of Down's Syndrome children. *American Journal of Mental Deficiency, 84,* 296–303.

Harrell, T., & Harrell, M. (1945). Army classification test scores for civilian occupations. *Educational and Psychological Measurement, 5,* 229–239.

Hill, P. M., & McCune-Nicholich, L. (1981). Pretend play and patterns of cognition in Down's Syndrome children. *Child Development, 52,* 1168–1175.

Hodapp, R., & Goldfield, E. (1983). The use of mother–infant games as therapy with delayed children. *Early Child Development and Care, 13,* 17–32.

Hodapp, R., & Goldfield, E. (1985). Self and other regulation during the infancy period. *Developmental Review, 5.*

Hodapp, R., Goldfield, E., & Boyatzis, C. (1984). The use and effectiveness of maternal scaffolding in mother–infant games. *Child Development, 55,* 772–781.

Hodapp, R., & Mueller, E. (1982). Early social development. In B. Wolman (Ed.), *Handbook of developmental psychology.* Englewood Cliffs, NJ: Prentice-Hall.

Honzik, M., & MacFarlane, J. (1973). Personality development and intellectual functioning from 21 months to 40 years. In L. Jarvik, C. Eisdorf, & J. Blum (Eds.), *Intellectual functioning in adults.* New York: Springer.

Johnson, R., & Abelard, R. (1969). The behavioral competence of mongoloid and nonmongoloid retardates. *American Journal of Mental Deficiency, 73,* 856–857.

Jones, O. (1977). Mother–child communication with prelinguistic Down's syndrome and normal infants. In H. R. Schaffer (Ed.), *Studies in mother-infant interaction.* New York: Academic Press.

Jones, O. (1980). Prelinguistic communication skills in Down's syndrome and normal infants. In T. Field, S. Goldberg, D. Stern, & A. Sostek (Eds.), *High-risk infants and children: Adult and peer interactions.* New York: Academic Press.

Kahn, J. (1977). Piaget's theory of cognitive development and its relationship to severely and profoundly retarded children. In P. Mittler (Ed.), *Research to practice in mental retardation* (Vol. 2). Baltimore: University Park Press.

Kaye, K. (1976). Infant's effects upon their mothers' teaching strategies. In J. C. Glidewell (Ed.), *The social context of learning and development.* New York: Gardner Press.

Kaye, K. (1982). *The mental and social life of babies.* Chicago: University of Chicago Press.

Kaye, K., & Furstenberg, F. (Eds.) (1985). Special issue: Family development and the child. *Child Development, 56* (whole no. 2).

Kessen, W. (1962). Stage and structure in the study of children. In W. Kessen and C. Kuhlman (Eds.), *Thought in the young child. Monographs of the Society for Research in Child Development, 27.*

Kessen, W. (1971). Early cognitive development: Hot or cold? In T. Mischel (Ed.), *Cognitive development and epistemology.* New York: Academic Press.

Kohlberg, L. (1976). Moral stages and moralization: The cognitive-developmental approach. In T. Lickona (Ed.), *Moral development and behavior: Theory, research and social issues.* New York: Holt, Rinehart & Winston.

Kopp, C. (1983). Risk factors in development. In P. Mussen (Ed.), *Handbook of Child Psychology.* Vol. 2: *Infancy and Developmental Psychobiology.* New York: Wiley.

Kopp, C., & McCall, R. (1982). Predicting later mental performance for normal, at risk, and handicapped infants. In P. Baltes & O. Brim (Eds.), *Lifespan development and behavior* (Vol. 4). New York: Academic Press.

Kounin, J. (1948). The meaning of rigidity: A reply to Heinz Werner. *Psychological Review, 55,* 157–166.

Krakow, J., & Kopp, C. (1982). Sustained attention in young Down syndrome children. *Topics in Early Childhood Special Education, 2,* 32–42.

Lamb, M. (1978). Influences of the child on marital quality and family interaction during the prenatal, perinatal, and infancy periods. In R. Lerner & G. Spanier (Eds.), *Child influences on marital and family interaction.* New York: Academic Press.

Lamb, M. (1981). *The role of the father in child development* (2nd ed.). New York: Wiley.

Leifer, J., & Lewis, M. (1984). Acquisition of conversational response skills by young Down Syndrome and nonretarded young children. *American Journal of Mental Deficiency, 88,* 610–618.

Lewin, K. (1935). *A dynamic theory of personality: Selected papers.* A. Adams & K. Zenner (Trans.). New York: McGraw-Hill.

Libb, J., Myers, G., Graham, E., & Bell, B. (1983). Correlates of intelligence and adaptive behavior in Down's Syndrome. *Journal of Mental Deficiency Research, 27,* 205–210.

Lubs, M., & Maes, J. (1977). Recurrence risk in mental retardation. In P. Mittler (Ed.), *Research to practice in mental retardation* (Vol. 3). Baltimore: University Park Press.

Luria, A. (1982). Psychological studies of mental deficiency in the Soviet Union. In E. Zigler & D. Balla (Eds.), *The delay-difference controversy.* Hillsdale, NJ: Erlbaum.

MacDonald, J., & Blott, J. (1974). Environmental language intervention: A rational for diagnostic and training strategy through rules, context, and generalization. *Journal of Speech and Hearing Disorders, 39,* 244–256.

MacTurk, R., Vietze, P., McCarthy, M., McQuiston, S., & Yarrow, L. (1985). The organization of exploratory behavior in Down Syndrome and nondelayed infants. *Child Development, 56,* 573–581.

Mahoney, G., Glover, A., & Finger, I. (1981). The relationship between language and sensorimotor development among Down syndrome and developmentally normal children. *American Journal of Mental Deficiency, 86,* 21–27.

McCall, R., Appelbaum, M., & Hogarty, P. (1973). Developmental changes in mental performance. *Mongraphs of the Society for Research in Child Development, 38.*

McCall, R., Eichorn, E., & Hogarty, P. (1977). Transitions in early mental development. *Monographs of the Society for Research in Child Development, 42.*

McLean, J., & Snyder-McLean, L. (1978). *A transactional approach to early language training.* Westerville, OH: Merrill.

Melyn, M. & White, D. (1973). Mental and developmental milestones of noninstitutionalized Down's syndrome children. *Pediatrics, 52,* 542–545.

Miller, J., & Yoder, D. (1974). An ontogenetic language teaching strategy for retarded children. In R. L. Schiefelbusch & L. L. Lloyd (Eds.), *Language perspectives: Acquisition, retardation and intervention.* Baltimore: University Park Press.

Motti, F., Cicchetti, D., & Sroufe, L. A. (1983). From infant affect expression to symbolic play: The coherence of development in Down syndrome children. *Child Development, 54,* 1168–1175.

Mundy, P., Seibert, J., & Hogan, A. (1984). Relationship between sensorimotor and early communication abilities in developmentally delayed children. *Merrill-Palmer Quarterly, 30,* 33–48.

Overton, W., & Reese, H. (1973). Models of development: Methodological implications. In L. R. Goulet & P. B. Baltes (Eds.), *Life-span developmental psychology.* New York: Academic Press.

Paradise, E., & Curcio, F. (1974). Relationship of cognitive and affective behaviors to fear of strangers in male infants. *Developmental Psychology, 10,* 476–483.

Parke, R. (1979). Perspectives in father–infant development. In J. D. Osofsky (Ed.), *Handbook of infant development.* New York: Wiley.

Piaget, J. (1952). *The origins of intelligence in children.* New York: International Universities Press.

Piaget, J. (1977). Problems of equilibration. In M. Appel & L. Goldberg (Eds.), *Topics in cognitive development* (Vol. 1). New York: Plenum.

Piaget, J. (1981). *Intelligence and affectivity.* Palo Alto, CA: Annual Reviews.

Plomin, R., & DeFries, J. (1980). Genetics and intelligence: Recent data. *Intelligence, 4,* 15–24.

Rondal, J. (1977). Maternal speech to normal and Down syndrome children. In P. Mittler (Ed.), *Research to practice in mental retardation* (Vol. 2). Baltimore: University Park Press.

Rosenberg, S. (1984). Disorders of first-language development: Trends in research and theory. In E. Gollin (Ed.), *Malformations of development: Biological and psychological sources and consequences.* New York: Academic Press.

Sameroff, A. (1975). Early influences on development: Fact or fancy? *Merrill-Palmer Quarterly, 21,* 267–294.

Scarr, S., & Carter-Saltzman, L. (1982). Genetics and intelligence. In R. Sternberg (Ed.), *Handbook of human intelligence.* Cambridge: Cambridge University Press.

Share, J. (1975). Developmental progress in Down's Syndrome. In R. Koch & F. F. de la Cruz (Eds.),

Down's Syndrome (mongolism): Research, prevention and management. New York: Brunner/Mazel.

Silverstein, A. (1982). Note on the constancy of the IQ. *American Journal of Mental Deficiency, 87,* 227–228.

Snyder, L. (1978). Communicative and cognitive abilities and disabilities in the sensorimotor period. *Merrill-Palmer Quarterly, 24,* 161–180.

Uzgiris, I., & Hunt, J. McV. (1975). *Assessment in Infancy: Ordinal scales of psychological development.* Urbana: University of Illinois Press.

Vernon, P. (1979). *Intelligence: Heredity and environment.* San Francisco: Freeman.

Wapner, S., & Kaplan, B. (Eds.) (1983). *Toward a holistic developmental psychology.* Hillsdale, NJ: Erlbaum.

Weisz, J., & Yeates, K. (1981). Cognitive development in retarded and nonretarded persons: Piagetian tests of the similar structure hypothesis. *Psychological Bulletin, 90,* 153–178.

Weisz, J., & Zigler, E. (1979). Cognitive development in retarded and nonretarded persons: Piagetian tests of the similar sequence hypothesis. *Psychological Bulletin, 86,* 831–851.

Werner, H. (1948). *Comparative psychology of mental development.* New York: Follett.

Werner, H., & Kaplan, B. (1963). *Symbol formation.* New York: Wiley.

White, S. (1984). Studies of developing mentality. Review of H. Werner, *Comparative psychology of mental development. Contemporary Psychology, 29,* 199–202.

Youniss, J. (1978). Dialectical theory and Piaget on social knowledge. *Human Development, 21,* 234–247.

Zeaman, D., & House, B. (1963). The role of attention in retardate discrimination learning. In N. R. Ellis (Ed.), *Handbook of mental deficiency.* New York: McGraw-Hill.

Zeaman, D., & House, B. (1979). A review of attention theory. In N. Ellis (Ed.), *Handbook of mental deficiency: Psychological theory and research* (2nd ed.). Hillsdale, NJ: Erlbaum.

Zigler, E. (1963). Metatheoretical issues in developmental psychology. In N. Marx (Ed.), *Theories in contemporary psychology.* New York: Macmillan.

Zigler, E. (1967). Familial mental retardation: A continuing dilemma. *Science, 155,* 292–298.

Zigler, E. (1969). Developmental versus difference theories of mental retardation and the problem of motivation. *American Journal of Mental Deficiency, 73,* 536–556.

Zigler, E. (1971). The retarded child as a whole person. In H. E. Adams & W. K. Boardman III (Eds.), *Advances in experimental clinical psychology* (Vol. 1). New York: Pergamon.

Zigler, E. (1984). A developmental theory on mental retardation. In B. Blatt & R. Morris (Eds.), *Perspectives in special education: Personal orientations.* Glenview, IL: Scott, Foresman.

Zigler, E., & Balla, D. (1977). Personality factors in the performance of the retarded. *Journal of the American Academy of Child Psychiatry, 16,* 19–27.

Zigler, E., & Hodapp, R. (1986). *Understanding mental retardation.* Cambridge: Cambridge University Press.

2 An organizational approach to the study of Down syndrome: contributions to an integrative theory of development

Dante Cicchetti and Marjorie Beeghly

During the past several decades, more and more investigators have focused their efforts on articulating the processes of ontogenesis in the perceptual, cognitive, socioemotional, linguistic, and representational domains of development in infants and children with Down syndrome. Recently, much of this work has been guided by the organizational perspective and has been conducted with the goal of expanding our knowledge of the normal developmental process (Cicchetti & Pogge-Hesse, 1982; Cicchetti & Sroufe, 1978). Studies of populations where varied patterns of development may occur as a consequence of the pervasive and enduring influences that mark the transaction between the child and the environment, such as with children with Down syndrome and their families, provide an appropriate basis for affirming, expanding, and challenging current development theory. Simultaneously, this approach allows for the formulation of a more comprehensive and integrative theory of normal development (Cicchetti, 1984, in press; Freud, 1965; Inhelder, 1966; Rutter, 1986; Werner, 1948). This ''developmental'' approach to Down syndrome is receiving increased attention in a variety of disciplines, including education, the neurosciences, pediatrics, psychiatry, and clinical and developmental psychology (see Hodapp & Zigler, Chapter 1, this volume).

Prior to these recent efforts, most investigators had conceptualized the developmental process of individuals with Down syndrome as necessarily being quantitatively and qualitatively different from that of mental-age-matched nonhandicapped children (for reviews, see Cicchetti & Pogge-Hesse, 1982; Hodapp & Zigler, Chap-

Writing of this chapter was supported by grants from the John D. and Catherine T. MacArthur Foundation Network on Early Childhood, the March of Dimes Birth Defects Foundation, and the Spencer Foundation. We are grateful to the many persons who have assisted us with data collection over the years of this research. Thanks are extended to Mary Breitenbucher, Dorothy Dittman, Michelle Gersten, Dan Nichols, Bedonna Weiss-Perry, and especially Linda Mans-Wagener, for their invaluable contributions to this work. We also would like to thank Sheree Toth for her feedback on an earlier draft of this manuscript. In addition, we would like to express our appreciation to Victoria Gill for typing the manuscript. Finally, Dante Cicchetti would like to thank Felicisima Serafica, Alexander Siegel, Alan Sroufe, and Edward Zigler for their support, guidance, and wise counsel throughout his development as a researcher in the area of mental retardation.

ter 1, this volume). Beginning with the publication of several important studies on the perceptual–cognitive and socioemotional development of infants and toddlers with Down syndrome (Cicchetti & Sroufe, 1976, 1978; Fantz, Fagan, & Miranda, 1975; Miranda & Fantz, 1974; Serafica & Cicchetti, 1976), researchers increasingly have demonstrated that the developmental process of children with Down syndrome is adaptive, organized, and meaningful–just as it is with nonhandicapped children. Despite the quantitative and qualitative differences that have been found between children with Down syndrome and cognitively comparable nonhandicapped children, a large body of empirical studies has revealed that children with Down syndrome manifest coherence in the organization of their behavioral and biological systems (in addition to the chapters in this volume, see: Beeghly & Cicchetti, 1987; Cicchetti & Mans-Wagener, 1987; Cicchetti & Pogge-Hesse, 1982; Cicchetti & Sroufe, 1976, 1978; Jasnow et al. 1988; Loveland, 1987; Mans, Cicchetti, & Sroufe, 1978; Motti, Cicchetti, & Sroufe, 1983; Mundy, Sigman, Kasari, & Yirmiya, 1988; Thompson, Cicchetti, Lamb, & Malkin, 1985).

Goals of this chapter

The organizational developmental psychopathology perspective, with its emphasis on the study of developing systems and on uncovering the relation between normal and atypical forms of ontogenesis, provides an excellent theoretical framework for conducting investigations of children with Down syndrome. The discipline of developmental psychopathology has been built upon the assumption that a developmental approach can be applied to any unit of behavior or discipline and to all cultures or populations, normal or otherwise atypical (Werner, 1948). Developmental psychopathologists emphasize the premise that we can learn more about the normal functioning of an organism by studying its pathology, and, likewise, more about its pathology by studying its normal condition (Cicchetti, 1984; Kaplan, 1966; Rutter, 1986). Due to its multidisciplinary perspective, the discipline of developmental psychopathology requires that multiple domains of development be examined, including perceptual–cognitive, socioemotional, linguistic-representational, and biological processes (Achenbach, in press; Cicchetti, 1984, in press; Rutter & Garmezy, 1983).

Within the discipline of developmental psychopathology, the investigation of normal and atypical patterns of ontogenesis requires a consideration of the different behavioral and biological systems within which advances are proceeding in parallel and exerting a mutual influence upon each other. To theorize about development without examining the interaction among multiple domains would lead to a diminished view of the complexity of the developmental process. Similarly, to formulate a developmental theory without considering the deviations that might be expected as a result of the prominent and wide-ranging intra- and/or extra-organismic disturbances, as well as the transactions that occur among them, would result in an incomplete or ambiguous account of ontogenesis that does not consider adequately individual differences, the continuity and quality of adaptation, or the various pathways by which the same developmental outcome may be achieved (cf. Werner, 1937, and Kaplan, 1983, for lucid discussions of the process–achievement distinction).

Accordingly, any approach to atypical patterns of early development needs to take into account the unique characteristics of the child, the age and stage-level of functioning, the experiences to which the child has been exposed, and the stability of environmental conditions. In addition, the characteristics of the caregiving environment, the compatibility of the infant–caregiver dyad, the continuity or discontinuity of adaptive or maladaptive behavioral patterns, and the advances or lags in different developmental domains must be considered (see Cicchetti & Schneider-Rosen, 1986, for an elaboration).

In this chapter, we illustrate how the study of Down syndrome can enhance our knowledge of normal development. Conversely, we demonstrate how an organizational approach to the investigation of children with Down syndrome can further our understanding of the process of development in these youngsters.

The organizational perspective

Up to the eighteenth century, the concept of development as qualitative change over time was hardly fathomable; however, by approximately 1850, it had blossomed into a major perspective. Most influential in bringing about this dramatic shift was the appearance of Herbert Spencer's ''Developmental Hypothesis'' (Spencer, 1862/ 1900), in which development was depicted as a uniform process that was governed by universal laws and principles. Most contemporary developmental models adhere to a similar organismic world view, stressing the dynamic role of the individual and conceptualizing the individual as an organized whole (Kaplan, 1967). Principles of behavior are seen in terms of the organization among parts and wholes, and of the dynamic interplay between the individual and the environment (Overton, 1976, 1984; Santostefano, 1978).

The organizational approach to development (Cicchetti & Sroufe, 1978; Sroufe, 1979a, 1979b) – also sometimes referred to as the ''organismic'' or ''structuralist'' approach – consists of a set of regulative principles that can guide research into and theorizing about human behavior (Santostefano, 1978; Sroufe & Rutter, 1984). In referring to these principles as ''regulative'' we follow Werner (1948), who denied that they are themselves to be seen as empirical laws or that, in research and theory, one should necessarily attempt to find laws that can serve as simple translations of these principles into empirical terms. Rather, such regulative principles are to be viewed as heuristic tools, by means of which one can look for meaningful patterns in the great variety and quantity of data often accumulated in contemporary studies of human development and developmental psychopathology (Cicchetti, 1984; Sroufe & Rutter, 1984). With the aide of this heuristic, investigators may formulate empirical laws with greater confidence that they have uncovered lawful relations rather than merely accidental correlations.

According to the organizational approach, development may be conceived as a series of qualitative reorganizations among and within behavioral and biological systems. Through development, these reorganizations reflect the further differentiation and hierarchical integration of abilities as well as the dynamic transaction of variables at many different levels of analysis (i.e., genetic, constitutional, neurobiological, biochemical, behavioral, cultural, psychological, environmental, and sociological).

"Normal" development is not defined in terms of the mean because it is not necessarily the case that the mean can be equated with mental health. Rather, it is defined in terms of the successful negotiation of a series of interlocking social, emotional, and cognitive competencies. Competence at one period of development, which tends to make the individual broadly adapted to his or her environment, paves the way for the formation of competence at the next (Sroufe & Rutter, 1984). In this regard, normal development is characterized by the integration of earlier competencies into later modes of functioning. It follows, then, that early adaptation tends to promote later adaptation and integration.

In contrast, pathological development may be viewed as the lack of integration of the social, emotional, and cognitive competencies important to achieving adaptation at a particular developmental level (Cicchetti & Schneider-Rosen, 1986; Kaplan, 1966; Sroufe, 1979a). Because early structures often are incorporated into later structures, an early deviation or perturbation in functioning may ultimately cause much larger perturbations to emerge subsequently.

According to the organizational approach, the qualitative reorganizations that accompany development are conceived as proceeding in accordance with the *orthogenetic principle* (Werner, 1948), which states that the developing organism moves from a relatively diffuse and globally undifferentiated state, by means of *differentiation* and *hierarchical integration,* to a state of greater articulation and organized complexity. The orthogenetic principle may be seen as a solution to the problem of the individual's continuous adaptation to the environment and to the question of how integrity of function may be maintained in the face of change. Continuity in functioning can be maintained via hierarchical integration despite the rapid constitutional changes and bio-behavioral shifts that characterize the process of development throughout the life course (Block, 1971; Block & Block, 1980; Brim & Kagan, 1980; Caspi, Elder, & Bem, 1987, 1988; Sackett, Sameroff, Cairns, & Suomi, 1981; Sroufe, 1979a).

In addition to orthogenesis, several related principles characterize the organizational framework: (1) with development, there is change in structure–function relationships over time; (2) the change that occurs is both qualitative and quantitative; and (3) developmental change is best conceived as a move toward increasing cortical control over the more diffuse, automatic behavioral centers.

Reasons why Down syndrome constitutes an interesting population for developmental research

Children with Down syndrome are an especially important population for developmentalists to study. As an "experiment in nature" (Bronfenbrenner, 1979), Down syndrome presents an excellent opportunity to answer critical questions in developmental theory that, on ethical grounds alone, would be impossible to manipulate experimentally. In addition, unlike most other groups of mentally retarded youngsters, children with Down syndrome are etiologically homogeneous, their condition is detectable at birth, and therefore their developmental processes can be monitored virtually from the beginning. Although their development unfolds at a delayed rate, children with Down syndrome are quite heterogeneous, ranging from severely mentally retarded to approximately normal intellectual functioning. The increased variability is a prominent characteristic of Down syndrome and also has been noted for growth in stature, skeletal maturation, tissue development, and dentition (Barden, 1983; Cronk, 1978; Roche, 1964, 1965; Shapiro, 1970, 1975). This combination of delayed, yet variable, development allows a more careful examination of the nature of developmental stages and sequences across different developmental domains and of the interrelations among behavioral and biological systems at a given point in development. Just as is true for cross-cultural research, the study of Down syndrome can inform us about which stages, sequences, and structures are logically necessary and what alternate pathways of ontogenesis are possible. Evidence concerning which factors (e.g., biological, psychological, cultural, sociological) contributing to the developmental process are most critical also can be provided.

Furthermore, their delayed pace of development, prolonged developmental transitions, and variability of functioning on different developmental domains (e.g., their productive language is far below their mental age – see Beeghly, Weiss-Perry, & Cicchetti, Chapter 10, and Fowler, Chapter 9, this volume) make the study of Down syndrome an ideal candidate for elucidating the understanding of sensitive periods in ontogenesis (Aslin, 1981; Bateson, 1979; Bornstein, 1989; Bronson, 1965; Curtiss, 1977; Gottlieb, 1983; Lenneberg, 1967). In particular, because of their heterogeneity the investigation of children with Down syndrome can advance our understanding of what is maturational and what is developmental about phenotypic change (see, for example, Cicchetti & Sroufe, 1976, 1978). For example, in his studies of normal children and children with Down syndrome, Lenneberg (1966, 1967) found that, even though the Down syndrome sample acquired their motor and language milestones later and at a slower rate, both groups progressed through the same developmental sequences in these domains. Moreover, Lenneberg discovered that there was a close correspondence between their motor development and language development. Consequently, Lenneberg argued that motor development and language acquisition were under the control of the maturation of the brain.

Children with Down syndrome possess many genetic and constitutional handicaps, including congenital heart and respiratory defects, an increased incidence of immunodeficiencies, hematopoietic dysfunction, leukemia and seizure disorders, and abnormalities of neuromuscular tone, visual acuity, and audiovestibular functioning. In addition, these children manifest morphologic and microscopic brain alterations, neuropsychological impairments, and neuropathological, neurochemical, and histological similarities to individuals with Alzheimer's disease (Courchesne, 1988; Coyle, Oster-Granite, & Gearhart, 1986; Petit, LeBoutillier, Alfano, & Becker, 1984; Purpura, 1974; Smith, 1985; Takashima, Becker, Armstrong, &

Chan, 1981; Thase, 1988). Nonetheless, we believe that the investigation of the psychological development of these youngsters can greatly enhance our knowledge of developmental processes. In particular, as progress on the biology and psychology of this condition continues to occur, we believe that Down syndrome may become a model for how the multidisciplinary study of the effects of chromosomal anomaly upon development can elucidate our understanding of brain–behavior relations during ontogenesis. This increased knowledge base should inevitably result in more rational, developmentally sensitive treatment interventions.

In the following sections of this chapter, we provide empirical illustrations of the nature of the interrelation among developmental domains in children with Down syndrome. Through these examples, we demonstrate both how the study of Down syndrome can augment our knowledge of normal ontogenetic processes and how an organizational analysis is helpful to understanding the coherence of development in children with Down syndrome.

The relation between motor control and visual proprioception

Developmental studies raise questions about the origins of the proprioceptive function of vision and about its role in the acquisition of motor control. An extensive animal research literature suggests that visual feedback is involved in the development of early motor skills (see, for example, Ganz, 1975; Hein, 1972). However, evidence derived from human infants is limited.

One approach utilized has been to study motor development in the congenitally blind. Fraiberg (1977) reported that blind babies were delayed in acquiring "static" postures such as sitting and standing and significantly impaired in acquiring "dynamic" postures such as crawling and walking. Because the major effects seem limited to self-initiated mobility, she argued that these deficits occur because the blind infant is deprived of external motivation to become mobile, such as the sight of attractive objects that are beyond reach. According to Fraiberg, visual feedback is not intrinsic to human motor development but rather is thought to serve a motivating function that elicits mobility.

Fraiberg's evidence is compatible with the theory that the lack of visual feedback may contribute to motor retardation in the blind, if it is indeed the case that the development of "dynamic" postures depends on the acquisition of control over "static" postures (Shirley, 1931). The absence of visual feedback may disrupt the developmental relation between motor control processes.

An alternative approach with sighted infants is made possible by use of an experimental procedure known as the "conflict" technique. When infants initially begin to stand without support, they use visual information to monitor their posture with respect to their external environment (Lee & Aronson, 1974). This has been demonstrated by putting mechanical-vestibular cues specifying a stable posture into conflict with visual cues specifying instability. The general procedure is to stand the infant on a stationary floor, inside a "movable room" consisting of three walls and a ceiling. The room is moved around the infant in such a way that the resulting provision of visual information coincides with that which would visually be contingent on body sway ("visual proprioception") (Gibson, 1966). Infants compensate for a perceived loss of balance and consequently they sway, stagger, or fall in a direction opposite to the plane of instability specified by the misleading visual information. The effect of discrepant visual information is not limited to the upright stance. Butterworth and Hicks (1977) found the conflict technique to disrupt the seated posture as much in the infants who could not stand as in infants who could sit or stand unsupported. Thus, vision is implicated in the control of standing and sitting and it may well be involved in the control of postures that occur even earlier in development.

Data obtained from the animal literature is again relevant. Findings suggest that motor experience within a structured visual space contributes to the development of skilled motor activity, although motor experience may not be required to establish basic visual–motor links (Ganz, 1975). The conflict technique can be used to establish whether changes in the effect of discrepant visual feedback occur with the advanced experience of a posture. Moreover, there exist populations of infants who are sighted but who are delayed in acquiring both static and dynamic postures. Infants with Down syndrome constitute one such group. We hypothesized that if vision were implicated in normal motor development, comparisons of the effects of discrepant visual feedback on postural stability in normal infants and infants with Down syndrome might reveal systematic differences between the groups.

Generally, infants with Down syndrome are delayed by 6 months in sitting unsupported and they evidence an even greater lag of approximately 10 months in standing unsupported (Cowie, 1970). The genesis of these delays is thought to be flaccidity (hypotonia) of the muscular system (Henderson, 1985). Extreme hypotonia is present in infants with Down syndrome from birth (McIntire & Dutch, 1964) and it can continue to be a severe problem throughout infancy (Cowie, 1970), thereby making it difficult for the infant to support his or her own weight. Thus, while it is possible that the locomotor retardation manifested by children with Down syndrome may be totally a function of poor muscle tone, failures of visual proprioception also may contribute to this state of affairs.

Two experiments were conducted in our laboratory in order to compare the effects of discrepant visual feedback on the control of sitting and standing in normal infants and in infants with Down syndrome (Butterworth & Cicchetti, 1978). The groups of babies were matched for the length of time they had achieved a given posture. This enabled us to examine simultaneously the effects of discrepant visual information on postural stability as a function of experience and motor delay.

In our initial study, we examined normal infants and infants with Down syndrome. Both samples of infants were divided into four subgroups matched according to how long they had been able to stand unsupported. The mean length of experience standing of the four subgroups of infants with Down syndrome was 1.2 months, 5.0 months, 8.7 months, and 19.5 months. The mean ages of these infants were 29.8, 26.6, 32.8 and 41.8 months respectively. The mean length of experience standing of the four normal subgroups was 1.25 months, 5.2 months, 8.5 months, and 22.9 months. The average ages of these groups were 14.0, 17.4, 18.8, and 34.1 months respectively. The Down syndrome group stood without support on an average of 24 months (range = 12 to 47 months). The age at which the normal infants stood unsupported was approximately 12 months (range = 8 to 16 months), congruent with the norms provided by the Bayley (1969) Motor Scale.

Infants were seen in an experimental ''room'' consisting of three walls and a ceiling, which was open at one end and mounted on wheels at each corner so that it could be moved backward and forward on its long axis. The inside of the room was painted white, and a brightly colored poster was hung on the interior end wall in order to provide contrast.

The first study included infants who could stand up supported for 1 minute without swaying, staggering, or falling. Following this pretest, infants were examined under conditions of discrepant visual feedback while standing and sitting, facing the interior end wall of the movable room. No physical support was provided, but an adult, usually the mother, knelt behind the infant a little to one side, ready to catch the infant if he or she fell. Trials were initiated when the infant was standing still, or sitting with legs extended and hands off the floor, while attending to the picture on the end wall. A counterbalanced design was used so that infants completed a maximum of six trials in each posture, with the room alternating in direction of movement on successive trials manually on its long axis. The closest the end came to the infant's marked position was 61 cm, the farthest was 122 cm. The side walls remained at a constant distance of 61 cm. The experiment was videotaped for subsequent analysis.

A rating scale devised by Lee and Aronson (1974) was used to score postural adjustments made by the infants. To be scored as a postural adjustment, the infant's response had to be contingent on movement of the room. The zero category included any response that could not be categorized as a postural adjustment, such as escaping from the room, as well as those trials on which no noticeable response occurred. The video recording was scored by two independent experimenters and only responses on which the raters agreed were included in the analyses (agreement was 98%).

Both normal infants and infants with Down syndrome made postural adjustments contingent on movement of the surround (Down syndrome on 90% of the trials and normals of 84% of the trials). The vast majority of responses were in the direction of movement of the room (95%). If the end wall approached, the infant reacted by moving backward, swaying, staggering, or falling, while, if it receded, the infant swayed, staggered, or fell forward. The remaining 5% of responses were ''mixed,'' in that the infant would initially move in the same direction as the room but would then compensate again so that the final response was in the direction opposite to the movement of the room. Data analyses were conducted on individual scores expressed as a proportion of trials completed and on a composite score reflecting the quality of response.

Although no significant difference emerged between the normal infants and the infants with Down syndrome in the total number of responses when standing in the moving room, there were differences between the groups in the magnitude of the response. Infants with Down syndrome fell over significantly more often than the normal infants. Although the Down syndrome group was delayed in the acquisition of the standing posture, they showed a greater qualitative effect of a discrepancy between visual and mechanical-vestibular proprioception than the normal infants. Falling was rare after 3 months experience of standing, whereas a comparable decline in falls was achieved by the infants with Down syndrome only after 7 to 12 months experience of the posture.

There was evidence of a decline in the total number of responses with experience of the posture among the normal infants. That is, the normal subgroup that had the greatest experience with the standing posture was least likely to make a postural adjustment when the room moved. By comparison, the distribution of responses among the infants with Down syndrome was homogeneous, with no overall difference among subgroups.

These results suggest that in the standing posture, infants with Down syndrome are more influenced by the discrepancy between visual and mechanical-vestibular cues than the normal infants, since infants with Down syndrome fall over more often when the room moves. Furthermore, with experience of the standing posture, there is a decline in the intensity of response to discrepant visual information in both groups. Normal infants, after 13 to 33 months of standing, become relatively independent of their surround to control standing, insofar as they make significantly fewer postural adjustments than any other group when the room moves.

Infants included in the second study were capable of sitting unsupported, yet were unable to stand alone. As in the first experiment, infants with Down syndrome and normal infants were divided into three subgroups matched on length of sitting experience: 0 to 3 months, 4 to 6 months, and 7 to 12 months. The mean experience sitting of the Down syndrome subgroups was 1.29 months, 4.94 months, and 10.33 months. The mean ages of these groups were 11.50, 14.80, and 17.66 months, respectively. The average experience sitting of the three normal subgroups was 1.45, 5.00, and 7.14 months, with average ages of 6.90, 11.90, and 12.60 months, respectively.

The apparatus and procedure were identical to those employed in the first experiment, except that there were eight trials (four approach and four recede) in which the infant sat facing the end wall of the moving room. The scoring procedure and response categories were the same as in Experiment 1. All infants were pretested on arrival at the laboratory in order to ensure that they could sit unsupported for 1 minute without swaying, staggering, or falling.

On average, movement of the room was less disruptive of the sitting posture, after any given period of experience, than it had been of the standing posture. Although these data replicate the results of Butterworth and Hicks (1977), they also extend previous findings, since it is clear that for the normal infants there was a decline in responding with experience paralleling that found for standing. In the 0 to 3 month group of normal infants, falls and staggers were observed, just as among the standing infants. Thus, discrepant visual feedback occurring shortly after the acquisition of the seated posture was sufficient to result in a complete loss of balance among normal infants. At times the seated normal infant was completely "bowled over" when the room moved, even though the infant was perfectly capable of maintaining a stable posture in the pretest.

This was true only for the normal infants. Whereas in Experiment 1 the infants with Down syndrome were significantly more likely than the normal infants to fall over, now the relative effect of discrepant visual feedback on the two groups was completely reversed. The normal infants made significantly more responses in total than the Down syndrome group and they made significantly more responses in each of the categories, sway, stagger, or fall. In the group of infants with Down syndrome, the usual response was a very slight sway in the direction of movement of the room or no response at all. Moreover, responses among the infants with Down syndrome remained at a constant basal level throughout the range of experience.

To summarize, the results of these two experiments present somewhat of a paradox. Infants with Down syndrome who recently have learned to sit unsupported are significantly less responsive to movements of the surround than normal infants. However, infants with Down syndrome who have recently learned to stand unsupported are somewhat more responsive to movements of the surround than normal infants. There is a decline in responding with increases in experience of the standing posture in both normal infants and infants with Down syndrome. In normal infants, control of sitting shows a similar developmental course to control of standing and the two processes appear to be interrelated. Among the Down syndrome group, however, the effect of experience on the stability of sitting under conditions of discrepant visual feedback is minimal. The infants with Down syndrome show a constant low basal level of response when sitting. In accord with the literature on animal motor development, the results suggest that experience of a posture in relation to the surround is an important component process in gaining motor control.

Regardless of the origin of the proprioceptive function of vision, the theory that seems best able to account for the results obtained is that postural control depends on congruence between mechanical-vestibular and visual indices of postural stability (Butterworth & Hicks, 1977). Elaborating upon this argument, a relatively unstable posture tolerates less of a discrepancy between visual and mechanical-vestibular proprioception before compensation is required. Hence, on average standing is more influenced by movement of the surround than sitting, although sitting also can be severely disrupted early in its history. This in turn suggests that the function of visual proprioception in postural development may be to "calibrate" or fine-tune the mechanical-vestibular system against the stable surround. As the infant gains motor control, the posture becomes increasingly independent of visual cues, so that eventually infants know that it is the surround that must be moving and they who are stable.

Analysis of infants' emotional reactions lends some support to this theory. In the first 2 months after standing unsupported, infants would usually cry when the room moved, if they showed an emotional reaction. However, 4 to 6 months after standing unsupported had emerged, infants would sometimes laugh, and by 12 months of standing experience their emotional reaction was always positive. That is, after a certain amount of experience of standing, infants behaved as if they interpreted the movement of the room as an incongruous event that was relatively independent of their own postural stability. Emotional reactions among the infants with Down syndrome were similar, but the frequency of response was only 15% that of normals.

The process of gaining autonomous control of posture may account for the differences obtained between normal and motorically delayed infants with Down syndrome. It is possible that obtaining some control over the sitting posture in the normal infant may have positive transfer to the upright stance. Among the Down syndrome group, however, there was little evidence that sitting was monitored closely with respect to the visual surround. Failure to calibrate sitting may lead to a correspondingly greater effect of proprioceptive discrepancy when the infant with Down syndrome finally becomes able to stand unsupported. If the sequence of postures preceding standing form part of a nested hierarchy of motor systems, failure to calibrate earlier postures might be expected to add an increment to the lag in acquisition of later postures.

Both the normal and the motor-delayed Down syndrome groups were able to utilize visual proprioception. When standing, the infants with Down syndrome were severely unbalanced by discrepant visual feedback and even when sitting they showed a constant basal level of response. It seems likely that differences between them and the normal infants may be due to the functioning of the mechanical-vestibular component of the postural control system. Infants with Down syndrome may need a higher level of vestibular stimulation before a significant discrepancy arises with information from the environment.

Thus, although the visual system had been considered merely to provide external motivation for motor development, through the study of infants with Down syndrome, it was demonstrated that visual information specifying postural instability may also play an intrinsic role in the normal achievement of motor control. In addition, these findings may have broader implications for understanding the development of infants with Down syndrome. Because the motor delays of infants with Down syndrome are generally accompanied by concomitant cognitive impairments (Cicchetti & Sroufe, 1976; Lenneberg, 1966, 1967), two possible interpretations seem likely. The co-occurrence of these problems may be a function of a common central deficit. Moreover, it is equally likely that intellectual development may depend on earlier motor achievements such as the acquisition of postural control. Failure to gain autonomous control of sitting may impede the development of fine motor skills, such as reaching and tool using, in which the trunk serves as a stable frame of reference while attention is focused on the task at hand (Trevarthen, 1968). Because fine motor skills of this kind are often conceived as precursors of cognitive activity, failure to acquire autonomous control over the postural subsystem involved may suggest an ontogenetic link between early motor retardation and subsequent intellectual retardation.

Contributions from the study of Down syndrome to the study of emotional development

One theoretical implication of the investigation of emotional development in "high-risk" populations underscores the importance of constructing a model of "normal" emotional development in order to differentiate between abnormal and well-adjusted emotional development. Underscoring the processes used for normal emotional development allows us to derive training procedures for the children expressing abnormalities in their emotional development. For example, now that we are beginning to learn more about the strategies employed in normal emotion language acquisition (Bretherton, Fritz, Zahn-Waxler, & Ridgeway, 1986), we will soon be able to develop therapeutic interventions that will facilitate the acquisition of emotional language and reduce the occurrence of acting-out behaviors (Cicchetti, Toth, & Bush, 1988).

The theoretical and practical impact of the investigation of emotional development is also important with respect to the formulation of an integrated theory of development. Only if we know, for example, how emotions relate to the other aspects of knowledge we have about children's development, will we be able to specify the necessary and/or sufficient conditions required to bring about change in the emotional domain.

In the following sections we explore how the study of Down syndrome can enhance our understanding of two aspects of the emotional domain: (1) the ontogenesis of emotion expression; and (2) the relation between emotion and cognition.

The development of emotion expressions

Although advances have been made in our understanding of the normal ontogenesis of the range of facial expressions exhibited at different developmental periods, many controversial problems remain to be solved. Any investigation into the organization of affective development must struggle with the fundamental question of what constitutes an emotion. Many researchers rely mainly on facial expressions as the major criterion for inferring the presence of an underlying emotion (Izard, 1977). Moreover, facial expressions are necessarily the primary index of emotion in infants because of their lack of verbal ability. However, investigators do not necessarily concur about such important issues as the exact age for the emergence of different emotions or the incentive events, eliciting conditions and contexts in which emotional expressions occur, or the mechanisms by which emotional differentiation unfolds (for example, compare Campos, Barrett, Lamb, Goldsmith, & Stenberg, 1983; Izard and Buechler, 1979; and Sroufe, 1979b). Similarly, it is not known whether there are qualitative differences that become manifest with age in the overt phenotypic expressions of certain emotions.

A general consensus does exist as to the order in which various emotional expressions emerge. Thus, pleasure, rage, disgust, wariness, interest, distress, and startle are present in the early months of life, while affects such as surprise, anger, and fear do not emerge until the second half of the first year of life (Bridges, 1932; Campos et al., 1983; Campos & Stenberg, 1981; Charlesworth, 1969; Izard & Buechler, 1979; Sroufe, 1979b). Shame, coyness, shyness, and guilt (the "self-conscious" reactions), as well as affection and defiance can be observed in the second year of life (Erikson, 1950; Kagan, 1981; Lewis & Brooks-Gunn, 1979; Lewis, Sullivan, Stanger, & Weiss, 1989; Sroufe, 1979b). Feelings of justice, pride, jealousy, envy, love, depression, and contempt do not appear to emerge until later in the developmental process (Arieti, 1967; Piaget, 1954/1981). In addition to their larger, more differentiated emotional repertoires, adults display these emotions in a wider ranger of contexts than either infants or children (Hesse & Cicchetti, 1982).

An important question that must be addressed is whether or not some emotions coincide with universal facial expressions. One way of approaching this question is to observe and compare a variety of populations of infants, including those who are developmentally deviant. If all samples of infants studied, regardless of differences in constitution, environment, or both, reveal the same facial expressions, this would provide compelling evidence for the universal existence of discrete affects. For example, Eibl-Eibesfeldt's (1979) work with blind and deaf children and congenitally deaf and blind thalidomide children found that the basic facial expressions, such as smiling, laughter, anger, and fear, occurred in the same situations as with normal children.

However, it is probable that differences in facial musculature, aberrant neural programs, and/or variations in speed of information processing may affect the actual appearance or delay the emergence of certain facial expressions. In Cicchetti and Sroufe's (1976, 1978) work with infants with Down syndrome, these infants were found to laugh far less at the incongruous stimulus items presented to them by their mothers than did their mental-age-matched normal counterparts. Emde, Katz, and Thorpe (1978) demonstrated that the onset of the social smile in infants with Down syndrome, although only slightly delayed in emergence, was characterized by dampened intensity, poor eye-to-eye contact, absence of crescendoing, and lack of activation of the arms and legs. Furthermore, Emde and colleagues (1978) have identified more uncertainty or "noise" in the emotional signaling system of the infant with Down syndrome. The signals of infants with Down syndrome may be less clear and more difficult to read as a result of their neuromuscular hypotonia (Cicchetti & Sroufe, 1978; Emde & Brown, 1978). Additionally, the range of facial expressions these infants are capable of displaying may be limited and/or may appear in distorted form. Cicchetti and Sroufe (1978) identified an inverse relationship between degree of hypotonia and both speed and amount of responding with laughter to visually presented stimuli. Gallagher, Jens, and O'Donnell (1983), studying a group of mentally retarded and multiply handicapped infants, including hydrocephaly, microcephaly, cerebral palsy, and seizure disorders of unknown etiology, found a decrease in laughter response in both hypotonic and hypertonic babies.

In addition, the characteristic slower rate of information processing in infants with Down syndrome may result in longer latencies to smile, to laugh, or to exhibit negative reactions such as distress or crying (Cicchetti & Sroufe, 1978). It also may result in the infrequent production of certain emotions (for example, surprise and fear) that require fast information processing and thus a strong arousal component (see, for example, Tomkins, 1962, 1963, 1980). These infants may express particular emotions in a qualitatively different way; that is, they may display fear, surprise, happiness, and so on, by means of different facial and gestural features, or only in terms of biologically based facial features, but never via characteristics that presuppose the acquisition of what Ekman (1972, 1977) has called "social display rules." Unfortunately, to date no research has addressed this important issue.

The developing child's ever-increasing capacities to monitor, modulate, and regulate his or her own emotional states also may play a role in the inhibition of what would previously have been an uncontrolled and disorganized outburst (see Cicchetti, Ganiban, & Barnett, in press; Gunnar, 1980). Mechanisms by which toddlers arrive at a particular emotional expression may be due primarily to their muscular ability to control affects and their capacity to identify their internal states, or to their cognitive and linguistic sophistication. Most likely, all of these factors are implicated in the process and interact in complex ways. Research on populations exhibiting deviant development can shed light on such issues by providing "natural" controls for these variables that may not be possible to attain with normal populations.

For example, research on infants with Down syndrome can help tease apart the role of cognition from the role of arousal modulation. Cicchetti and Sroufe (1978) found that even when infants with Down syndrome and normal infants were matched on level of cognitive development (mental age), the infants with Down syndrome showed less fear (crying, heart rate acceleration) on the "visual cliff" or with looming objects than their normal counterparts. Moreover, when infants with Down syndrome did show fear reactions, they experienced greater difficulty calming themselves than the nonhandicapped infants. These data suggest that infants with Down syndrome may have basic arousal modulation problems, and underscore the importance of arousal factors in emotional expression (Thompson et al., 1985). A likely explanation for these results is that infants with Down syndrome have difficulties with forebrain inhibitory control (see also Ganiban, Wagner, & Cicchetti, Chapter 3, this volume). This raises the question as to the role inhibitory mechanisms play in emotional expression in general. The answer possibly may be found through research on infants with localized brain damage. For example, expressions of disgust have been found in anencephalic and hydrocephalic infants suggesting that they originate in the brain stem (Steiner, 1973). Whether specific sites are associated with certain emotional functions and whether particular areas of the brain are implicated in emotional expression and behavior continues to be an important question (Pribram, 1967, 1980).

While Cicchetti and Sroufe's (1976) results on smiling and laughter in infants with Down syndrome again illuminate the role of arousal factors in emotional expression, several other issues surface when reviewing this work. Even though the infant with Down syndrome could not generate enough *tension* ("cognitively produced arousal" – Cicchetti & Sroufe, 1978) to laugh, information-processing factors were clearly implicated, as was neuromuscular hypotonia. Cicchetti and Sroufe (1976) argued that babies with Down syndrome could not process the incongruity of the stimulus presentations with sufficient speed to generate the "arousal jag" (Berlyne, 1969) required for laughter. Moreover, the infants with Down syndrome who smiled and laughed least and latest to the incongruous stimuli were the most hypotonic. Thus, these experiments point out that all three factors – cognition, physiology, and muscle tone – played an important role in producing the results and underscore the intricate relationship that exists among these three systems. Clearly, the individual differences and developmental heterogeneity of infants with Down syndrome have enabled researchers to gain insight into a complex issue that might not be as readily accessible through the study of normal populations alone.

The relationship between emotion and cognition

During the past fifteen years, the organizational perspective (Cicchetti & Sroufe, 1978; Sroufe, 1979b; Sroufe & Waters, 1976), has influenced research on normal emotional development (Barrett & Campos, 1987; Izard, 1977; Izard, Kagan, & Zajonc, 1984; Izard & Malatesta, 1987; Lewis & Michalson, 1983). Contemporary conceptions of the nature of the relation between emotion and cognition are based upon the sequence or emergence of new cognitive or affective qualities or characteristics (Cicchetti & Hesse, 1983). Emotions may be regarded as developing ontogenetically earlier than cognition, thereby providing the context within which cognitive development may occur (*cognitive epiphenomenalism*). The emergence of new emotions may be dependent upon cognitive advances that must be made before various emotions may be expressed (*emotional epiphenomenalism*). Emotions may develop along a separate pathway from cognitive advances so that the sequence, rate, and quality of change must be considered distinctly within each domain (*parallelism*). Finally, emotions may emerge in interaction with cognitive advances, thereby suggesting a progression that necessitates a consideration of developmental changes that occur across domains and that exert a reciprocal influence upon each other (*interactionism*).

In a longitudinal investigation of the development of smiling and laughter, Cicchetti and Sroufe (1976, 1978) studied 25 infants with Down syndrome from 4 through 24 months of age. These infants were visited in their homes twice monthly and were presented with a standard series of incongruous stimuli by their mothers. In addition, each infant was administered the Bayley (1969) and Uzgiris-Hunt (1975) scales of cognitive development several times during the course of this investigation by experimenters blind as to the infant's performance on the affect-eliciting items. Cicchetti and Sroufe (1976, 1978) found that even though infants with Down syndrome showed a later onset of laughter, these babies laughed at the incongruous stimulus items *in the exact order as normal infants* – first to intrusive auditory and tactile items, and next, during the second year of life, to the more complex social and visual items. This sequencing suggests a link between cognitive development and laughter on the more sophisticated items. Moreover, just as was true of nonhandicapped infants, with increasing cognitive sophistication it was the infant with Down syndrome's effortful assimilation of the stimulus content or participation in the event that generated the tension necessary for laughter and smiling, rather than mere quantity of stimulation. In effect, as schema formation becomes increasingly important in the elicitation of positive affect, it is no longer stimulation per se that produces the affective response, but the babies' *effort* in processing the stimulus content. Infants with Down syndrome and normal infants both progress from smiling and laughing, to intrusive stimulation, to stimulation mediated by active attention, to smiling and laughing in response to stimulus content, and, finally, toward an *ever more active participation* in producing affectively effective stimulation.

Cognitive test results provide the most compelling data on the affect – cognition interchange. In these observations, level of cognitive development paralleled level of affective development. For example, infants who laughed earliest or smiled and laughed most to the more cognitively sophisticated social and visual items were those who obtained the highest level of cognitive development on the assessment scales. Laughter was also found to be an excellent predictor of later cognitive development. The babies with Down syndrome who laughed before 10 months had higher developmental quotients at 2 years of age on the Bayley scales than those babies who did not begin to laugh until later. Even more surprisingly, early laughter was a better predictor of later cognitive development than was the infant's early level of cognitive development. In other words, affect predicted cognition better than cognition predicted cognition.

In a cross-sectional study of a group of multiply handicapped infants, Gallagher, Jens, and O'Donnell (1983) found that the smiling responses of babies were significantly related to their mental age. Gunn, Berry, and Andrews (1981) likewise provide evidence for a close association between affective and cognitive development. They followed ten infants with Down syndrome longitudinally, assessing their affective reactions to a repeated auditory–visual event – the squeaking of a baby doll. Gunn and colleagues (1981) found that the majority of affective responses were elicited after the first year of life. Moreover, the onset of affective responsiveness was significantly positively correlated with level of cognitive development on the Bayley scales.

Cicchetti and Sroufe (1978) have also studied the ontogenesis of negative reactions in infants with Down syndrome. They found that the infants with Down syndrome exhibited delayed negative emotions (crying, distress, heart-rate acceleration, and so on), both to direct placement on the "visual cliff" and in response to looming shadows approaching them on a "collision" course. Similar to their studies of positive affect, Cicchetti and Sroufe (1978) showed that there was a close relationship between negative reactions and cognitive development. Thus, babies with Down syndrome who showed early fear and distress reactions were more advanced in their cognitive development, obtaining higher Bayley and Uzgiris–Hunt scores.

In a further examination of affect and cognition in infants with Down syndrome, Mans, Cicchetti, and Sroufe (1978) explored visual self-recognition of these infants. In normal infants, at approximately 18 to 24 months, visual self-recognition and the development of shame have been found to coincide with the emergence of the autonomous self and positive valuation of the self (Lewis & Brooks-Gunn, 1979). When shown their rouge-marked noses in a mirror, most normal infants manifest their self-knowledge by touching their own noses while examining their reflections in the mirror. The emergence of self-directed behaviors is first observed at 15 to 18 months and is common by 21 to 24 months of age. Mans and colleagues (1978) found that when infants with Down syndrome achieved the appropriate cognitive developmental level, they, too, showed the emergence of self-recognition. Thus, self-recognition was not the coincidental result of a particular chronological age but, rather, was closely tied to and emerged with cognitive development. Before 23 months of age, for example, only those infants with Down syndrome having nearly normal cognitive functioning showed evidence of self-recognition by touching their rouge-marked noses when observing themselves in a mirror. It was not until at least the age of 34 months that virtually all toddlers with Down syndrome showed self-recognition. Similarly, the affective reactions of these infants to their rouge-marked reflections mirrored those of normal infants. The predominant affective reaction of the younger infants with Down syndrome was a change from positive affect before the application of the rouge, to one of being serious or puzzled afterward. Older toddlers with Down syndrome evidenced surprise reactions or an increase in positive affect after the rouge. Thus, their affective reactions, such as nose touching, reflected their differential understanding of this event.

Hill and Tomlin (1981) observed two groups of preverbal retarded toddlers' responses to watching marked or unmarked television images of themselves. One group was made up of toddlers with Down syndrome, while the other was made up of a multihandicapped group including toddlers with anoxia, rubella, and seizure disorders. Hill and Tomlin found that the toddlers with Down syndrome all evidenced the curiosity and self-conscious behaviors that characterize nonhandicapped babies during the second year of life. Moreover, 11 of the 12 toddlers with Down syndrome recognized their television images. In sharp contrast, fewer than half of the multiply handicapped group recognized themselves, and their affective reactions were similar to those of normal 1-year-olds. In both groups of toddlers, Hill and Tomlin (1981) reported that of those who evidenced self-recognition all had attained mental ages comparable to normal toddlers who manifested that aspect of self-knowledge.

Several investigators have studied cognitive–affective links in the play of children with Down syndrome (see Beeghly, Weiss-Perry, & Cicchetti, Chapter 10, this volume). The literature on normal children has identified relationships between cognitive and affective development within the domain of object play. This has been thought to index "mastery motivation" or "play style" (Fein & Apfel, 1979; Jennings, Harmon, Morgan, Gaiter, & Yarrow, 1979). The persistence and enthusiasm of children during object play has been found to be significantly correlated with the complexity and maturity of object play in these studies.

Similar interrelationships between cognitive and affective dimensions of object play have been observed in children with Down syndrome. For example, in a longitudinal study of children with Down syndrome, Motti, Cicchetti, and Sroufe (1983) found that both symbolic play maturity and affective play behavior at 3 to 5 years of age were significantly correlated with indices of cognitive and affective development assessed during the first and second years of these children's lives. Specifically, affect ratings of these children at 10 months and scores from the Bayley mental scales at 24 months both predicted children's symbolic play maturity and affective–motivational behavior during a free play episode at 3 to 5 years. Coherence among cognitive and affective behavior also was observed in this sample throughout infancy. In addition, cognitive development at 16 months was predicted by affective ratings made at several prior developmental periods during the first year of life (Cicchetti & Sroufe, 1976, 1978). Similarly to other investigators of symbolic play, Motti and colleagues (1983) found that the symbolic play behavior of children with Down syndrome was qualitatively similar to that reported for normally developing children (Nicolich, 1977). Marked individual differences existed for these children such that children with higher levels of cognitive development engaged in more mature levels of symbolic and social play, engaged in more active and thorough exploration of toys, were more enthusiastic during play, and exhibited more positive affect than that seen in less cognitively advanced children. Thus, close correspondences among affective and cognitive dimensions of behavior were observed during the first five years of life for these children with Down syndrome (see also Beeghly, Weiss-Perry & Cicchetti, Chapter 10, this volume, for a description and discussion of findings that have replicated and extended those reported by Motti and her colleagues).

In view of these findings, we can further explore the nature of the relationship between affect and cognition. Based on the significant intercorrelations obtained between affective and cognitive indices in a developmentally heterogeneous sample of infants, it is clear that cognitive and emotional development are inextricably intertwined. However, when the infants with Down syndrome were matched on mental age with samples of normal infants (Sroufe & Wunsch, 1972), they showed less affect, both positive and negative, than would be predicted based on a purely cognitive interpretation. We interpret these data as demonstrating that affect and cognition are indeed separate developmental systems and as a refutation of both a cognitive and an emotional epiphenomenalist position. However, it is difficult to choose between a parallelist and an interactionist viewpoint. Because affect and cognition predicted later cognitive and symbolic development (Motti et al., 1983), we lean toward an interactionist explanation, although additional data is needed to resolve this question. Furthermore, while interactionism may characterize the nature of the affect–cognition relationship during infancy, it is conceivable that discrepant results may emerge at later stages of development.

Investigations of other atypical populations of infants and children may provide an important contribution toward furthering our understanding of the temporal relationship between advances in the affective and cognitive domains. Their study may allow for an understanding of the relative contribution of emotion and cognition for the development of particular competencies throughout ontogenesis. Because the development of normal children is generally more rapid than that evidenced by youngsters with developmental deviations, the study of atypical children (such as those with Down syndrome) will permit us to examine more closely the unfolding of various domains of development. Additionally, it will contribute to our current theoretical conceptions of the relationship between cognitive and affective development in both normal and atypical populations of children.

In the preceding sections, we addressed how the study of infants and children with Down syndrome could contribute to the understanding of normal developmental processes as well as the formulation of an integrative and comprehensive developmental theory. Next, we explore how children with Down syndrome negotiate the crucial developmental tasks of the early years of life. A developmental scheme is necessary for tracing the etiology and processes of maladaptation so that therapeutic interventions may be appropriately timed and guided (Cicchetti, Toth, Bush, & Gillespie, 1988; Spiker, Chapter 13, this volume). Furthermore, a developmental perspective may prove useful for uncovering the nature and etiology of the maladaptation and the development of compensatory mechanisms in the face of deficiencies.

Stage-salient issues of early development

In recent years, there has been a great deal of agreement concerning the presence of a sequence of stage-salient issues that are characteristic of the early years of life (Sroufe, 1979a; see also Erikson, 1950). Rather than construe the ontogenetic process as a series of unfolding tasks that must be accomplished and then decrease in importance, we view development as comprising a number of important age- and stage-appropriate tasks that, upon emergence, remain critical to the child's present and future adaptation. As new tasks emerge, old issues may decrease in relative importance. Nonetheless, each issue represents a life-span developmental task that requires ongoing coordination with and integration into the child's adaptation to the environment and to the stage-salient developmental issue of the period. There also are corresponding tasks for caregivers that increase the likelihood that their children will successfully resolve each stage-salient issue (see Sroufe, 1979a).

The transactional model

Inherent in the organizational perspective on development and the notion of stage-salient issues is the recognition of the importance of transactions among genetic, constitutional, neurobiological, biochemical, psychological, and social factors in the determination of behavior (Sameroff, 1983). Advocates of the transactional model contend that the various factors operating in normal or pathological conditions do not occur in isolation, but together impact upon the developmental process through a hierarchy of influence (Cicchetti, 1987). According to Sameroff and Chandler (1975), the multiple transactions among parental, child, and ecological characteristics contribute to child development in a reciprocal, dynamic fashion. Accordingly, if a child evidences pathological development over time, it is presumed that the child has been involved in a *continuous* maladaptive transactional process. The ongoing manifestation of child maladaptation is shaped by parental and environmental support, while the child's characteristics help to determine the nature of the "environment." Because the child and the environment are seen as exerting mutual influence on each other, it follows that development at a later point reflects not only the quality of earlier adaptation but also the intervening environmental effects. Over time and as development progresses, both the match between child and parent, as well as salient parent characteristics, may become modified. Under these circumstances, declining quality of adaptation would demonstrate continuity of development. Moreover, the emergence of adaptive or maladaptive outcomes may be influenced by the presence of long-term protective factors and transient buffers (cf. Cicchetti & Rizley, 1981).

It follows, then, that a transactional analysis incorporates conceptions of stability and change over time, while simultaneously attempting to account for those factors that may maintain, or lead to alterations in, the child's capacity to resolve developmentally salient tasks. In extending this analysis to the assessment of early competence (i.e., successful resolution of the stage-salient issues), several points need to be emphasized:

1. Positive adaptation at one developmental period will exert a positive influence toward achieving successful adaptation at the next period.
2. Early competence also exerts a subtle influence toward adaptation throughout the life-span because each developmental issue, although perhaps *most salient* at one developmental period, is of importance *throughout* the life cycle.
3. The failure to achieve adaptation at one period makes adaptation that much more difficult at the next, and, in a lesser way, more difficult throughout the course of life because each issue continues to be important throughout the individual's development.
4. Many mediating factors between early and later adaptation or maladaptation may permit alternative outcomes to occur; that is, early problems or deviations in the successful resolution of a developmental task may be countered by major changes in the child's experience that could result in the successful negotiation of subsequent developmental tasks.

We now examine how infants and young children with Down syndrome negotiate these early stage-salient issues, which include: (1) homeostatic regulation and the development of a reliable signaling system; (2) management of tension and the differentiation of affect; (3) development of a secure attachment relationship; (4) development of an autonomous self; and (5) symbolic representation and self–other differentiation.

*Homeostatic regulation and the development of a reliable signaling
system (0–3 months)*

The initial developmental task facing the newborn infant involves issues related to neurophysiological organization, regulation, and homeostasis (Emde, Gaensbauer

& Harmon, 1976; Greenspan, 1981; Sander, 1962, 1975). During the early months of life, the infant must establish basic cycles and rhythms of sleep and wakefulness and of feeding and elimination. Increased stabilization of these processes allows the infant to interact more extensively with the outside environment and to begin developing a reliable signaling system.

Caregivers play a critical role in facilitating the development of this regulatory system (Cicchetti, Ganiban, & Barnett, in press). They must be able to provide a physical and emotional environment in which the infant can balance inner state and external stimuli. Adaptive patterns of homeostasis and the emergence of a reliable signaling system result from a protective, predictable, and engaging environment. A chaotic, arbitrary, hypo/hyperstimulating environment contributes to problems in the successful resolution of this task.

As discussed earlier in this chapter, infants with Down syndrome have a variety of neurological, biochemical, physiological, and psychophysiological problems that may stress the caregiving system and result in homeostatic failure. For example, their delayed maturation of reflexes and of organ systems impairs the development of reliable sleep–wake patterns. Moreover, the confluence of neuromuscular hypotonia, minimal eye contact, dampened affect intensity, higher arousal thresholds, "noise" in the emotion signaling system, and absence of crescendoing during face-to-face interaction places significant stressors on the caregiver–infant communicative system (Berger, Chapter 4, this volume; Cicchetti & Sroufe, 1978; Emde et al., 1978). Despite the difficulties that occur in the early months, most caregivers of infants with Down syndrome are able to accommodate to their infants' behavioral and physiological anomalies and to facilitate the development of a mutually adaptive signaling system over the course of their child's first year of life (Sorce & Emde, 1982).

Management of "tension" (cognitively produced arousal) and the differentiation of affect (4–6 months)

A qualitatively new phase of development and behavioral organization accompanies the emergence of the social smile (Emde et al., 1976). Mastery of homeostatic regulation and the development of reliable patterns of signaling contribute to an increased capacity for sustained attention to the environment. Consequently, the infant begins to engage with both the animate and inanimate world in a more organized manner (Sroufe & Waters, 1976). Behaviors that were previously endogenously stimulated and primarily reflexive in nature become replaced by contingent responses to exogenous stimulation. This state is characterized by increased intensity and differentiation in the expression of affect (Sroufe, 1979b). During this stage, the infant first laughs in response to vigorous stimulation and exhibits frustration and/or rage in response to failed expectations. The infant's ability to elicit maternal responsivity, as well as maternal sensitivity to infant cues, are critical for successful negotiation of this issue.

Once again, the biological system difficulties that exist in infants with Down syndrome present special challenges for the caregiver. Cicchetti and Sroufe (1976) have documented that infants with Down syndrome are slower to develop laughter to a variety of stimuli presented by their mothers, and that these infants cannot process the incongruity of these stimuli with the speed necessary to promote the *tension* required for laughter. Cicchetti and Sroufe (1978) also have demonstrated similar lags in the emergence of full-blown fear expressions. The delays of the appearance of these displays may affect the caregiver's cognitive perception or interpretation of the infant's cues, causing caregivers to misread the emotional messages of these infants, or to react with less affective involvement to their less arousable infants.

The decreased responsivity of infants with Down syndrome and the dampened affective tone displayed by these infants necessitate adequate compensatory mechanisms on the part of the caregiver in order to initiate or maintain interactions or to be successful in the interpretation of, and response to, affective states. Just as with homeostatic regulation, over time the caregivers of infants with Down syndrome become increasingly able to negotiate patterns of communication that facilitate the successful resolution of this task (Jasnow et al., 1988; Sorce & Emde, 1982).

Cicchetti and Sroufe (1976, 1978) state that mothers of infants with Down syndrome appear to be able to compensate for morphological and psychophysiological deviations in their infants by exerting themselves more strenuously to initiate interaction and to elicit affective responses. Although an observer may perceive what appears to be overstimulation or intrusiveness in the behavior and affective responsiveness of a parent interacting with an atypical infant, this behavior may actually be the overt manifestation of a sensitive and contingently responsive caregiver who is employing compensatory adjustments in order to encourage the harmony of the interaction and the adaptation of the infant.

Bridges and Cicchetti (1982) demonstrate that in rating their infants with Down syndrome, mothers do not ascribe a greater degree of difficulty in interacting with these infants. However, classification of infants according to Carey's (1970) criteria for assigning infants to different types of temperament categories reveals that a greater percentage of the infants with Down syndrome are difficult to manage relative to Carey's original standardization sample. This finding indicates that the caregiver is successful in altering perceptions of, and attitudes toward, the infant in a manner that promotes harmonious interaction within the dyad (see Ganiban, Wagner, & Cicchetti, Chapter 3, this volume).

The development of a secure attachment relationship (6–12 months)

The development of a secure, adaptive attachment relationship with the primary caregiver is a stage-salient issue that has generated considerable research (Ainsworth, Blehar, Waters & Wall, 1978; Bowlby 1969/1982). Although the capacity for attachment originates in earlier stages, behavioral manifestations of this issue reach ascendancy in the latter half of the first year of life (Sroufe, 1979a). During this period, the infant learns to coordinate a broad variety of behavioral responses into an adaptive and flexible goal-corrected response repertoire. Dyadic interactions, marked by relatedness and synchrony, resiliency to stress, and appropriate affective interchange, are associated with successful adaptation during this stage (Sroufe, 1979b). Also critical is the knowledge that a caregiver is reliable and responsive. Inadequate response contingent stimulation is likely to exert a negative impact on the infant's ability to master the tasks of this stage. In the absence of regular contingent responsivity, neither infant nor caregiver develops feelings of efficacy and the development of a secure attachment relationship may be hindered (Ainsworth et al., 1978; Belsky, Rovine, & Taylor, 1984; Lamb, Thompson, Gardner, Charnov, & Estes, 1984).

Despite their constitutional anomalies, the attachment system of infants with Down syndrome is organized in a manner similar to that of mental-age-matched nonhandicapped youngsters. The majority of these children form secure attachment relationships with their caregivers (Thompson et al., 1985). In addition, research on infants with Down syndrome demonstrates that a relationship similar to that seen in normal infants may be found between early attachment with the primary caregiver and the control of emotions. Cicchetti and Serafica (1981) found the attachment, affiliation, and fear–wariness systems of infants with Down syndrome to be organized in a manner similar to that in normal infants (Bretherton & Ainsworth, 1974). Specifically, the intensity of emotional responses in the infants with Down syndrome varied with the context and the behaviors of both mother and stranger, thereby suggesting an awareness of, and sensitivity to, different eliciting conditions, and a capacity for the modulation and control of emotional states. Cicchetti and Serafica's (1981) analysis of qualitative and quantitative differences in responsivity to mother and stranger for the fear–wariness, affiliation, and attachment behavioral systems allowed for a clearer understanding of the complexity of the potential conclusions that could be drawn regarding the emotional control of the infants with Down syndrome. Thus, for example, the increased latency to crying during separation from the mother and the greater difficulty in soothing and calming the distressed infant with Down syndrome reflect the influence of the higher arousal threshold in these infants. This psychophysiological disturbance mediates the overt display of affective responsiveness, but does not minimize the need for attributing importance to the control that infants with Down syndrome must learn to exert over their emotional displays. Berry, Gunn, and Andrews (1980) observed babies with Down syndrome in a sequence of episodes similar though not identical to the "strange situation" (Ainsworth et al., 1978). These babies displayed greater distress upon separation from the mother than the infants studied by Cicchetti and Serafica (1981). However, the infants in the investigation conducted by Berry and his colleagues (1980) were younger in mental and chronological age than those included in Cicchetti and Serafica's (1981) sample, thereby indicating the potential influence of increased socialization experiences upon the capacity for emotional control.

The development of an autonomous self (18–24 months)

The toddler's emerging acquisition of a sense of self, seen as encompassing both affective and cognitive dimensions, is a significant developmental task (Lewis &

Brooks-Gunn, 1979; Stern, 1985) that allows the toddler to more fully comprehend environmental occurrences. Moreover, a well-differentiated sense of self provides the toddler with an enhanced understanding of personal functioning as a separate and independent entity. Issues related to body management begin to emerge from the context of the mother–infant relationship into the realm of autonomous function. The infant becomes increasingly invested in self-managing due to new cognitive and motor achievements, as well as to more sophisticated notions about self and other. Empathic acts also begin to emerge at this time, again a manifestation of the realization that the self can have an impact on others (Zahn-Waxler & Radke-Yarrow, 1982). Caretaker sensitivity and ability to tolerate the toddler's strivings for autonomy, as well as the capacity to set age-appropriate limits, are integral to the successful resolution of this issue. In contrast, intolerance of infant initiative may impede the development of autonomy. Caretakers who tend to feel rejected by the infant's increasing independence and/or overwhelmed by their infant's actively initiated demands may inhibit the emergence of age-appropriate independence (Mahler, Pine & Bergman, 1975).

Toddlers with Down syndrome evidence visual self-recognition in the mirror-and-rouge paradigm (Lewis & Brooks-Gunn, 1979) when they reach a mental age of approximately 2 years (Hill & Tomlin, 1981; Loveland, 1987; Mans et al., 1978). In this procedure, infants observe their reflections in a mirror for a brief period of time in the presence of their mothers and an experimenter. After a short inspection, the experimenter surreptitiously wipes a dot of rouge onto the infant's nose. Visual self-recognition is inferred when the infant touches his or her nose while watching himself or herself in the mirror. In addition to self-recognition, the toddlers with Down syndrome show the concomitant positive affective changes observed in cognitively equivalent nonhandicapped infants. The positive affect accompanying their visual self-recognition suggests that children with Down syndrome "feel positively" about themselves. In contrast, the affective responses of abused and/or neglected toddlers (Schneider-Rosen & Cicchetti, 1984) and autistic youngsters (Spiker & Ricks, 1984) are predominately neutral or negative in nature.

Symbolic representation and further self–other differentiation (24–36 months)

Between 24 and 36 months, toddlers begin to construct increasingly differentiated mental representations of animate and inanimate objects (Greenspan & Porges, 1984). Concomitantly, the use of language and play as a means of representing the growing awareness of self and other emerges. Children become increasingly able to label emotions, intentions, and cognitions and manifest their developing social awareness through symbolic play (Beeghly & Cicchetti, 1987; Cicchetti & Beeghly, 1987). Investigations of play, language, and cognition have burgeoned in recent years (Bretherton, 1984; Rubin, Fein, & Vandenberg, 1983).

Unfortunately, as in other studies of Down syndrome, much of the play data involving children with Down syndrome contains serious methodological flaws (see

Quinn & Rubin, 1984). More recently, however, researchers have applied a developmental perspective to investigations of play in children with Down syndrome. This has served to clarify and refine theories of normal play development, as well as to increase our knowledge of the development of children with Down syndrome. The results of these studies have revealed that the course and content of symbolic play development in children with Down syndrome is remarkably similar to that observed in normal children. Additionally, similar relationships with cognitive, affective, and social development also have been observed in both children with Down syndrome and cognitively comparable nondisordered children (see Beeghly, Weiss-Perry, & Cicchetti, Chapter 10, this volume, for a review).

In normal groups of children, the use of language and play to represent early conceptions of relationships is an age-appropriate reflection of children's growing awareness of self and other (Bretherton, 1984). These abilities usually emerge and become more sophisticated during the child's second and third years. Self-descriptive utterances are used more often as children provide verbal descriptions of their actions (Kagan, 1981). In addition, children also become more able to label the emotional states, intentions, and cognitions of both themselves and others (Bretherton & Beeghly, 1982), and begin to use their own name and personal pronouns appropriately. Moreover, the use of self-related language becomes less context dependent, with children initially speaking mainly about themselves in the present, and then discussing the behaviors and internal states of other nonpresent individuals or of hypothetical contexts.

Children's developing social understanding also is manifested in symbolic play. As with other forms of symbolization, the representation of self and other in play proceeds through a sequence of decentration, decontextualization, and integration (Fenson, 1984). Initially, toddlers play at being themselves and then project their actions onto other objects, such as dolls. By the end of the third year, children are able to represent the behavior of several interacting replicas in an integrated manner, and to be involved in sociodramatic play requiring elementary roletaking capacities (Watson and Fischer, 1977).

Beeghly and Cicchetti (1987) found that children with Down syndrome evidenced similar sequences of language and play development to that observed in nonhandicapped children, but that those abilities emerged at a delayed rate. In both language and play, children with Down syndrome first represented themselves symbolically. With increasing cognitive maturity, the language and play of children with Down syndrome became more decentered, integrated, and decontextualized. Only the most cognitively mature children used language and play to represent self and other in hypothetical contexts. Children with Down syndrome were significantly more advanced in symbolic play maturity than their Mean Length of Utterance (MLU)–matched controls, but not than their MA–matched controls. However, the children with Down syndrome did differ from their language controls when *linguistic* representatives were analyzed. These results suggest that, despite the similarity in developmental sequence in both domains, children with Down syndrome may be more advanced in nonlinguistic domains of symbolic representation. However, both linguistic and nonlinguistic variables are significantly correlated with mental age for children with Down syndrome. These findings underscore the coherence of symbolic development in children with Down syndrome (see Beeghly, Weiss-Perry, & Cicchetti, Chapter 10, this volume, for an elaboration).

Further confirmation of the ontogenetic sequencing of symbolic abilities in children with Down syndrome is revealed in relation to self-knowledge. Children with Down syndrome show increasingly differentiated concepts of self and other during their play. When observed while playing, their self-related language (e.g. talking about their ongoing activities and internal states, using personal pronouns, etc.) was related to advances in both symbolic and cognitive development. Furthermore, parallel advances were found in their ability to use language as a means of enhancing social communication (Beeghly & Cicchetti, 1987).

In summary, even though children with Down syndrome possess a large number of reproductive casualties, they successfully negotiate the early stage-salient issues of development. These findings emphasize the vicissitudes of parenting in facilitating the positive resolution of developmental tasks. At least during the early years of life, parents of children with Down syndrome avoid caretaking casualties and help to foster positive developmental outcomes in their progeny.

Conclusion

Guided by the organizational, developmental psychopathology perspective, it is apparent that the study of young children with Down syndrome can contribute to the understanding of both normal and atypical forms of ontogenesis. Because children with Down syndrome do not have a normal nervous system, we cannot claim that the study of Down syndrome is identical to observing the unfolding of normal development in "slow motion." In fact, as we demonstrate and as other contributors to this volume note, there are indeed some quantitative and qualitative differences in the developmental process of mental-age-matched normal children and youngsters with Down syndrome. Most importantly, we have illustrated that despite their constitutional anomalies, children with Down syndrome are amenable to a "developmental analysis." Earlier, Cicchetti and Pogge-Hesse (1982) documented that the development of infants with Down syndrome was organized, adaptive, and coherent. Much of the work reported in this chapter, in addition to that described elsewhere in this volume (see, for example, Beeghly, Weiss-Perry, & Cicchetti, Chapter 10, this volume; Fowler, Chapter 9, this volume; Mervis, Chapter 8, this volume), confirms and extends these conclusions throughout the period of early childhood. Consequently, we believe that Zigler's position on the "developmental–difference" controversy in the field of mental retardation (Zigler, 1969; Zigler & Balla, 1982), when viewed from a broad-band developmental "world view" (Pepper, 1942), also can be generalized to organically retarded children. Even though young children with Down syndrome do not function identically to their cognitively matched nonhandicapped counterparts, the application of a developmental approach reveals both the organization and coherence characteristic of their early development (cf. Cicchetti & Ganiban, in press). Contributions derived from this approach to the study of Down syndrome can enhance our knowledge of developmental theory.

Several important tasks await developmental researchers investigating Down syndrome.

Increasing work must be conducted with older children, adolescents, and adults with Down syndrome. Research on older individuals with Down syndrome, guided by a developmental perspective, is crucial (cf. Rondal, 1988). In its absence, we cannot be certain whether existing developmental principles could be applicable to explain the functioning of children with Down syndrome at later periods of the life cycle. In order to formulate more precise statements about the processes and mechanisms underlying these later achievements, it would be ideal if such studies were longitudinal. Recently, Carr (1988, 1989) has published the results of a long-term follow-up of a cohort of children with Down syndrome from 6 weeks to 21 years. Work such as this is essential. We wish to add that future prospective longitudinal studies must adopt an organizational approach and focus on the coherence of development across biological and psychological domains.

Multidisciplinary longitudinal research, in which multiple biological and behavioral domains are investigated, is sorely needed. As we have argued, a developmental approach can be applied to any discipline and to any population. We can no longer afford to dissect the child with Down syndrome into separate psychological and biological organisms. Now that exciting findings have occurred in the genetics, biochemistry, and neurophysiology of Down syndrome, the developmentalist studying Down syndrome can assess the interrelation between brain and behavioral development throughout the course of ontogenesis (Coyle et al. 1986; Ganiban et al., Chapter 3, this volume; Nadel, 1988).

In order to ascertain whether or not the reported similarities and differences found between children with Down syndrome and cognitively comparable normal children are specific to Down syndrome, research with mentally retarded populations, both organic and cultural–familial, must be conducted from an organizational developmental perspective. Although the implementation of such research programs looms as a difficult task owing to problems associated with the early identification of many of the other forms of mental retardation, it is critical to the advancement of our knowledge of Down syndrome. Along similar lines, Burack, Hodapp, and Zigler (1988) have argued persuasively that if additional advances in the developmental understanding of mental retardation are to be made, then studies of different organic groups, as well as organic–cultural familial comparisons, must be initiated.

Research linking family functioning and child developmental outcome must be implemented. In the field of normal child development, a growing literature has documented that individual differences in family functioning can impact the child's developmental status (Belsky, 1984). Because the presence of a child with Down syndrome can place a great burden upon the family at virtually any point in the life cycle, research is sorely needed on families with a child with Down syndrome (see Carr, 1988, 1989; Crnic, Chapter 12, this volume; Gath & Gumley, 1984).

Alternative approaches to the assessment of children with Down syndrome must be developed and implemented. Children with Down syndrome are typically administered conventional assessment batteries. Because the outcome of these assessments often results in major decisions being made about the child with Down syndrome (e.g., type of school placement), we recommend that traditional psychometric tests be conducted in conjunction with alternative methods of evaluating diverse domains of development (see Cicchetti & Wagner, in press).

Now that we possess a great deal more knowledge about the development of children with Down syndrome, we believe that interventions with these children should be guided by the transactional model and the organizational perspective. Consequently, the parent, child, and environment must all be a part of the specific intervention for a given child with Down syndrome. Ideally, intervention should focus upon multiple developmental domains, age- and stage-appropriate areas of functioning, and on the risk and protective factors characteristic of the particular parent–child–environment constellation at hand (Cicchetti, 1987; Cicchetti & Toth, 1987; Cicchetti, Toth, & Bush, 1988; Spiker, Chapter 13, this volume).

References

Achenbach, T. (in press). What is "developmental" about developmental psychopathology? In J. Rolf, A. Masten, D. Cicchetti, K. Neuchterlein, & S. Weintraub (Eds.), *Risk and protective factors in the development of psychopathology.* New York: Cambridge University Press.

Ainsworth, M.D.S., Blehar, M. C., Waters, E., & Wall, S. (1978). *Patterns of attachment: A psychological study of the strange situation.* Hillsdale, NJ: Erlbaum.

Arieti, S. (1967). *The intrapsychic self.* New York: Basic Books.

Aslin, R.N. (1981). Experiential influences and sensitive periods in perceptual development: A unified model. In R. N. Aslin, J. R. Alberts, & M. R. Peterson (Eds.), *Development of perception: Psychobiological perspectives* (Vol. 2, pp. 45–93). New York: Academic Press.

Barden, H. (1983). Growth and development of selected hard tissues in Down syndrome: A review. *Human Biology, 55,* 539–576.

Barrett, K. C., & Campos, J. (1987). Perspectives on emotional development II: A functionalist approach to emotions. In J. Osofsky (Ed.), *Handbook of infant development* (2nd ed., pp. 555–578). New York: Wiley.

Bateson, P. (1979). How do sensitive periods arise and what are they for? *Animal Behavior, 27,* 470–486.

Bayley, N. (1969). *The Bayley scales of infant development.* New York: Psychological Corporation.

Beeghly, M., & Cicchetti, D. (1987). An organizational approach to symbolic development in children with Down syndrome. *New Directions for Child Development, 36,* 5–29.

Belsky, J. (1984). The determinants of parenting: A process model. *Child Development, 55,* 83–96.

Belsky, J., Rovine, M., & Taylor, D. G. (1984). The Pennsylvania infant and family development project, III: The origins of individual differences in infant–mother attachment: Maternal and infant contributions. *Child Development, 55*(3), 718–728.

Berlyne, D. (1969). Laughter, humor, and play. In G. Lindzey and E. Aronson (Eds.), *Handbook of social psychology* (2nd ed. vol. 3). Boston: Addison-Wesley.

Berry, P., Gunn, P., & Andrews, R. (1980). Behavior of Down's syndrome infants in a strange situation. *American Journal of Mental Deficiency, 85,* 213–218.

Block, J. (1971). *Lives through time*. Berkeley, CA: Bancroft.

Block, J. H., & Block, J. (1980). The role of ego-control and ego resiliency in the organization of behavior. In W. A. Collins (Ed.), *Minnesota Symposium on Child Psychology* (Vol. 13). Hillsdale, NJ: Erlbaum.

Bornstein, M. H. (1989). Sensitive periods in development: Structural characteristics and causal interpretations. *Psychological Bulletin, 105*(2), 179–197.

Bowlby, J. (1969/1982). *Attachment and loss* (Vol. 1). New York: Basic.

Bretherton, I. (Ed.), (1984). *Symbolic play*. Orlando, FL: Academic Press.

Bretherton, I., & Ainsworth, M. (1974). Response of 1-year-olds to a stranger in a strange situation. In M. Lewis & L. Rosenblum (Eds.), *The origins of fear*. New York: Wiley.

Bretherton, I., & Beeghly, M. (1982). Talking about internal states: The acquisition of an explicit theory of mind. *Developmental Psychology, 18*, 906–921.

Bretherton, I., Fritz, J., Zahn-Waxler, C., & Ridgeway, D. (1986). Learning to talk about emotion: A functionalist perspective. *Child Development, 57*, 530–548.

Bridges, F., & Cicchetti, D. (1982). Mothers' ratings of the temperament characteristics of Down syndrome infants. *Developmental Psychology, 18*, 238–244.

Bridges, K. M. (1932). Emotional development in early infancy. *Child Development, 3*, 324–341.

Brim, O. G., & Kagan, J. (Eds.) (1980). *Constancy and change in human development*. Cambridge, MA: Harvard University Press.

Bronfenbrenner, U. (1979). *The ecology of human development: Experiments by nature and design*. Cambridge, MA: Harvard University Press.

Bronson, G. (1965). The hierarchical organization of the central nervous system: Implications for learning processes and critical periods in early development. *Behavioral Science, 10*, 7–25.

Burack, J., Hodapp, R., & Zigler, E. (1988). Issues in the classification of mental retardation: Differentiating among organic etiologies. *Journal of Child Psychology and Psychiatry, 29*, 765–780.

Butterworth, G., & Cicchetti, D. (1978). Visual calibration of posture in normal and motor retarded Down's syndrome infants. *Perception, 7*, 513–525.

Butterworth, G., & Hicks, L. (1977). Visual proprioception and postural stability in infancy: A developmental study. *Perception, 6*, 255–262.

Campos, J. J., Barrett, L., Lamb, M., Goldsmith, H. L., & Stenberg, C. R. (1983). Socioemotional development. In M. Haith & J. Campos, *Handbook of child psychology;* Vol. 2: *Infancy and developmental psychology*. New York: Wiley.

Campos, J. J., & Stenberg, C. R. (1981). Perception, appraisal and emotion: The onset of social referencing. In M. Lamb & L. Sherrod (Eds.), *Infant social cognition*. Hillsdale, NJ: Erlbaum.

Carey, W. (1970). A simplified method for measuring infant temperament. *Journal of Pediatrics, 77*, 188–194.

Carr, J. (1988). Six weeks to twenty-one years old: A longitudinal study of children with Down's syndrome and their families. *Journal of Child Psychology and Psychiatry, 29*, 407–431.

Carr, J. (1989). Erratum. *Journal of Child Psychology and Psychiatry, 29*, 187.

Caspi, A., Elder, G., & Bem, D. (1987). Moving against the world: Life-course patterns of explosive children. *Developmental Psychology, 23*, 308–313.

Caspi, A., Elder, G., & Bem, D. (1988). Moving away from the world: Life-course patterns of shy children. *Developmental Psychology, 24*, 824–831.

Charlesworth, W. R. (1969). The role of surprise in cognitive development. In D. Elkind & J. Flavell (Eds.), *Studies in cognitive development: Essays in honor of Jean Piaget*. New York: Oxford University Press.

Cicchetti, D. (1984). The emergence of developmental psychopathology. *Child Development, 55*, 1–7.

Cicchetti, D. (1987). Developmental psychopathology in infancy: Illustration from the study of maltreated youngsters. *Journal of Consulting and Clinical Psychology, 55*, 837–845.

Cicchetti, D. (in press). An historical perspective on the discipline of developmental psychopathology. In J. Rolf, A. Masten, D. Cicchetti, K. Neuchterlein, & S. Weintraub (Eds.), *Risk and protective factors in the development of psychopathology*. New York: Cambridge University Press.

Cicchetti, D., & Beeghly, M. (1987). Symbolic development in maltreated youngsters: An organizational perspective. In D. Cicchetti & M. Beeghly (Eds.), *Atypical symbolic development* (pp. 47–68). San Francisco: Jossey-Bass.

Cicchetti, D., & Ganiban, J. (in press). The organization and coherence of developmental processes in infants and children with Down syndrome. In R. M. Hodapp, J. A. Burack, & E. Zigler, *Issues in the developmental approach to mental retardation*. New York: Cambridge University Press.

Cicchetti, D., Ganiban, J., & Barnett, D. (in press). Contributions from the study of high risk populations to understanding the development of emotion regulation. In K. Dodge & J. Garber (Eds.), *The development of emotion regulation*. New York: Cambridge University Press.

Cicchetti, D., & Hesse, P. (1983). Affect and intellect: Piaget's contributions to the study of infant emotional development. In R. Plutchik & H. Kellerman (Eds.), *Emotion: Theory, research and experience* (Vol. 2, pp. 115–169). New York: Academic Press.

Cicchetti, D., & Mans-Wagener, L. (1987). Sequences, stages, and structures in the organization of cognitive development in infants with Down syndrome. In I. Uzgiris & J. McV. Hunt (Eds.), *Infant performance and experience: New findings with the ordinal scales* (pp. 281–310). Urbana: University of Illinois Press.

Cicchetti, D., & Pogge-Hesse, P. (1982). Possible contributions of the study of organically retarded persons to developmental theory. In E. Zigler & D. Balla (Eds.), *Mental retardation: The developmental–difference controversy* (pp. 277–318). Hillsdale, NJ: Erlbaum.

Cicchetti, D., & Rizley, R. (1981). Developmental perspectives on the etiology, intergenerational transmission, and sequelae of child maltreatment. *New Directions for Child Development*, *11*, 31–55.

Cicchetti, D., & Schneider-Rosen, K. (1986). An organizational approach to childhood depression. In M. Rutter, C. Izard, & P. Read (Eds.), *Depression in young people: Clinical and Developmental perspectives* (pp. 71–134). New York: Guilford.

Cicchetti, D., & Serafica, F. (1981). The interplay among behavioral systems: Illustrations from the study of attachment, affiliation and wariness in young Down syndrome children. *Developmental Psychology*, *17*, 36–49.

Cicchetti, D., & Sroufe, L. A. (1976). The relationship between affective and cognitive development in Down syndrome infants. *Child Development*, *47*, 920–929.

Cicchetti, D., & Sroufe, L. A. (1978). An organizational view of affect: Illustration from the study of Down's syndrome infants. In M. Lewis & L. Rosenblum (Eds.), *The development of affect* (pp. 309–350). New York: Plenum.

Cicchetti, D., & Toth, S. (1987). The application of a transactional risk model to intervention with multi-risk maltreating families. *Zero to Three*, 1–8.

Cicchetti, D., Toth, S., & Bush, M. (1988). Developmental psychopathology and incompetence in childhood: Suggestions for intervention. In B. Lahey & A. Kazdin (Eds.), *Advances in clinical child psychology* (pp. 1–73). New York: Plenum.

Cicchetti, D., Toth, S., Bush, M. A., & Gillespie, J. F. (1988). Stage-salient issues in infancy and toddlerhood: Implications for a transactional model of intervention. *New Directions for Child Development*, *39*, 123–145.

Cicchetti, D., & Wagner, S. (in press). Alternative assessment strategies for the evaluation of infants and toddlers: An organizational perspective. In S. Meisels & J. Shonkoff (Eds.), *Handbook of early intervention*. New York: Cambridge University Press.

Courchesne, E. (1988). Physioanatomical considerations in Down syndrome. In L. Nadel (Ed.), *The psychobiology of Down syndrome* (pp. 291–313). Cambridge, MA: MIT Press.

Cowie, V. A. (1970). *A study of the early development of mongols*. Oxford: Pergamon Press.

Coyle, J., Oster-Granite, M., & Gearhart, J. (1986). The neurobiologic consequences of Down syndrome. *Brain Research Bulletin, 16*, 773–787.

Cronk, C. (1978). Growth of children with Down syndrome: Birth to age 3 years. *Pediatrics, 61*, 564–568.

Curtiss, S. (1977). *Genie: A psycholinguistic study of a modern-day "wild child."* New York: Academic Press.

Eibl-Eibesfeldt, I. (1979). Human ethology: Concepts and implications for the science of man. *Behavioral and Brain Sciences, 2,* 1–57.

Ekman, P. (1972). Universals and cultural differences in facial expressions of emotion. *Nebraska symposium on Motivation.* Lincoln: University of Nebraska Press.

Ekman, P. (1977). Biological and cultural contributions to body and facial movement. In J. Blacking (Ed.), *The anthropology of the body.* London: Academic Press.

Emde, R. N., & Brown, C. (1978). Adaptation to the birth of Down syndrome infants. *Journal of the American Academy of Child Psychiatry, 17,* 299–323.

Emde, R. N., Gaensbauer, T., & Harmon, R. (1976). *Emotional expression in infancy: A biobehavioral study.* New York: International Universities Press.

Emde, R. N., Katz, E. L., & Thorpe, J. K (1978). Emotional expression in infancy: II. Early deviations in Down syndrome. In M. Lewis & L. A. Rosenblum (Eds.), *The development of affect.* London: Plenum.

Erikson, E. (1950). *Childhood and society.* New York: Norton.

Fantz, R. L., Fagan, J. F., & Miranda, S. B. (1975). Early visual selectivity. In L. B. Cohen & P. Salapatek (Eds.), *Infant perception: From sensation to cognition,* Vol. 1: *Basic Visual Processes* (pp. 249–346). New York: Academic Press.

Fein, G., & Apfel, N. (1979). The development of play: Style, structure, and situation. *Genetic Psychology Monographs, 99,* 231–250.

Fenson, L. (1984). Developmental trends for action and speech in pretend play. In I. Bretherton (Ed.), *Symbolic play.* Orlando, FL: Academic Press.

Fraiberg, S. (1977). *Insights from the blind.* New York: International Universities Press.

Freud, A. (1965). *Normality and pathology in childhood: Assessments of development.* New York: International Universities Press.

Gallagher, R., Jens, K., & O'Donnell, K. (1983). The effect of physical status on the affective expression of handicapped infants. *Journal of Infant Behavior and Development, 6,* 73–77.

Ganz, L. (1975). Orientation in visual space by neonates and its modification of visual deprivation. In A. H. Riesen (Ed.), *Developmental psychology of sensory deprivation.* New York: Academic Press.

Gath, A., & Gumley, D. (1984). Down's syndrome and the family: follow-up of children first seen in infancy. *Developmental Medicine and Child Neurology, 26,* 500–508.

Gibson, J. J. (1966). *The senses considered as perceptual systems.* Boston: Houghton Mifflin.

Gottlieb, G. (1983). The psychobiological approach to developmental issues. In M. M. Haith & J. J. Campos (Vol. Eds.), *Infancy and developmental psychobiology* (Vol. 2). P. H. Mussen (Ed.), *Handbook of child psychology* (pp. 1–26). New York: Wiley.

Greenspan, S. I. (1981). *Psychopathology and adaptation in infancy and early childhood.* New York: International Universities Press.

Greenspan, S. I., & Porges, S. W. (1984). Psychopathology in infancy and early childhood: Clinical perspectives on the organization of sensory and affective-thematic experience. *Child Development, 55,* 49–70.

Gunn, P., Berry, P., & Andrews, R. (1981). The affective response of Down's syndrome infants to a repeated event. *Child Development, 52,* 745–748.

Gunnar, M. (1980). Control, warning signals, and distress in infancy. *Developmental Psychology, 16,* 281–289.

Hein, A. (1972). Acquiring components of visually guided behavior. In A. Pick (Ed.), *Minnesota Symposium on Child Psychology, 6.* Minneapolis: University of Minnesota Press.

Henderson, S. (1985). Motor skill development. In D. Lane & B. Stratford (Eds.), *Current approaches to Down's syndrome* (pp. 187–218). New York: Praeger.

Hesse, P., & Cicchetti, D. (1982). Toward an integrative theory of emotional development. *New Directions for Child Development, 16,* 3–48.

Hill, S., & Tomlin, C. (1981). Self recognition in retarded children. *Child Development, 52,* 145–150.

Inhelder, B. (1966). Cognitive development and its contribution to the diagnosis of some phenomena of mental deficiency. *Merrill-Palmer Quarterly, 11,* 299–319.

Izard, C. (1977). *Human emotions*. New York: Plenum.

Izard, C., & Buechler, S. (1979). Emotion expressions and personality integration in infancy. In C. Izard (Ed.), *Emotions in personality and psychopathology*. New York: Plenum.

Izard, C., Kagan, J., & Zajonc, R. (Eds.) (1984). *Emotions, cognition and behavior*. New York: Cambridge University Press.

Izard, C., & Malatesta, C. (1987). Perspectives on emotional development I: Differential emotions theory of early emotional development. In J. Osofsky (Ed.), *Handbook of infant development* (2nd ed., pp. 494–554). New York: Wiley.

Jasnow, M., et al. (1988). Coordinated interpersonal timing of Down's syndrome and nondelayed infants with their mothers: Evidence for a buffered mechanism of social interaction. *Biological Bulletin, 174*, 355–360.

Jennings, K., Harmon, R., Morgan, G., Gaiter, J., & Yarrow, L. (1979). Exploratory play as an index of mastery motivation: Relationships to persistence, cognitive functioning, and environmental measures. *Developmental Psychology, 15*, 386–394.

Kagan, J. (1981). *The second year*. Cambridge: Harvard University Press.

Kagan, J. (1982). *Psychological research on the human infant: An evaluative summary*. New York: W. T. Grant Foundation.

Kaplan, B. (1966). The study of language in psychiatry: The comparative developmental approach and its application to symbolization and language in psychopathology. In S. Arieti (Ed.), *American handbook of psychiatry*. New York: Basic.

Kaplan, B. (1967). Meditations on genesis. *Human Development, 10*, 65–87.

Kaplan, E. (1983). Process and achievement revisited. In S. Wapner & B. Kaplan (Eds.), *Toward a holistic developmental psychology*. Hillsdale, NJ: Erlbaum.

Kopp, C. (1982). Antecedents of self-regulation: A developmental perspective. *Developmental Psychology, 18*, 199–214.

Lamb, M., Thompson, R., Gardner, W., Charnov, E., & Estes, D. (1984). Security of infantile attachment as assessed in the strange situation: Its study and biological interpretation. *Behavioral and Brain Sciences, 7*, 124–147.

Lee, D. N., & Aronson, E. (1974). Visual proprioceptive control of standing in human infants. *Perception and Psychophysics, 15*(3), 529–532.

Lenneberg, E. H. (1966). The natural history of language. In F. Smith & G. Miller (Eds.), *The genesis of language*. Cambridge, MA: MIT Press.

Lenneberg, E. H. (1967). *Biological foundations of language*. New York: Wiley.

Lewis, M., & Brooks-Gunn, J. (1979). *Social cognition and the acquisition of self*. New York: Plenum.

Lewis, M., & Michalson, L. (1983). *Children's emotions and moods: Developmental theory and measurement*. New York: Plenum.

Lewis, M., Sullivan, M. W., Stanger, C., & Weiss, M. (1989). Self-development and self-conscious emotions. *Child Development, 59*, 146–156.

Loveland, K. (1978). Behavior of young children with Down syndrome before the mirror: Finding things reflected. *Child Development, 58*, 928–936.

Mahler, M., Pine, F., & Bergman, A. (1975). *The psychological birth of the human infant*. New York: Basic.

Mans, L., Cicchetti, D., & Sroufe, L. A. (1978). Mirror reactions of Down's syndrome infants and toddlers: Cognitive underpinnings of self-recognition. *Child Development, 49*, 1247–1250.

McIntire, M., & Dutch, J. (1964). Mongolism and generalized hypotonia. *American Journal of Mental Deficiency, 68*, 669–670.

Miranda, S. B., & Fantz, R. L. (1974). Recognition memory in Down's syndrome and normal infants. *Child Development, 45*, 651–660.

Motti, F., Cicchetti, D., & Sroufe, L. A. (1983). From infant affect expression to symbolic play: The coherence of development in Down syndrome children. *Child Development, 54*, 1168–1175.

Mundy, P., Sigman, M., Kasari, C., & Yirmiya, N. (1988). Nonverbal communication skills in Down syndrome children. *Child Development, 59*, 235–249.

Nadel, L. (1988) (Ed.). *The psychobiology of Down syndrome*. Cambridge, MA: MIT Press.

Nicolich, L. (1977). Beyond sensorimotor intelligence: Assessment of symbolic maturity through analysis of pretend play. *Merrill-Palmer Quarterly, 23*, 89–99.

Overton, W. (1976). The active organism in structuralism. *Human Development, 19*, 71–86.

Overton, W. (1984). World views and their influence on psychological theory and research: Kuhn–Lakatos–Laudan. In H. Reese (Ed.), *Advances in child development and behavior* (Vol. 18, pp. 191–226). New York: Academic Press.

Pepper, S. (1942). *World hypotheses.* Berkeley: University of California Press.

Petit, T., LeBoutillier, J., Alfano, D., & Becker, L. (1984). Synaptic development in the human fetus: Amorphometric analysis of normal and Down's syndrome neocortex. *Experimental Neurology, 83*, 13–23.

Piaget, J. (1954/1981). *Intelligence and affectivity: Their relationship during child development.* Palo Alto: CA: Annual Reviews.

Pribram, K. (1967). The new neurology and the biology of emotion: A structural approach. *American Psychologist, 22*, 830–838.

Pribram, K. (1980). The biology of emotions and other feelings. In R. Plutchik & H. Kellerman (Eds.), *Emotion: Theory, research and experience* (Vol. 1). New York: Academic Press.

Purpura, D. (1974). Dendritic spine "dysgenesis" and mental retardation. *Science, 186*, 1126–1128.

Quinn, J., & Rubin, K. (1984). The play of handicapped children. In T. Yawkey & A. Pelligrini (Eds.), *Child's play: Developmental and applied.* Hillsdale, NJ: Erlbaum.

Roche, A. (1964). Skeletal maturation rates in mongolism. *American Journal of Roentgenology, 91*, 979–987.

Roche, A. (1965). The stature of mongols. *Journal of Mental Deficiency Research, 9*, 131–145.

Rondal, J. (1988). Language development in Down's syndrome: A lifespan perspective. *International Journal of Behavioral Development, 11*, 21–36.

Rubin, K., Fein, G., & Vandenberg, B. (1983). Play. In P. Mussen (Ed.), *Handbook of child psychology,* Vol. 4: *Socialization.* New York: Wiley.

Rutter, M. (1986). The developmental psychopathology of depression: Issues and perspectives. In M. Rutter, C. Izard, & P. Read (Eds.), *Depression in young people, clinical and developmental perspectives.* New York. Guilford.

Rutter, M., & Garmezy, N. (1983). Developmental psychopathology. In P. Mussen (Ed.), *Handbook of child psychology.* New York: Wiley.

Sackett, G., Sameroff, A., Cairns, R., & Suomi, S. (1981). Continuity in behavioral development: Theoretical and empirical issues. In K. Immelmann, G. Barlow, L. Petrinovich, & M. Main (Eds.), *Behavioral development.* Cambridge: Cambridge University Press.

Sameroff, A. (1983). Developmental systems: Contexts and evolution. In P. Mussen, *Handbook of child psychology* (4th ed.), Vol. 1: *Infancy* (pp. 237–294). New York: Wiley.

Sameroff, A., & Chandler, M. (1975). Reproductive risk and the continuum of caretaking casualty. In F. Horowitz (Ed.), *Review of child development research* (Vol. 4). Chicago: University of Chicago Press.

Sander, L. (1962). Issues in early mother–child interaction. *Journal of the American Academy of Child Psychiatry, 1*, 141–166.

Sander, L. W. (1975). Infant and caretaking environment: Investigation and conceptualization of adaptive behavior in systems of increasing complexity. In E. J. Anthony (Ed.), *Explorations in child psychiatry.* New York: Plenum.

Santostefano, S. (1978). *A bio-developmental approach to clinical child psychology.* New York: Wiley.

Schneider-Rosen, K., & Cicchetti, D. (1984). The relationship between affect and cognition in maltreated infants: Quality of attachment and the development of visual self-recognition. *Child Development, 55*, 648–658.

Serafica, F. C., & Cicchetti, D. (1976). Down's syndrome children in a strange situation: Attachment and exploratory behaviors. *Merrill-Palmer Quarterly, 21*, 137–150.

Shapiro, B. L. (1970). Prenatal dental anomalies in mongolism: Comments on the basis and implications of variability. *Annals of the New York Academy of Science, 171*, 562–577.

Shapiro, B. L. (1975). Amplified developmental instability in Down's syndrome. *Annals of Human Genetics, 38*, 429–437.

Shirley, M. (1931). *The first two years* (Vol. 1). Minneapolis: University of Minnesota Press.

Smith, G. (Ed.) (1985). *Molecular structure of the number 21 chromosome and Down syndrome*. [Special issue of the *Annals of the New York Academy of Science, 450*]

Sorce, J. F., & Emde, R. N. (1982). The meaning of infant emotional expressions: Regularities in caregiving responses in normal and Down syndrome infants. *Journal of Child Psychology and Psychiatry, 22*, 145–158.

Spencer, H. (1900). *First principles* (6th ed.). New York: Appleton. (Originally published 1862.)

Spiker, D., & Ricks, M. (1984). Visual self-recognition in autistic children: Developmental relationships. *Child Development, 55*, 214–225.

Sroufe, L. A. (1979a). The coherence of individual development. *American Psychologist, 34*, 834–841.

Sroufe, L. A. (1979b). Socioemotional development. In J. Osofsky (Ed.), *Handbook of infant development* (1st ed.). New York: Wiley.

Sroufe, L. A., & Rutter, M. (1984). The domain of developmental psychopathology. *Child Development, 55*, 1184–1199.

Sroufe, L. A., & Waters, E. (1976). The ontogenesis of smiling and laughter: A perspective on the organization of development in infancy. *Psychological Review, 83*, 173–189.

Sroufe, L. A., & Wunsch, J. (1972). The development of laughter in the first year of life. *Child Development, 43*, 1326–1344.

Steiner, J. (1973). The gustofacial response: Observation on normal and anencephalic newborn infants. In J. Bosma (Ed.), *Fourth symposium on oral sensation and perception*. Bethesda, MD: U.S. Department of Health, Education, and Welfare.

Stern, D. (1985). *The interpersonal world of the infant: A view from psychoanalysis and developmental psychology*. New York: Basic.

Takashima, S., Becker, L., Armstrong, D., & Chan, F. (1981). Abnormal neuronal development in the visual cortex of the human fetus and infant with Down's syndrome: A quantitative and qualitative Golgi cell study. *Brain Research, 225*, 1–21.

Thase, M. (1988). The relationship between Down syndrome and Alzheimer's disease. In L. Nadel (Ed.), *The psychobiology of Down syndrome* (pp. 345–368). Cambridge, MA: MIT Press.

Thompson, R., Cicchetti, D., Lamb, M., & Malkin, C. (1985). The emotional responses of Down syndrome and normal infants in the Strange Situation: The organization of affective behavior in infants. *Developmental Psychology, 21*, 828–841.

Tomkins, S. (1962). *Affect, imagery, consciousness* (Vol. 1). New York: Springer-Verlag.

Tomkins, S. (1963). *Affect, imagery, consciousness* (Vol. 2). New York: Springer-Verlag.

Tomkins, S. (1980). Affect as amplification: Some modifications in theory. In R. Plutchik & H. Kellerman (Eds.), *Emotion: Theory, research, and experience* (Vol. 1). New York: Academic Press.

Trevarthan, C. (1968). Two visual systems in primates. *Psychologische Forschung, 31*, 299–377.

Uzgiris, I., & Hunt, J. (1975). *Assessment in infancy*. Urbana: University of Illinois Press.

Watson, M., & Fischer, K. (1977). A developmental sequence of agent use in late infancy. *Child Development, 48*, 828–836.

Werner, H. (1937). Process and achievement: A basic problem of education and developmental psychology. *Harvard Educational Review, 7*, 353–368.

Werner, H. (1948). *Comparative psychology of mental development*. New York: International Universities Press.

Zahn-Waxler, C., & Radke-Yarrow, M. (1982). The development of altruism: Alternative research strategies. In N. Eisenberg (Ed.), *Development of social behavior*. New York: Academic Press.

Zigler, E. (1969). Developmental versus differences theories of mental retardation and the problem of motivation. *American Journal of Mental Deficiency, 73*, 536–556.

Zigler, E. & Balla, D. (Eds.) (1982). *Mental retardation: The developmental–difference controversy*. Hillsdale, NJ: Erlbaum.

3   Temperament and Down syndrome

Jody Ganiban, Sheldon Wagner, and Dante Cicchetti

Temperament and Down syndrome

The characteristic manner in which individuals engage their world is typically referred to as temperament. This concept describes the approach to the world as well as the nature and affective tone of interactions that occur. In recent years, interest in temperament has been spurred by reports of the importance of understanding individual characteristics of infants and children and subsequent caretaking needs. For example, Bell's (1968) model of reciprocal influences in mother–infant interactions has underscored the importance of the infant's effect upon the mother's behavior. Additional reports by Thomas and Chess (1977, 1980) have indicated that problems in the goodness of fit between a child's characteristics and environmental demands may lead to maladaptive behavior later in life. These findings are in accord with the transactional model set forth by Sameroff and Chandler (1975), who viewed development as the product of continuous interaction between individuals and their caretaking environment. Within this theoretical framework, developmental ''casualties'' are poor or nonoptimal outcomes that result when the characteristics of the individual are not congruent with the expectations of the environment.

Lastly, recent research has also pointed toward the theoretical and pragmatic importance of exploring the concept of temperament. Kagan (1982; cited by Sroufe, 1985) has suggested that difficult temperament profiles in infancy may adversely affect parent–child interactions, while Cutrona and Troutman (1986) have proposed that temperament may affect parents' perceptions of self-efficacy, inducing feelings of helplessness. Additionally, researchers have also found that infant temperament is modestly related to later behavior disorders (Thomas & Chess, 1980; for a re-

The writing of this chapter was supported by grants from the John D. and Catherine T. MacArthur Foundation Network on Early Childhood, the March of Dimes Foundation, the National Center on Child Abuse and Neglect (90-C-1929), the National Institute of Mental Health (R01 = MH37960-01), and the Spencer Foundation to author Cicchetti and by a grant from the National Institute of Mental Health (1 R03 MH 42189-01) to author Wagner. Special thanks are due to Doug Barnett, Bonnie Bitran, Walter Murphy, and Sheree Toth for their valuable help, feedback, and suggestions, and to Victoria Gill for typing this manuscript.

view, see Bates, 1987). Others have suggested that difficult temperament patterns may delay the attainment of cognitive milestones such as object permanence (Wachs & Gandour, 1983) as well as performance on standard developmental tests.

Research with infants with Down syndrome also has drawn attention to understanding individual differences in behavioral capacities and the impact these capacities have upon temperament perceptions. For example, Emde, Katz, and Thorpe (1978) have emphasized the importance of parents establishing appropriate expectations for their children's development in order to relieve parental stress and feelings of disappointment. Vietze, McCarthy, McQuiston, MacTurk, and Yarrow (1983) have also discussed the importance of parents understanding the reactive limitations of children with Down syndrome in order to create an environment that will adequately meet the needs of these children.

In this chapter, we review studies that have explored the manner in which individuals approach and respond to their environment. This review includes two themes. The overall aim of the chapter is to examine how Down syndrome affects the temperament of infants and children. In what ways do children with Down syndrome differ from nonhandicapped and other mentally retarded populations (see also Wagner, Ganiban, & Cicchetti, Chapter 5, this volume)? Do individuals with Down syndrome differ in their rate of development of abilities that underlie temperament, or is the organization of these abilities unique to individuals with Down syndrome? The second goal of our review is to provide a multidomain approach to the study of temperament in infants and children with Down syndrome. In the following sections, we explore the impact of constitution, physiological maturation, cognitive level, emotionality and self-regulation upon temperament in Down syndrome.

Approaches to the study of temperament

The initial construct of temperament emphasized intraindividual differences in behavioral style. Through extensive interviews with parents and children within the New York Longitudinal Study, Thomas and Chess (Thomas & Chess 1977; Thomas, Chess, & Birch, 1968) originally identified nine behavioral dimensions they felt captured the core characteristics of temperament: tendency to approach or withdrawal from the world, activity level, general emotional tone, intensity of response, distractibility, adaptability, reactive threshold, rhythmicity, and soothability characteristics among individuals. Additionally, Thomas and Chess further described three temperament profiles that were present in their sample: easy, difficult, and slow to warm up. While easy infants and children were predominantly positive in mood, highly adaptable to situations, and only mild to moderate in their intensity of response, difficult children were arrhythmic, prone to withdraw from new situations, low in adaptability, and generally of negative affect. Similarly, slow to warm up children demonstrated initial withdrawal from new situations, responses of mild to moderate intensity and slow adaptability. Although most children in the New York Longitudinal Study were classified as easy, approximately 25% of the children were described as slow to warm up or difficult (Thomas, Chess, & Birch, 1968).

In recent years, various research groups have delineated alternative definitions and dimensions of temperament (for reviews see Bates, 1987; and Goldsmith et al., 1987). The trend in each case has been to refine the definition of temperament and to identify more fundamental behavioral tendencies that represent and shape individual differences. In this light, Buss and Plomin have argued that the core characteristics that define one's temperament are emotionality, sociability, and overall activity level (Buss & Plomin, 1975; Plomin, 1987). Goldsmith and Campos (1982, 1986) define temperament in terms of individual differences in the temporal and intensive aspects of affect expression. Lastly, Rothbart and her colleagues (Derryberry & Rothbart, 1984; Rothbart & Derryberry, 1981; Rothbart & Posner, 1985) conceptualize temperament as individual differences in emotional and physiological arousability and regulation. Similar to Goldsmith and Campos, Rothbart describes temporal and intensive aspects of responsivity as important components of temperament.

Two additional themes are also apparent across these approaches: First, each framework argues that individual differences in temperament are rooted in one's genetic makeup or integrity of neurological systems. Second, with development, changes in the expression of behaviors that constitute temperament are expected. These changes may be a function of genetically guided maturation coupled with interaction with the environment or by the development of abilities that underlie and shape the expression of temperament (Plomin, 1987; Rothbart & Derryberry, 1981; Wilson & Matheny, 1986).

A genetic predisposition to temperament implies that the range of temperament characteristics expressed by individuals at any point in development may be constrained by their genotypes. Evidence for a genetic component to individual differences in temperament has been gathered by several groups (Goldsmith & Campos, 1986; Plomin, 1987; Wilson & Matheny 1986). Studies that have compared the concordance rates of emotionality, activity, and sociability among monozygotic and dizygotic twins or between the biological parents of adopted children generally indicate that a significant portion of variance associated with the expression of these characteristics, at least in infancy, is accounted for by genetic predispositions. These findings are apparent whether objective behavioral observations are made or when parent report measures are used (see Plomin, 1987, for a review). Additionally, Wilson and Matheny (1986) have found that changes in temperament over time may also be genetically influenced. This finding suggests that temperament characteristics may unfold as one matures.

However, although there appears to be a genetic influence upon the expression and development of temperament characteristics, intact, discrete traits are not transmitted from generation to generation. Rather, only the *potential* or *probability* of demonstrating a particular characteristic is constrained by one's genotype; the phenotypic expression of a specific behavior style is influenced by myriad psychological and environmental factors (Plomin, 1987).

The range of possible characteristics delineated by one's genotype may be expressed through the sensitivity and reactivity of individuals to stimulation. In their conceptualization of temperament, Rothbart and Derryberry (1981) and others (Garcia Coll, Kagan, & Reznick, 1984; Goldsmith & Campos, 1986; Kagan, Reznick, & Snidman, 1987) have focused upon qualitative differences among infants and children in the integrity, responsivity, and organization of the central (CNS) and peripheral (PNS) nervous systems. Such differences are likely to influence one's subjective experience of the world by affecting one's arousal threshold, as well as temporal and intensive aspects of arousability and reactivity to the environment: how long it will take for one to become aroused, arousal duration, susceptibility to overstimulation, and the magnitude of arousal. Consequently, at a very basic level these systems work in concert to shape the individual's emotionality or reactivity to the world.

Importantly, however, the expression of emotionality, is modified as nervous systems mature and differentiate and as individuals interact with their environment and develop self-regulatory and coping skills. Therefore, as development proceeds, initial differences in arousability to stimulation interact with one's self-regulatory abilities and experiences to specify temperament characteristics. Following Werner's conception of development (1957), biological and genetic predispositions form the undifferentiated state from which the individual's characteristic behavior will be fashioned. One's temperament will be within the range established by genetic restrictions, yet specified by experience and the interaction of additional abilities as one develops and matures (cf. Dobzhansky, 1955).

Through the first years of life, changes in expressed temperament characteristics are expected. Although physiological responsivity or sensitivity of central, autonomic and somatic nervous systems may remain constant, the regulation, organization and expression of these characteristics change. Given this framework, changes are expected to result from the reorganization and integration of cognitive abilities, self-regulation, and reactivity as one matures and interacts with the world (Rothbart & Derryberry, 1981). In this light, change may be genetically determined to some extent (Wilson & Matheny, 1986). One's genotype may specify the rate of maturation and development of qualities that underlie temperament. However, the exact characteristics that will be expressed again will be determined by experience and how these abilities are organized.

In the newborn period and during early infancy, in the absence of object permanence or strong self-regulatory abilities, responses to the environment are thought to be reflexive and guided by the capacity of the individual to perceive and react (Cicchetti, Ganiban, & Barnett, in press). That is, the individual reacts to stimuli in the world without cognitive mediation. Thus, temperament at this time reflects the inherent reactivity of the infant, as governed by the sensitivity of perceptual and arousal systems. At this level, the direct effects of subtle differences in the neurochemical systems and the integrity of perceptual and arousal systems mediate reactivity and thus should be apparent in the emotionality of the infant. Individual differences in response threshold, intensity, duration, and affective tone are expected to be highly influenced by the arousability and reactivity of biological systems. For example, Gunnar (1986) reports that newborn infants exhibit individual differences in their sensitivity to being washed and weighed. While some infants become only slightly aroused, other infants become distressed. These behavioral reactions were associated with individual differences in adrenocortical activity, as indexed by adrenocorticotropic hormone (ACTH) and cortisol levels. The infants who become most distressed to handling had more highly active adrenocortical systems than those who did not exhibit distress. Thus, hypersensitivity of this arousal system may be related to the behavioral distress expressed by individual infants.

However, during the first year of life, behavior becomes less reflexive as self-regulatory and cognitive skills develop. In this stage of development, the responsivity of the individual reflects the interaction between emotionality, cognitive capacity, and self-regulation. The rudiments of self-regulation lie in neurological maturation. Rothbart and Derryberry (1981) highlight the development of forebrain inhibition through the strengthening of cortical tracts that control forebrain structures such as the limbic system (see also Cicchetti & Sroufe, 1978). As the brain continues to mature after birth, forebrain inhibitory tracts enable the infant to gain control over arousal states and reflexive behaviors. Additionally, the development and strengthening of interhemispheric tracts also promote inhibitory control of emotionality (Fox & Davidson, 1984).

Although these developments rely upon maturational processes, the environment also plays an important part. Caregivers may serve as the organizers of experience for infants. In this role, caregivers support the development of self-regulation within the infant by aiding them in maintaining physiological homeostasis and organization. This support acts as a scaffold upon which the infant builds his or her own self-regulatory abilities (Kopp, 1982). In this regard, although the development of inhibitory tracts are highly canalized, their full development is experience expectant; a minimum of environmental responsivity is needed for their optimal development (Cicchetti et al., in press; Greenough, Black, & Wallace, 1987). Kopp (1982; Chapter 7, this volume) proposes that this type of "neurophysiological modulation" develops within the first 3 months of life.

After this period, infants start to develop the ability to modify their reactivity in response to environmental demands and changes ("sensorimotor modulation"). With the development of refined representational and symbolic skills, the child's reactions to the world become dependent upon his or her understanding of events, in addition to his or her immediate physiological response: In this regard, one's reactivity to experiences is increasingly moderated by memory, thought, and intention. Children's expressed temperament characteristics reflect the interaction between their understanding of an event and their emotionality (Rothbart & Derryberry, 1981). For example, following Kagan's (1970) discrepancy hypothesis (see also Rothbart & Derryberry, 1981) new experiences that are only moderately discrepant from an infant's past experiences may promote arousal, motivating exploration and interest. However, events that are extremely discrepant from one's previous experiences may be arousing, but also overwhelming and distressing. In each case, the child's evaluation of a current event promotes arousal or "psychological tension" within the child (Cicchetti & Sroufe, 1976, 1978). In turn, such tension may motivate specific types of behavior such as approach toward or withdrawal from further stimulation.

The development of memory and the ability to categorize experiences also enables one to perceive consistencies in the environment and to evaluate new experiences and choose appropriate responses on the basis of past experiences. In this sense, evaluation drives self-regulatory behaviors and, again, affect one's reactivity or emotionality to an experience. An event might first spark a high level of arousal in a highly reactive person. However, if the individual associates the experience with positive feelings, he or she will approach the experience willingly. In contrast, if past experiences were negative, the person's arousal level may further increase, prompting tension, anxiety, and eventual withdrawal from the situation. For example, Kagan and colleagues (1987) have noted that some extremely inhibited infants become relatively uninhibited in later years. They argue that this shift in responsivity to the world reflects the adoption of coping strategies that enable one to recognize arousal levels and to control arousal states in an adaptive manner.

The impact of cognition upon self-regulation of one's emotionality or reactivity is also apparent within atypical populations such as maltreated children or children with emotionally unavailable caregivers (Cicchetti et al., in press). In these cases, children's anticipation of their caregivers' responses is expected to alter the way in which they react to events. For example, children who expect their caregivers to respond negatively to emotions (i.e., crying or smiling) may inhibit or dampen their affect expressiveness to such an extent that they appear to be depressed or nonreactive. Temperamentally, these children may seem to be extremely withdrawn and nonresponsive to their world.

Thus, ultimately, the responses emitted by a person and the behavioral tendencies that characterize the temperament of each person, reflect a combination of evaluative, self-regulative, and reactive processes. Individual differences in temperament arise from variation within each capacity, as well as from variation in their interaction. Ironically, the same factors that promote variability between individuals also promote stability within individuals. Temperament characteristics are expected to be somewhat stable for each person because they rely upon the past history of the individual, in addition to fundamental, stable differences in the biological makeup of the individual.

Temperament in Down syndrome

Studies of temperament in individuals with Down syndrome are warranted for several reasons. One pragmatic reason is to gain more information about the response characteristics of this unique population. Additional research can only aid caregivers in forming appropriate expectations for the interactive capacities and responsivity of the individual with Down syndrome. Second, the early identifiability and unique features of Down syndrome may enable one to make inferences about the possible contribution of genetic and biological influences to behavior characteristics (see Cicchetti & Beeghly, Chapter 2, this volume). Third, as others have argued, the discordance between intellectual development and chronological age affords the opportunity to look at the coherence of organization of different capacities and their impact upon behavioral responsivity (see Cicchetti & Sroufe, 1976).

In a review of temperament and personality studies with the Down syndrome population, Gibson (1978) reported that individuals with Down syndrome are commonly stereotyped as obstinate, but affectionate and easy in temperament. Uniformity, presumably, is attributed either to a common genetic syndrome or to the effect of mental retardation. However, when this stereotype is subjected to empirical investigation, Gibson argues, it is inconsistently supported. In several studies discussed by Gibson, the majority of children and adults with Down syndrome fit the stereotype. Yet in many cases a subgroup of individuals with Down syndrome seemed restless, aggressive, and generally difficult to manage. Gibson concludes that temperament in the individual with Down syndrome is not uniform. Rather, a large variety of temperament profiles exist within this population, as with other mentally retarded and normal populations. Like Rothbart and Derryberry in their conceptualization of temperament (1981), Gibson attributes temperament variability to karyotype (genetic makeup), reactivity, neurological maturation, and intellectual status.

In the following sections, this chapter takes a multidomain approach. Guided by the theoretical framework of Rothbart and Derryberry (1981), we examine the impact of Down syndrome upon reactive systems and the interaction and organization of abilities that serve as the foundation for temperament. Consequently, we review studies that have explored physiological maturation and reactivity, affect expression, self-regulation, and their interactions with evaluative capacities. Finally, in the last section, studies that have utilized parental ratings of temperament are discussed in light of the organization of these abilities. Implicit in this approach is the examination of how individuals with Down syndrome differ from nonhandicapped, nonretarded populations and the uniqueness of temperament characteristics to Down syndrome. We also briefly outline the extent to which Down syndrome and mental retardation affect temperament and discuss reasons for the variability in temperament characteristics within the Down syndrome population.

Biological underpinnings of temperament

Given the framework described by Rothbart and Derryberry (1981), the origins of individual differences are presumed to lie in the biological constitution of the individual. At this level, minute differences in central (neurotransmitter systems) and peripheral (autonomic nervous system) nervous systems are thought to underlie the range of potential response characteristics observed across individuals. Rothbart and others (Goldsmith & Campos, 1986; Rothbart & Derryberry, 1981; Rothbart & Posner, 1986) have highlighted four neurological systems that they feel determine the underlying reactivity or emotionality of the individual to stimulation: (1) the reticular activating system (RAS); (2) the autonomic nervous system (ANS); (3) endocrine response systems; and (4) somatic response systems. Additionally, recent studies in the area of affect development have started to explore the role of hemispheric lateralization of neurotransmitters and reactivity upon individual differences in emotionality as well (Fox & Davidson, 1984; Tucker & Williamson, 1984).

The RAS is often described as the alerter of the central nervous system (CNS), which mediates consciousness (Kandel & Schwartz, 1985). The RAS pathway arises in the brain stem and projects to the cortex. In recent years, serotonin has been targeted as the primary neurotransmitter of this system. Brain lesions that severely damage the locus coeruleus, an area of the CNS that contains serotenergic producing cells, result in insomnia. In contrast, chronic activation of serotonergic systems leads to unconsciousness (Kandel & Schwartz, 1985).

Within the CNS, hemispheric asymmetries and the lateralization of neurotransmitter systems may also influence arousability to stimulation and individual differences in temperament. Tucker and Williamson (1984) have proposed that the right hemisphere is associated with the general arousal or *activation* of the brain. Through the interaction of noradrenergic and serotonergic systems, this hemisphere is particularly sensitive to change and helps alert the brain to novelty in the environment. In contrast, they argue, the left hemisphere is dominated by dopaminergic and cholinergic motor systems that seem to be relatively nonresponsive to novelty. Rather, through the interaction of both neurotransmitter systems, the left hemisphere appears to be biased toward *redundancy*; novel environmental occurrences do not disrupt their activation, thereby enabling one to carry out motor acts within a changing environment.

At birth, since interhemispheric connections are poorly developed, some have argued that behavior may be characterized by a simple continuum of approach (i.e., redundancy) or withdrawal (i.e., activation) behaviors (e.g., Fox & Davidson, 1984). The infant's position on this continuum is dependent upon which hemisphere is activated and the intensity of its response. Thus, in terms of temperament, one's emotionality may reflect individual differences in the relative dominance and reactivity of the left and right hemispheres to stimulation. For example, infants with greater right brain activation may be more prone to overstimulation and distress than other infants (Cicchetti & White, 1988). As such, they may be extremely sensitive and distracted by changes in their environment. Conversely, infants with greater left brain activation may be perceived as less distressed by change in their environment and more persistent. This latter group of infants may also demonstrate difficulties in shifting and or refocusing attention.

Within the PNS, the ANS is tied to arousal level as well, but primarily functions during times of physiological stress (Gilman & Newman 1987). This system is divided into two branches, the parasympathetic (PSNS) and sympathetic (SNS) nervous systems, which operate in a reciprocal fashion. The SNS is activated in times of stress and uses norepinephrine and acetylcholine as its primary transmitters. Activation of the SNS prompts increased heart rate and production of blood cells. These changes have been described as the ''fight or flight response'' (Gilman & Newman, 1987) – that is, activation of this system places the individual in an alert state, ready to flee from danger or meet challenges. The PSNS, in contrast, is mediated by acetylcholine and is antagonistic to the SNS. This system reduces heart rate and returns one to a relaxed state.

The SNS is also related to endocrine systems that moderate physiological responses to stress (Gunnar, 1986). Specifically, this system enervates the adrenal glands, prompting the production and release of catecholamines (i.e., epinephrine) in the body. Once in the bloodstream, catecholamines act as hormones that promote cardiac acceleration, the breakdown of organic compounds necessary for energy, as well as affect the action of other hormones (Gunnar, 1986). Another endocrine system that mediates physiological arousal is the hypothalamo–pituitary–adrenal axis (Axelrod & Reisine, 1984). This system reflects the interaction of the CNS (hypothalamus) and glands in the periphery (the anterior pituitary and adrenal glands). Activation of this circuit during times of stress leads to transient increases in adrenocorticotropic hormone (ACTH) and cortisol. Both compounds have been used as indicators of physiological stress (e.g., Gunnar, 1986).

The fourth response system described by Rothbart and Derryberry (1981) pertains to the somatic or bodily responsivity of the individual. These systems include motor activity, vocal activity and facial expressions. Motor activity in some regards will reflect the arousability and reactivity of other systems, such as the ANS. For example, children who are hypersensitive to stimulation may be less active than their peers because they become easily overaroused (e.g., Kagan et al., 1987). Another factor affecting motor activity is integrity of motor areas within the CNS. For example, problems in maintaining proper muscle tone or difficulties in coordinating motor schemes may make it difficult for a child to engage the world actively (cf. Butterworth & Cicchetti, 1978). Vocal activity and facial expression will also affect interaction with the world in similar ways. In both cases, however, each determines the child's ability to express reactions and to emit readable cues to their caregivers (Cicchetti & Pogge-Hesse, 1982; Hesse & Cicchetti, 1982). Infants who cannot be consistent in their ability to express a need or perhaps displeasure may be perceived as unadaptable or irritable by caretakers simply because the caretakers are not able to soothe or satisfy such children consistently (McGehee & Eckerman, 1983).

Together, the sensitivity and integrity of these reactive systems will establish thresholds and arousal levels to stimulation within the CNS and, consequently, regulate one's perception of the world at a very basic level. These systems influence what will arouse a person, how long it will take for a person to become aroused, how much a person will become aroused, and the ease with which one will find stimulation aversive or overstimulating (Rothbart & Derryberry, 1981).

Several studies have described differences between individuals with and without Down syndrome in the activity of central and peripheral transmitter systems that are thought to regulate reactivity to stimulation. However, most research in this area is plagued by methodological and interpretive limitations. First, many studies have centered upon postmortem examinations of a small number of patients with Down syndrome. In such studies, findings may be biased by the sample size and by commonalities between subjects that might have led to their premature deaths but that might not characterize persons with Down syndrome as a group. Second, several studies have also depended upon noninvasive measurements of different compounds in blood or urine. In the latter case, peripheral measurements of neurotransmitters may reflect the activity of both the CNS and PNS. Because of the nonspecificity of such measurements it is impossible to determine where anomalies reside. Relatedly, often studies report main effects of the Down syndrome genotype upon neurotransmitter levels and activity or upon the cytoarchitecture of the brain (see Coyle, Oster-Smith, & Gearhart, 1986). However, given the diffuseness and widespread impact of each neurotransmitter system, it is impossible to pinpoint the origin of these differences and to determine the significance and impact of these differences upon behavior and temperament. Consequently, the interpretations or conclusions we offer should be couched within these weaknesses and regarded as only speculative.

In one study, Casanova, Walker, Whitehouse, and Price (1985) examined the nucleus basalis of Meynart in a postmortem examination of five adolescent and adult patients with Down syndrome (age range 16 to 56 years) and five normal patients of the same chronological age. This neuroanatomical structure contains acetylcholine-producing neurons that project to the cortex. In the patients with Down syndrome, the nucleus basalis contained fewer neurons and consequently fewer projections than the non-Down syndrome brains at each age examined. These data imply that there may be decreased acetylcholine enervation in the brains of individuals with Down syndrome. Consistent with these findings, Yates, Simpson, Maloney, Gorden, and Reid (1980) have presented evidence of decreased acetylcholine levels within the CNS. This study found a decrease in brain tissue choline acetyltransferase and acetylcholinesterase in individuals with Down syndrome. Both enzymes facilitate the synthesis and breakdown of acetylcholine. Lastly, additional research reported by Courchesne (1988) suggests that the evoked potentials of infants with Down syndrome may reflect decreased cholinergic-basalis projections to the frontal cortex. Within this study, such deficiencies may have resulted in the poor selective attention of 6- to-30-month-old infants with Down syndrome to a novel sound.

Therefore, taken together, these studies imply that within the CNS there is a decreased number of cholinergic cells and levels and, additionally, these differences may be reflected in decreased reactivity of at least cholinergic systems originating from the nucleus basalis of Meynart. Casanova et al. (1985) indicate that such differences either may be a result of nervous system degeneration or reflect a fundamental characteristic of the brains of individuals with Down syndrome that are present at birth. Although the significance of these findings is not known, it is possible that decreases in acetylcholine within the CNS may be reflected in differences between individuals with and without Down syndrome in their general responsivity and orientation to their environment. For example, one may speculate that decreased cholinergic enervation may affect an individual's ability to sustain a motoric response (Tucker & Williamson, 1984), to modulate distress (Fox & Davidson, 1984), or to attend to the environment (Courchesne, 1988).

Another neurotransmitter that may be affected by the Down syndrome genotype is serotonin. Scott, Becker, and Petit (1983) discuss several studies that point toward decreased serotonin levels within this population. In these studies, decreased levels of serotonin were found in the blood platelets and whole blood of children with Down syndrome, relative to the normal population. Because serotonin is almost exclusively produced in the CNS, such quantitative differences reflect CNS differences between individuals with and without Down syndrome. An overall decrease in serotonin levels implies that individuals with Down syndrome may have difficulties in regulating sleep–wake cycles, with a tendency toward demonstrating more "wakefulness" than other individuals. However, although these children may be more alert to their environment, they still may be deficient in perceiving and selectively attending to novelty and change within their world.

Another neurotransmitter that may be affected by the Down syndrome genotype is noradrenaline. For example, Weinshilbaum, Thoa, Johnson, Kopin, and Axelrod (1971) found decreased concentrations of dopamine-beta-hydroxylase (DBH) in the blood of children with Down syndrome relative to normal children. This enzyme facilitates conversion of dopamine to noradrenaline. Thus, low DBH levels may indicate a decrease in noradrenaline production. Unfortunately, it is difficult to determine whether this reflects anomalies of the CNS or PNS, or of both. If decreased noradrenaline levels are present within the CNS, this might lead to an overall decrease in sensitivity to novelty within the environment (Tucker & Williamson, 1984). If, however, decreased norephinephrine levels represent functioning within ANS, one would expect overall decreased activation of the SNS, and thus a higher threshold to stress.

The Down syndrome genotype may also affect the release of transmitters into the bloodstream by endocrine systems. For example, Keele, Richards, Brown, and Marshall (1969) report decreased levels of adrenaline metabolites in the urine of individuals with Down syndrome. Because the release of adrenaline from the adrenal glands is activated by the SNS, these findings also indirectly suggest decreased SNS activity.

These possible differences in the activity of neurotransmitter systems, as well as neuroanatomical structures, suggest the presence of fundamental constitutional differences in the reactivity of individuals with Down syndrome. Given Rothbart and Derryberry's (1981) model of temperament, differences within central and peripheral nervous systems are expected to be reflected in the underlying emotionality of these individuals. Quantitative differences in noradrenaline suggest decreased activity of the ANS and, perhaps, decreased sensitivity to novelty in the world. Evidence of decreased cholinergic enervation and serotonergic levels within the CNS also suggests that responsivity to the environment may be affected by Down syndrome. In the latter case, lowered serotonergic activity may increase the alertness of individuals with Down syndrome; however, such individuals still may not be sensitive to novel events that occur within the environment.

Thus, in terms of temperament characteristics, infants with Down syndrome are expected to be responsive to their environment. However, qualitative differences between infants and children with and without Down syndrome in how they react to their environment are expected. Given possible decreased noradrenergic and adrenergic activity, the intensity with which individuals with Down syndrome respond to events may be dampened relative to others. Additionally, decreased sensitivity to novelty (as suggested by decreases in cholinergic and noradrenergic levels) may render these infants less sensitive to change, causing them to perseverate or to approach a large range of experiences that others might find too discrepant from past experiences and thus too anxiety-provoking.

Accordingly, the results of the preceding studies suggest possible overall differences between individuals with Down syndrome and the normal population that may affect reactivity to the world and emotionality. Nonetheless, these studies do not indicate to what extent such differences are unique to individuals with Down syndrome versus being characteristic of individuals who are mentally retarded or immature in their development. Unfortunately, studies that explore the main effect of mental retardation upon reactivity and emotionality throughout development do not exist. Moreover, such studies would be difficult to carry out in infancy and early childhood because most forms of other organically mentally retarded children are not viable or possess a limited range of phenotypic expressiveness. In addition, cultural-familial mentally retarded children are identified much later than mentally retarded children with organic etiologies. Nonetheless, studies at later ages that compare mentally retarded adults with and without Down syndrome may answer this question.

Behaviorally, the emotionality of an infant is perceived through the infant's facial expressions, body movements (e.g., cuddliness versus squirming), approach, and vocalizations. One study completed by Sorce and Emde (1982) provides support for decreased emotionality in 4-month-old infants with Down syndrome relative to 4-month-old normal infants. In this study, 20 infants with Down syndrome and 20 nonhandicapped infants were photographed during interactions with their mothers and experimenters. These pictures were subsequently rated by the mothers of the infants and college students. Both groups of raters found that the facial expressions of infants with Down syndrome were less intense (particularly in enjoyment) than those of the normal infants. However, the infants with Down syndrome were also described as demonstrating more low- and high-intensity interest facial expressions than the nonhandicapped infants. Thus, the babies born with Down syndrome responded to stimulation in a manner qualitatively different from that of the normal infants. The dampened emotionality and passive interaction with the world on the part of the infants with Down syndrome reported by Sorce and Emde (1982) are congruent with the hypothesis that Down syndrome is characterized by a decreased reactivity of arousal systems to stimulation.

In the first years of life, changes in reactivity are expected as the CNS and PNS mature. The growth and further development and differentiation of these systems underlie one's ability to voluntarily regulate arousability and emotionality. During the first months of life, the development of forebrain inhibition and neurotransmitter systems support self-regulation. Additionally, self-regulation is also dependent upon the development of interhemispheric inhibitory tracts. Forebrain and transhemispheric inhibitory tracts provide the neurological "hardware" necessary for self-regulation.

Numerous studies have also indicated that Down syndrome is associated with abnormalities in the growth and elaboration of neuronal networks postnatally (for reviews, see Courchesne, 1988; Kemper, 1988). In most studies, measurements of the growth and structure of dendrites and extensions of neurons are used as indices of neurological maturation. Throughout development, as the individual interacts with the world, these structures grow and branch out to make contact with the axons and dendrites of other neurons, creating elaborate neural networks (Greenough, Black, & Wallace, 1987). Becker, Armstrong, and Chan (1986) point out that the development of dendrites appears to be a major feature of postnatal maturation. Postmortem studies of infants and children with Down syndrome have found evidence of an overall decrease in neurons and dendritic spine abnormalities in limbic structures (Purpura, 1975) and in the visual cortex (Takashima, Becker, Armstrong, & Chan, 1981). In these studies, the brains of individuals with Down syndrome appeared to have shorter dendrites with less branching than those of normal individuals of the same chronological age. Developmentally, Becker and collaborators (1986) have found that in individuals with Down syndrome, such elaborate branching of neurons occurs in the neocortex within the first four months of life to the extent that infants with Down syndrome actually appear to have more elaborate dendritic trees than normal infants. However, by the end of infancy there is a decrease in arboritization and consequently less elaborate and differentiated neuronal networks in the brains of infants and children with Down syndrome relative to the brains of normal individuals. Thus, Becker and colleagues propose that although the neuronal networks of persons with Down syndrome grow quickly in early development, by late infancy this process slows down significantly. Consequently, the brains of the individuals with Down syndrome mature less rapidly and extensively.

Such findings of decreased neuronal development are suggestive of "premature aging" in individuals with Down syndrome, which, if persistent, could appear to lead to degeneration of the brain as connections between neurons are not strengthened, rebuilt, or restructured. This suggestion is congruent with other studies that have found an abnormally high incidence of Alzheimer's disease in middle-aged patients with Down syndrome (for reviews, see Scott, et al., 1983; Thase, 1988). In Alzheimer's disease, patients usually demonstrate loss of memory and mental faculties, becoming easily confused and disoriented. Thase, Liss, Smeltzer, and Maloon (1982), in a survey of institutionalized adults with Down syndrome, found that of patients with Down syndrome over the age of 30 years, a significantly larger percentage demonstrated signs of dementia than did institutionalized nonhandicapped patients of the same age, race, and length of hospitalization. One possible link between Alzheimer's disease and Down syndrome resides in the brain abnormalities common to Alzheimer's patients and older individuals with Down syndrome. In dementia, poorly developed, degenerated neuronal networks, and dendritic plaques and tangles, are usually observed. Scott and colleagues (1983) indicate that both qualities are more prevalent in middle-aged individuals with Down syndrome than in the nonhandicapped population. This relationship has been strengthened as well by growing evidence of neurotransmitter abnormalities that are common to both conditions (Scott et al., 1983).

The implications of decreases or cessation in maturation of the brain are widespread. First, decreased maturation may inhibit the full development of important inhibitory tracts that act to control behavioral systems accurately such as motor or reactive systems. This may account for the persistence of primitive reflexes beyond the early months of life and poor muscle tone in individuals with Down syndrome (Cicchetti & Sroufe, 1978; Cowie, 1970). One might also hypothesize that decreased branching of dendrites in the neocortex might affect communication between different brain areas, or perhaps different sensory modalities. Thus, the ability to synthesize various pieces of information about the world quickly and efficiently might be impaired (O'Connor & Hermelin, 1970; Wagner, Ganiban, & Cicchetti, Chapter 5, this volume). In addition, biological constraints upon the maturation of the brain may influence developmental changes in temperament (Rothbart and Derryberry, 1981; Wilson and Matheny, 1986). If changes in temperament across time reflect the maturation of the CNS, as prescribed by the qualities of the system, individuals with Down syndrome would not be expected to demonstrate shifts or changes in temperament characteristics at the same time as the normal population. Further research must be conducted to determine whether these differences in dendritic maturation are an effect of mental retardation or a consequence of Down syndrome per se.

In summary, neurochemical and neuroanatomical studies presented thus far have documented that there are differences in the emotionality, regulatory, and maturational components of temperament between individuals with Down syndrome and normal individuals. These differences imply that the reactive capacity of individuals with Down syndrome and the nonhandicapped population may be qualitatively different. Specifically, although infants and children with Down syndrome are alert, their sensitivity to novelty and change in their environment may be decreased relative to other children. In turn, children with Down syndrome may seem less reactive or interactive with their environment and be perceived as passive or less interested and engaged within their environment than other children. In addition, studies have pointed toward possible restrictions upon the growth and maturation of capacities that underlie and guide temperament. In this regard, anomalies within the CNS may influence the evaluative and regulatory components of the child's temperament.

When considering these studies it is important to keep in mind several caveats. The investigations conducted to date have focused on the comparison of group means, thereby ignoring the within- and between-group variability characteristic of most samples. In the future, more attention must be paid to the study of individual differences and on uncovering the sources of this variability. First, although individuals with Down syndrome share a genetic disorder, they might differ genetically in countless other ways. For example, the family history of a person with Down syndrome may contain the genes for supersensitivity to stimulation or above-average intelligence. This person might seem less affected by Down syndrome than other individuals with Down syndrome because his or her threshold of reactivity may be muted, but still relatively low, or his or her developmental level may be higher than usually expected of a person with the condition. Thus, the effects of Down syndrome at this level may differ from child to child as genetic makeup differs from child to child. Consequently, great variability would be expected to exist between individuals with Down syndrome as well as between groups of individuals with and without Down syndrome.

When interpreting the findings of these studies, the limitations we outlined at the beginning of this section must also be kept in mind. First, techniques for measuring neurotransmitter activity are not precise (Gunnar, 1986; Rose, 1984). Although peripheral measurements of transmitters are noninvasive, they yield only estimates of transmitter activity. Second, our knowledge of brain and behavior relations has not reached the point at which undisputed conclusions can be drawn about the effects of many anatomical and neurochemical anomalies. For example, one cannot argue that smaller neuroanatomical structures always have a specific effect upon the functioning of the brain and behavior. Third, the small sample size of many of these studies may accentuate spurious relations between brain or neurochemical abnormalities and Down syndrome. Therefore, conclusions and inferences drawn from such data should be regarded as speculative, inviting further research rather than as definitive assertions. Finally, as previously discussed, differences in maturation and neurochemical activity between individuals with and without Down syndrome may not be unique to Down syndrome but, rather, may be a more general characteristic of mental retardation.

Evaluative capacity, attention and self-regulation

Differences in the reactivity of arousal systems and neurological maturation constitute the most basic level of temperament. However, these characteristics establish only a possible range of responses by influencing the perception of events and arousal level. The ultimate response emitted by the individual will be shaped by the development, refinement, and reorganization of additional abilities. One ability that modifies reactivity and shapes responses to the world is the capacity to interpret and analyze an event (Cicchetti & Sroufe, 1976; Rothbart & Derryberry, 1981).

The evaluation of an event may attenuate or accentuate one's arousal level. In this case, when persons are initially confronted with an unfamiliar event, they are placed in a state of uncertainty in which the SNS is activated and their arousal level increases. Analysis and recognition of the event as similar to past experiences may, however, decrease arousal by removing uncertainty. In contrast, if the event is extremely discrepant from past experiences, they may remain in a state of uncertainty in which their level of arousal increases.

Arousal level or reactivity caused by one's evaluations may also fuel affective responses to the world. A highly aroused person may react to an event with great intensity, while an individual who is only minimally aroused may seem indifferent or respond only slightly. Additionally, as one matures the affective tone of his or her response, be it positive or negative, is related to the meaning he or she attaches to the event.

Finally, evaluative capacity may also affect the temporal dimensions of responses. For example, a person who is slow in interpreting an event may react more slowly than an individual who interprets an event quickly. In the latter case, individuals who interpret events slowly may appear to approach or engage the world reluctantly, perhaps seeming detached or disinterested as they attempt to make sense of the world. In contrast, an individual who can rapidly analyze a situation will formulate a response readily, appearing to engage the world quickly.

In this section, we briefly discuss studies that have examined the evaluative capacity of infants with Down syndrome (for more comprehensive reviews, see Dunst, Chapter 6, this volume; and Wagner et al., Chapter 5, this volume). Although these studies concentrate on primarily cognitive abilities, we attempt to relate their findings to differences in attention and approach to the world that have been observed between infants and children with and without Down syndrome and how these differences may affect temperament perceptions.

Miranda and Fantz (1973, 1974) completed the first studies to examine the visual-information processing capacities of infants with Down syndrome. Using a preferential looking paradigm, this research group examined the development of the ability to analyze and distinguish between black and white patterns (see also Wagner et al., Chapter 5, this volume). In their initial study, Miranda and Fantz (1973) showed 8-month-old normal infants and infants with Down syndrome 13 stimulus pattern pairs that differed in pattern (i.e., striped vs. plain surface), dimensionality, curvature, element arrangement, and brightness. Throughout the testing sessions, the infants with Down syndrome appeared to be more attentive to the patterns than the nonhandicapped infants. However, the nonhandicapped infants were able to discriminate between patterns more consistently than the infants with Down syndrome. Although the poorer performance on the part of infants with Down syndrome may have been affected by acuity differences, differences independent of acuity were also found. Consequently, these findings indicate less efficient processing of visual information by the infants with Down syndrome than by the nonhandicapped infants. Although infants with Down syndrome may have the ability to detect differences (i.e., acuity), they utilize early visual experiences to a lesser extent than the nonhandicapped infants (Miranda & Fantz, 1973).

In a second study, Miranda and Fantz (1974) utilized a recognition memory test (see Wagner et al., Chapter 5, this volume). Within this paradigm infants were first familiarized with a pattern. Following familiarization, the old pattern was paired with a novel pattern of similar complexity and luminance. Evidence of recognition memory on the part of the infant is provided if infants selectively attend to the novel pattern. In this cross-sectional study, nonhandicapped infants and infants with Down syndrome were tested at three ages: 8 to 16 weeks, 17 to 29 weeks, and 30 to 40 weeks.

As in the previous study, differences between the infants with Down syndrome and normal infants emerged. In this case, the Down syndrome infants seemed to lag behind normally developing infants. Whereas the nonhandicapped infants started to demonstrate novelty preference at 8 to 16 weeks of age, the infants with Down syndrome as a group did not show novelty preference until 17 to 29 weeks. Additionally, the infants with Down syndrome in the two older age groups also required significantly more time to familiarize themselves with a pattern than their nonhandicapped peers. Thus, in the initial "familiarization" phase of the study, the infants with Down syndrome looked at the test stimuli more than the normal infants. However, despite these differences, the infants with Down syndrome as a group still demonstrated recognition at a relatively young age and followed a developmental pattern that was similar to the nonhandicapped infants.

Taken together, these results suggest that delay and lack of distinction between some patterns reflect delays in the ability of infants with Down syndrome to process or to encode visual information. Miranda and Fantz propose that infants with Down syndrome do not make use of their visual experiences to the same extent as nonhandicapped infants of the same chronological age. Rather, they may need "longer periods of neural maturation" and more experience with the world in order to encode and interpret information than nonhandicapped infants (Miranda & Fantz, 1973). These conclusions are consistent with neuroanatomical studies completed by Becker et al. (1986) and Takashima et al. (1981). Both groups of researchers found evidence of decreased maturation of tissue in the visual cortex of patients with Down syndrome relative to nonhandicapped patients of the same age. Additionally, these studies are consistent with those reported by Courchesne (1988) and Weinshilbaum et al. (1971), which were suggestive of decreased sensitivity of the CNS to novelty.

Difficulties in visual information processing coupled with possible low physiological reactivity to novelty in children with Down syndrome may be reflected in their approach and engagement of the world. In a longitudinal study, Vietze et al. (1983) focused upon the play interactions of infants with Down syndrome. In the Vietze et al. study, infants with Down syndrome were observed at 6, 8, and 12 months chronological age as they engaged in 12 play tasks designed to assess affect production, sensorimotor skills, and problem solving. Their patterns of behaviors were analyzed and additionally compared to those of a group of 6-month-old nonhandicapped children. In general, infants with Down syndrome spent a large proportion of their time looking at toys rather than interacting with them. As they became older, visual attention decreased significantly, whereas object manipulation increased. When compared to the 6-month-old nonhandicapped infants, the 6- and 12-month-old infants with Down syndrome demonstrated significantly more visual attention and less manual exploration and manipulation. Consequently, the infants with Down syndrome seemed to rely upon visual exploration of toys rather than active manipulation. However, as they became older, they demonstrated more active engagement with the toys and less visual attention.

Similarly, MacTurk, Vietze, McCarthy, McQuiston, and Yarrow (1985) have found that play and social interactions for 9-month-old infants with Down syndrome center upon visual attention: infants with Down syndrome tend to look at objects or people a great deal before approaching or engaging an event or task. In contrast, the interactions of nonhandicapped infants of the same developmental level (as assessed by the Bayley Mental Scales of Development, Bayley, 1969) center upon social interactions. Consistent with the work of Miranda and Fantz (1973, 1974), one reason for such reliance upon visual attention may be the need for a longer time to interpret a situation or objects and a delay in the ability to interpret subtle and complex information (i.e., social signals). These infants require a longer time than nonhandicapped infants to assess a situation and cannot rely upon the cues of others to frame responses. Difficulties in these areas, in addition to possible delays in motor skills and low physiological reactivity, may initially decrease immediate approach to and engagement with the world, leading to perceptions of infants with Down syndrome as initially noninteractive, nonapproaching, but highly attentive once oriented to a task or event.

Visual processing capacities also affect another ability: self-regulation. Many self-regulatory capacities are supported and learned through interactions with caretakers. Within Kopp's framework (Kopp, 1982, and Chapter 7, this volume), infants initially learn to regulate physiological states, such as arousal level. In the next stage of development, as infants develop cognitively, they learn to interpret and use cues produced by their caretakers to modify their own behaviors. At this stage infants may look to or "reference" their caretakers when confronted with a situation that is unfamiliar to them and subsequently use their caretakers' reactions to guide their own responses.

The development of "maternal referencing" of nonhandicapped and infants with Down syndrome has been followed longitudinally by Sorce and his colleagues (Sorce, Emde, & Frank, 1982). Starting at 6 months, chronological age, Sorce et al. videotaped 13 nonhandicapped infants at 1-month intervals and 6 infants with Down syndrome at 3-month intervals. At each time the infants were confronted by a male stranger in the presence of their mothers.

In this study, Sorce et al. found that the greatest portion of nonhandicapped infants started to demonstrate maternal referencing at 7 to 10 months of age. However, the infants with Down syndrome did not demonstrate maternal referencing until several months later (approximately 10 to 12 months of age). They suggest that this delay may reflect a more general delay in distinguishing unfamiliar faces from familiar faces on the part of infants with Down syndrome. Alternatively, this delay may also result from difficulties on the part of these babies in decoding subtle but important information from their mother's expressions and reactions. Thus, although they may be able to distinguish between familiar and unfamiliar faces, they may not be able to abstract information from faces with which they can guide their own behavior. In both cases, deficits in visual-information processing skills would account for delays in maternal referencing.

These data are consistent with observations made by MacTurk and colleagues (1985). In this study, nonhandicapped infants by 6 months of age tended to seek social reinforcement (a form of maternal referencing) before engaging in further play, whereas infants with Down syndrome of the same developmental level did not. Thus, in this study, as in the Emde et al. study, infants with Down syndrome may not derive the same type of information or impetus from social interactions as nonhandicapped infants, even when developmental level, as assessed by the Bayley Mental Developmental Index (MDI; Bayley, 1969), is controlled for. Rather, in both cases visual-information processing skills, which are not always accessed by the Bayley, may distinguish the two groups of infants (Wagner et al., Chapter 5, this volume). Infants with Down syndrome may need to rely more upon their ability to interpret the simpler, unchanging characteristics of objects in their environment, rather than the more abstract cues provided by their mothers' facial expressions and reactions. Consequently, they attend to the object world more during infancy than nonhandicapped infants.

In summary, therefore, these studies suggest that the capacity to evaluate information may affect one's approach to and engagement of the world, as well as the development of self-regulatory skills. Studies with infants with Down syndrome have indicated that individuals in this population are delayed in their ability to process visual information. In turn, difficulties in this area may make individuals with Down syndrome seem less interactive with their environment. Behaviorally, they may be extremely visually attentive but take longer to approach a situation and to interact actively with the world than nonhandicapped infants. Given Rothbart and Derryberry's (1981) construction of temperament, each aspect of temperament is influenced by the amount of time required to evaluate an event and formulate an appropriate response.

However, although these investigations point to such a relationship, there are no studies that have directly examined both evaluative processes and differences in temperament characteristics. Accordingly, further work that assesses evaluative skills and behaviors such as approach and engagement concurrently needs to be conducted. The adoption of a multidomain approach in the exploration of behavioral responsivity would provide insight into the organization of abilities that underlie perceived temperament characteristics such as approach and attention to the world for both individuals with Down syndrome and nonhandicapped individuals at a very early age.

Studies also should focus upon individual differences. Unfortunately, however, the studies discussed in this section have not examined individual differences in evaluative capacity and the impact of such differences upon responsivity to the world within the Down syndrome population as well as between the Down syndrome population and other handicapped and nonhandicapped groups. A multidomain approach is essential in the exploration of individual differences. For example, at the level of the individual, are there differences in the way abilities are organized that account for differences in approach and engagement with the world? Or, perhaps, do individual differences in the strengths and weaknesses of specific abilities prompt differences across infants and between infants with Down syndrome and normal infants?

In addition, longitudinal studies similar to the study of Vietze and his colleagues

(1983) need to be conducted to examine the coherence and organization of abilities that underlie responsivity through development. Only longitudinal studies can elucidate the extent to which individuals with Down syndrome are unique in their interactions with the world or perhaps delayed in the manner in which they approach and engage the world.

Affect and cognition

Within the Rothbart and Derryberry (1981) temperament framework, emotionality is influenced by the individual's capacity to interpret an event and to coordinate this evaluation with appropriate behaviors. This section reviews the organization of abilities that underlie the affective component of individuals with Down syndrome. Studies that have adopted a multidomain and developmental approach in understanding the behavioral responsivity of individuals with Down syndrome are also discussed.

Cicchetti and Sroufe (1976, 1978) have examined the expression of positive and negative affect in infants with Down syndrome from a developmental perspective. In their first study, they examined the affective reactions of babies with Down syndrome to intrusive (auditory and tactile) and to nonintrusive (visual and social) stimulation. Across the first 2 years of life, these infants demonstrated the same developmental stages as the normal infants, but progressed through each stage at a delayed rate. Similar to normal infants, the infants with Down syndrome responded to intrusive stimuli first with positive affect, followed by smiling and laughter to the more subtle and complex social–visual stimulation. Interestingly, differences in the onset of these responses were related to the infant's degree of muscular hypotonia and to the infant's developmental status, as assessed by the Bayley MDI (Bayley, 1969). Infants with the most flaccid tone were also the most delayed in the expression of smiling and laughter across all forms of stimulation (see also Gallagher, Jens, and O'Donnell, 1983). Additionally, infants with the lowest MDIs (i.e., less than 50 points) were also the most delayed in their expression of positive affect. Accordingly, it seems that motoric ability and developmental level, not chronological age, are related to the capacity to express positive and negative emotion. These findings are consistent with reports of delayed or arrested neurological maturation in individuals with Down syndrome, which may affect both motor control and cognitive development (cf. Cowie, 1970).

In a subsequent series of studies, Cicchetti and Sroufe (1978) examined the expression of fear to the visual cliff (Gibson & Walk, 1960) and to a looming stimulus on an apparent collision course (Bower, Broughton, & Moore, 1970). In one study, infants with Down syndrome were placed at the deep end of a visual cliff. Placement at the deep end occurred within 1 month after these infants started to crawl. Once placed on this side of the cliff, only approximately half of the infants with Down syndrome (47%) demonstrated negative affect. Of this group, only 20 (29%) of the infants with Down syndrome had heart-rate decelerations and crawled to the shallow end of the cliff, toward their mothers. Ten of these infants also cried.

An additional 8 infants (11%) held on to the sides of the visual cliff, with 4 infants crying. The remaining 5 infants (7%) demonstrated negative reactions to the cliff and simply seemed to freeze with uncertainty when placed on the visual cliff.

In a second study, responses by infants with Down syndrome and normal infants to a looming stimulus were observed (Cicchetti & Sroufe, 1978). The normal infants were tested at 4, 8, and 12 months of age, while the infants with Down syndrome were tested at 4, 8, 12, and 16 months of age. At each age examined, quantitative differences distinguished the infants with Down syndrome and the normal infants. At each age examined more infants with Down syndrome responded to the looming stimulus with multiple blinks than was the case for the normal infants. This difference persisted after attempts were made to control for developmental level. Differences between the groups were also found in the amount of crying exhibited by the infants. At 8 and 12 months of age, significantly fewer infants with Down syndrome also cried when confronted with the looming stimulus than normal babies. Again, this difference persisted when the developmental levels of both groups of infants were similar.

In general, there was great consistency in an infant's expression of negative affect across the two tasks. This consistency, however, may be rooted in developmental level. In both studies, developmental status again seemed to be related to the expression of negative affect. Infants with Down syndrome who demonstrated negative affect in the visual cliff and looming studies as a group had higher Bayley MDI scores than infants who did not. These data concur with the previous study of positive affect (Cicchetti & Sroufe, 1976).

Thus, quantitative differences in the expression of affect between infants with Down syndrome and normal infants seem at least partially dependent upon cognitive status and motoric ability (see also Cicchetti & Beeghly, Chapter 2, this volume). Importantly, despite a delayed rate of development, infants with Down syndrome demonstrate the same organization of affect and cognitive abilities and undergo the same developmental stages as normal infants.

However, infants with Down syndrome also demonstrate some qualitative differences in their responsivity that cannot be accounted for by developmental level solely. Two such characteristics are multiple blinking and crying. Cicchetti and Sroufe (1978) describe blinking as a reflexive response to stimulation that comes under the control of forebrain inhibitory mechanisms early in development. Therefore, they argue, increased blinking in infants with Down syndrome may reflect poorly developed inhibitory systems of the CNS. In addition, Cicchetti and Sroufe propose that the stimulation threshold of the infant with Down syndrome may be high relative to other infants due to dysfunctions in the SNS. They argue that low-intensity responses to stimulation (such as smiling instead of laughter, or blinking instead of crying) may reflect dampened reactivity of response systems.

Accordingly, it is not the objective qualities of an object or event that prompts the expression of affect. Rather, one's ability to interpret an experience, reactivity to stimulation, and ability to regulate a response will shape the expression of affect. At a basic level, reactivity of response systems will set one's arousal level. However, further interpretation of a stimulus as pleasant or aversive may potentiate or diminish arousal. Likewise, self-regulatory abilities such as the inhibition of reflexes will affect the pairing of event appraisals with appropriate responses. If arousal is dampened from the beginning, one should expect low-intensity responses, such as smiling instead of laughing. This effect may be accentuated by failure to appreciate the qualities of the stimulus fully, leading either to inappropriate affect or to a more diminished affect than one would expect. This effect may also be accentuated by the interference of reflexes that cannot be controlled.

In a study of 19-month-olds, Thompson, Cicchetti, Lamb, and Malkin (1985) focused upon the expression of affect by infants with Down syndrome during the "strange situation" (Ainsworth & Wittig, 1969) and its relation to developmental level. Comparisons were made between infants with Down syndrome and normal infants of the same chronological age and of the same mental age. In both comparisons, the infants with Down syndrome were less intensely distressed by separation and needed a longer time to respond to separation than normal infants of the same chronological and mental age. In addition, the infants with Down syndrome expressed only a limited range of emotional intensity to separation and thus significantly less "emotional lability" than normal infants matched for developmental level and age. In keeping with the results of prior studies, responsivity characteristics and expressed affect by babies with Down syndrome are both delayed and qualitatively different from the normal population. These data indicate that fundamental differences between Down syndrome and normal populations again cannot be accounted for solely by cognitive delay. Although mental retardation may exert a large effect, underlying "constitutional" factors might exist that limit the manner in which the individual with Down syndrome can respond to the world. Again, this fundamental difference may lie in reactive capacity.

In the toddler years, affect also interacts with cognitive development. Motti, Cicchetti, and Sroufe (1983) compared affect expression to the level of symbolic play engaged in by 31 children (ages 3 to 5 years) with Down syndrome. Children in this study had Bayley MDIs that ranged from 50 to 116 points. As found in samples of normal children, developmental quotient and level of symbolic play were significantly correlated to the expression of positive affect and the manifestation of enthusiasm in interaction with toys (Beeghly & Cicchetti, Chapter 2, this volume). The investigators also examined the children's previous responses to visual cliff, looming objects, and playful interactions (Cicchetti & Sroufe, 1976, 1978). Again children who cried as infants in response to a looming object or laughed at subtle stimuli before 10 months of age, engaged in higher levels of symbolic play and at an earlier age than children with Down syndrome whose affect responses were more delayed. These findings further demonstrate consistency and coherence in development, as well as the close relationship between cognitive systems and expressed affect (Cicchetti & Beeghly, Chapter 2, this volume).

The series of studies reviewed in this section suggest that infants and children with Down syndrome differ from normal youngsters along several dimensions relevant to temperament. As the individuals with Down syndrome develop, their capacity to respond to the environment is affected by the interaction of cognitive ability and reactivity, again given restrictions specified by genetic makeup. Thus, changes in temperament, or responsivity, are due to myriad factors. The studies of Cicchetti and Sroufe (1976, 1978) suggest a main effect of mental retardation in the expression of affect. The exhibition of affect seems to be related to the extent to which a person can appropriately evaluate an event. However, the intensity of expression (e.g., blinking vs. crying) seems related to noncognitive factors. Given possible constitutional and maturational differences between Down syndrome and normal groups at different points in development, the inherent reactivity of Down syndrome may affect the sensitivity to stimulation and the intensity qualities of emotions as well. These relationships between appraisal processes, reactivity, and constitution are central to Rothbart and Derryberry's (1981) conceptualization of temperament. Further studies with different mentally retarded and Down syndrome groups are needed to specify the effect of mental retardation upon the early expression of affect and the uniqueness of Down syndrome in this area.

Temperament research: parental perceptions of the temperament characteristics of infants and children with Down syndrome

The preceding sections have considered the interaction of abilities thought to underlie temperament. Qualitative and quantitative differences were found between individuals with Down syndrome and normal individuals in emotionality and response capacity. However, we have not explored the overall temperament profiles of persons with Down syndrome. In this section we examine parental perceptions of temperament of children with Down syndrome.

Until the late 1970s, most studies of the personality of mentally retarded persons depicted individuals with Down syndrome as uniformly placid, stubborn, affectionate, and of generally "easy" temperament (for a review, see Gibson, 1978). In short, individuals with Down syndrome were perceived to be a temperamentally homogeneous group. Current research has attempted to address three basic questions. Are infants or children with Down syndrome perceived as temperamentally different from individuals without Down syndrome? Second, is there homogeneity or variability in the temperament profiles and characteristics within groups of Down syndrome individuals? Finally, the third question often asked is whether mental retardation has an impact upon behavioral tendencies.

Parental questionnaires typically are used to describe the behavioral characteristics of infants and children. These measures contain questions about the typical behavior of one's infant or child in different situations. One of the most widely used inventories is the Carey Infant Temperament Questionnaire (ITQ; Carey, 1973). The responses provided by parents are used to characterize the infant's perceived temperament along the dimensions specified in the New York Longitudinal Study (Thomas and Chess, 1977): activity level, rhythmicity, willingness to approach new situations, adaptability, threshold of stimulation, reaction intensity, quality of mood, distractibility, attention span, and persistence. These ratings also are used to classify infants as temperamentally "difficult," "easy," or "slow to warm up." Similarly, the Toddler Temperament Scale (TTS) (Fullard, McDevitt, & Carey, 1978, 1984) is also based upon the behavioral dimensions and profiles described in the New York Longitudinal Study, and yields "difficult," "slow to warm up," and "easy" temperament classifications for this age group. The Rothbart Infant Behavior Questionnaire (IBQ; Rothbart, 1981) is another parent report measure of perceived temperament. However, this report measure contains questions relevant to six temperament characteristics: activity level, positive affect (smiling and laughter), negative affect (fear), distress to limitations, soothability, and duration of orienting.

Recently, the extent to which parents accurately report the temperament of their children on such measures has become an issue of debate. Specifically, because these questionnaires rely upon *parental perceptions* of their children's characteristics, they might not yield objective measures of children's temperament. Not surprisingly, most current research has found that temperament questionnaires reflect characteristics of both the mother and the child, as well as the interaction of these characteristics (Bates & Bayles, 1984; Crockenberg & Acredelo, 1983; and Zeanah, Keener, & Anders, 1986).

Thus, to some extent temperament ratings may reflect the fit between maternal feelings and expectations and their children's actual behavior. For example, if a mother becomes easily upset by crying, she might perceive her own infant as inordinately difficult, irritable, or fussy if he or she cries at all. In contrast, if a mother expects that all infants within the first 3 months are unpredictable or irritable, she might rate her own infant as average along these dimensions even if he or she demonstrates these behaviors to an extreme. The impact of parental expectations upon temperament ratings is particularly important with handicapped populations. The birth of an infant with Down syndrome may be a stressful event for parents. In some cases, parents may have feelings of disappointment or mourning (Emde & Brown, 1978). Such feelings may subsequently color their perceptions of their infant. Additionally, Emde, Katz, and Thorpe (1978) note that parents of infants with Down syndrome may not completely accept that their child will not be "normal" until he or she fails to negotiate several developmental milestones. Consequently, early in development, parents may establish inappropriate expectations for the reactive capacity of their infant. Thus, in the following section the potential influence of parental qualities and expectations must always be kept in mind as we discuss parental ratings of temperament.

Using the ITQ, Bridges and Cicchetti (1982) explored the existence of a temperament stereotype in individuals with Down syndrome as well as qualitative differences between normal infants and infants with Down syndrome. To address these questions, Bridges and Cicchetti administered the ITQ in addition to a questionnaire that taps the mothers' overall impressions of their children's temperament (the General Impression Inventory, GII; Carey, 1973). Thirty-nine infants with Down syndrome (mean age = 10.6 months, range 6 to 18 months) were rated with the ITQ by their mothers. This age range was chosen because the mental level of the infants with Down syndrome was roughly equivalent to that of Carey's original standardization sample of normal infants (chronological age = 5.9 months, range 3.5 to 8.5 months) to which infants with Down syndrome were compared.

Overall, the infants with Down syndrome were rated by their mothers as low in approach to objects, low in threshold to stimulation, and highly persistent. On the basis of ratings of approach to objects, rhythmicity, adaptability, intensity, and mood, Bridges and Cicchetti classified infants as "difficult" (including high intermediate as well as difficult profiles) or "easy" (including easy and low intermediate characteristics). When classifications were made on the basis of the distribution of only the sample with Down syndrome, approximately 25% of the infants with Down syndrome were classified as difficult. However, when classifications were made on the basis of the means and standard deviations of Carey's standardization sample, almost 40% of the infants with Down syndrome were classified as difficult, whereas within the distribution of normal infants, only approximately 25% of the infants fell in this extreme category. Thus, in addition to qualitative differences in approach, threshold, and persistence between infants with Down syndrome and normal infants, the infants with Down syndrome were also rated more frequently as difficult. These data demonstrate variability in the temperament profiles of individuals with Down syndrome in addition to contradicting an "easy" stereotype for individuals with Down syndrome at this age.

The GII results, however, indicate that such ratings may not reflect the overall perceptions of the parents. Significantly, the GII responses and ITQ ratings were not strongly correlated. Thus, either qualities that are considered as difficult in normal populations are not viewed as difficult in Down syndrome populations, or perhaps the measures of parents' ratings of temperament and overall impressions are not tapping the same experiences. Bridges and Cicchetti opted for the latter explanation. They argued that responses given to the ITQ might reflect mother–infant interactions, rather than the mothers' overall impressions of their infants (see Berger, Chapter 4, this volume). For example, low approach to objects might really reflect low-intensity affect or passive responses rather than active engagement with the world. Likewise, ratings of low threshold might reflect the parent's natural adjustment to low responsivity by being intrusive or engaging in prolonged interactions or perhaps, infants' inability to maintain joint attention (e.g., Landry & Chapieski, 1989). These types of interactions would give the impression of low tolerance owing to the nature and strength of the stimulation within a specific situation – but not to the actual characteristics of the child.

Rothbart and Hanson (1983) used the Infant Behavior Questionnaire (IBQ; Rothbart, 1981) in addition to laboratory observations to assess temperament in infants with Down syndrome. In this case, laboratory observations included vocal activity, motor development, and tendency to startle to stimulation. Ratings of 15 infants with Down syndrome were compared to the ratings of the standardization sample at 6, 9, and 12 months of chronological age. At all three ages, the infants with Down syndrome demonstrated less positive affect, motor development, and vocal activity than the normal sample. At 6 and 9 months of age, the infants with Down syndrome were rated as less fearful but also as showing greater duration of orienting. Finally, at 6 and 12 months of age, the infants with Down syndrome were startled less than the normal infants. Therefore, infants with Down syndrome were consistently rated as low in affect expression when compared to normal infants of the same chronological age.

However, decreased affect does not imply a general decreased response. The Down syndrome group was rated as highly attentive and average in their activity level, soothability, and distress at these ages. Rothbart and Hanson's (1983) findings coincide with the implications of Bridges and Cicchetti (1982): For parents of infants with Down syndrome, differences in affect expressiveness and attention persistence between their infants and normally developing infants are very salient. Such differences appear early in development and are present through the first year of life. Moreover, these data again concur with previous studies that have found differences in the amount and quality of affect expressed by infants with Down syndrome and normal infants, in which infants with Down syndrome were delayed in their expression of affect as well as in affect intensity. In these studies, developmental level, motoric ability, and reactive capacity were proposed as qualities that mediate differences in the expression of emotions (Cicchetti & Sroufe, 1976, 1978).

Gunn, Berry, and Andrews (1981) have also completed several temperament studies with infants and toddlers with Down syndrome. Using the Carey ITQ and GII, Gunn and colleagues examined the maternal ratings of 15 infants at 14 months of age (average developmental level = 10 months) and 13 toddlers at 30 months of age (average developmental level = 17 months). Overall, mothers tended to rate their infants as average on the ITQ. In addition, consistent with other reports, the distribution of temperament profiles ranged from easy to difficult. However, more infants in the younger group received difficult ratings in specific dimensions than the infants in the older group.

Similar to Bridges and Cicchetti (1982), Gunn and collaborators also found that the mothers' GII ratings did not always coincide with their ITQ ratings. In this case, the general impressions of the mothers were slightly more positive and in the direction of easy temperament than the ITQ at both ages. Differences in ratings again suggest that the different questionnaires may not be assessing the same behaviors.

Lastly, although the effect of age upon the presence of difficult characteristics was small, Gunn and associates argue that this difference reflects a transition to easy temperament perceptions from infancy to the toddler years for individuals with Down syndrome. They attributed this transition to the development of more appropriate expectations on the part of the mothers for the behavioral capacities of their infants, rather than to objective changes in the characteristics of their infants.

In a longitudinal study, Gunn, Berry, and Andrews (1983) further explored the issue of stability in parental temperament ratings from infancy to toddlerhood. At the approximate age of 3 years and developmental level of 14 months, mothers of the preceding study were asked to rate their children's temperament characteristics with the Toddler Temperament Scale (TTS; Fullard, et al., 1978). Gunn and colleagues found very little stability in the temperament ratings from infancy to tod-dlerhood. Of the nine behavioral dimensions included in the TTS, only rhythmicity and mood were significantly correlated across the two time periods. Easy, difficult, and slow-to-warm-up classifications were also unstable. However, at the level of the individual child, when changes occurred, they were usually in the direction of difficult to easy characteristics, rather than easy to difficult. Although Bridges and Cicchetti (1982) similarly report shifts in temperament classifications for infants with Down syndrome during a 6-month interval, they failed to find significant trends in the direction of change. Thus, it is difficult to evaluate the significance of change in Gunn and Berry's study.

Gunn and collaborators (1981, 1983), however, claim that these data support a transition from difficult to easy temperament from infancy to early childhood in infants with Down syndrome. However, the presence of change in temperament characteristics may mean several things. For example, it may reflect normal matu-rational processes, parents' changing reactions and expectations toward a handi-capped child, or both qualities. Unfortunately, whether this change is because of parental expectations or true changes in the children's behaviors is at best ambigu-ous. To answer this question, additional measures of the parents' expectations and the child's developmental level at each point measured are needed. Additionally, it would be informative if the stability of temperament ratings of a normally devel-oping control group were also assessed. In this way, one would be able to examine whether such changes in temperament profiles are apparent in nonhandicapped pop-ulations as well. If this is the case, then Gunn and Berry's argument would be weakened.

Aside from these concerns, change in temperament characteristics also may be an artifact of the methods of the study, rather than a veridical finding. First, it is unclear whether Gunn and collaborators used chronological age or developmental level as a basis of comparison with the normal standardization sample: This is an important point since each child's ratings are considered relative to those of a nor-mative sample. Toddlers with Down syndrome may be less oppositional, and thus perceived as less difficult than normal toddlers of the same age. Second, changes in temperament ratings from one period to the next might reflect differences between the two measures used, rather than true changes in temperament. Clearly, more studies that assess developmental changes in temperament characteristics need to be conducted.

Currently, there are only a few studies which examine the perceived temperament characteristics of toddlers with Down syndrome. Within their continuing research program with individuals with Down syndrome, Gunn and Berry (1985) adminis-tered the TTS to parents of 37 toddlers with Down syndrome (chronological age = approximately 30 months; developmental level = approximately 18 months). Gunn and Berry compared the average Down syndrome TTS ratings to the stan-dardization means of toddlers of the same chronological age and toddlers of the same developmental level. Comparisons to peers of the same chronological age indicated that the group with Down syndrome was high in rhythmicity, low in response intensity, predominantly positive in mood, low in persistence and high in threshold. When compared to a group of toddlers with the same mental age, the toddlers with Down syndrome were rated as high in approach and adaptability, low in response intensity, positive in mood, and low in threshold. In contrast, however, they were perceived as having low thresholds to stimulation and to be highly approaching and adaptable relative to their peers. Thus, in both comparisons, the groups with Down syndrome differed in threshold, mood, and intensity. It is interesting, however, that comparisons based on developmental level and chronological age yield different results. These data suggest that qualitative difference between individuals with Down syndrome and normal infants may not simply be attributable to delayed cognitive development. Rather, reactivity level may be related to one's inherent capacity to respond to the environment.

Most studies, however, do not examine groups of Down syndrome individuals in isolation. Rather, children with Down syndrome often are placed within a broader group of "developmentally delayed" children, and are not treated separately. Heffernan, Black, and Poche (1982), for example, obtained TTS ratings of 17 children with Down syndrome and 46 children with a wide variety of neurological impairments. The average mental age of all 63 children was 21 months. Because Heffernan et al. failed to find statistically significant differences between the ratings of children with Down syndrome and the children with neurological impairments, she combined both groups to form one "delayed" group. When compared to the normal standardization sample, the delayed group was generally perceived as less active, low in attention and persistence, withdrawing from stimulation, and having a high sensory threshold. Generally, however, the distribution of easy to difficult profiles did not vary significantly from the standardization sample. Thus, the delayed group may be described as less interactive than nondelayed children, but they represent a range to temperaments. Because the number of neurologically impaired children in this study is greater than the number of children with Down syndrome examined, it is difficult to determine how much qualitative differences between the overall group and the standardization group are applicable to the children with Down syndrome. Separate comparisons between the groups with Down syndrome and the standardization sample were not reported. Consequently, some genuine differences may have been obscured inadvertently.

Marcovitch, Goldberg, MacGregor, and Lojkasek (1986) also used the TTS (revised TTS; Fullard et al., 1984) to rate the temperament of 96 developmentally delayed children. The age range of this sample was from 2 to 4 1/2 years, with a developmental delay of at least 6 months. This population consisted of 32 children with Down syndrome, 29 children with neurological disorders, and 35 children with delay of unknown etiology. The TTS was completed by 96 mothers and fathers and the scale means for 2- to 3-year-olds were used. Again, significant differences were found between the different delayed groups. These trends indicated that the toddlers with Down syndrome were slightly more active than other delayed groups, less distractible and approaching than the neurological impairment group, but more approaching and distractible than the unknown etiology group. The comparison of the

Down syndrome to the standardization sample also indicated that the children with Down syndrome were more approaching, less persistent, and had higher thresholds than the average and nondelayed child. These differences are very similar to the differences that emerge between the combined delayed groups and the standardization means. When the delayed group was compared to the standardization sample, the overall delayed sample was rated as more approaching, less intense, less persistent, and higher in threshold than the nondelayed sample.

These data indicate that toddlers with Down syndrome are similar to other groups of delayed children, with some qualitative differences in approach, activity, and distractibility. However, the Down syndrome and overall delayed groups seem to share characteristics of increased approach to the world, decreased persistence, and high threshold to stimulation. All these differences lie in the direction of the easy temperament profile.

This brief review of current temperament research with infants and toddlers with Down syndrome reiterates many of the themes first discussed by Gibson (1978). Consistent with Gibson's review, most temperament studies with individuals with Down syndrome indicate that a variety of temperament profiles exists within this group. Thus, the stereotype of "easy temperament" and temperament homogeneity across individuals with Down syndrome is not supported. Although individuals with Down syndrome share a common genetic syndrome, homogeneity in behavioral characteristics should not be assumed. Thus this population is expected to demonstrate a wide range of characteristics and profiles.

A second theme Gibson touched upon was change in temperament as a function of maturation of certain capacities, such as neurological inhibition of behaviors and cognitive development. Gibson argued that changes in temperament for individuals with Down syndrome were usually in the direction of difficult characteristics to easy characteristics. Given Rothbart and Derryberry's (1981) framework, changes in the expression of temperament are expected to occur owing to brain maturation and to the development, refinement, and organization of cognitive and self-regulatory capacities. Both qualities are expected to exhibit increasing control over reactivity. Through development, however, the direction of change may also be influenced by factors such as the expectations of the environment.

A transition from easy to difficult temperament during the early toddler years is tentatively supported by the work of Gunn and colleagues (1983, 1985) in their cross-sectional and longitudinal studies. Both investigations describe changes in the direction of "easiness." Additionally, when one compares the findings of other studies reviewed in this paper, the trend is again tentatively supported. For example, infants with Down syndrome, as well as other forms of handicaps, were generally perceived as demonstrating less affect, less approach, decreased threshold, and increase in attention when compared to the normal standardization group of the same chronological age. Often these characteristics are described as difficult. In contrast, although the attention level and persistence of toddlers with Down syndrome are perceived as low, these toddlers are also rated as high in approach and threshold, as well as low in intensity of response, positive in mood, and high in rhythmicity, relative to normal toddlers of the same chronological age. Many of these characteristics are typically described as temperamentally easy.

However, the underlying reasons for change are ambiguous. It is questionable whether changes in parents' reports of their children's temperament are because of changing expectations on the parents' part, or because of the maturation and development of cognitive or self-regulatory skills. Further research is needed to specify the mechanism of change.

Despite difficulties associated with parent report measures, temperament questionnaires have also provided evidence for some qualitative differences in the response characteristics of individuals with and without Down syndrome. These studies indicate that infants and children with Down syndrome generally differ from the nonhandicapped population in the amount and quality of affect expressed, in the duration of attention and persistence, and in general approach to objects. Given the Rothbart and Derryberry (1981) view of temperament, these behavioral differences should be rooted in more fundamental differences that are unique to Down syndrome (constitution and reactivity of response systems), and perhaps spurred by delayed maturation and cognitive development.

One example of the interaction of the features unique to Down syndrome and mental retardation is the difference in the expression of affect and emotionality found between children with Down syndrome and normal children. Throughout the first year of life, Rothbart and Hanson (1983) have indicated that maternal ratings of infants with Down syndrome differ from those of normal infants of the same age in the amount of positive and negative affect expressed. In the toddler years, however, children with Down syndrome are rated as more positive than the standardization sample of normal toddler of the same age.

Decreased affect in infancy may be partially accounted for by developmental level. Both Cicchetti and Sroufe (1976, 1978) and Sorce et al. (1982) have found that when developmental level is not accounted for, infants with Down syndrome are perceived as showing less affect and response intensity than normal infants of the same age. When ratings of infants with Down syndrome are compared to normal infants of the same developmental level, no differences are noted between the two groups (Gunn et al., 1981). However, the same research group reports that in the toddler years, children with Down syndrome are still perceived as more positive in affect than normal youngsters of the same developmental level. Thus, these data are consistent again with the work of Cicchetti and Sroufe (1976, 1978) who found that affect expression interacts with developmental level during infancy.

However, a surprising finding is that in the toddler years developmental level does not account for differences between toddlers with Down syndrome and those in the normal standardization sample. This effect might be because of the impact of the Down syndrome genotype upon response threshold and intensity. The ratings Gunn and Berry (1985) obtained also describe the toddlers with Down syndrome as more approaching to objects and situations and low in their response intensity when developmental level is controlled for. Thus, similar to when these toddlers are compared to toddlers of the same age, an increase in approach to situations and dampened affect might prompt parents to rate their children as positive in mood because they are not volatile or as fearful as normal toddlers. Observations of children with Down syndrome in the "strange situation" in fact describe these toddlers as less emotionally labile and upset when separated from their mothers than groups of normal infants the same mental age (Cicchetti & Serafica, 1981; Serafica & Cicchetti, 1976; Thompson et al., 1985).

Although developmental level did not seem to account for qualitative differences between individuals with and without Down syndrome in affect, studies that have included other groups of mentally retarded subjects implied that mental retardation may affect temperament. Two studies with mentally retarded and Down syndrome groups failed to find qualitative differences between them in terms of characteristic affect or mood, whereas differences were found between the delayed groups and normally developing individuals (Heffernan et al., 1982; Marcovitch et al., 1986). These data suggest, therefore, that an aspect of mental retardation that is not being tapped by conventional infancy tests may influence the expression of emotion in individuals.

These qualities may have their foundation in the sensitivity of response systems of individuals with Down syndrome relative to individuals without this syndrome. Research on the biological aspects of Down syndrome has implied that, in general, the response systems of individuals with Down syndrome may be less reactive to stimulation than those of individuals in the normal population. Decreases in noradrenergic, serotonergic, and cholinergic activity imply decreased activity of CNS and PNS arousal and reactive systems. Thus, caretakers might describe their children as less intense in their reactions to the world, but decreased intensity may also be perceived as general complacency, and thus, general positiveness. However, to determine whether such constitutionally based differences are unique to Down syndrome, further research is needed with groups of other mentally retarded individuals.

As noted earlier in the chapter, approach to the world also seems to differentiate individuals with Down syndrome from normal individuals in infancy and early childhood. When chronological age comparisons are made, infants with Down syndrome approach their worlds as often as their same-age peers. However, when developmental level is used as the basis of comparison, infants with Down syndrome are rated as less approaching. In the toddler years, children with Down syndrome are described as more approaching in both chronological and developmental age comparisons. The discrepant findings in infancy may reflect the diversity of this characteristic in the Down syndrome population or may perhaps reflect the cognitive and attentional difficulties of children with Down syndrome. However, one might expect that infants with Down syndrome would be rated as less approaching to the world than their normal peers, given the research findings of the play style of infants with Down syndrome. Vietze and colleagues (1983) and MacTurk and colleagues (1985) report that infants with Down syndrome in the first year of life tend to look at objects more, but manipulate objects less than normal infants. Additionally, Landry and Chapieski (1989) have noted that owing to problems in regulating attention, infants with Down syndrome may have difficulty attending to both caregivers and toys simultaneously. In this case, the attentional capacity of these children might become easily overloaded, leading them to withdraw from play to attend to caregivers solely. To some parents all these qualities may seem to be a decrease in approach.

In toddlerhood, the predominant finding of increased approach to objects across several studies indicates that this characteristic is particularly salient to most parents. Marcovitch and colleagues (1986) and Heffernan and colleagues (1982) have both found that this quality characterizes other mentally retarded groups of children as well. In their studies, groups of delayed infants, including children with neurological disorder, Down syndrome, and delays of unknown origin, also were rated as qualitatively different from nonretarded children in their approach to objects. However, the developmentally delayed groups differed with the neurologically impaired children being most approaching, followed by children with Down syndrome and children with delays of unknown origin. When mental age comparisons are drawn between Down syndrome and normal individuals, toddlers with Down syndrome are still rated as more approaching to objects. Thus, delayed development does not account for qualitative differences between normal individuals and individuals with Down syndrome. Down syndrome may in this way contribute some qualities that accentuate approach to objects. One possibility is increased threshold levels (Gunn & Berry, 1985). If constitutional differences in neurotransmitter systems (i.e., the noradrenergic, serotonergic and cholinergic systems) that mediate arousability and reactivity (e.g., ANS, RAS) exist, individuals with Down syndrome may be more insensitive to novelty and discrepant events or perhaps less liable to be overstimulated or distracted, and may approach the world demonstrating less inhibition and withdrawal than would be expected in the normal population.

A third qualitative difference between infants and toddlers with and without Down syndrome is ratings of attention level and persistence. When chronological age comparisons are made, toddlers with Down syndrome are rated as more persistent and attentive than normal toddlers (Gunn & Berry, 1985; Marcovitch et al., 1986). Likewise, Rothbart and Hanson (1983) have found that mothers rated their infants with Down syndrome as more attentive (i.e., they showed a larger duration of orienting) than normal babies at 6 and at 12 months of age. These findings are consistent with the findings of Cohen (1981). In the Cohen study, infants with Down syndrome tended to fixate on a visual target for longer time periods than did normal infants. In addition, the work of Vietze and his colleagues (1983) also proposes that infants with Down syndrome visually attend to objects in place of active manipulation. Both qualities reflect an increased attention level, at least in infancy. Cohen argues that infants with Down syndrome may need more time to encode or retrieve information in the visual modality (see also Miranda & Fantz, 1973, 1974; and Wagner et al., Chapter 5, this volume). This would account for their increased looking behavior and longer time-trials for habituation. These findings are consistent with anatomical studies of the visual cortex that have found decreased maturation in individuals with Down syndrome relative to normal persons. In addition, consistent with the possibility of poorly inhibited reflex and self-regulation, elevated attention levels in this population may also reflect an impaired ability to shift and refocus attention to new events (Courchesne, 1988; Wagner et al., Chapter 5, this volume). Further research is required to determine whether children with other forms of mental retardation also demonstrate similar neurological abnormalities.

In this regard, studies conducted with other delayed groups have found that they also differ from normal toddlers on this dimension, implying perhaps differences attributable to mental retardation (Heffernan et al., 1982; Marcovitch et al., 1986). When ratings of persons with Down syndrome are compared to those of normal individuals of the same developmental level, differences in attention level are not apparent (Gunn & Berry, 1985). This pattern further supports that differences in attention may be due to developmental delay rather than to qualitative differences in responsivity unique to the Down syndrome population. Again, increments in visual attention may reflect a need for more time to process information relative to nonretarded individuals.

The last qualitative difference in responsivity between infants and toddlers with Down syndrome and normal youngsters lies in threshold. Chronological age comparisons show that mothers rate toddlers with Down syndrome as higher in threshold of responsivity than nonretarded toddlers. This difference in threshold is also observed between developmentally delayed toddlers and nonretarded toddlers. In contrast, when mental age comparisons are drawn, infants and toddlers with Down syndrome are rated as lower in threshold than normal toddlers (Bridges & Cicchetti, 1982; Gunn & Berry, 1985). These findings are contrary to the experimental observations of high thresholds in the Down syndrome population and inconsistent with the implications of biological findings. Bridges and Cicchetti argue that these ratings are dependent upon mothers' perceptions of interactions rather than upon the infant's true characteristics. Alternatively, low thresholds might reflect the poor development of inhibitory systems that control states of arousal. These characteristics may contribute to perceptions of low threshold to stimulation.

Conclusion and future directions

The Rothbart and Derryberry (1981) conceptualization describes temperament as reflective of the development and organization of reactive capacities, emotionality, cognitive and self-regulatory abilities. Therefore, one's current temperament is determined by the status of capacities in various domains. Examination of the temperament characteristics of individuals with Down syndrome provides the opportunity to test this model by enabling researchers to start to tease apart the influence of neurological integrity and reactivity and cognitive skills upon one's expressed temperament characteristics.

Biological studies have indicated that individuals with Down syndrome may be inherently less reactive to stimulation than individuals without Down syndrome. Studies with neurotransmitters have pointed toward decreased reactivity of the CNS and ANS to stimulation (particularly to novelty). These biological differences may predispose infants with Down syndrome to be more passive or less reactive than other children of their chronological age. In addition, neuroanatomical studies have provided evidence for delayed or arrested neurological maturation.

In spite of the qualitative differences between Down syndrome persons and other individuals, the organization of abilities that underlie temperament in Down syndrome is similar to that found in individuals without Down syndrome. The questions of "uniqueness" and "normalcy" in temperament have started to be examined within Down syndrome; however, most studies have focused upon the normalcy question and examined the impact of a single domain upon temperament – namely, cognition.

In addition, little research has been conducted that directly addresses whether the processes that underlie temperament in the normal population are organized in the same manner in Down syndrome or other mentally retarded groups. Further research assessing different developmental domains and their interaction and perceptions of temperament may provide insight into this question. Studies measuring self-regulation and attention, or affect, reactivity, and cognitive ability, in addition to ratings of temperament, would be two examples of such an approach.

Assumed in the multidomain approach to the study of temperament is the importance of the development of different abilities. Thus, another direction of research would include longitudinal studies of temperament in the Down syndrome group. In this manner, one may start to ask not only how different abilities interact, but also how they influence each other through development, and how this interaction promotes change or stability in how the child engages the world.

Future temperament research utilizing questionnaires must also determine the impact of parental biases upon ratings of their children. To what extent does a parent's ability to cope with a handicapped child affect his or her ability to perceive the child objectively or to establish realistic expectations for the child? These questions may be answered by concomitant measurements of parents' expectations for and acceptance of a handicapped child, the amount of stress they feel they are under, and, finally, the amount of emotional support they receive.

A second related difficulty with parent report measures concerns the ambiguity about what these ratings actually mean. It is difficult to control how parents interpret questions and draw upon their experiences in generating their answers. Therefore, as in research with groups of other mentally retarded and normal persons, objective measures also must be collected in order to establish the concurrent validity of the parental report.

Finally, the formation of multidisciplinary research teams to investigate common areas of functioning must be encouraged. For example, the neurobiology of behavior is evolving to the point at which meaningful relationships between brain and behavior have been established. The behavioral psychologist is in the position of being able to orient the neurobiological efforts to the study of fundamental psychological processes. One case in which this would be important is in the investigation of neurotransmitters and behavior. Those few studies that have demonstrated a relationship between mental retardation, emotionality, and level of neurotransmitter have not yet done so in a dose-dependent manner. For example, if it could be shown that level of neurotransmitter (e.g., noradrenaline) was related to *degree* of mental retardation, there would be an unequivocal relationship demonstrated between noradrenaline and intelligence. Likewise, collateral efforts of the neurochemists, temperament researchers, and cognitive psychologists are now possible.

References

Ainsworth, M., & Wittig, B. (1969). Attachment behaviors of one-year-olds in a strange situation. In B. Foss (Ed.), *Determinants of infant behavior* (Vol. 4, pp. 11–136). New York: Wiley.

Axelrod, J., & Reisine, T. (1984). Stress Hormones: Their interaction and regulation. *Science, 224*, 452–458.

Bates, J. E. (1987). Temperament in infancy. In J. D. Osofsky (Ed.), *Handbook of infant development* (2nd Ed., pp. 1101–1149). New York: Wiley.

Bates, J., & Bayles, K. (1984). Objective and subjective components in mothers' perceptions of their children from age 6 months to 3 years. *Merrill-Palmer Quarterly, 30*, 111–129.

Bayley, N. (1969). *Bayley Scales of Infant Development: Birth to 2 Years.* New York: Psychological Corporation.

Becker, L., Armstrong, D., & Chan, F. (1986). Dendritic atrophy in children with Down's syndrome. *Annals of Neurology, 20* (4), 520–526.

Bell, R. (1968). A reinterpretation of the direction of effects in studies of socialization. *Psychological Review, 75*, 81–95.

Bower, T., Broughton, J., & Moore, T. (1970). Demonstration of intent in the reaching behavior of human neonates. *Perception and Psychophysics, 8*, 51–53.

Bridges, F., & Cicchetti, D. (1982). Mothers' ratings of temperament characteristics of Down Syndrome infants. *Developmental Psychology, 18*, (2), 238–244.

Buss, A., & Plomin, R. (1975). *A temperament theory of personality development.* New York: Wiley.

Butterworth, G., & Cicchetti, D. (1978). Visual calibration of posture in normal and motor retarded Down syndrome infants. *Perception, 7*, 513–525.

Carey, W. (1973). Measurement of infant temperament in pediatric practice. In J. C. Westman (Ed.) *Individual differences in children,* (pp. 298–304). New York: Wiley.

Casanova, M., Walker, L., Whitehouse, P., & Price, D. (1985). Abnormalities of the nucleus basalis in Down's syndrome. *Annals of Neurology, 18*, 310–313.

Cicchetti, D., Ganiban, J., & Barnett, D. (in press). Contributions from the study of high risk populations to understanding the development of emotion regulation. In K. Dodge & J. Garber (Eds.), *The development of emotion regulation.* New York: Cambridge University Press.

Cicchetti, D., & Pogge-Hesse, P. (1982). Possible contributions of the study of organically retarded persons to developmental theory. In E. Zigler & D. Balla (Eds.), Mental retardation: The developmental–difference controversy (pp. 277–318). Hillsdale, NY: Erlbaum.

Cicchetti, D., & Serafica, F. (1981). The interplay among behavioral systems: Illustrations of the study of attachment, affiliation, and wariness in young children with Down's syndrome. *Developmental Psychology, 17*, 36–49.

Cicchetti, D., & Sroufe, L. A. (1976). The relationship between infants. *Child Development, 47*, 920–929.

Cicchetti, D., & Sroufe, L. A. (1978). An organizational view of affect: Illustrations from the study of Down's syndrome infants. In M. Lewis and L. Rosenblum (Eds.), *The development of affect* (pp. 309–350). New York: Plenum.

Cicchetti, D., & White, J. (1988). Emotional development and the affective disorders. In W. Damon (Ed.), *Child development today and tomorrow* (pp. 177–199). San Francisco: Jossey-Bass.

Cohen, L. B. (1981). Examination of habituation as a measure of aberrant infant development. In S. L. Friedman & M. Sigman (Eds.), *Preterm birth and psychological development* (pp. 241–253). New York: Academic Press.

Courchesne, E. (1988). Physioanatomical considerations in Down syndrome. In L. Nadel (Ed.), *The psychobiology of Down syndrome* (pp. 291–314). Cambridge, MA: MIT Press.

Cowie, V. (1970). *A study of the early development of mongols.* Oxford: Pergamon Press.

Coyle, J., Oster-Smith, M., & Gearhart, J. (1986). The neurobiology of Down syndrome. *Brain Research Bulletin, 16,* 773–787.

Crockenberg, S., & Acredolo, C. (1983). Infant temperament ratings: A function of infants, of mothers, or both? *Infant Behavior and Development, 6,* 61–72.

Cutrona, C. E., & Troutman, B. R. (1986). Social support, infant temperament, and parenting self-efficacy: A mediational model of postpartum depression. *Child Development, 57,* 1507–1518.

Derryberry, D., & Rothbart, M. K. (1984). Emotion, attention and temperament. In C. E. Izard, J. Kagan & R. Zajonc (Eds.), *Emotion, cognition, and behavior* (pp. 132–166). New York: Cambridge University Press.

Dobzhansky, T. (1955). *Evolution, genetics and man.* New York: Wiley.

Emde, R., & Brown, C. (1978). Adaptation to the birth of Down syndrome infants. *Journal of American Academy of Child Psychiatry, 17,* 299–323.

Emde, R., Katz, E., & Thorpe, J. (1978). Emotion expression in infancy: II. Early deviations in Down's Syndrome. In M. Lewis & L. Rosenblum (Eds.) *The development of affect* (pp. 351–360). New York: Plenum.

Fox, N., & Davidson, R. (1984). Hemispheric substrate of affect: A developmental model. In N. A. Fox & R. J. Davidson (Eds.), *The psychobiology of affective development* (pp. 353–382). Hillsdale, NJ: Erlbaum.

Fullard, W., McDevitt, S., & Carey, W. (1978). *Toddler Temperament Scale.* Philadelphia: Temple University Press.

Fullard, W., McDevitt, S., & Carey, W. (1984). Assessing temperament in one- to two-year-old children. *Journal of Pediatric Psychology, 9,* 205–217.

Gallagher, R., Jens, K., & O'Donnell, K. (1983). The effect of physical status on the affective expressions of handicapped infants. *Infant Behavior and Development, 6,* 73–77.

Garcia Coll, C., Kagan, J., & Reznick, S. (1984). Behavioral inhibition in young children. *Child Development, 53,* 1005–1019.

Gibson, D. (1978). *Down's syndrome: The psychology of mongolism.* Cambridge: Cambridge University Press.

Gibson, E., & Walk, R. (1960). The "visual cliff." *Scientific American, 202,* 2–9.

Gilman, S., & Newman, S. (1987). *Manter and Gatz's essentials of clinical neuroanatomy and neurophysiology* (7th ed). Philadelphia: F. A. Davis.

Goldsmith, H., et al. (1987). Roundtable: What is temperament? Four approaches. *Child Development, 58,* 505–529.

Goldsmith, H. H., & Campos, J. J. (1982). Toward a theory of infant temperament. In R. N. Emde & R. J. Harmon (Eds.), *The development of attachment and affiliative systems* (pp. 161–194). New York: Plenum.

Goldsmith, H. H., & Campos, J. J. (1986). Fundamental issues in the study of early temperament: The Denver Twin Temperament Study. In M. Lamb, A. Brown, & B. Rogoff (Eds.), *Advances in developmental psychology* (Vol. 4, pp. 231–283).

Greenough, W., Black, J., & Wallace, C. (1987). Experience and brain development. *Child Development, 58,* 539–559.

Gunn, P., & Berry, P. (1985). The temperament of Down Syndrome toddlers and their siblings. *Journal of Child Psychology and Psychiatry, 26,* 973–979.

Gunn, P., Berry, P., & Andrews, R. (1981). The temperament of Down syndrome infants: A research note. *Journal of Child Psychology and Psychiatry, 22,* 189–194.

Gunn, P., Berry, P., & Andrews, R. (1983). The temperament of Down syndrome toddlers: A research note. *Journal of Child Psychology and Psychiatry, 24,* 601–605.

Gunnar, M. (1986). Human developmental psychoneuroendocrinology: A review of research on neuroendocrine responses to challenge and threat in infancy and childhood. In M. Lamb, A. L. Brown, & B. Rogoff (Eds.), *Advances in developmental psychology* (Vol. 4, pp. 51–103). Hillsdale, NJ: Erlbaum.

Heffernan, L., Black, F., & Poche, P. (1982). Temperament patterns in young neurologically impaired children. *Journal of Pediatric Psychology, 7,* 415–423.

Hesse, P., & Cicchetti, D. (1982). Toward an integrative theory of emotional development. *New Directions for Child Development, 16,* 3–48.

Kagan, J. (1970). The determinants of attention in the infant. *American Scientist, 58,* 298–305.

Kagan, J., Reznick, S., & Snidman, N. (1987). The physiology of behavioral inhibition in children. *Child Development, 58,* 1459–1473.

Kandel, E., & Schwartz, J. (1985). *Principles of neuroscience* (2nd ed.). New York: Elsevier.

Keele, D., Richards, C., Brown, J., & Marshall, J. (1969). Catecholamine metabolism in Down's syndrome. *American Journal of Mental Deficiency, 74,* 125–129.

Kemper, T. L. (1988). Neuropathology of Down syndrome. In L. Nadel (Ed.), *The psychobiology of Down syndrome* (pp. 270–189). Cambridge, MA: MIT Press.

Kopp, C. (1982). The antecedents of self regulation. *Developmental Psychology, 18,* 199–214.

Landry, S. H., & Chapieski, M. L. (1989). Joint attention and infant toy exploration: Effects of Down syndrome and prematurity. *Child Development, 60,* 103–118.

MacTurk, R., Vietze, P., McCarthy, M., McQuiston, S., & Yarrow, L. (1985). The organization of exploratory behavior in Down Syndrome and non-delayed infants. *Child Development, 56,* 573–587.

Marcovitch, S., Goldberg, S., MacGregor, D., & Lojkasek, M. (1986). Patterns of temperament variation in three groups of developmentally delayed preschool children: Mother and father ratings. *Developmental and Behavioral Pediatrics, 7,* 247–252.

McGehee, L., & Eckerman, C. (1983). The preterm infant as a social partner: Responsive, but unreadable. *Infant Behavior and Development, 6,* 461–470.

Miranda, S. B., & Fantz, R. L. (1973). Visual preferences of Down syndrome and normal infants. *Child Development, 45,* 651–660.

Miranda, S. B., & Fantz, R. L. (1974). Recognition memory in Down's syndrome and normal infants. *Child Development, 54,* 1168–1175.

Motti, F., Cicchetti, D., & Sroufe, L. A. (1983). From infant affect expression to symbolic play: The coherence of development in Down syndrome children. *Child Development, 54,* 1168–1175.

O'Connor, N., & Hermelin, B. (1978). *Seeing and hearing and space and time.* New York: Academic Press.

Plomin, R. (1987). Developmental behavioral genetics and infancy. In J. D. Osofsky (Ed.), *Handbook of infant development,* (2nd ed., pp. 363–414). New York: Wiley.

Purpura, D. (1975). Dendritic differentiation in human cerebral cortex: Normal and aberrant developmental patterns. In G. Kretzberg (Ed.), *Advances in neurology* (Vol. 12, pp. 91–116). New York: Raven Press.

Rose, S. (1984). Disordered molecules and diseased minds. *Journal of Psychiatric Research, 18,* 351–360.

Rothbart, M. (1981). Measurement of temperament in infancy. *Child Development, 52,* 569–578.

Rothbart, M., & Derryberry, D. (1981). The development of individual differences in temperament. In M. Lamb & A. L. Brown (Eds.), *Advances in developmental psychology* (Vol. 1, pp. 37–86). Hillsdale, NJ: Erlbaum.

Rothbart, M., & Hanson, M. (1983). A caregiver report comparison of temperament characteristics of Down Syndrome and normal infants. *Developmental Psychology, 19,* 766–769.

Rothbart, M. K., & Posner, M. (1985). Temperament and the development of self-regulation. In L. C. Hartlage & C. F. Teltzrow (Eds.), *The neuropsychology of individual differences: A developmental perspective* (pp. 93–123). New York: Plenum.

Sameroff, A., & Chandler, M. (1975). Reproductive risk and the continuum of caretaking casualty. In F. Horowitz (Ed.), *Review of child development research* (Vol. 4, pp. 187–243). Chicago: University of Chicago Press.

Scott, B., Becker, L., & Petit, T. (1983). Neurobiology of Down's syndrome. *Progress in Neurobiology, 21,* 199–237.

Serafica, F., & Cicchetti, D. (1976). Down's syndrome children in a strange situation: Attachment and exploratory behaviors. *Merrill-Palmer Quarterly, 21,* 137–150.

Sorce, J., & Emde, R. (1982). The meaning of infant emotion and expression: Regularities in caregiving responses of normal and Down's syndrome infants. *Journal of Child Psychology and Psychiatry, 23,* 145–158.

Sorce, J., Emde, R., & Frank, M. (1982). Maternal referencing in normal and Down's syndrome infants: A longitudinal analysis. In R. Emde & R. Harmon (Eds.), *The development of attachment and affiliative systems* (pp. 283–294). New York: Plenum.

Sroufe, L. A. (1985). Attachment classification from the perspective of infant–caregiver relationships and infant temperament. *Child Development, 56,* 1–14.

Takashima, S., Becker, L., Armstrong, D., & Chan, F. (1981). Abnormal neuronal development in the visual cortex of the human fetus and infant with Down's syndrome: A quantitative and qualitative Golgi Study. *Brain Research, 225,* 1–21.

Thase, M. (1988). The relationship between Down syndrome and Alzheimer's disease. In L. Nadel (Ed.), *The Psychobiology of Down Syndrome,* (pp. 345–368). Cambridge, MA: MIT Press.

Thase, M., Liss, L., Smeltzer, D., & Maloon, J. (1982). Clinical evaluation of dementia in Down syndrome: A preliminary report. *Journal of Mental Deficiency Research, 26,* 249–254.

Thomas, A., & Chess, S. (1977). *Temperament and development.* New York: Brunner/Mazel.

Thomas, A., & Chess, S. (1980). *The dynamics of psychological development.* New York: Brunner/Mazel.

Thomas, A., Chess, S., & Birch, H. (1968). *Temperament and behavior disorders in children.* New York: New York University Press.

Thompson, R., Cicchetti, D., Lamb, M., & Malkin, K. (1985). The Emotional responses of Down syndrome and normal infants in the Strange Situation: The organization of affective behavior in infants. *Developmental Psychology, 21,* 828–841.

Tucker, D. M., & Williamson, P. A. (1984). Asymmetric neural control systems in human self-regulation. *Psychological Review, 91* (2), 185–215.

Vietze, P., McCarthy, M., McQuiston, S., MacTurk, R., & Yarrow, L. (1983). Attention and exploratory behavior in infants with Down Syndrome. In T. Field & A. Sostek (Eds.), *Infants born at risk: Perceptual and physical processes* (pp. 251–268). New York: Grune & Stratton.

Wachs, T. D., & Gandour, M. J. (1983). Temperament, environment, and six-month cognitive-intellectual development: A test of organismic specificity hypothesis. *International Journal of Behavioral Development, 6,* 135–152.

Weinshilbaum, R., Thoa, N., Johnson, D., Kopin, I., & Axelrod, J. (1971). Proportional release of norepinephrine and dopamine-beta-hydroxylase from sympathetic nerves. *Science, 174,* 1349–1351.

Werner, H. (1957). The concept of development from a comparative and organismic point of view. In D. Harris (Ed.), *The concept of development.* Minneapolis: University of Minnesota Press.

Wilson, R., & Matheny, A. (1986). Behavior–genetics research in infant temperament: The Louisville Twin Study. In R. Plomin & J. Dunn (Eds.), *The study of temperament: Continuities and challenges.* Hillside, NJ: Erlbaum.

Yates, C., Simpson, J., Maloney, A., Gorden, A., & Reid, A. (1980). Alzheimer-like cholinergic deficiency in Down's syndrome. *Lancet, ii,* 979.

Zeanah, C., Keener, W., & Anders, T. (1986). Developing perceptions of temperament and their relation to mother and infant behavior. *Journal of Child Psychology and Psychiatry, 27,* 499–512.

4 Interactions between parents and their infants with Down syndrome

Jiri Berger

Introduction

This chapter attempts to provide a fairly comprehensive review of research into interactions between infants with Down syndrome and their parents. As suggested by the word "infants," the focus will be primarily on studies involving children up to about 2 years of age. Nevertheless, because of the generally much slower developmental progress of these children, studies of older children with Down syndrome will also be considered occasionally, especially when their developmental ages were not higher than those of average 2-year-old infants.

Scientific research into interactions between infants with Down syndrome and their parents dates back only about a decade and the data available so far are more fragmentary than one would wish. Although the consistency of some of the findings is encouraging, there are also contradictions and inconsistencies that are not always easy to explain. It is an aim of this chapter to examine at least some of these, and to consider a wider perspective within which they may be understood and even resolved.

In studying that which is in some way exceptional, we are often caught in a dilemma. Should we try to see the unusual in its own right, or should we try to compare it with the norm? There is, in fact, a need and place for both of these, and our understanding of the "exceptional" as well as of the "normal" is advanced through the to-and-fro process of making distinctions as well as finding similarities and analogies. A mature appreciation and understanding of what is unique, and of what is common, are based on such a process. Indeed, it is difficult to imagine even beginning to understand something that is new to us without referring to that which we already understand at least a little, and with which we can compare the "new."

I wish to thank my ex-colleagues at the Hester Adrian Research Centre, particularly Dr. Cliff Cunningham, with whom I collaborated on the research in this area most closely. The cooperation of the many families with young infants living in the Manchester area, both those with Down syndrome and nonretarded ones, was of course invaluable. I want to express my gratitude to all of them, both for what they taught me about babies, their development, problems and joys, and for being such patient and supportive participants in our studies.

101

The research on infants with Down syndrome has been so far characterized mainly by such a comparative approach. Therefore, the first part of the chapter is given to a discussion of what the author sees as some of the central issues and ideas within the area of parent–infant interactions generally, from both the theoretical and the methodological viewpoints. It is hoped this will help the reader appreciate the evidence about infants with Down syndrome in a more useful and critical way.

PCIs: What are they and why are they important?

For most developmental psychologists it is almost an axiom that early interactions between infants and their primary caregivers are among the most powerful formative influences on a child's development. Nevertheless, although much clinical as well as the rapidly accumulating ''scientific'' evidence seems to support this assumption, we are still far from having a sufficiently clear and comprehensive framework of knowledge about exactly why and how the parent–child interactions (PCIs) exert their influence on the growing child. The complexity of the problem is reflected, among other places, in the many different perspectives currently found among developmental psychologists concerning these questions; attributing different weights to behavioral, biogenetic, cognitive, social, or wider environmental factors. Despite such differences in opinion and emphasis, broad agreement exists on at least two central points: First, that a child's overall development is the result of interactions among many such factors; second, and more to the point here, that PCI is a bidirectional process in which the behaviors of each partner are influencing and shaping the future responses, expectations, and conceptions of the other participant, as well as the nature of the interactive process itself. The term ''interactionist approach'' is thus used to refer to the interactions between organismic and environmental variables, as well as to the more specific case of interactions between children and caretakers.

But what precisely do we mean by ''parent–child interactions''? As used in this chapter, the definition of PCI encompasses any situation in which a behavior or action by either the parent or the child can be seen (or assumed) to be contingent upon an immediately preceding behavior or action (intentional and unintentional) by the other partner. This definition covers a very wide range of interpersonal phenomena, ranging from a verbal dialogue between a mother and her 5-year-old son, to a father's unintentionally dropping a plate that by its noise awakens the interest of his 2-month-old daughter lying on the floor. It should be noted that the inclusion of unintentional acts and influences is crucial, as it is these which can sometimes have the greatest impact on the other partner, and the nature of the interactions.

How, and in what form, do parents behave and respond to their infants? How is their behavior influenced by the infant? How do different aspects of parental behavior affect and synchronize with different aspects of the infant's behavior and development? These are some of the most frequently researched questions among the hundreds of interaction studies reported during the last decade or so. Increasingly prominent among them are studies of PCI where the infant is considered to be at risk from a developmental disability. The reason behind this is well encapsulated by Lipsitt (1979): "The view of the infant, even the newborn, as a reciprocating social creature necessitates that we try to understand learning disabilities and other developmental problems in terms of their earliest origins" (p. 126).

Infants with Down syndrome have been probably the most frequently studied group, at least where the earliest stages of development are concerned. This seems to be due to several interrelated factors. In particular, Down syndrome, the most common genetically caused condition, which carries a virtually 100% risk of learning disability, can at the same time be usually diagnosed at birth and is associated with a fairly high survival rate. Moreover, because children with Down syndrome develop in most cases at a significantly slower rate than their nonretarded peers, it is often possible to study and discern more clearly the nature of developmental processes and the relative contributions of its various aspects and components (e.g., Cicchetti, & Sroufe, 1976; Cunningham, 1979; Motti, Cicchetti, & Sroufe, 1983).

When investigating PCI, we are dealing with two distinct, if closely interrelated, types of phenomena. One could be described as "pure" social interaction in the sense that the interpersonal transactions are conducted entirely by means of "social signaling" behaviors such as facial expressions, vocalizations, and gestures (i.e., behaviors that have no meaning or function outside a social, interpersonal context). The other category of interactive phenomena are those conducted through and focused on inanimate objects, and whose meaning and form is defined, more or less, by actions related to such objects. Although most real PCI transactions combine, in various proportions and forms, both the social–subjective level and the objective physical reality, the infant's learning how to use, respond to, and understand people and the physical world poses a number of very different requirements, problems, and possibilities. It is perhaps because in nonhandicapped children's development these two aspects of interactions become inseparably and effortlessly intertwined at a fairly early stage, that not enough attention has been paid to their differences. With constitutionally handicapped infants a recognition of such distinctions is especially important for a deeper understanding of their behavioral and developmental difficulties. The question of the interrelationships between emotional and communicative development on one hand, and the child's cognitive, "practical," and linguistic abilities on the other, has been, of course, a major theme in developmental psychology (e.g., Kagan, 1971; Lewis & Coates, 1980; Motti et al., 1983; Ravenette, 1973). Precisely how these two areas of functioning interact and influence each other is, however, still relatively little understood, especially in the context of PCIs and their various abnormalities. In an attempt to highlight some of the differences as well as continuities between these two kinds of interactions, the chapter is organized in terms of a developmental transition from one into the other. For this purpose the conceptualization of the development of "normal" social interactions in terms of two stages put forward by Trevarthen (1977, 1979) will be used as an overall framework. The first stage of a so-called primary intersubjectivity lasts approximately over the first 6 to 9 months and is characterized by purely social transactions between the infant and a caregiver. This is followed by the "secondary intersubjectivity" stage during which interactions become much more object-oriented.

The emergence of secondary intersubjectivity requires the formation of functions combining performed intentions to object and performed intentions of persons. It would thus seem obvious that such a level of functional synthesis will require for its adequate accomplishment not only relatively well-established prerequisite abilities (i.e., understanding of objects and people, and a range of related actions and uses), but also a degree of synchronization between the rate and quality of their development and the salient environmental conditions and responses. In view of this complexity of interrelationships among maturational, developmental, and environmental factors, it is not surprising that for infants with Down syndrome, the secondary intersubjectivity stage is apparently associated with more serious developmental problems than the preceding primary intersubjectivity period. Consequently, a major emphasis will be given in this chapter to examining evidence pertaining to the interphase between parent interactions and object interactions in infants with Down syndrome.

Infant's early developing ability to engage in social interactions through their relatively mature and functional visual, facial, and vocal behaviors is by now well documented (e.g., Robson, 1967; Vine, 1973; Wolff, 1963, 1969). It is clear that at least from the second or third month after birth there is also a considerable degree of behavioral synchrony, turn-taking, and reciprocity between the parent and her infant (e.g., Brazelton, Koslowski & Main, 1974; Fogel, 1977; Schaffer, 1977a, 1977b; Stern, 1974a, 1974b, 1977). The temporal organization appears to be at first determined primarily by the infant's physiological, behavioral, and attentional rhythms according to which the parent tunes and phases her own responses and stimulation (e.g., Brazelton et al., 1974; Field, 1977; Kaye, 1977). Under normal circumstances it is mainly her ability to do this sensitively that facilitates and determines the maintainance of progressively longer, well-meshed, and more varied exchanges. Caretakers' failure to "read" and respect the changes in the infants' state, interests, or readiness to engage in interactions, as signaled by their various behaviors, can lead to a disruption of smooth and enjoyable interactions (e.g., Field, 1977; Richards, 1974; Spitz, 1964; Stern, 1971). Research and clinical evidence suggest that this is more likely to happen when the infant has a difficult temperament, or is in the at-risk category (e.g., Fraiberg, 1975; Greene, Fox, & Lewis, 1983; Neubauer, 1967).

Moreover, there are indications that such interactive difficulties may persist and perhaps even worsen as the handicapped children enter the second year of life, that is, the stage of secondary intersubjectivity (Berger & Cunningham, 1983b; Mogford, 1979).

There is also, however, a growing body of evidence showing that many such interactive difficulties can be substantially reduced through preventative or remedial intervention, or a combination of the two (e.g., Berger & Cunningham, 1983b; Cunningham, 1983; Field, 1977; Fraiberg, 1975; Mogford, 1979). The last part of the chapter considers studies and approaches to therapeutic intervention. It is surely such practical applications to alleviating people's problems that best justify research in this area and are the best reason for its further continuation.

Methodological background

Research methods are determined by what we want to find out (e.g., Yarrow and Anderson, 1979), but it is also true that we can find out and establish with any degree of certainty only that for which we have adequate methods. It is therefore imperative to be aware of methodological possibilities and limitations if we are to understand properly what the evidence presented in this chapter means, and in particular to what extent it is likely to reflect the real parent–child interactions. Fortunately, the major methodological issues and approaches formulated in relation to general PCI research also apply in the case of handicapped populations. Certain aspects, such as the effects of being under observation, the influence of attitudes and personality traits of the parents, or their distinct interactive style, may, however, have amplified effects.

The contemporary view of PCI has become crystallized in terms of the system model and approach (e.g., Mitchell, 1980; Newson, 1977; Parke, 1978), a significant departure from the now outdated causalistic, linear view. The application of the systemic approach has again taken place at: (1) the parent–infant dyad level itself (e.g., Denneberg, 1979; Thoman, Acebo, Dryer, Becker, & Freese, 1979), and (2) at the level of wider ecological systems within which the parent–infant dyad is functioning and of which it is a part (e.g., Bronfenbrenner, 1979). Despite this progress in the general conceptualization of PCIs, the appropriate methodologies are still in very early stages of development. This is not surprising given the potentially vast range of variables that are involved in and influence the PCI systems. Whether it will ever be possible to devise methods that could adequately monitor and quantify all such multiple factors and their interrelationships, and to find theoretical models that could accurately and reliably anticipate and predict future states and changes of such systems, is an open question. As yet, probabilistic methods such as path analysis, structural equation models, and Markov chains have been employed only with a limited range of variables and predictive efficacy (e.g., Jaffe, Stern, & Peery, 1973; Martin, 1981; Stern, 1974a). An excellent example of a less formal methodology within the spirit of the systems approach can be found in the study of early parental adaptation to the birth of an infant with Down syndrome by Emde and Brown (1978). This involved detailed and systematic observations and descriptions of the PCIs in the home, supplemented by interviews with parents, data about the family situation, and information concerning infants' medical, neurological, behavioral, and temperamental characteristics. In addition to giving a very vivid picture of the role played by many different variables, it demonstrates clearly that even a severe deficiency in one or more elements of the system can in some cases be compensated for by its other parts and mechanisms. Such built-in redundancy and self-correcting potential are defining features of all organic systems. This is particularly relevant when considering interactions with at-risk or handicapped infants, where such compensatory processes are likely to be called for (e.g., Broussard, 1980; Sax, 1981).

The changing nature of the PCIs both in time and in different contexts means that interactions should be studied longitudinally as well as in different situations, so as to discover any continuities in their development and to understand the longer-term influences of different variables and contextual factors. As yet, only a handful of interaction studies on infants with Down syndrome appear to have attempted this (e.g., Berger & Cunningham, 1981, 1983a, 1983b; McConkey & Martin, 1984; Motti et al., 1983) and then mainly with regard to the temporal factor.

As pointed out by Yarrow and Anderson (1979), another important feature of parent–infant interactions inherent in this systemic nature and posing serious methodological problems is the "meaning" of the infant's various states and behaviors as perceived and interpreted by the parents. Thus the same infant behavior can be perceived and responded to quite differently depending on the parental expectations, time of day, context, cultural milieu, or personality dispositions. Similarly, the effects of parental stimulation can vary considerably according to the infant's state, sensory threshold, developmental level, context in which it occurs, timing, and other factors. Consequently, a new generation of conceptual categories, which would allow for psychologically more meaningful measures and descriptions, needs to be developed. There has, in fact, been a marked shift toward using more "interactive" variables over the past decade, but categories such as "responds appropriately to the infant's vocalization," or "allows the infant enough time to respond" are only the first steps in the right direction. In general, however, the use of such composite, relatively subjective, and dyadic variables is necessary at least at the present, because it is still extremely difficult, if not impossible, to capture the atmosphere and quality of interactions through the use of purely molecular and discrete behavioral categories alone.

One way to tackle the problem of discovering and establishing with any degree of certainty not only the immediate short-term effects of particular interactional variables but also their more important long-term influence on the child's development, is to compare dyads with naturally different interactive styles. Another way is experimentally to induce temporary modifications in the parent's interactive behavior and observe any accompanying changes in the infant's behavior. The problem can also be approached through interventions designed to bring about more permanent changes in the PCI and by monitoring over a longer period the interactive processes and the child's development. Whereas the experimental approach allows for drawing inferences about genuine causal effects of the manipulated variables, the other two are inevitably confounded by a range of possible intervening variables to such an extent that often no direct causal inferences are possible. Rather, a systemic analysis is required if one is to capture and comprehend the true nature of any changes. Although this is bound to be a difficult task, it is likely to prove more rewarding and valuable by virtue of reflecting more faithfully the real nature of the processes involved.

Studies representing all three methodological approaches are reviewed in this chapter. Because in all of them some degree of manipulation of, or at least control over, the interactive situation is involved, there is also always a danger of reducing the richness of the interactions as they normally are, if only because it is impossible in practice to observe PCIs in all the variety of forms, moods, contexts and times, and because the presence of an outside observer is likely to affect at least the parents' feelings and behaviors. Thus at best we may obtain a fairly representative approximation to and reflection of the real thing, and at worst a totally distorted and false picture. Although most studies take precautions to minimize such danger, this is done with a varying degree of success, and it is never possible to eliminate the danger completely. It is therefore essential that great caution also be taken in interpreting all the research findings presented later in this chapter and in making generalizations from them.

Interactional studies involving infants with Down syndrome will be presented in a chronological order, according to the infants' age. As noted in an earlier section, the developmental perspective will be further emphasized by organizing and interpreting the evidence primarily within a developmental framework proposed by C. Trevarthen (1974, 1977, 1979). In his descriptions and analyses of nonretarded infants' social development, Trevarthen makes a distinction between the earliest stage, during which some of the most fundamental forms of interpersonal awareness, expression, and responsivity emerge and are practiced, usually within the context of interactions with primary caretakers (i.e., primary intersubjectivity), and a subsequent stage of secondary subjectivity, during which more elaborate and mature forms of communication begin to take shape, particularly transactions involving objects and gradual crystallizations and elaborations of shared symbolic meaning.

Moreover, Trevarthen maintains that the infants' earliest expressions of sociability are due to innate "intentionality" toward other people, which, in turn, is based on neuromaturational processes. It is also clear, however, that with age, learning and experience gradually begin to play an important role in early social development (e.g., Stern & Gibbon, 1979). And perhaps partly as a result of the basic interactive rules' becoming well established and mastered by the infant, a temporary shift in interest away from people occurs at around 6 months of age. The following period of relative social disinterest (quiescence), which last usually from about 6 to 9 months of age, is characterized by the infant's intense preoccupation with exploring and manipulating inanimate objects and the space that contains them. This, however, seems to serve a very important purpose from the point of further social development. By enlarging the infant's understanding of a vitally important new area of functioning and reality, it also helps enrich and expand the realm of potential social interactions and of shared meanings and interests.

That this period of social quiescence can be in fact seen as a preparation, or transition, phase of development is substantiated by the subsequent appearance of secondary intersubjectivity. Now the infant's social and object-related abilities begin to combine in functional and communicatively novel ways. For example, we can see for the first time the infant's ability to follow mother's pointing or gaze direction (Scaife & Bruner, 1975), or to give and take objects (Gray, 1978; Trevarthen & Hubley, 1978). The importance of a rudimentary understanding of objects, space, and movements, as well as of social abilities is clearly apparent in such interpersonal transactions.

In addition to the relevance of such general developmental and experimental factors in considering the early social interactions of infants with Down syndrome, the neuromaturational perspective of Trevarthen's model has a particular and added significance for infants with a biogenetic disorder such as Down syndrome.

The presentation of research evidence will begin, however, with a short section about the first three to four weeks of life. Although this earliest period seems to predate the generally agreed dawn of infants' "real" social interactions, it can be seen as an important preparation for the emergence of primary intersubjectivity. During this period the infants' basic "reflexive" behaviors are tested and exercised, and thus gradually mastered and brought under voluntary control (e.g., Zelazo, 1976). This includes various facial expressions, as well as limb, hand, head, and trunk movements, all of which constitute the basic behavioral repertoire in subsequent social interactions.

Moreover, it is during these early weeks that parents begin to get to know their newly born babies and learn to recognize and adapt to their individual characteristics. Indeed, it could be argued that vitally important social interactions are taking place from the very first contact between the parents and their infant. Interactions are mediated primarily through tactile, olfactory, gustatory and vestibular sense (e.g., Klaus & Kennell, 1976; Sander, Stechler, Burns, & Julia, 1970; Spitz, 1965), rather than the more widely recognized and studied interactions conducted mainly through distal senses of vision, hearing, and through gestural and vocal expression. Nevertheless, it is interesting that already during the first few hours of life, infants show organized movement patterns in response to adult speech (Condon & Sander, 1974). Surely, this is compelling evidence for innate responsivity to even the more distal social behaviors and signals.

The first month: before eye contact and smiling

This earliest period is often considered particularly important and formative for later PCIs and relationship, and it has been suggested that the first few days, or even hours, of contact are most favorable for the establishment of positive maternal feelings and mother's attachment to the newborn infant (e.g., Kennell et al., 1974; Leifer, Leiderman, Barnett, & Williams, 1972). There is some evidence, for example, that a lack of contact between mother and her infant in the hours and days immediately after birth (usually because of special care procedures in prematurity or other complications), is associated with increased danger of maternal depression and of difficulties in the establishment of affectionate maternal behavior (Kennell, Gordon, & Klaus, 1970; Klaus & Kennell, 1976; Leifer et al., 1972). Several studies also indicate that an enhancement of early postpartum contact tends to have marked beneficial effects on maternal caretaking and interactive behaviors in the short term, as well as on the mother–infant interactions over the first few years of life, when compared to dyads who had only the fairly sporadic contacts prescribed by hospital routines (Kennell et al., 1974; Klaus & Kennell, 1976; Ringler, Kennell, Jarvella, Navojsky, & Klaus, 1975). Other studies (e.g., Scarr-Salapatek & Williams, 1972; Weintraub, Sokoloff, Yaffe, & Blase, 1969) suggest that extra stimulation enrichment itself improves the infants' condition and responsiveness, which, in turn, is likely to have beneficial effects on the mother and the interactions between her and the infant. Yet, the question of how critically important the duration and quality of the first contact is for later development remains open. For example, in a comprehensive review of studies in this area, Goldberg (1983) concluded that there was insufficient evidence for any strong and unequivocal causal effects of early mother–infant bonding, or postpartum contact. She did, nevertheless, also suggest that more modest claims concerning the importance of these early influences may be justified. In her own words, "the notion of early contact as critical rather than beneficial needs to be dispelled," and "the parent–infant relationship is a complex system with many fail-safe or alternative routes to the same outcome. Its success or failure does not hinge on a few brief moments in time" (Goldberg, 1983, 1379). Such a position has, of course, important implications, especially for infants with Down syndrome and their parents, who are often separated (for medical, emotional, or practical reasons) after birth more than nonhandicapped infants. In particular, it offers more hope and grounds for optimism, despite the frequent difficulties in the earliest stages of parent–infant interactions.

Unfortunately, in the case of infants with Down syndrome we have much less, and then mainly anecdotal, evidence about the effects associated with the frequent postpartum separation, and of the shock, depression, and grief that usually follow the disclosure of the diagnosis (e.g., Cunningham & Sloper, 1977; Emde & Brown, 1978). Nevertheless, some of these reports describe the often dramatic effects which the first contact with her newborn Down syndrome infant can have on the mother's feelings of attachment, as well as on her nurturant behavior. Emde and Brown (1978), for example, describe how at the moment when a mother held her baby for the first time, her feelings of unreality, and that "he may be better off dead" were suddenly replaced by feelings of love and care. However, these authors also emphasize the real grief over the "loss" of a wanted and expected normal baby and the resulting emotional and behavioral trauma that can make the task of caring for the newborn Down syndrome infant very difficult.

Another source of early interactive difficulties may be the Down syndrome infant's reported delays in the onset of various rhythmic behavioral patterns (Kravitz & Boehm, 1971; Wolff, 1966, 1967). These are among the infant's first responses used by mothers to establish interactions and a primitive form of reciprocity (e.g., Gunther, 1961; Kaye, 1977; Sander et al., 1970). This possibility is also substantiated by reports of impairments in the development of early "reflexive" behaviors (e.g., rooting, postural, grasping, etc.) in infants with Down syndrome (Cowie, 1970; Haraldsdottir, 1983). Furthermore, there are some indications that, for example, feeding-related interactions, and particularly the breast-feeding of the infant with Down syndrome, may be adversely affected by sucking difficulties (e.g., Aumonier & Cunningham, 1983). It is also clear, however, that there are enormous variations in the parents' early adaptation to, and interactions with, their newborn infant with Down syndrome. These have been well illustrated by Emde and Brown (1978). It is apparent that whereas some parents can adopt a positive and loving attitude to their infant, and cope well with even the most severe physical complications, other parents find this extremely difficult even when the baby is healthy and responsive and external support is available. The large number of factors that may lie behind these differences still awaits a systematic investigation. Among these, the manner in which the diagnosis is disclosed to the parents and the immediate emotional and practical support certainly appears to have a considerable influence on the parents' feelings and attitudes toward the infant (Cunningham, Morgan, & McGucken, 1984), and probably also on the nature of their care and interactions. In particular, a sympathetic, positive, yet realistic attitude by doctors and other professionals toward the infant with Down syndrome and his or her future development is important in helping parents. Thus, reports of some recent home intervention studies (e.g., Cunningham, 1983; Emde and Brown, 1978) indicate that through honest but sensitive professional support parents can be effectively helped in resolving and overcoming the initial shock, rejection, disappointment, and grief, and in releasing their energy for more positive attachment and interactions.

Primary intersubjectivity stage: 1–6/9 months

Eye contact

Although PCIs begin as soon after birth as there is contact, a significant change seems to occur in the interactions once the infant is able to establish genuine eye-to-eye contact (e.g., Robson, 1967; Wolff, 1963). At this time mothers report that they feel as if the infant recognized and knew them, and often begin to spend more time playing with their infant. Robson (1967) suggests that when young infants persistently avoid looking at their mothers' eyes and thus preempt reciprocal maternal eye contact, mothers are likely to feel anxious, inadequate, and frustrated.

There is some evidence that this behavior is both impaired in its quality, and slower in making its first appearance in infants with Down syndrome. Thus, Emde and Brown (1978) described it as lacking "the crescendo of sparkling eyes" for several infants in their study, although in some it appeared to be less impaired than in others. However, their descriptions were not particularly systematic nor accurate as to the exact age of emergence, frequency, and durations. A longitudinal study by Berger and Cunningham (1981), employed a combination of direct observational methods and experimental manipulations of the mothers' behavior during home-based face-to-face interactions, to investigate the onset and early development of eye contact and other signaling behaviors in five infants with Down syndrome. The results suggested that : (1) The first mutual eye contact as observed and reported by the mothers was delayed on average by about 2.5 weeks when compared to a group

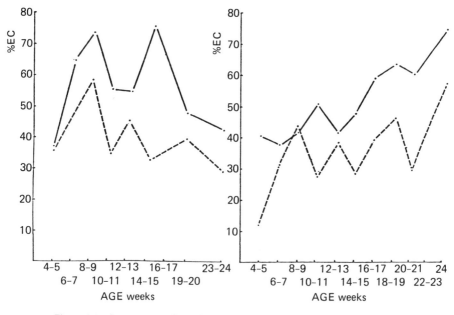

Figure 4.1. Group means of % EC recorded during the mobile and the immobile conditions over the first 6 months of life (mobile = ▬▬▬▬▬▬▬; immobile = ▬ ▬ ▬ ▬ ▬ ▬). (a) Nonhandicapped, on the left side of the figure; (b) Down syndrome, on the right side of the figure.

of seven nonhandicapped infants; (2) the amount of eye contact by infants with Down syndrome increased more slowly during the first three or four months, reaching a peak at least seven to ten weeks later than in nonhandicapped infants; and (3) once a peak was attained at about 4 to 5 months of age, the infants with Down syndrome maintained much higher levels of mutual eye contact (both in overall duration and the durations of individual gazes) than nonhandicapped infants who showed a significant decrease on both these measures between the fourth and sixth months of age. (see Figure 4.1) These findings indicate that although infants with Down syndrome engage in eye contact with their mothers from a relatively early age, there are also some significant deviations from the norm. Of particular interest from the point of view of longer-term interactive development appears to be the absence of a decline in the amount of gazing at the mother's eyes toward the end of the first half of the first year. A more detailed analysis of the data also indicated that already during the first four to six months, infants with Down syndrome remained fixated almost exclusively on the mother's eyes rather than using the episodes of face-to-face gazing to explore other facial features, as did the nonretarded infants (Berger, 1980). This is indicative of the Down syndrome infant's lower level of visual exploration of other aspects of their environment and of visual switching generally. Several other studies help to set these findings within a longer-term developmental perspective. Thus, a study of 6- to 9-months-old infants with Down syndrome (Gunn, Berry, & Andrews, 1982) reported twice as much interpersonal looking during interactions with mothers than by a chronologically matched sample of nonhandicapped infants. Jones (1977, 1980) found significantly more 'personal' but less referential eye contact with mothers by 13- to 23-months-old Down syndrome infants when compared to a developmentally matched group of nonhandicapped infants. And for 2- to 3-year-old children with Down syndrome observed during free play with toys, Krakow and Kopp (1983) reported significantly less visual monitoring of their mothers, and of the room in which they were playing, when compared to a group of developmentally matched nonretarded children.

All these findings provide compelling evidence that at least during the first three years of life, children with Down syndrome tend to show considerable deviations in their attentional development, particularly in distributing their visual attention between people and other foci of interest. Moreover, they indicate that the socially quiescent period reported for nonhandicapped infants (and used primarily for learning about inanimate objects and space – see preceding section) is either missing or greatly delayed. Unfortunately, there appear to be no longitudinal studies documenting longer-term shifts in interest in infants with Down syndrome. The earliest origins of such atypical developmental and behavioral patterns may be related to perceptual and cognitive deficits and less efficient information-processing (Berger & Cunningham, 1981; Cicchetti and Sroufe, 1978; Miranda, 1976). Its apparent maintenance over the first two or three years is, however, probably related also to the nature of parental behavior during interactions and the kinds of infants' learning experiences occasioned by these. Such processes will be discussed later in the chapter, particularly in the context of interactions involving objects and their relationship with sensorimotor and affective development.

Vocal interactions

While mutual eye gaze provides an underlying setting signal and "frame" (Fogel, 1977) for intimate social interactions, vocalizing and smiling are usually seen as the infant's other two most important "social" behaviors (e.g., Vine, 1973). Although it is somewhat artificial to consider these various aspects separately, because they all form part and parcel of a single interactive flow (e.g., Brazelton et al., 1974; Trevarthen, 1974, 1977; Wolff, 1963, 1969), there are as yet no observational data describing this process as a whole in infants with Down syndrome. With regard to vocal behaviors it has been demonstrated that phonological and temporal vocalization patterns (both cry and non-cry) of newborn infants with Down syndrome differ from those of nonhandicapped infants (Fisichelli & Karelitz, 1966; Karelitz & Fisichelli, 1969). If, as suggested, for example, by Wolff (1969), there is a functional and morphological continuity between early and later vocal behaviors, it would seem likely that the development of later vocal interactions in infants with Down syndrome could also be affected.

Undoubtedly, one of the developmentally most important features of early vocal interactions is turn-taking, which can be seen as one of the major precursors of mature linguistic interactions. These reciprocal interactions characterized by alternate vocalizing and listening, have been observed during mother–infant interactions already from about the third month after birth (e.g., Bateson, 1975; Bullowa, 1979; Stern, Jaffe, Beebe, & Bennett, 1975). Although in the first few months it is the parent who takes the main responsibility for ensuring that the respectively active/ vocal and passive/listening acts are smoothly interphased, the infant's capacity to vocalize in relatively regular and predictable rhythms is very important for a successful maintenance of turn-taking sequences.

Recently, Jasnow and his colleagues have examined the rhythmic or temporal patterning of vocal exchanges between infants with Down syndrome and their mothers (Jasnow, Crown, Feldstein, Taylor, Beebe, & Jaffe, 1988). They similarly propose that coordination between the rhythmic qualities of mother and infant vocalizations constitutes a "buffered" mechanism which facilitates social interaction and communication. Within this study, Jasnow and his collaborators recorded the vocal interactions of nine pairs of infants with Down syndrome and their mothers and nine pairs of normally developing infants and mothers at 4 and 9 months of age. Careful analyses of these interactions indicated that dyads within both groups demonstrate temporal coordination in their vocalizations. Specifically, infants with and without Down syndrome appeared to be sensitive to the temporal qualities of their mothers' vocalizations (e.g., turns, pauses) and modified their own vocalizations to match those of their mothers. However, despite this similarity, infants with Down syndrome differed from the normally developing infants in the magnitude of coordination they demonstrated. Generally, at 4 months the infants with Down syndrome evidenced less coordination than the other infants. However, by 9 months this difference attenuated, with the interactions of infants with Down syndrome being just as coordinated as those of normals.

These data suggest that the rhythmicity of the vocalizations of infants with Down syndrome is influenced by the characteristics of maternal vocalizations, and also the infants' abilities to perceive these characteristics and to modify their own behavior. Coordination in the temporal qualities of vocalizations of mothers and infants seems to be slightly delayed within the Down syndrome population. However, at early ages these infants demonstrate some coordination and seem to improve over time.

In another study, Berger and Cunningham (1983) also examined the coordination of mother–infant vocal interactions with infants with Down syndrome. However, in this study, the investigators focused upon turn-taking within exchanges, rather than whether the overall patterning of each member's vocalizations matched. Specifically, Berger and Cunningham used frequency and durations of vocal behaviors in addition to dyadic categories of vocal switches and vocal clashes as the basic units of turn-taking.

To summarize, this study showed: (1) a slower initial increase in the amount of vocalizing by the infants with Down syndrome as compared to a matched group of nonhandicapped infants; (2) once the infants with Down syndrome "caught up," at about the fourth month of age, their overall vocal output continued to increase, whereas that of the nonhandicapped infants showed a marked decrease between the

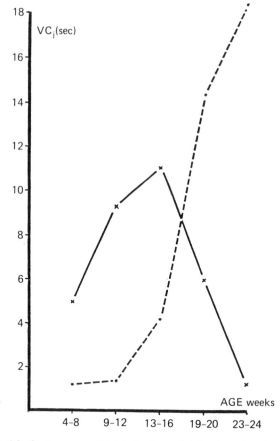

Figure 4.2. Group means of total durations of infants' vocalizations (VC_1) (Nonhandi-capped = ⸻; Down syndrome = ▬ ▬ ▬ ▬)

fourth and six month (see Figure 4.2). These trends are analogous to those presented for the infants' eye contact earlier. (3) With age the infants with Down syndrome and their mothers, showed an increasing tendency to be involved in vocal clashes as compared to the nonhandicapped dyads. When this was expressed as a ratio between clashes and switches, the difference became statistically significant at six months of age (see Figure 4.3). (4) The overall durations of maternal vocalizations were very similar for the two groups during the first four months, but during the fifth and sixth months the vocal output of the Down syndrome infants' mothers became significantly higher (see Figure 4.4).

What can be inferred from these results about the nature of the mother–infant vocal interactions in the first six months? First, it is clear that such interactions do take place although the infants with Down syndrome vocalize considerably less during the first two or three months of life. Second, the increases in their vocal

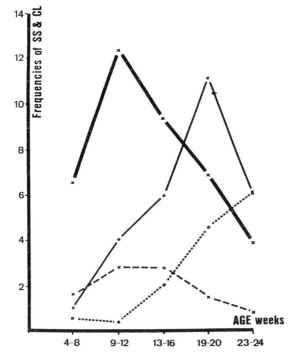

Figure 4.3. Group mean frequencies of speaker-switches (SS) and vocal clashes (CL). (Nonhandicapped, SS = ▬▬▬▬▬, CL = ▬ ▬ ▬ ▬; Down syndrome, SS = ▬▬▬▬; CL = ••••••••••)

output after this age, (reaching levels well above those shown by nonhandicapped infants at any time during the six-month period), suggest that a lack of vocalization is not likely to be a cause of interactive difficulties. On the contrary, it may be that the Down syndrome infants vocalize too much. In particular, they may not be making sufficient pauses between individual bursts to allow mothers to phase and take turns to the extent mothers of nonhandicapped can. That this may be so is suggested by findings on older infants with Down syndrome reported by Jones (1977, 1980). They were found to vocalize more randomly, densely, and repetitively, leaving fewer and less predictable spaces for the maternal vocalizations. Finally, the mothers of Down syndrome infants appeared to be matching the increasing vocal output of their babies, which, in turn, may have contributed to the observed age-related increase in the proportion of vocal clashes. Unfortunately, it was not possible to distinguish from these data to what extent the so-called positive unison vocalizations (Stern et al., 1975) or other non-clash overlaps were represented in the measures of vocal clashes. This issue was, however, investigated recently in a study of naturalistic vocal interactions of four 3-year-old children with Down syndrome (Peskett & Wootton, 1985). Their findings indicate that at least for this age group, the ma-

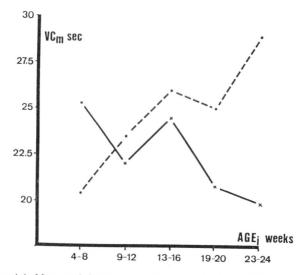

Figure 4.4. Mean total durations of maternal vocalizations (VC^m) plotted against infants' age (AGE$_1$) (Nonhandicapped = ⎯⎯⎯⎯⎯; Down syndrome = ▬ ▬ ▬ ▬)

jority of such overlaps did not lead to a breakdown in interactions and could not therefore be regarded as communicative clashes. Overall, the findings by Berger and Cunningham (1983a) are consistent with those reported by older infants with Down syndrome (e.g., Buckhalt, Rutherford, & Goldberg, 1978; Jones, 1980) and for infants and children with other handicaps (e.g., Davis & Oliver, 1980). The high levels of maternal stimulation and poorer reciprocity are among the most consistently noted features.

The results of Berger and Cunningham's (1983a) study also suggest that such interactive anomalies can be traced back to the first six months of life, long before any "performance" related to objects or language could possibly be expected by even the most optimistic or impatient of parents. Sorce and Emde (1982), who found that mothers of infants with Down syndrome indicated a significantly heightened tendency to initiate stimulation when compared with mothers of nonhandicapped infants, put forward a compensation hypothesis to explain this phenomenon. They argue that due to a history of interactive experiences in which their infants have consistently manifested low levels of "invitations" and a depressed intensity of facial signals and expressions (e.g., Emde, Katz, & Thorpe, 1978), these mothers are likely to have activated the so-called lower limit control behaviors. In effect this is an attempt to compensate for the infant's deficit and leads to a tendency to intervene more often. As the study of Sorce and Emde used maternal verbal reports of their likely reactions to photographs of their infants, their findings provide some evidence to counter the argument that the high levels of stimulation recorded in observational studies could be merely due to the mothers' greater anxiety and desire to "show off" their infants with Down syndrome. The suggested absence of a vocally quiescent period may also be significant as this in nonhandicapped infants is thought to be a period of transition between phonetically and semantically non-discriminate babbling and the beginnings of speech proper (e.g., Crystal, 1976; Lewis, 1959).

Smiling

The expressive deficits of infants with Down syndrome and their link with other developmental domains have been so far most clearly highlighted by studies of smiling, generally considered to be one of the most potent signals for eliciting and reinforcing caretaking and affectionate responses (e.g., Klaus & Kennell, 1976; Spitz & Wolff, 1946; Stechler & Carpenter, 1967; Wolff, 1963). It is thus likely to play an important role in early infant–parent interactions. It is perhaps for this reason, as well as due to the close connection between infants' smiling and percep-tual–cognitive functioning (e.g., Haith, 1972; Kagan, 1971; Piaget, 1952; Watson, 1972; Zelazo, 1972; Zelazo & Komer, 1971) that it has been among the most fre-quently studied behavior in young infants with Down syndrome (Berger, 1980; Berger & Cunningham, 1986; Buckhalt, Rutherford, & Goldberg, 1978; Carr, 1975; Cicchetti & Sroufe, 1976; Cytryn, 1975; Emde & Brown, 1978). There is a consen-sus among these authors that smiling in these infants appears later, is dampened, and is less frequent than in nonhandicapped infants. Again, the study by Emde and Brown (1978) provides a most vivid account of the qualitative aspects of smiling infants with Down syndrome, and of its role in the interactions with parents. They noted that its dampened form was mainly due to a lack of general activation and enhanced eye-to-eye contact, yet they illustrated how in most cases it nevertheless generated warm and joyful feelings in the parents.[1] This concurs well with our findings that mothers often spontaneously commented about how rewarding it was for them to see their babies smile (Berger & Cunningham, 1986). The main purpose of this study was, however, to record the infants' smiles during face-to-face inter-actions with mothers over the first six months of life, and to examine the temporal relationship between smiling and eye contact. While the onset of smiling, as re-ported by the mothers, was on average three weeks later for the infants with Down syndrome than for the nonhandicapped infants, the mean difference was more than five weeks for the smiles recorded by the authors in the course of mother–infant interactions. Moreover, the discrepancy between the first mother-reported and first author-recorded smiles was significantly greater for the mothers of infants with Down syndrome than for the nonhandicapped infant–mother pairs. This may have reflected their greater eagerness, as compared to the nonhandicapped infants' moth-ers, to see their babies smile, since this in turn may diminish their subjective per-ception of the infants' handicap. It could, however, be also related to the more fleeting and dampened nature of the smile. Furthermore, over the whole first six months the frequencies of smiling by infants with Down syndrome were signifi-cantly lower, and the durations of their individual smiles were significantly shorter. Their smiles were, however, temporally associated with episodes of eye contact to about the same extent as those of the nonhandicapped infants. Although the brevity of the smiles may be one of the factors contributing to the impression of their dampened character, these findings indicate that at least its timing within the interactive process was relatively unimpaired.

In this study the mothers were instructed not to use tactile or kinesthetic stimulation during the recording of face-to-face interactions so that the effects of the mothers' vocal behaviors, their facial expressions, and the face stimulus generally could be separated from the effects of physical stimulation. We then asked the mothers also to try and get the baby to smile in any way they liked. Under these freer conditions, the mothers of infants with Down syndrome were found to use considerably more tactile and kinesthetic stimulation than mothers of the nonhandicapped infants. This suggests that intuitively they were employing a stimulation strategy that is probably most effective in eliciting the smiles of infants with Down syndrome in this age group (Cicchetti & Sroufe, 1976). In their study Cicchetti and Sroufe also found positive and significant correlations between Down syndrome infants' affective responsivity at 10 months, as reflected in smiling and laughing, and measures of cognitive functioning at 2 years. In a follow-up study significant positive correlations were found between several of the infants' affective measures at 10 months of age and their levels of symbolic play with objects at 3 to 5 years of age (Motti et al., 1983). Such findings are consistent with, and supportive of, the reported links between affective responding, such as smiling, and cognitive functioning in nonhandicapped infants (e.g., Kagan, 1971; Piaget, 1952; Zelazo, 1972).

The findings of Berger and Cunningham (1981, 1983a, 1986) and by others indicate that during the first six months, smiling appears to be the most defective among the Down syndrome infants' major social signaling behaviors. Considering that smiling is also closely related to the infants' recognition of the contingencies between their own behavior and the environmental responses to these (e.g., Watson, 1967, 1972), it is possible that one reason for the smiling deficiency may be a lack of effective contingent experiences during the infants' social interactions. A combination of their slower information processing and response capacity (e.g., Berkson, 1960a; Miranda, 1976), the high levels of maternal stimulation, and the apparently impaired turn-taking during vocal interactions all seem to point to this eventuality. Additional support for the notion that the usual interactive behavior of mothers of infants with Down syndrome may be less than optimal for the eliciting of their infants' social responses came also from the following findings by Berger and Cunningham (1983a, 1985): (1) Infants with Down syndrome showed significantly less differential vocalizing and smiling (than the nonhandicapped infants) between conditions when their mothers were interacting "naturally" (Mobile condition) and when the mothers remained silent and held their faces immobile, at the experimenters' instructions (Immobile condition); (2) after the nonhandicapped infants' vocalization (during the Mobile condition) has started to decrease toward the end of the fourth month, their vocal output in the Immobile condition registered dramatic increases and became for the first time significantly higher, indicating the infants' strong reaction to the perceptual incongruity and violation of expectations represented by the immobile face. By contrast, no such developmental changes in the pattern of vocalization were noted for the infants with Down syndrome; (3) over the whole six-month period, the Down syndrome infants showed more crying and distress vocalizations in the Mobile condition while the nonhandicapped infants cried more during the Immobile condition, suggesting again a greater negative response to the discrepancy in the mothers' behavior.

To examine the hypothesis that the low levels of smiling and apparent lack of preferential responding by infants with Down syndrome could be at least in part due to a lack of functionally effective contingent properties of their mothers' interactive behaviors, the following study was carried out by Cunningham & Berger (in press). Twelve mothers of infants with Down syndrome (5 to 7 months old) were each given three sets of instructions by the experimenters on how to behave during their face-to-face interactions with their infants. Central to this study was an Imitation condition during which the mothers were asked only to imitate their infant's facial and vocal behaviors, but not to initiate or attempt to elicit any themselves. In addition, mothers were also asked to interact as naturally as possible (Smile-eliciting condition). Each condition lasted 2 minutes and their order was counterbalanced so as to control for any possible order effect bias. The main objective was to compare the infants' smiling, vocalization and looking at mother during the three conditions. We hypothesized that the Imitation condition would be associated with higher levels of infants' smiling and vocalization because during it the mothers' responses and stimulation would be more clearly contingent upon the infants' behaviors, allowing more opportunities and time for the infant to respond and initiate interactive behaviors. In this way, the mothers' behavior would also become more manageable relative to their infants' processing and response capacities. The imitation strategy was chosen also because it appears to be a common and natural feature of early mother–infant interactions (Papousek & Papousek, 1977; Pawlby, 1977; Sylvester-Bradley and Trevarthan, 1977). Papousek and Papousek (1977) argue: "From the first day she [the mother] offers her infant what we call a biological mirror. By imitating him she gives him a chance to associate his introceptive information about his own movements with their visual representation," and "he may detect that his act elicits a response in his mother with a certain regularity, and the contingency of this response may be enough first to initiate operant learning in him." (p. 82). By virtue of creating longer spaces in between the mothers' responses, the imitation strategy is also likely to facilitate turn-taking and interactive reciprocity. Studies by Stern (1971) and Spitz (1964) indicate that when mothers do not allow sufficient opportunities for the infant to respond or to withdraw temporarily from the face-to-face situation, the interactive process becomes distorted and unsatisfactory. Field (1977) used such imitation strategy successfully to improve aspects of interactions between mothers and their young "at risk" infants.

The main findings of our study confirmed the original hypothesis. While frequencies of smiling and vocalizing by infants with Down syndrome were significantly higher in the Imitation condition than in the Natural condition, a comparison group of 12 developmentally matched nonhandicapped infants did not show such difference between these two conditions. The analysis of the maternal behavior showed that in terms of frequencies of contingent responses and response opportunities, the two groups of mothers did not differ significantly. The mothers of infants with Down syndrome showed, however, significantly higher levels of stimulation in the Natural condition. This was also reflected in the finding that for them, these measures were not significantly different in the Natural and Smile-eliciting conditions, whereas the mothers of the nonhandicapped infants showed significantly higher stimulation levels in the latter. These results suggest that although the Down syndrome infants' mothers were more active during face-to-face interactions, their phasing did not seem to be impaired. Nevertheless, in view of their infants' significantly lower levels of smiling and vocalizing in the Natural condition and the significant increase in the frequencies of these behaviors in the Imitation condition, the imitation strategy appeared to be associated with a more optimal form of stimulation for the infants with Down syndrome. Although their mothers may have been providing adequate stimulation and responses by "normal" standards, the considerably longer response opportunities, more clearly contingent responses, and significantly lower levels of maternal activity in the Imitation condition were more effective for enhancing the infants' social responsivity.[2]

A somewhat surprising result was that the infants with Down syndrome smiled significantly more in the Smile-eliciting than in the Natural condition. No such differences were, however, found for either the infants' vocalizations or their looking at the mothers' faces. This suggests that the different maternal instructions and the resulting strategies had specific effects on the infants' responses. Unfortunately, at present we can only speculate as to the reasons for this. Since the overall amounts and the phasing of their mothers' activity were not different in the Natural and Smile-eliciting conditions, it seems likely that some of its other aspects differed. For example, the mothers may have used more tactile and proprioceptive stimulation in the Smile-eliciting condition, as suggested by the findings of our previous study (Berger & Cunningham, 1986). The heightened arousal associated with such a form of vigorous and physical stimulation could be one of the reasons behind the increase in smiling, but not in the other two behaviors.

Finally, it is worth noting that the measures of maternal reciprocity as expressed in terms of contingent phasing and response opportunities were compared with more subjective ratings of this aspect of maternal behavior. Using videotapes recorded during the interaction experiment, seven statements concerning each of the mothers' sensitivity, confidence, timing of stimulation, and enjoyment or anxiety (as manifested during the interactions) were scored independently along a 6-point scale by three raters who were otherwise not involved in any of the other data analyses. Spearmen rank–order correlations between these ratings and those obtained by the microanalysis of contingent phasing and response opportunities carried out by the experimenters, were all positive and statistically significant (mean $= +.677$, $p < .01$, range: .590 to .860). On one hand this supports the validity of the fine-grain measures of maternal reciprocity and on the other hand suggests that more global and less time-consuming assessment of the quality of maternal interactive behaviors is feasible.

A longitudinal study aiming to explore the applicability of the imitation strategy within a home setting and its use as a practical basis for improving interactions between mothers and their Down syndrome infants was carried out subsequently (see note 3). Seven mother–infant pairs took part, the infants' age ranging from 14 to 32 weeks (mean = 21 weeks) at the beginning of the study and 21 to 43 weeks (mean = 31 weeks) at the end. The mean number of home visits per dyad was four (range 3 to 6 visits). In addition to comparing the infants social behaviors during a Natural and Imitation condition (the same instructions were given to the mothers as in the preceding study), an investigation of the mother–infant interactions using toys was also included. This was done partly because most of the infants began to show interest in, and reached toward objects during the course of this study and partly because the mothers themselves liked to use objects such as rattles, bells, and squeezy toys. After observing the natural interactions of this kind for about 5 minutes (Natural object play = NOP) we asked mothers to present the objects more slowly so the infants could have more time to explore them visually, to reach for and get hold of them (Phased object play = POP). The comparison between Imitation and Natural conditions showed no significant differences for any of the seven infant behaviors rated (i.e., smiling, vocalizing, laughing, positive facial expressions, negative facial expressions, looking at mother's face, visual avoidance of mother's face). Again, however, the infants showed great individual differences in their social responding under the two conditions. This is illustrated by figures shown in Table 4.1. Thus, the findings of the previous laboratory-based study using the imitation strategy were not confirmed under more realistic home conditions. Although some of the infants showed more smiling and vocalizing in the Imitation condition in the home study as well, others smiled and vocalized more in the Natural condition. Some of the mothers also found the Imitation condition unnatural and even disturbing. This negative effect was particularly strong with one mother whose infant was extremely passive during this condition (and, according to the mother, appearing more "Downlike"), whereas in the Natural condition the mother was able to elicit quite a lot of smiling and vocalizing and both she and the infant appeared to enjoy their interactions.

Effects of the intervention into object–play interactions proved to be more beneficial (see Table 4.2). Under the Slowed-down conditions the infants' positive behaviors toward the toys increased considerably, in particular because of higher levels of grasping, simple play, and looking at the objects. Nevertheless, even here some of the infants show more responding and simple play in the Natural condition. We are still in the process of analyzing the finer-grained aspects of the interactions, searching for clues to help us account for the various idiosyncratic patterns of responding and interaction under the different conditions.[3]

While the overall findings of this study so far indicate that a beneficial intervention strategy into the mother–infant interaction should involve an emphasis of some

Table 4.1. *Means of infant behaviors across all sessions. Face-to-face interactions: percentage duration measures*

	EJ (pair 1)		DG (pair 2)		DL (pair 3)		AM (pair 4)		LW (pair 5)		KJ (pair 6)		MS (pair 7)	
Total	SIN n=2	SII	SIN n=4	SII	SIN n=4	SII	SIN n=5	SII	SIN n=5	SII	SIN n=3	SII	SIN n=3	SII
SM	2.5	2.5	12.5	1.5	12.5	6.3	12.6	11	7.6	6.4	6.3	13.6	2.7	1.3
SD	3.5	3.5	11.3	1.9	9	4.6	10	12.2	4.8	3.1	5.5	4.8	1.9	1.2
VC	23	28	14.8	10.3	8.3	6.3	28	17.6	2.8	9.4	14.7	18.7	14	17
SD	21	24	14	13.6	4.3	4.6	18.2	18.8	4.1	10.9	1.7	13.6	9.9	10.7
LG	0	1	1.3	0	0.3	0	4.6	7.8	0	.6	0	1	0	0
SD	0	1.4	1.5	0	0.5	0	4.7	9.6	0	1.2	0	1.4	0	0
FE	21	30	12.5	15.8	29.3	26.3	14.6	32.6	25.2	22	12.3	12.3	10.3	27
SD	2	13	2.9	12.6	23.7	11.3	6.3	32.8	8.2	11.6	10.3	6.6	8.2	5.4
FR	5.5	1.5	1.5	0	0	0	0	0	4.2	.6	7.3	21.3	.7	0
SD	7.7	2.1	1.9	0	0	0	0	0	8.4	1.2	5.2	23.9	.9	0
LM	48	43.5	70.5	63.8	68.5	43.3	74.6	78.4	43.8	37.4	41.3	48.7	24	39.7
SD	11.3	23	7.6	24.3	6.9	22.9	19.5	23.6	21.4	37.4	25.9	14.4	24.7	35.1
LA	20.5	27.5	14.5	16.3	27.5	25.5	16.2	17.6	17.4	1.2	6.3	17	.8	.6
SD	20.5	21.9	10.9	15.6	1.9	18	12.2	24.2	15.2	1.6	4.5	15.6	.5	.5

Note: SIN = natural; SII = imitation; LM = imitation; LM = looking at mother; LA = avoidance look from mother; SM = smiling; VC = vocalizing; LG = laughing; FE = facial expression; FR = upset, negative facial expressions, and crying.

Table 4.2. *Means of infant behaviors across all sessions. Object Interactions: percentage duration measures*

	EJ (pair 1)		DG (pair 2)		DL (pair 3)		AM (pair 4)		LW (pair 5)		MS (pair 7)	
Total	NOP n = 5	POP	NOP n = 4	POP	NOP n = 1	POP	NOP n = 3	POP	NOP n = 3	POP	NOP n = 1	POP
RC	16	15.2	16.2	23.3	4	10	21	21	34.7	27.3	25	48
SD	10.5	8.2	12.2	16			10.4	8.8	25.7	15.1		
SG	20.6	30.4	33	15.8	33	5	7.7	8	6.7	29	17	20
SD	10.6	11.2	15.7	9.6			5.9	11.3	9.4	12.6		
SP	29.8	40.2	6.3	35	23	11	58	28	18	23.3	3	7
SD	11.5	15.4	9.1	13.6			24	19.1	25.5	24.7		
MP	2.2	2.6	0	4	7	0	3.3	0	0	1.7	0	0
SD	3.9	5.2	0	6.9			2.9	0	0	1.7	0	0
IT	10.2	6.8	9	12.8	17	28	6	32	6.7	3.3	15	13
SD	10.3	6.1	9	12.7			8.4	18	5.3	2.5		
SM and LG	0	0	9.5	1.3	2	0	1.3	3	2.3	4.7	1	0
SD	0	0	10.4	2.1			1.9	3.5	3.3	5.2		
VC	16.6	19	2.5	11.3	0	0	6.7	12.7	0	0	0	4
SD	16.2	21.8	4.2	6.6			7.4	13.9	0	0		
LO	73.4	79.4	63	64.3	49	65	42.3	62.3	57	68.3	64	80
SD	15.2	10.1	10.6	25.1			17.9	22.9	9.4	27.8		

Note: NOP = natural; POP = phased; RC = reaching; SG = simple grasp; SP = simple play; MP = mutual play with mother; IT = intentionality toward object; SM & LG = smiling and laughing; VC = vocalizing; LO = looking at object.

aspects of maternal imitation and slower pacing of the mother's behavior, they also suggest caution. It seems that in some cases such a strategy's effects could be detrimental to the mother's feelings, the infant's responsiveness, and the interactive process as a whole.

As demonstrated by this last study, mothers often used objects quite naturally as part of interactions with their infants with Down syndrome already during the first 6 months, and the infants showed occasional interest reaching and even simple play with these. Although they were not as yet making any manifest connection between the object and the mother, and responded as if they were quite separate and unrelated, such early play with objects was clearly an important preparation for making a transition into the next stage of interactive development.

From 9 months till the 3rd year of life: secondary intersubjectivity

This transition marks, in fact, the beginning of a long process in which the two most important areas of the children's understanding and functioning begin manifestly to interact. Namely, at this period of developmental transition, infants are capable of coordinating their understanding and use of the physical environment and their ability to interact and communicate with other people. While the former constitutes the basis of important areas of cognitive and practical functioning – such as understanding of spatial relations between objects and their various other properties, use of tools, operational and logical thought, classification abilities, conceptual thought, and constructional skills – the growth of communicative competence is indispensable for the ability to receive and share information with other people, and for becoming a fully functioning member of a social group and of the human community.

Recent studies show that the infants' growing interest and competence with objects are instrumental in transferring the focus of parent–infant interactions exclusively from the participants themselves toward transactions and actions related to objects. The joint attention of the participants and their respective demands, expectations, messages, and activities thus become increasingly influenced and dominated by the objective reality (e.g., Crawley et al., 1978; Gray, 1978; Pawlby, 1977; Schaffer, Collis, & Parsons, 1977; Trevarthen, 1977; Winnicott, 1971).

Landry and Chapieski (1989) have started to explore the joint attentional abilities and object exploration of infants with Down syndrome. In one study, Landry and Chapieski (1987) found that 6-month-old infants with Down syndrome had more difficulty in attending to both toys and their mothers than normally developing infants of the same chronological age. They noted, however, that the joint-attentional abilities in the infants with Down syndrome could be enhanced by their mothers' responsivity. For example, when mothers attempted to maintain their infants' attention to the toys rather than to redirect their attention to new toys, the infants demonstrated more joint attention.

At 12 months, difficulties in joint attention were present in addition to diminished interest in the object world (Landry & Chapieski, 1989). Within this study, infants with Down syndrome as a group manipulated toys less than other infants of the same developmental level. Parents of infants with Down syndrome, however, appeared to compensate for their infants' low responsivity through their actions. For example, mothers of infants with Down syndrome tended physically to orient their infants to toys and to present more toys to their infants more often than mothers of premature infants.

Additionally, at this age, when mothers attempted to direct their infants' attention to a toy, the infants with Down syndrome seemed to become distracted and tended either to look at their mothers or to cease playing with the toys. Landry and Chapieski argue that the mothers' attempt to direct their infants' attention overtaxes the infants' attentional capacity: They cannot simultaneously attend to the toys and interact with the caregiver. Thus, they withdraw from playing. Landry and Chapieski note that this response is also apparent in premature infants of similar chronological age and developmental level who have had various neurological insults. However, infants with Down syndrome seem to be more susceptible to being overtaxed than the premature infants – even when developmental level is controlled.

Thus, these studies suggest that infants with Down syndrome demonstrate less interest in the object world than other infants. When they do explore their environment, however, their attention can be easily overtaxed and disrupted. Mothers' attempts to direct or redirect their infants' attention during play interactions in most cases decreased the infants' manipulation of objects. This type of response indicates that infants with Down syndrome have marked difficulty in maintaining joint attention to their caregivers and objects at 12 months.

Researchers into the early development of retarded children have also begun to realize that many of the communicative and linguistic problems of these children may be related to their difficulties in playing with and understanding objects (e.g., Filler, Bricker, & Smith, 1973; Krakow & Kopp, 1983; McConkey & Martin, 1983, 1985; Mitchell, 1976, 1980; Mogford, 1979). Probably the most comprehensive study to date addressing itself to the exploration of the different interactive strategies during such interactions was carried out by Mogford (1979). Her sample, which consisted of several etiologically and functionally distinct groups of handicapping conditions (e.g., cerebral palsy, mental handicap, speech and language handicap), also included five children with Down syndrome between 1 and 5 years of age. Her study centered around a detailed analysis of children's play episodes with a range of toys, both with and without the participation of their mothers.

Mogford's theoretical position assumed that play was of fundamental importance for children's intellectual and adaptive development. Moreover, in her review of literature she drew attention to the number of findings that indicate that with handicapped children, play may often be hampered rather than facilitated through parental participation. For example, Shere and Kastenbaum (1966) found that mothers of severely handicapped children tended to be so preoccupied with mobility and speech that they almost totally ignored play activities. Even when play did occur, Jeffree and Cashdan (1971) and Terdal, Jackson, and Gardner (1976) observed unusually high rates of maternal commands and questions that were, more often than not, ineffective and gave these transactions a noncontingent controlling character. A quoted report by Corrigal also showed that whereas infants with Down syndrome were not less sociable during interactions with mothers in the first year of life, by 15 months of age there was still no evidence of social reciprocal games involving objects.

Mogford thus focused much of her analysis on identifying the nature of various parental, social, and interactive behaviors and their negative as well as positive effects on the children's play.

The results concerning the five subjects with Down syndrome (who were, incidentally, among the least retarded and showed more even developmental profiles than the other children in her sample) indicated great individual differences in the mothers' interactive styles, ranging from very child-dependent and responsive to highly controlling and mother-dominated ones. Although she was not able to find any significant correlations between the different maternal styles and the children's degree of developmental handicap (which would have been questionable in any case because of the small size of the sample), she noted that the children of mothers with the strongest controlling and explicitly "pedagogic" styles were rated lowest on initiative and independence of play. Mogford also found that at least some of the mothers tried hard to extend the children's activity by imitative elaborations and demonstrations, which apparently were usually successful.

Although it is difficult to gain any clear picture from these findings about the relationships between the mothers' interactive strategies and their children's age, play, and communicative functioning, the interactive problems related to excessive maternal control and directiveness appeared to be on the whole less serious in the case of children with Down syndrome than with most of the other dyads in her sample. Nevertheless, Mogford described a number of instances of non-mesh controlling interventions by the mothers of children with Down syndrome, such as when a mother tried hard to make her son say something while he appeared either unable or unwilling to do so. Another mother was trying to elicit a social response while the child was involved in a constructive object play, which was thus disrupted. She also found that during so-called nonparticipant sessions (i.e., mothers asked not to interact with children), some children demonstrated higher levels and more varied play behaviors, which during the mothers' participation sessions were often persistently but unsuccessfully urged by the mothers. Generally, instances of non-mesh interventions were associated with an apparent attempt by the mothers to bring about a particular end result, and her consequent failure to monitor the child's own activity. This led eventually in most such cases to a breakdown of smooth interactions. Despite its limitations with respect to data about infants with Down syndrome, Mogford's study represents a valuable contribution to our understanding of the different kinds of transactions associated with "remedial" play between mothers and their young handicapped children. Therefore, it seems worthwhile to summarize some of her main conclusions:

1. Specific teaching goals appeared to detract from the mothers' supportive role in the interactions, and a repeated failure to achieve such a goal led usually to a

rejection of the relevant toy. This was often due to the mother's pitching her demands too high.

2. Mothers of handicapped children appeared to interpret play-session and any other remedially oriented interactions as requiring them to "work harder." This again seemed to be counterproductive.

3. There was often a discrepancy between the perception of play success by the mothers and the quality of play as observed by the researcher. This "underevaluation" by mothers may have resulted from comparisons with nonhandicapped children, although the play may have in fact included a number of positive features, such as a smooth flow of cooperative activities, communication, and extension of the child's behavior into areas and forms hardly possible if unaided.

4. The type of experience handicapped children received during remedial play with mothers verged on being "more and different" rather than "more of the same or similar." There was also much greater determination and control of their play activities than in nonhandicapped children, and in this sense the remedial play exercises did not appear to "normalize" the handicapped children's experience.

5. Repetitions of play routines, when they occurred, led to increased participation by the child and were almost never stereotyped, but rather were progressive in nature in that they tended to facilitate new elements of the child's participation. Overall, the mother's participation was associated with longer play episodes by the handicapped children.

As will become apparent, many of these observations are consistent with the findings reported by Olwen Jones regarding infants with Down syndrome only. In her home-based study Jones (1977, 1980) investigated several features of play interactions between six infants with Down syndrome (13 to 23 months old) and of six developmentally matched nonhandicapped infant–mother pairs (8 to 18 months old). During the recording sessions the mothers were instructed to play with their children as they normally would and to use either their child's favorite toys or a standard set provided by the investigator. Some of the main findings were as follows:

1. There were significantly more unsuccessful invitations to interact from the mothers of the Down syndrome infants.

2. Although the overall interactive time was about the same for the two groups, the infants with Down syndrome were involved in a larger number of separate interactive episodés, indicating that these were on average shorter than those of the nonhandicapped infants.

3. The mothers of Down syndrome infants were more directive and less child-dependent during the interactive exchanges and consequently the infants experienced relatively less responsive interpretations and support of their own activities.

4. The vocalizations of the infants with Down syndrome were more repetitive, dense, and randomly spaced, thus allowing mothers fewer and less predictable spaces for their own responses. This apparently also contributed to the mothers' feeling of being "left out."

5. As noted earlier, Jones also reported less referential but more personal eye contact by the infants with Down syndrome.

Several conclusions were drawn by Jones. First, she argued that the children with Down syndrome were not as often as their nonhandicapped counterparts in situations where the mother allowed them the freedom to choose the topic of "conversation." Second, the data on eye contact suggest that the children with Down syndrome were not drawing out feedback from their mothers to the same extent as did the nonhandicapped children. Third, while the infants with Down syndrome produced as much and varied vocal output as the nonhandicapped children, the context in which it was employed was more often inconsiderate of the requirements of vocal dialogue.

Although Jones offered a number of (speculative) suggestions as to the reasons for these interactive deviations, she avoided allocating blame for them to either partner. The only exception was the poor vocal turn-taking skill of the infants with Down syndrome. She suggested that the apparently greater frequency of vocal clashes seemed to be the children's "fault" in that their vocalizations usually started when the mother had already started speaking. The earlier mentioned study of 3-year-old children with Down syndrome by Peskett and Wootton (1985) suggests, however, that more thorough analyses of the precise nature of such vocal overlaps are needed. Their results showed that even in the worse case, less than 6% of all the infant's communicative vocalizations could be considered as genuine clashes. Furthermore, the amount of such "midunit" overlaps (i.e., clashes) were related to the children's general level of communicative development, as was also the variety and use of repair, overlap-sensitive techniques. As no comparison group was used in this study it is unfortunately not possible to ascertain how these findings compare to vocal interactions by nonhandicapped children. It should also be noted that the data in this study were recorded by the parents themselves under a variety of ordinary home situations. The discrepancies between these and other findings underline the need for replications of studies, regard for situational and age variables, and a careful analysis of data, before any generalizations are made.

As to the greater directiveness of the mothers of infants with Down syndrome, Jones speculated that this might have developed because of the children's relative passivity, for example, in that they initiated sequences less frequently than their nonhandicapped counterparts, or because the mothers believed them to be so and were more concerned to "help" their child's development. This is similar to the argument by Sorce and Emde (1982) noted earlier.

In discussing the infants' lack of referential eye contact, Jones argues that this was probably not due to their not having reached a sufficient level of cognitive competence to cope with a three-way reference situation (i.e., Self–Other–Object), as they all showed referent looking occasionally, and no correlation was found between its frequency and the developmental age. Although not offering any explanation for this deficiency, Jones argues that through it the children with Down syndrome were depriving themselves of a powerful and important communicative signal, one that is a prelinguistic form of later question–comment, and which already at this early stage is instrumental in eliciting a contingent explanation, elaboration, interpretation, or affirmation from the mother. Other reports of deficient referential gazing both in younger (i.e., Gunn et al., 1982), and older (Krakow & Kopp, 1983) children with Down syndrome, were considered earlier, together with some of their developmental implications (see section on the first month). In addition, this lack of referential gazing is also a likely factor in the mothers' reported difficulties in "reading" and interpreting their infants' signals and needs (Jones, 1980). Among other problems mentioned by mothers in this study were not knowing whether the children were addressing their vocalizations to them, difficulties in interpreting the child's needs because of a limited number of cues, confusion as to the child's participation in interactive exchanges because of lack of eye contact, and difficulties in attracting the child's attention.

Interviews with the mothers of these infants with Down syndrome also revealed a strong tendency to refer repeatedly to "teaching" their child during verbal interactions and to enjoying most of all their successes in teaching situations. By contrast, the comparison group of mothers of the nonhandicapped infants referred more often to enjoying their children for themselves and their company. Furthermore, the mothers of the Down syndrome children expressed more anxiety about their children's various behaviors being socially unacceptable, although the same behaviors when observed in nonhandicapped children were seen by their mothers as being quite normal. It is likely that such excessive concern and anxiety over the child's performance and behavior is often transmitted onto the children (e.g., Winnicott, 1971) and affect adversely their interactions and relationship. David and Appell (1969) noted how "the anxiety and frustration of the mother lead over and over again to interactions which are frustrating for both infant and mother and which increase the handicap" (p. 181). This in fact may also lie behind the infants' lack of referential looking at mothers. Because eye contact does not appear to be deficient in situations not involving play with objects, it seems quite possible that the children may be actively avoiding eye contact in anxiety-laden situations associated with excessive demands on their understanding and performance (e.g., Jones, 1980; Mogford, 1979), and with stressful interactions generally (e.g., Kogan, 1980). It is probably the interaction between these children's inherent difficulties in coping both with objects and with the mothers' attempts to "teach" them to cope better and respond more, which gradually leads to any increasingly intense, directive, and intrusive interactive style. Unfortunately, this appears to be counterproductive in that it tends further to increase the child's emotional discomfort, hinders the opportunities for both play with objects and reciprocal communication, and reduces the likelihood of enjoyment and learning within the context of rewarding interactions. Circumstantial and clinical evidence point to the role of an object or, more precisely, to demands on the handicapped child's performance with objects, as one of the critical factors in setting up such a self-perpetuating spiral of negative interactions. For example, as noted earlier in this section, Mogford (1979) found that handicapped children often played better when their mothers were not directly involved. Dunst (1981) reported more smiling by children with Down syndrome when performing tasks that were well familiarized and within their competence than those more novel and difficult. We have observed in a number of home situations that siblings who were evidently not as anxious as parents about the performance of their brother or sister with Down syndrome, were more often much more effective in eliciting play behaviors than were the parents (Berger & Cunningham, 1983a, 1983b). And Jones (1977, 1980) found relatively normal "personal" eye contact, but a deficient one when object-related activities were involved. It is likely that the Down syndrome infants' difficulties with reaching and other fine manipulative and tactile actions (e.g., Cunningham, 1979; Frith & Frith, 1974; Gibson, 1978; O'Connor & Hermelin, 1961), as well as their early perceptual cognitive impediments (e.g., Cicchetti & Sroufe, 1976; Johnson & Olley, 1971; Miranda & Fantz, 1973, 1974), make their object-related activities inherently more frustrating and less rewarding. By contrast, such relatively "easy" social behavior as smiling, vocalizing, and personal eye contact probably also attract more pleasurable parental responses and reinforcements. Consequently, the latter will compete with the former for the children's interest, increasingly becoming the preferred mode of interaction, mainly through the effects of selective instrumental conditioning and learning. That such learning mechanisms operate within PCIs has been demonstrated in a study by Gewirtz and Boyd (1977), in which maternal interactive behaviors were systematically changed through experimental manipulations of their infants' behavioral contingencies, using video-recording techniques.

Conversely, infants' social behaviors such as smiling and vocalizing can be brought under stimulus control through reinforcement techniques (e.g., Brackbill, 1958, 1967; Etzel & Gewirtz, 1967; Rheingold, Gewirtz, & Ross, 1959; Weisberg, 1963). The initial increase in smiling and other social behaviors during mother–infant interactions has also been attributed, at least in part, to the contingencies between maternal responses and those of the infant (e.g., Watson, 1972), that is, in an operant learning process under a different name. Indeed, a number of microanalytic studies of mother–infant interactions (e.g., Brazelton et al., 1974; Stern, 1974a, 1974b; Trevarthen, 1974; Tronick, Als, & Brazelton, 1980) have clearly demonstrated how typical such contingencies are.

When considered from the perspective of fundamental adaptive processes (Papousek & Papousek, 1979), and in particular of the functional significance of approach and avoidance behaviors, some of the above described anomalies in the handicapped infants' interactions with their parents become even more understandable. Lipsitt (1979) outlined a view of the infant as an approaching–avoiding organism vis-à-vis pleasurable and unpleasurable stimuli, and argued that pleasure and pain serve as a screen through which all sensory stimulation passes and by which it is either appreciated and perpetuated (through further approach or repetition) or censured and rejected (through various forms of avoidance behaviors). An ambivalent and potentially stressful situation arises when a particular stimulus event becomes associated with both pleasurable and unpleasurable sensations. This generates a conflict between attraction and repulsion, approach and avoidance. Some evidence indicates that unpleasant feelings and avoidance responses can arise not only in the face of physically painful and noxious stimuli but also when the infant is exposed to information that is too incongruous, complex, and difficult to assimilate or that is merely inappropriately timed (e.g., Lipsitt, 1979; Papousek & Papousek, 1979; Stern, 1971; Stern & Gibbon, 1979). Thus, an adult who presents stimulation and demands that are consistently beyond the infant's ability to assimilate and fulfill can in effect become an ambivalent and stressful stimulus. The reported preferences and willingness of infants with Down syndrome to engage in only some types of interactions (e.g., personal but not referential eye contact, boisterous physical play but not cognitively demanding interactions with objects) can then be viewed as a basic adaptive strategy partly conditioned by inappropriately pitched demands. The infants' constitutional impediments certainly play a part in such preferences and avoidance tendencies.[4]

An important recent study by Crawley and Spiker (1983) investigated individual variations in the interactions between infants with Down syndrome and their mothers, focusing particularly on the dimensions of maternal sensitivity and directiveness, and their relationship with the infants' interactive behaviors and play maturity. Through a multivariate analysis of interactive behaviors of eighteen mothers and their 2-year-old children with Down syndrome, the authors were able to highlight great individual differences as well as the makeup of the mothers' individual styles. Their most important findings were those showing that (1) maternal directiveness is not incompatible with sensitivity to the infants' behaviors and needs, although they represent separable dimensions of maternal style; (2) of all the maternal variables the dimension called "stimulation value" (i.e., degree to which mother's participating in play provides optimal cognitive stimulation) was most highly correlated with the child's developmental level (Bayley Mental Development Index scores), play maturity, and social responsiveness; (3) mothers who were highly sensitive and highly directive were also rated high on stimulation value; (4) only 44% of the mothers were rated as being consistently appropriate with respect to intrusiveness; (5) directiveness was the only maternal dimension showing a statistically significant negative correlation with infants' object initiative; (6) the infants' social responsivity was positively correlated with the MDI scores, play maturity, and social initiative; (7) the dyadic rating of mutuality was also positively correlated with these infants' variables; and (8) almost 50% of the mothers were rated as being appropriate on all the subcomponents of sensitivity and directiveness. Crawley and Spiker (1983) concluded that "these observations were in marked contrast, however, to the picture usually portrayed in the literature of mothers of handicapped children as being highly directive and intrusive" (p. 1320). Nevertheless, the relatively great proportion of the mothers who scored highly on the intrusiveness subscale is indicative of, and consistent with, the type of maternal style reported by other studies. Unfortunately, as no comparison group of nonhandicapped infant–mother pairs was included in the Crawley and Spiker study, it is difficult to judge to what extent the intrusiveness of the mothers of the children with Down syndrome deviated from the norm. Another important conclusion drawn from these findings is that sensitivity and elaborativeness alone do not correlate significantly with the infants' measures of play maturity, initiative, or developmental age, nor does maternal directiveness alone necessarily inhibit the infant's development. It would seem, however, that a combination of high sensitivity, elaborativeness, and directiveness may constitute the most optimal maternal style conducive to these infants' development, but that directiveness without such ingredients does interfere with social and cognitive growth.[5]

Language and parent–child interactions

Probably the largest group of studies on PCIs concerning infants with Down syndrome are those focusing on various aspects of linguistic interactions, language stimulation, and functioning. This is partly a reflection of the marked and apparently disproportionate deficits in their language relative to the other aspects of their development (e.g., Carr, 1975; Cheseldine, 1977; Gibson, 1978; Johnson & Olley, 1971) and in comparison to other retarded children (e.g., Lyle, 1959, 1960), and partly due to the recognition that early linguistic environment can have a considerable long-term influence on the child's linguistic development (e.g., Bateson, 1975; Birrer, 1977; Bruner, 1977; Cross, 1976).

The rationale for much of the research into prelinguistic interactions generally is thus embedded in the notion that such interactions are an important prerequisite for later linguistic communications (e.g., Bruner, 1975; Bullowa, 1979; Lewis & Freedle, 1973; Mahoney, 1975; Roe, McClure, & Roe, 1982).

A number of studies investigating maternal speech during interactions with their prelinguistic infants with Down syndrome have reported consistently higher densities and rates of speech directed at the infant (Berger & Cunningham, 1983a; Buckhalt et al., 1978; Buium, Rynders, & Turnure, 1974; Davis & Oliver, 1980). The only exception has been a study with somewhat older children (3 to 12 years) by Rondal (1977), which found no significant difference in the mothers' word rate as compared to a group of mothers of nonhandicapped children matched on the mean length of utterance (MLU). Some of these studies have also identified a higher directive quality of the mothers' speech, particularly as related to the infants activities with objects (e.g., Cunningham, Reuler, Blackwell, & Deck, 1981; McConkey & Martin, 1984). These findings are thus in line with those discussed in an earlier section, documenting further the apparent tendency of mothers to dominate the interactions and direct the activities of their children with Down syndrome.

The findings concerning several other characteristics of maternal speech, such as its grammatical complexity and MLU, are less consistent but in general appear to indicate a relatively "normal" pattern (Buckhalt et al., 1978; Gunn, Clark, & Berry, 1980; McConkey & Martin, 1984; Rondal, 1978). On the basis of such "grammatical" data analyses McConkey and Martin concluded that there was little evidence to show that some of the delays in the language acquisition of Down syndrome children could in general be attributed to an atypical linguistic environment provided by the parents, even though it may be so for certain individuals. In their longitudinal study of 12- to 24-month-old infants with Down syndrome, McConkey and Martin (1984) recorded mothers' language and analyzed its relationship to the infants' vocalizations as well as to their actions with a standard set of toys. They found significant age-related increases in the proportion of maternal commands, although no changes were registered in the infants' vocal behaviors, but only in the frequency of their play with objects. The authors suggest that the mothers seemed to be estimating the children's ability to understand language from the way they played with toys, and were adjusting their speech accordingly. Consequently, they argued, more attention should be paid to the infants' sensorimotor functioning and their overall nonverbal understanding of the physical world in order to understand and optimize their social interactions and communicative development. This is consistent with some findings that nonverbal understanding may be an essential prerequisite to the development of linguistic competence, at least during the first few years of life (e.g., Bretherton, Bates, Benigni, Camaioni, & Voltera, 1980; Lobato, Barrera, & Fieldman, 1981).

In a study focusing on what mothers actually do rather than say, McConkey and Martin (1983) showed that during free play, mothers of 1- to 2-year-old infants with Down syndrome used far more physical prompting in the course of play with a ring-stacking toy than with a doll set. Because the former represents a relatively more structured situation with a clearly defined end point, this finding provides a useful indication about the mothers' spontaneous adaptations and involvement under marginally different play contexts. This study also shows that as the infants became older and their play more mature, the mothers' actions also changed. In particular the modeling of more simple relational play decreased and was gradually replaced by more advanced sequence-pretend models in the doll play situation. Similarly, in the ring-stacking situation, the mothers were using increasingly more gestural prompts as the children became more competent, while their use of physical prompts decreased correspondingly. In this respect, at least, mothers appeared to adapt their interactive style quite appropriately both to the child's level of play and to the nature of the play materials. One shortcoming was, however, noted by McConkey and Martin (1984). Namely, the mothers seemed to have fairly fixed, if reasonable, expectations concerning the types of activities the children should carry out with the different toys. This, in the authors' opinion, unduly and unnecessarily restricted the range of potentially beneficial use of the materials. It is suggested that this may stem, at least in part, from the mothers' not being aware of the requisite skills and behaviors that lead to particular "landmarks" on which they choose to concentrate. This is an important point, as an encouragement of a varied practice of such requisite skills and abilities may be necessary for the infants with Down syndrome in view of the reported lack of stability in their developmental attainments on cognitive tasks (Morss, 1983) as well as the relatively stereotyped and restricted nature of their play with toys (e.g., Krakow & Kopp, 1983). In making such suggestions we should, however, also be aware of the possible danger for parent–child interactions, associated with an emphasis on "education goals."

PCI research and its implications for remedial intervention

In conclusion, some implications of the reviewed research evidence for remedial intervention with parents and their infants with Down syndrome will be considered.

The prevailing trend toward delegating back to parents the primary responsibility for their handicapped infants' early "education," and the view that satisfying reciprocal interactions between them is a vital feature of successful remedial intervention (e.g., Affleck, McGrade, McQueeny, & Allen, 1982; Berger & Cunningham, 1983b; Bromwich, 1976), make this a topical and important issue.

Moreover, as noted in an earlier section, there appear to be particular dangers as well as benefits stemming from parental involvement in early intervention, in particular for parent–infant interactions (e.g., Cunningham, 1983; Kogan, 1980; Mogford, 1979).

Once the parents overcome the initial shock and grief over the birth of an infant with Down syndrome and begin to mobilize their energies and resources toward doing something to help their baby's development, it is not uncommon for some of them to become caught up in a conflict between stimulating and exercising the infant as much as possible, and feeling that they also want to treat her or him as just a "normal" baby. In following either course, they can feel guilt either for not seeming to be doing enough or for pushing the baby too hard. A main function of early intervention should be to help parents with such conflicting emotions, and enable them to reconcile and harmonize their own intuitive style and preferences with their infant's needs for optimal or at least "good enough" stimulation.

There is a wide consensus about the need for, and benefits of, such early intervention, both for parents and for infants (e.g., Affleck et al., 1982; Cunningham, 1983; Sax, 1981). It has been noted, for example, that practical advice concerning early sensory and motor stimulation often helps parents overcome their initial uncertainties and inhibitions about handling their young infants with Down syndrome, and thus facilitates more positive all-round interactions. Furthermore, the feeling by parents that they can do something helpful for the baby, and the positive attitude implied within such an intervention approach, are certainly also beneficial. Among the main principles of early intervention should, however, be an emphasis on providing infants with only as much as they can cope with and respond to, whether in the form of social or general sensorimotor stimulation. An approach tempered by such a commonsense guideline is more likely to facilitate reciprocal interactions, the infant's active involvement, and enjoyment by both partners.

This is especially important in view of the findings that mothers of infants with Down syndrome often begin to manifest unusually high levels of vocal activity when their babies are only about 3 or 4 months old; and that such excessive activity seems to become a characteristic feature of the mothers' interactive behavior from then on. It would thus seem desirable to start helping mothers to adopt a more relaxed and reciprocal attitude as early as possible, and before this overly intense mode has become too strongly established. If successful, such help should also reduce the infants' need to rely on various avoidance and defensive maneuvers in order to protect themselves from a "flood" of stimulation that they cannot, or at least feel they cannot, cope with. The available evidence indicates that such avoidance behaviors may become an integral part of the infants' interactive style, perhaps already by the end of the first year of life (e.g., the lack of referential eye contact).[6]

There is, however, also some encouraging evidence that mothers of infants with Down syndrome are quite able to employ appropriate and effective interactive strategies that seem to facilitate the infants' constructive play with objects and more adaptive and enjoyable social transactions. Let us briefly summarize some of the main features of such adaptive strategies. Entering a hypothetical flow of interactive behaviors at the parent input stage, consider a situation involving play with objects. If the main goal is to activate and maintain the infant's motivation to play with the materials provided and cooperate with the adult, it is essential that the materials and the parent allow the infant to carry out activities already within his or her sphere of competence and understanding (e.g., Dunst, 1981; Harter, 1978; Harter, Schultz, & Blum, 1974). The task–material arrangement appears to be also of utmost importance, particularly for a handicapped infant (e.g., Filler et al., 1973). In the case of some infants with Down syndrome, however, a mere presentation of even highly familiar and attractive materials may not be enough to ensure optimal and active involvement of sufficient variety and intensity. In order to compensate for their constitutional difficulties with object-directed activities such as reaching, manipulation, and relational play (e.g., Cunningham, 1979; Firth & Firth, 1974), a considerable amount of prompting and guidance may often be required (e.g., Cicchetti & Sroufe, 1978; Cunningham & Sloper, 1977).

Considering the degree to which a parent can make his or her presence felt to the child during such guidance, there is a continuum from an almost impersonal presentation of materials and guidance to a very social intense presentation involving eye contact, speech, gestures, and physical prompting or guidance of the child. It would seem that a reduction in the mother's verbal attention bids, imperatives, questions, and demands with which the child evidently cannot cope, would be highly beneficial.[7] Nevertheless, a degree of directive intervention in the form of modeling of activities, and even physical guidance and prompting can at the same time be also usefully employed, if pitched at the appropriate developmental level and conducted in a socially unobtrusive manner. For example, as shown by McConkey & Martin (1985), play of 2-year-old children with Down syndrome can be facilitated by their mothers, particularly when they play with the toys themselves and the demonstrated behaviors are well matched to the child's current level of play. However, although these authors suggest that such matching involves modeling activities just above the infants' ability level, other authors (e.g., Mogford, 1979) suggest that repetition of play routines already within the child's repertoire may be more beneficial. Probably both of these approaches are important and should be part of "good enough" strategies. Whereas the latter tends to facilititate essential practice consolidation and generalization of already existing abilities, the former strategy can, if done sensitively, introduce the infant to less familiar and developmentally important "new" areas.

Let us now consider some aspects of parental feedback to the various forms of infant activity.

In wider terms the parental feedback strategies are probably determined by their general perception of, and attitude to, play interactions. As noted by Mogford (1979), parents can conceive of them either as a medium for didactic teaching, characterized by rigorous correcting of "mistakes," and close adherence to the parsimony of the materials, or they can be seen as an opportunity to allow the child to experiment, make mistakes, struggle a bit, and have a good time.[8]

More specifically, the infant can either (1) comply fully with the parent's explicitly communicated or implicitly held expectation; (2) she or he can comply only partially; or (3) she or he can respond in a way that is either entirely at odds or unrelated to the parent's expectations. Although all of these possible responses can be potentially beneficial for the child's learning and the interactive process itself, their actual value is probably determined to the greatest extent by the parent's response to it.

In the first two instances, parental strategies involving further facilitation, modeling, elaboration, and extension of the child's actions are probably best. On the other hand, if the parent either rebukes the child for a partially compliant response, or begins to intrude into the child's activity the consequences for the interaction and for the infant's further play are more likely to be negative. The principles of taking up the child's lead, providing sufficient response opportunities to behave autonomously, and giving positive and reciprocal feedback when requested, would in general seem to be paramount.

When the infant's response is clearly noncompliant, but could still be seen as adaptive and appropriate in more general terms, the same guidelines as those given above should apply. The parental response could then be evaluated according to whether it facilitated or hindered further positive interactions and constructive activity by the infant.

When the infant exhibits a "problem" behavior that is clearly inappropriate even by the most generous standards, a different kind of parental response strategy may be called for. These can range from physical restraint and forceful reprimand to a gentle distraction by introducing a new activity or toy. There appear to be, however, no reported studies concerning such types of interactions in the case of infants with Down syndrome, and therefore the area will not be pursued further here.

Finally, let us consider a briefly common form of parental feedback, namely, praise and other approving reactions such as clapping and cheering the infant's "successful" performances. Although these are often emphasized and recommended by professionals involved in early intervention, their value and possible consequences are dubious when used too liberally during play interactions. On the theoretical level, several questions come to mind. First, as "normal" play is characterized primarily by intrinsic reinforcement and motivation, what are the likely effects of consistently using extrinsic reinforcers within such contexts? Second, in view of the fact that "success" (as defined by external criteria and rewards) is not a usual feature of young children's play and spontaneous exploratory activities, what are the likely effects of imposing and emphasizing such adult criteria in these contexts? Third, are not the combination of the cognitive and functional fragility and instability of infants with Down syndrome, and the tendency of parents to have unrealistic expectations, likely to result in stressful experiences, especially when the child desires the parent's approval and praise but feels at the same time unable to get it? Moreover, we have often noted that parent's praise or clapping also tend to disrupt the child's attention and fragment the continuity of his or her play. This was especially noticeable when the praise was used very often and without an apparent regard for the nature of the activity. Frequently the children themselves started to interrupt the flow of their activity and demand parental praise after having performed the tiniest segments of "appropriate" behavior. Although these observations have not been properly recorded, they were common and rather typical. They are indicative of a possible origin of an excessive and counterproductive dependence on extrinsic reinforcement. Inasmuch as one of the paramount aims of remedial intervention should be the fostering of independence, autonomy, and "normal" communications, the strategy appears to be anomalous and inappropriate. The use of systematic and liberal parental reinforcement may, however, be better and more appropriately used in other types of interactions, such as those concerned with encouraging particular social or self-help skills.

Conclusions

Let us conclude by summarizing some of the main points and issues that have emerged from the preceding review and discussion of research findings.

1. In the majority, infants with Down syndrome are able to enter into reciprocal interactions with their parents soon after birth. Their main social signaling behaviors such as smiling, eye contact, and vocalizing usually emerge with only minor delays and distortions. This also seems to help parents to establish and continue more positive attitudes and feelings toward their baby, and to begin overcoming the initial shock and despair. Nevertheless, there is also little doubt that while such early interactions are possible and play an important role for both the parents in the infants' development, they also tend to be in some ways different from those enjoyed by nonretarded infants and their parents. The ever-present, if not always manifest, feelings of sadness, inner conflict, and doubt on the part of the parents seem to be often among such difficulties coloring the early interactions. There are considerable individual differences, both in the infants' social and general ability, and in the parents' emotional resilience and acceptance of their handicapped babies. Consequently, the nature and quality of the parent–infant interactions also vary considerably, according to these and other, more peripheral, factors. It would therefore be inappropriate to make any broad generalizations about them. Rather, each individual case should be seen and considered in its own right, as a complex and open system with many different influences, regulatory mechanisms, and a potential for self-repair and change.

2. There can be little doubt, however, that even the least retarded infants and the most robust of parents are likely to encounter many difficulties, both during the period of initial adaptation after the birth, and later on throughout the different phases of development. Sympathetic yet realistic and well-informed professional help can play an invaluable role in aiding parents to come to terms with and resolve

their personal difficulties, to begin to take positive measures in facilitating their infants' development, and to establish more enjoyable and beneficial interactions.

3. The main problems in the area of parent–infant interactions seems to stem on the whole not from a lack of time spent in interpersonal contact, but rather in certain qualitative aspects of the interactions. It would appear that especially during the second year of life, parents often begin to make too great demands on their children's performance and understanding. Much of the interaction seems to be colored and dominated by misguided if well-meant educational expectations, rather than being enjoyed for its own sake. Rather than helping the infant or the parent, this tends to lead to frustration, stress, and breakdowns of the natural flow of activity, both individual and interpersonal. It has been argued that there are probably several reasons for such interactive problems, some of them related to the children's developmental and functional difficulties, and some to the parents' natural and legitimate concerns and worries.

Unfortunately, some problems also seem to be related to the prevailing emphasis on early stimulation and parental responsibility in facilitating the children's learning and development. Thus, it may be that in their eagerness to help these children and their families, professional workers have been instrumental in creating a new kind of problem. The pendulum seems to have swung too far from doing too little, to perhaps doing too much, or not quite what is always needed or most beneficial.

4. It has also been shown that many parents of children with Down syndrome are able to estimate their child's functional and competence level quite accurately, and pitch their own behavior appropriately to this. In such cases, interactions tend to be characterized by a smooth flow of interpersonal behaviors as well as of the children's play, and by a positive atmosphere of enjoyment of, and respect for the child's individuality. It has also been shown in a few studies that when interactions are less enjoyable and more stressful, it is at least sometimes possible to improve their quality through professional intervention. The cornerstone of such intervention is to help the parents to observe, appreciate, and respond to their children's current behaviors and abilities, rather than to worry about what they should be doing and learning next. The emphasis on understanding, encouraging, and building on current abilities, both of the child and of the parent, should, in our opinion, be the main guiding principle of remedial intervention as well as of parent–child interactions generally (see Cunningham, 1982; Spiker, Chapter 13, this volume).

Notes

1 Emde & Brown also noted the frequently biphasic nature of the grieving process due to the Down syndrome infants' defects and delays in early signaling behaviors such as eye contact and smiling. This apparently often leads to newly felt disappointment after the initial shock has been overcome.

2 Despite this, and the frequent remarks by the mothers as to how much their Down syndrome infants smiled during the Imitation condition, they showed no significant change in their interactive behavior during the immediately following Natural condition, reverting back to their usual style.

3 In particular, this will include an examination of the timing of maternal stimulation, its phasing with the infants' behaviors, the modalities used in stimulating and responding to the infants, and the dif-

ferential effectiveness of the Imitation and Slowed-down object play conditions in relation to the infants' movement and other developmental problems.

4 Some research findings can help us appreciate how difficult it must be for these mothers to estimate accurately their handicapped children's real levels of understanding and competence. Thus, for example, Krakow and Kopp (1983) reported that although children with Down syndrome show types of play superficially similar (e.g., with dolls, cars, bricks, etc.) to those of their developmentally matched nondelayed peers, the quality of their play was significantly different. In particular, they showed much more stereotyped and regressive patterns of play, more throwing behavior and longer periods of nonengagement. Together with other reports of performance-related problems and instabilities (e.g., Cunningham, 1979; Morss, 1981), these findings suggest a serious impoverishment of basic behavioral and cognitive patterns or schemas (Kephart, 1971; Piaget, 1952). And this would inevitably make it more difficult to cope with external demands, partly because of the children's likely insecurity stemming from the fragility and deficiency of their own abilities, and partly because such demands would be more often likely to fall above the child's real level of competence.

5 Similar differential effects of particular features of maternal styles on different areas of infants' development have been reported by Bretherton et al. (1980). Specifically, mothers' affective readiness and responsivity appeared to be related to the infant's sense of competence and confidence, whereas the content of the mother's mediation between the infant and his or her environment was more strongly associated with his or her actual competence and cognitive functioning.

6 In a study of developmental changes in infants' preferences for various kinds of auditory stimuli, Glenn and Cunningham (1983) reported that while at around 1 year of age Down syndrome infants chose to listen significantly more to mother's "baby talk" than to her adult talk, as did developmentally matched nonhandicapped infants, by about 2 years of age this preference for mother's baby talk disappeared in the Down syndrome but increased in the nonhandicapped subjects. The reasons for this finding are not clear, but it could be argued that the decline in the attractiveness of "motherese" for the Down syndrome infants may have been seen in some way related to the changes in maternal speech taking place during the second year of life. In particular, if the marked shift from maternal requests for the infant's attention to imperatives and requests for the child to carry out particular actions (McConkey & Martin, 1984) was also taking place during this period, this may have increased the frequency of unpleasurable interactions.

7 A language intervention study with 4- to 6-year-old Down syndrome children (Cheseldine & McConkey, 1979) showed that when parents were asked to teach their child during play certain phrases that were at the appropriate developmental level (e.g., two-word pivot open utterances) most of the parents were successful in that the children increased their spontaneous use of the target utterances during play. Moreover, the parents of the more "improved" children showed more significant decreases in their mean length of utterances, used altogether fewer words during play interactions, decreased their use of questions, made fewer demands on the child's verbal or nonverbal response, used more statements and fewer initiations, and responded more consistently to the child's behavior.

8 There are some indications that the so-called hovering behavior by mothers during the child's play with objects may be detrimental to even a "normal" child's interpersonal and play development (Trevarthen, personal communication) and that such a hovering style, characterized by the parent's inopportune and persistent interference in the child's activities, may be particularly common during interactions with handicapped children. Indeed, it would not be surprising to find this style. Overprotectiveness and excessive concern have been reported even for mothers who were separated from their infants only during the first few hours after delivery because of minor neonatal complications such as jaundice, slow feeding, or mild respiratory distress (Kennell, Voos, & Klaus, 1979). Furthermore, such maternal attitude often persisted over the first year of life, or even longer, although the infant's medical problem had been completely resolved before discharge from the hospital.

References

Affleck, G., McGrade, J. B., McQueeny, M., & Allen, D. (1982). Promise of relationship-focused early intervention in developmental disabilities. *Journal of Special Education, 16,* 413–430.

Aumonier, M. E., & Cunningham, C. C. (1983). Breast feeding in infants with Down Syndrome. *Child: Care, Health and Development, 9,* 357–376.

Bateson, M. C. (1975). Mother–infant exchanges: The epigenesis of conversational interaction. In D. Aronson & W. Rieber (Eds.), *Developmental psycholinguistics and communication disorders.* New York: Academy of Science.

Berger, J. 1980). *Early development of social signaling, attentional and communicative behaviors in Down syndrome and non-retarded infants.* Unpublished doctoral dissertation, University of Manchester.

Berger, J. (1983). *Home-based intervention study of interactions between mothers and their infants with Down syndrome.* Final report, Hester Adrian Research Centre, Manchester.

Berger, J., & Cunningham, C. C. (1981). Development of eye contact between mothers and normal versus Down syndrome infants. *Developmental Psychology, 17,* 678–689.

Berger, J., & Cunningham, C. C. (1983a). The development of early vocal behaviors and interactions in Down syndrome and non-handicapped infant–mother pairs. *Developmental Psychology, 19,* 322–331.

Berger, J., & Cunningham, C. C. (1983b). Early social interactions between infants with Down syndrome and their parents. *Health Visitor, 56,* 58–60.

Berger, J., & Cunningham, C. C. (1985). Aspects of the development of smiling in young infants with Down syndrome. *Child: Care, Health and Development, 12,* 13–24.

Berkson, G. (1960). An analysis of reaction time in normal and mentally deficient young men: I, II, III. *Journal of Mental Deficiency Research, 4,* 51–77.

Birrer, C. (1977). Fundamental education: Towards a theory of learning in infancy. *Genetic Psychology Monographs, 96,* 247–335.

Bowlby, J. (1969). *Attachment and loss,* Vol. 1: *Attachment.* New York: Basic Books.

Brackbill, Y. (1958). Extinction of the smiling response in infants as a function of reinforcement schedule. *Child Development, 29,* 115–124.

Brackbill, Y. (1967). The use of social reinforcement in conditioning smiling. In Y. Brackbill & G. G. Thompson (Eds.), *Behavior in infancy and early childhood.* New York: Free Press.

Brazelton, T. B., Koslowski, B., & Main, N. (1974). The origins of reciprocity: The early mother–infant interactions. In M. Lewis & L. A. Rosenblum (Eds)., *The effects of the infant on its caregiver.* New York: Wiley.

Bretherton, I., Bates, E., Benigni, C., Camaioni, L., and Voltera, V. (1980). Relationship between cognition, communication and quality of attachment. In E. Bates (Ed.), *Cognition and communication: The emergence of symbols.* London: Academic Press.

Bromwich, R. M. (1976). Focus on maternal behavior in infant intervention. *American Journal of Orthopsychiatry, 46,* 439–446.

Bronfenbrenner, U. (1979). *The ecology of human development.* Cambridge, MA: Harvard University Press.

Broussard, E. R. (1980). Assessment of the adaptive potential of the mother–infant system: The neonatal perception inventories. In P. M. Taylor (Ed.), *Parent–infant relationship.*

Bruner, J. (1975). From communication to language – A psychological perspective. *Cognition, 3,* 255–287.

Bruner, J. (1977). Early social interaction and language acquisition. In R. H. Schaffer (Ed.), *Studies in mother–infant interaction.* London: Academic Press.

Buckhalt, J. A., Rutherford, R. B., & Goldberg, K. E. (1978). Verbal and nonverbal interaction of mothers with their Down syndrome and nonretarded infants. *American Journal of Mental Deficiency, 82,* 337–343.

Buium, N., Rynders, J., & Turnure, J. (1974). Early maternal linguistic environment of normal and Down syndrome language-learning children. *American Journal of Mental Deficiency, 79,* 52–58.

Bullowa, M. (1979). Infants as conversation partners. In T. Myers (Ed.), *The development of conversation and disclosure.* Edinburgh: Edinburgh University Press.

Carr, J. (1975). Young children with Down syndrome. *IRMMH Monograph No. 4.* London: Butterworth.

Cheseldine, S. E. (1977). *Parent–child interaction and language facilitation schemes with the mentally handicapped.* Unpublished doctoral dissertation, University of Manchester.

Cheseldine, S. E., & McConkey, R. (1979). Parental speech to young Down syndrome children: An intervention study. *American Journal of Mental Deficiency, 83,* 612–620.

Cicchetti, D., & Sroufe, L. A. (1976). The relationship between affective and cognitive development in Down syndrome infants. *Child Development, 47,* 920–929.

Cicchetti, D., & Sroufe, L. A. (1978). An organizational view of affect: Illustration from the study of Down syndrome infants. In M. Lewis & L. A. Rosenblum (Eds.), *The development of affect.* New York: Plenum.

Condon, W. S., & Sander, L. W. (1974). Neonate movement is synchronized with adult speech: Interactional participation and language acquisition. *Science, 183,* 99–101.

Cowie, V. A. (1970). *A study of early development of mongols,* IRMR Monograph 1. Oxford: Pergamon.

Crawley, S. B., Rogers, P. P., Friedman, S., Iacobo, M., Criticos, A., Richardson, L., & Thompson, A. (1978). Developmental changes in the structure of mother–infant play. *Developmental Psychology, 14,* 30–36.

Crawley, S. B., & Spiker, D. (1983). Mother–child interactions involving two-year-olds with Down syndrome: A look at individual differences. *Child Development, 54,* 1312–1323.

Cross, T. G. (1976). Motherese: Its association with rate of syntactic acquisition in young children. In N. Waterson & C. Snow (Eds.), *The development of communication: Social and pragmatic factors in language acquisition,* New York: Wiley.

Crystal, D. (1976). *Child language, learning and linguistics.* London: E. Arnold.

Cunningham, C. C. (1979). *Aspects of early development in Down syndrome infants.* Unpublished doctoral dissertation, University of Manchester.

Cunningham, C. C. (1982). *Down syndrome: Introduction for parents.* London: Souvenir Press.

Cunningham, C. C. (1983). Early support and intervention: The Hester Adrian Research Centre infant project. In P. J. Mittler & H. R. McConachie (Eds.), *Parents, professionals and mentally handicapped people: Approaches to partnership.* London: Croom Helm.

Cunningham, C. C., & Berger, J. (in press). The effects of experimental manipulation on the mother-infant interactions of Down syndrome and non-handicapped dyads. Hester Adrian Research Centre, University of Manchester.

Cunningham, C. C., Morgan, P., & McGucken, R. B. (1984). Down syndrome: Is dissatisfaction with disclosure of diagnosis inevitable?, *Developmental Medicine and Child Neurology, 26,* 33–39.

Cunningham, C. C., Rueler, E., Blackwell, J., & Deck, J. (1981). Behavioral and linguistic development in the interactions of normal and retarded children with their mothers. *Child Development, 52,* 62–70.

Cunningham, C. C., & Sloper, P. (1977). *Helping your handicapped baby.* London: Souvenir Press.

Cytryn, L. (1975). Studies of behavior in children with Down syndrome. In E. J. Anthony (Ed.), *Explorations in child psychiatry.* New York: Plenum.

David, M., & Appell, G. (1969). Mother–child interaction and its impact on the child. In A. Ambrose (Ed.), *Stimulation in early infancy.* London: Academic Press.

Davis, H., & Oliver, B. (1980). A comparison of aspects of the maternal speech environment of retarded and non-retarded children. *Child: Care, Health and Development, 6,* 135–145.

Denneberg, V. H. (1979). Paradigms and paradoxes in the study of behavioral development. In E. B. Thoman (Ed.), *Origins of infant's social responsiveness.* Hillsdale, NJ: Erlbaum.

Dunst, C. J. (1981). Social concomitants of cognitive mastery in Down syndrome infants. *Infant Mental Health Journal, 2,* 144–154.

Emde, R. N., & Brown, C. (1978). Adaptation to the birth of Down syndrome infants. *Journal of American Academy for Child Psychiatry, 17,* 299–323.

Emde, R. N., Katz, E. L., & Thorpe, J. K. (1978). Emotional expression in infancy: Early deviations in Down syndrome. In M. Lewis & L. A. Rosenblum (Eds.), *The development of affect.* London: Plenum.

Etzel, B. C., & Gewirtz, J. L. (1967). Experimental modification of caretaker-maintained high-rate operant crying in 6- and 20-week-old infants: Extinction of crying with reinforcement of eye-contact and smiling. *Journal of Experimental Child Psychology, 3,* 303–317.

Field, T. M. (1977). Effects of early separation, interactive deficits, and experimental manipulation of infant–mother face-to-face interaction. *Child Development, 48,* 763–771.

Filler, J., Bricker, W., & Smith, R. (1973). Modification of maternal teaching style: The effects of task arrangement on the match-to-sample performance of delayed children. In D. Bricker & W. Bricker (Eds.), *Infant, toddler and preschool research and intervention project report–Year 3.* Institute on Mental Retardation and Intellectual Development, Nashville, TN.

Fisichelli, V. R., & Karelitz, S. (1966). Frequency spectra of the cries of normal infants and those with Down syndrome. *Psychonomic Science, 6.*

Fogel, A. (1977). Temporal organization in mother–infant face-to-face interaction. In H. R. Schaffer (Ed.), *Studies in mother–infant interaction.* London: Academic Press.

Fraiberg, S. (1975). Intervention in infancy: A program for blind infants. In B. Z. Friedlander, G. M. Sterritt, & G. E. Kirk (Eds.), *Exceptional infant* (Vol. 3). New York: Brunner/Mazel.

Frith, U., & Frith, C. D. (1974). Specific motor disabilities in Down syndrome. *Journal of Child Psychology and Psychiatry, 15,* 293–301.

Gewirtz, J. L., & Boyd, E. F. (1977). Experiments in mother–infant interaction underlying mutual attachment acquisition: The infant conditioning the mother. In T. Alloway, L. Pliner, & P. Krames (Eds.), *Attachment behavior.* New York: Plenum.

Gibson, D. (1978). *Down syndrome: The psychology of mongolism.* New York: Cambridge University Press.

Glenn, S. M., & Cunningham, C. C. (1983). What do babies listen to most? Development study of auditory preferences in nonhandicapped infants and infants with Down syndrome. *Developmental Psychology, 19,* 332–338.

Goldberg, S. (1983). Parent–infant bonding: Another look. *Child Development, 54,* 1355–1382.

Gray, H. (1978). Learning to take an object from the mother. In A. Lock (Ed.), *Action, gesture and symbol,* London: Academic Press.

Greene, J. G., Fox, N. A., & Lewis, M. (1983). The relationship between neonatal characteristics and three-month mother–infant interaction in high-risk infants. *Child Development, 54,* 1286–1296.

Gunn, P., Berry, P., & Andrews, R. J. (1982). Looking behavior of Down syndrome infants. *American Journal of Mental Deficiency, 87,* 344–347.

Gunn, P., Clark, D., & Berry, P. (1980). Maternal speech during play with a Down syndrome infant. *Mental Retardation Research, 18,* 15–18.

Gunther, M. (1961). Infant behavior at the breast. In B. M. Foss (Ed.), *Determinants of infant behavior.* London: Methuen.

Haith, M. M. (1972). The forgotten message of the infant smile. *Merrill-Palmer Quarterly, 18,* no. 4.

Haraldsdottir, G. (1983). *Early stimulation and reflexes in Down syndrome infants.* Unpublished doctoral dissertation, University of Manchester.

Harter, S. (1978). Effectance motivation reconsidered. *Human Development, 21,* 36–64.

Harter, S., Schultz, T., & Blum, B. (1974). Smiling in children as a function of their sense of mastery. *Journal of Experimental Child Psychology, 12,* 396–404.

Jaffe, J., Stern, D. N., & Peery, J. C. (1973). "Conversational" coupling of gaze behavior in prelinguistic human development. *Journal of Psycholinguistic Research, 2,* 321–330.

Jasnow, M., Crown, C. L., Feldstein, S., Taylor, L., Beebe, B., & Jaffe, J. (1988). Coordinated interpersonal timing of Down-syndrome and nondelayed infants with their mothers: Evidence for a buffered mechanism of social interaction. *Biological Bulletin, 175,* 355–360.

Jeffree, D. M., & Cashdan, A. (1971). Severely subnormal children and their parents: An experiment in language improvement. *British Journal of Educational Psychology, 41,* 184–193.

Johnson, J. T., & Olley, J. G. (1971). Behavioral comparisons of mongoloid and nonmongoloid retarded persons: A review. *American Journal of Mental Deficiency, 75,* 546–559.

Jones, O. H. M. (1977). Mother–child communication with pre-linguistic Down syndrome and normal infants. In H. R. Schaffer (Ed.), *Studies in mother–infant interaction.* London: Academic Press.

Jones, O. H. M. (1980). Prelinguistic communication skills in Down syndrome and normal infants. In T. Field, D. Goldberg, D. Stern, & A. Sostek (Eds.), *High-risk infants and children: Interactions with adults and peers.* New York: Academic Press.

Kagan, J. (1971). *Change and continuity in infancy.* New York: Wiley.

Karelitz, S., & Fisichelli, V. R. (1969). Infants' vocalizations and their significance. *Proceedings of the Children's Hospital, 25,* no. 11.

Kaye, K. (1977). Toward the origin of dialogue. In H. R. Schaffer (Ed.), *Studies in mother–infant interaction.* London: Academic Press.

Kennell, J. H., Gordon, D., & Klaus, M. (1970). The effects of early mother–infant separation on later maternal performance. *Pediatrics Research, 4,* 473–474.

Kennell, J. H., Jerauld, R., Wolfe, H., Chesler, D., Kreger, N. C., McAlpine, W., Steffa, N., & Klaus, M. H. (1974). Maternal behavior one year after early and extended post-partum contact. *Developmental Medicine and Child Neurology, 16,* 172–179.

Kennell, J. H., Voos, D. K., & Klaus, M. H. (1979). Parent–infant bonding. In J. D. Osofsky (Ed.), *Handbook of infant development.* New York: Wiley.

Kephart, N. C. (1971). *The slow learner in the classroom* (2nd ed.). Westerville, OH: Merrill.

Klaus, M. H., & Kennell, J. H. (1976). *Maternal–infant bonding.* St. Louis, MO: Mosby.

Kogan, K. L. (1980). Interaction systems between preschool handicapped or developmentally delayed children and their parents. In T. M. Field, S. Goldberg, D. Stern, & A. Sostek (Eds.), *High-risk infants and children: Interactions with adults and peers.* New York: Academic Press.

Krakow, J. B., & Kopp, C. B. (1983). The effects of developmental delay on sustained attention in young children. *Child Development, 54,* 1143–1155.

Kravitz, H., & Boehm, J. J. (1971). Rhythmic habit patterns in infancy, their sequence, age of onset and frequency. *Child Development, 42,* 399–414.

Landry, S., & Chapieski, M. L. (1989). Joint attention and infant toy exploration: Effects of Down syndrome and prematurity. *Child Development, 60,* 103–118.

Leifer, A. D., Leiderman, P. H., Barnett, C. R., & Williams, J. A. (1972). Effects of mother–infant separation on maternal attachment behavior. *Child Development, 43,* 1203–1218.

Lewis, M. M. (1959). *How children learn to speak.* New York: Basic Books.

Lewis, M., & Coates, D. L. (1980). Mother–infant interaction and cognitive development in twelve-week-old infants. *Infant Behavior and Development, 3,* 95–105.

Lewis, M., & Freedle, R. (1973). Mother–infant dyad: The cradle of meaning. In M. Lewis (Ed.), *Communication and affect: Language and thought.* New York: Academic Press.

Lipsitt, L. T. (1979). The pleasure and annoyance of infants: Approach and avoidance behavior. In E. B. Thoman (Ed.), *Origins of the infant's social responsiveness.* Hillsdale, NJ: Erlbaum.

Lobato, D., Barrera, R. D., & Fieldman, R. S. (1981). Sensorimotor functioning and prelinguistic communication of severely and profoundly retarded individuals. *American Journal of Mental Deficiency, 85,* 489–496.

Lyle, J. G. (1959). The effect of institution environment upon the verbal development of imbecile children: 1. Verbal intelligence. *Journal of Mental Deficiency Research, 3,* 122–128.

Lyle, J. G. (1960). The effect of institution environment upon the verbal development of imbecile children: 2. Speech and language. *Journal of Mental Deficiency Research, 4,* 1–13.

Mahoney, G. J. (1975). Etiological approach to delayed language acquisition. *American Journal of Mental Deficiency, 80,* 138–148.

Martin, J. A. (1981). Longitudinal study of the consequences of early mother–infant interaction: A microanalytic approach. *Monograph of the Society for Research in Child Development, 46,* no. 190.

McConkey, R., & Martin, H. (1983). Mother's play with toys: A longitudinal study with Down syndrome infants. *Child: Care, Health and Development, 3,* 215–226.

McConkey, R., & Martin, H. (1984). A longitudinal study of mother's speech to preverbal Down syndrome infants. *First Language, 5,* 41–55.

McConkey, R., & Martin, H. (1985). The development of object and pretend play in Down syndrome infants: Longitudinal study involving mothers. *Trisomy 21.*

Miranda, S. B. (1976). Visual attention in defective and high-risk infants. *Merrill-Palmer Quarterly*, 22, 201–228.

Miranda, S. B., & Fantz, R. L. (1973). Visual preferences of Down syndrome and normal infants. *Child Development*, 44, 555–561.

Miranda, S. B., & Fantz, R. L. (1974). Recognition memory in Down syndrome and normal infants. *Child Development*, 45, 651–660.

Mitchell, D. R. (1976). *Mentally handicapped children in structured dyadic communication situations with their parents.* Unpublished doctoral dissertation, University of Manchester.

Mitchell, D. R. (1980). Down syndrome children in structured dyadic communication situations with their parents. In J. Hogg & P. Mittler (Eds.), *Advances in mental handicap research* (Vol. 1). New York: Wiley.

Mogford, K. P. (1979). *Interaction and communication between handicapped children and their parents: A study of remedial play.* Unpublished doctoral dissertation, University of Nottingham.

Morss, J. R. (1983), Cognitive development in the Down syndrome infant: Slow or different? *British Journal of Educational Psychology*, 53, 40–47.

Motti, F., Cicchetti, D., & Sroufe, L. A. (1983). From infant affect expression to symbolic play: The coherence of development in Down syndrome children. *Child Development*, 54, 1168–1175.

Neubauer, P. B. (1967). The deviant infant: Perceptual misinformation. In J. Hellmuth (Ed.), *Exceptional infant* (Vol. 1). New York: Brunner/Mazel.

Newson, J. (1977). A general approach to the systematic description of mother–infant interaction. In R. H. Schaffer (Ed.), *Studies in mother–infant interaction.* London: Academic Press.

O'Connor, N., & Hermelin, B. F. (1961). Visual and stereognostic shape recognition in normal children and mongol and non-mongol imbeciles. *Journal of Mental Deficiency Research*, 5, 63–66.

Papousek, H., & Papousek, M. (1977). Mothering and the cognitive head-start: Psychobiological considerations. In H. R. Schaffer (Ed.), *Studies in mother–infant interaction.* London: Academic Press.

Papousek, H., & Papousek, M. (1979). The infant's fundamental adaptive response system in social interactions. In E. B. Thoman (Ed.), *Origins of the infant's social responsivity.* Hillsdale, NJ: Erlbaum.

Parke, R. D. (1978). Parent–infant interaction: Progress, paradigms and problems. In G. P. Sackett (Ed.), *Observing behavior*, Vol. 1: *The theory and application in mental retardation.* London: University Park Press.

Pawlby, S. J. (1977). Imitative interaction. In H. R. Schaffer (Ed.), *Studies in mother–infant interaction.* London: Academic Press.

Peskett, R., & Wootton, A. J. (1985). Turn-taking and overlap in the speech of young Down syndrome children. *Journal of Mental Deficiency Research*, 29, 263–274.

Piaget, J. (1952). *The origins of intelligence in children.* New York: International University Press.

Ravenette, A. T. (1973). Planning treatment programs for school-age children. In P. Mittler (Ed.), *Assessment for learning in the mentally handicapped* (Study Group 5). Edinburgh: Churchill Livingstone.

Rheingold, H. L., Gewirtz, J. L., & Ross, H. W. (1959). Social conditioning of vocalizations in the infant. *Journal of Comparative and Physiological Psychology*, 52, 69–73.

Richards, M.P.M. (1974). The development of psychological communication in the first year of life. In K. Connolly & J. Bruner (Eds.), *The growth of competence.* London: Academic Press.

Ringler, N. M., Kennell, J. H., Jarvella, R., Navojsky, B. J., & Klaus, M. H. (1975). Mother to child speech at 2 years: Effects of early postnatal contact. *Behavioral Pediatrics*, 86, 141–144.

Robson, K. S. (1967). The role of eye-to-eye contact in maternal–infant attachment. *Journal of Child Psychology & Psychiatry*, 8, 13–25.

Roe, K. V., McClure, A., & Roe, A. (1982). Vocal interaction at 3 months and cognitive skills at 12 years. *Developmental Psychology*, 1, 15–16.

Rondal, J. A. (1977). Maternal speech in normal and Down syndrome children. In P. Mittler (Ed.), *Research to practice in mental retardation* (Vol. 2). London: University Park Press.

Rondal, J. A. (1978). Patterns of correlations for various language measures in mother–child interactions for normal and Down syndrome children. *Language and Speech*, 242–252.

Sander, L. W., Stechler, G., Burns, P., & Julia, H. (1970). Early mother–infant interaction and 24-hour patterns of activity and sleep. *Journal of American Academy of Child Psychiatry, 9,* 103–123.

Sax, P. (1981). *Facilitating communication between mothers and infants with special needs: A rationale and guidelines for professions.* Master's thesis, University of British Columbia.

Scaife, M., & Bruner, J. The capacity for joint visual attention in the infant. *Nature, 253,* 265–266.

Scarr-Salapatek, S., & Williams, M. C. (1972). A stimulation program for low-birth-weight infants. *American Journal of Public Health, 62,* 662–667.

Schaffer, H. R. (1974). Early social behavior and the study of reciprocity. *Bulletin of British Psychological Society, 27,* 209–216.

Schaffer, H. R. (1977a). Early interactive development. In H. R. Schaffer (Ed.), *Studies in mother–infant interaction.* London: Academic Press.

Schaffer, H. R. (1977b). *Mothering.* Cambridge, MA: Harvard University Press.

Schaffer, H. R., Collis, G. M., & Parson, G. (1977). Vocal interchange and visual regard in verbal and pre-verbal children. In H. R. Schaffer (Ed.), *Studies in mother–infant interaction.* London: Academic Press.

Shere, E., & Kastenbaum, R. (1966). Mother–child interaction in cerebral palsy: Environmental and psychological obstacles to cognitive development. *Genetic Psychology Monographs, 73,* 255.

Sokoloff, N., Weintraub, D., Yaffe, S., & Blase, B. (1969). Effects of handling on the subsequent development of premature infants. *Developmental Psychology, 1,* 765–768.

Sorce, J. F., & Emde, R. N. (1982). The meaning of the infant emotional expressions: Regularities in caregiving responses in normal and Down syndrome infants. *Journal of Child Psychology and Psychiatry, 22,* 145–158.

Spitz, R. A. (1964). The derailment of dialogue: Stimulus overload, action cycles and the completion gradient. *Journal of American Psychoanalytic Association, 12,* 752–775.

Spitz, R. A. (1965). *The first year of life.* New York: International Universities Press.

Spitz, R. A., & Wolfe, R. M. (1946). The Smiling response: A contribution to the ontogenesis of social relations. *Genetic Psychology, Monograph 34,* 57–125.

Stechler, G., & Carpenter, G. (1967). A viewpoint on early affective development. In J. Hellmuth (Ed.), *Exceptional infant* (Vol. 1). New York: Brunner/Mazel.

Stern, D. N. (1971). A microanalysis of mother–infant interaction. *Journal of American Academy of Child Psychiatry, 10,* 501–517.

Stern, D. N. (1974a). Mother and infant at play: The dyadic interaction involving facial, vocal and gaze behaviors. In M. Lewis & L. A. Rosenblum (Eds.), *The effects of the infant on its caregiver.* New York: Wiley.

Stern, D. N. (1974b). The goal and structure of mother–infant play. *Journal of American Academy of Child Psychiatry, 13,* 402–421.

Stern, D. (1977). The first relationship. Cambridge, MA: Harvard University Press.

Stern, D. N., & Gibbon, J. (1979). Temporal expectancies of social behaviors in mother–infant play. In E. B. Thoman (Ed.), *Origins of infant's social responsiveness.* Hillsdale, NJ: Erlbaum.

Stern, D. N., Jaffe, J., Beebe, B., & Bennett, S. L., (1975). Vocalizing in unison and in alternation: Two models of communication within the mother–infant dyad. In D. Aaronson & W. Reiber (Eds.), *Developmental psycholinguistics and communication disorders.* New York: Academy of Science.

Sylvester-Bradley, B., & Trevarthan, N. C. (1977). Baby talk as an adaptation to the infant's communication. In N. Waterson & C. Snow (Eds.), *The development of communication.* New York: Wiley.

Terdal, L., Jackson, R. H., & Garner, A. M. (1976). Mother–child interactions: A comparison between normal and developmentally delayed groups. In E. J. Mash, L. A. Hamerlynk, & L. C. Handy (Eds.), *Behavior modification and families.* New York: Brunner/Mazel.

Thoman, E. B., Acebo, C., Dryer, C. A., Becker, P. T., & Freese, M. P. (1979). Individuality in the interactive process. In E. B. Thoman (Ed.), *Origins of the infant's social responsiveness.* Hillsdale, NJ: Erlbaum.

Trevarthen, C. (1974). Conversation with a two-month-old. *New Science* May, 230–236.

Trevarthen, C. (1977). Descriptive analyses of infant communicative behavior. In H. R. Schaffer (Ed.), *Studies in mother–infant interaction*. London: Academic Press.

Trevarthen, C. (1979). Communication and cooperation in early infancy: A description of primary intersubjectivity. In M. Bullowa (Ed.), *Before speech*. New York: Cambridge University Press.

Trevarthen, C., & Hubley, P. (1978). Secondary intersubjectivity: Confidence, confiding, and acts of meaning in the first year. In A. Lock (Ed.), *Action, gesture and symbol: The emergence of language*. London: Academic Press.

Tronick, E., Als, H., & Brazelton, T. B. (1980). Monadic phases: A structural descriptive analysis of infant–mother face-to-face interaction. *Merrill-Palmer Quarterly, 26*, 3–24.

Vine, I. (1973). The role of facial–visual signaling in early social development. In M. von Cranach & I. Vine (Eds.), *Social communication and movement*. London: Academic Press.

Watson, J. S. (1967). Memory and "contingency analysis" in infant learning. *Merrill-Palmer Quarterly, 13*, 55–76.

Watson, J. S. (1972). Smiling, cooing and "The Game." *Merrill-Palmer Quarterly, 18*, 324–339.

Weisberg, P. (1963). Social and non-social conditioning of infant vocalizations. *Child Development, 34*, 377–388.

Whitt, J. K., & Casey, P. H. (1982). The mother–infant relationship and development: The effects of pediatric intervention. *Child Development, 53*, 948–956.

Winnicott, D. W. (1971). *Playing and reality*. London: Pelican.

Wolff, P. H. (1963). Observations on the early development of smiling. In B. M. Foss (Ed.), *Determinants of infant behavior* (Vol. 1). London: Methuen.

Wolff, P. H. (1966). The causes, controls and organization of behavior in the neonate. *Psychological Issues, 5*, no. 1 (Monograph no. 7).

Wolff, P. H. (1967). The role of biological rhythms in early psychological development. *Bulletin of the Menninger Clinic, 31*, no. 4.

Wolff, P. H. (1969). The natural history of crying and other vocalizations in early infants. In B. M. Foss (Ed.), *Determinants of infant behavior* (Vol. 4). London: Methuen.

Yarrow, L. J., & Anderson, B. J. (1979). Procedures for studying parent–infant interactions: A critique. In E. B. Thoman (Ed.), *Origins of the infant's social responsiveness*. Hillsdale, NJ: Erlbaum.

Zelazo, P. R. (1972). Smiling and vocalizing: A cognitive emphasis. *Merrill-Palmer Quarterly, 18*, 349–365.

Zelazo, P. R. (1976). From reflexive to instrumental behavior. In L. P. Lipsitt (Ed.), *Developmental psychobiology–the significance of infancy*. Hillsdale, NJ: Erlbaum.

Zelazo, P. R., & Komer, J. M. (1971). Infant smiling to nonsocial stimuli and the recognition hypothesis. *Child Development, 42*, 1327–1339.

5 Attention, memory, and perception in infants with Down syndrome: a review and commentary

Sheldon Wagner, Jody M. Ganiban, and Dante Cicchetti

In recent years, interest in the development of perceptual, memory, and attentional processes in infants and children has burgeoned. A great deal of this work has been spurred by technological advances and by the development of new experimental paradigms that have made it possible to explore infants' abilities and limitations in these areas (Cicchetti & Wagner, in press). Such research has underscored the importance of examining these basic capacities in elucidating how individuals perceive and understand their world. As a result, our knowledge of the processes and mechanisms that underlie cognitive development during these periods has increased dramatically.

In this chapter, we focus upon perception, attention, and memory in infants and children with Down syndrome. Consequently, we review studies that have utilized nontraditional assessments of these abilities. We have adopted a developmental framework in our discussion of these abilities because we are interested in the ontogenesis and interactions of psychological processes over developmental time. Historically, most of the previous reviews and research on Down syndrome has been characterized by an *a-developmental* approach. In general, Down syndrome samples and normal or other mentally retarded groups of similar mental or chronological age have been compared at a single point in time. True developmental studies have been infrequently conducted because it is difficult to collect data from sufficient numbers of children with Down syndrome at several different ages and to examine them longitudinally. Additionally, another difficulty in longitudinal studies with this population resides in the controls: Over time normal controls become inappropriate owing to their accelerated rate of development. Although individuals may be matched along a specific dimension at one age (e.g., cognitive developmen-

The writing of the chapter was supported by grants from the John D. and Catherine T. MacArthur Foundation Network on Early Childhood, the March of Dimes Foundation, the National Center on Child Abuse and Neglect (90-C-1929), the National Institute of Mental Health (R01-MH37960-01), and the Spencer Foundation to author Cicchetti and by a grant from the National Institute of Mental Health (1 R03 MH 42189-01) to author Wagner. Special thanks are due to Sheree Toth for her valuable help, feedback, and suggestions and to Victoria Gill for typing this manuscript.

tal level or language skills), the rate of normal development so exceeds that of a retarded child that different controls may be necessary for each age point studied.

In this review we also discuss two fundamental issues that are often addressed in the literature with Down syndrome: (1) whether there are differences between children with Down syndrome and normally developing, nonretarded children; and (2) whether there are differences between children with Down syndrome and other mentally retarded children, organic or cultural–familial.

We will refer to the former question as the "Normalcy Question" and to the latter as the "Uniqueness Question." We have chosen "normalcy" and "uniqueness" so as to distinguish them from developmental and difference approaches to mental retardation (Cicchetti & Pogge-Hesse, 1982; Hodapp & Zigler, Chapter 1, this volume; and Zigler, 1969). The issues are in a sense independent of each other. Normalcy and uniqueness have to do with the specific effect of Down syndrome. For example, do the processes that underlie the development of children with Down syndrome differ from those of normally developing children (normalcy) or from those of other retarded children (uniqueness)? In contrast, researchers who adopt the developmental–difference approach have examined whether the development of retarded children without evidence of central nervous system dysfunctions is best understood by the same principles and mechanisms that apply to nonretarded individuals or whether it is necessary to invoke specific differences over and above a generally lower rate and asymptote of cognitive development. Those who maintain that the same mechanisms apply take a "developmental" position, while those who posit other mechanisms for retarded individuals assume a "difference" position (see Cicchetti & Beeghly, Chapter 2, this volume; Cicchetti & Ganiban, in press; Cicchetti & Pogge-Hesse, 1982; Cicchetti & Sroufe, 1978; Weisz & Yeates, 1981; Weisz & Zigler, 1979).

In general, the few infancy studies that have been conducted with the Down syndrome population have focused upon the Normalcy Question. In fact, our own view is that one of the principal justifications for conducting psychological research on Down syndrome is that it homogenizes the causal factors involved in retardation. That is, most studies that have examined the psychological development of retarded individuals have used groups of people with widely varying problems and etiology. As a result, the findings of such studies are difficult to interpret. Within these studies it is impossible to determine whether the presence or absence of group differences between retarded and normally developing samples are due to the qualities of a specific subgroup of retarded individuals with similar etiologies or are characteristic of *all* retarded individuals. Accordingly, by studying individuals with Down syndrome it becomes possible to study experiential effects on cognitive, linguistic, representational, and socioemotional development and to examine whether these ontogenetic domains manifest the same or different levels of functioning.

The slower pace of development found in Down syndrome can also be useful for examining similar stage-sequence hypotheses (see Hodapp & Zigler, Chapter 1, this volume). For example, Cicchetti and Sroufe (1978) have observed that the slower pace of development in Down syndrome can also be useful for the examination of whether the correlations among diverse domains found in studies with normal infants (such as fear on the visual cliff and Stage 4 object permanence) are truly dependent on a single underlying competence (as Piaget believed) or are just spuriously related. Because the slower pace of development in Down syndrome will better reveal "asynchronies" at the onset, researchers can demonstrate true convergences and discontinuities in functioning.

In contrast, the Uniqueness Question has been largely neglected in infancy. At least two reasons explain the absence of such studies. First, most forms of organic retardation are nonviable (Gibson, 1975). In addition, when these children do survive, they are generally profoundly retarded. Second, cultural–familial retardation is inordinately difficult to diagnose in infancy. Consequently, it is an exceedingly hard task to isolate groups of nonorganic, retarded infants.

Despite such difficulties in the infancy period, the Uniqueness Question has been a major theme in the child and adult literature. In these studies, however, individuals with Down syndrome are often compared to other retarded groups that are either etiologically heterogeneous or diagnostically undifferentiated. Conducting studies that include unspecified groups of retarded subjects seems to be justified only if the guiding view of intelligence and cognition is such that retardation is conceptualized as a homogeneous entity. That is to say, an individual is viewed as either "normal" or retarded. Such studies have implicitly concluded that the developmental processes underlying organic and nonorganic types of retardation do not differ.

Another theme of this chapter will be to examine main effects versus interactions in the attentional, memory, and perceptual capacities of individuals with Down syndrome. In any study of the differences between Down syndrome and any normal or mentally retarded group, the claim that *different* cognitive processes are involved requires the demonstration of a main effect for mental retardation (or type of retardation). To attribute a *specific* deficit to the retarded on the basis of inferior performance on one or more tasks is to confuse correlation with causation (Stanovitch, 1978). There are any number of non-task-specific factors that might produce uniformly lower performance on the part of the retarded. Such factors might include motivation, fatigue, familiarity with the stimuli, and so on. Postulating the role of a specific factor producing the delay requires the demonstration of an interaction with some stimulus condition. If children with Down syndrome are uniformly "slower" than other mentally retarded children (i.e., they score lower means), or if they get uniformly lower means than normally developing children, this does not support a Difference claim (Zigler, 1969). For a veridical difference statement to be made, the child with Down syndrome must be differentially better or worse as a function of some manipulated variable (e.g., auditory vs. visual presentation, stimulus complexity, etc.).

Additionally, we will also discuss variability in development. There seems to be an implicit notion in much of the research with older children that Down syndrome is somehow a "unitary, invariant" psychological condition, or that all children with Down syndrome of equal chronological age (CA) are the same. Investigators have sometimes ignored variability *within* Down syndrome in favor of comparisons with normal samples. Although it is true that no one truly believes that all children with Down syndrome are the same, historically there has been a lack of research concern in exploring individual differences in the cognitive, linguistic, representational, and socio-emotional functioning of children with Down syndrome. The developmental performance of children with Down syndrome – like any genotypically specified trait – has a "reaction range" of variability. For most variables, the distribution of performance within children with Down syndrome is likely to demonstrate some overlap with the distribution of scores on the same measure in normal children, even when there is a significant difference between the means of the distributions. Some infants with Down syndrome are likely to perform better than some normal, CA-matched infants on almost any measure. Indeed, it is the range and kind of variability found on a particular measure that are the most psychologically meaningful for our purposes.

Attention and memory research in infants and toddlers with Down syndrome

The vast majority of research concerning cognitive processes in children with Down syndrome has been confined to the age range from childhood to adulthood. The principal reason for this has been the unavailability of sensitive and valid intelligence and cognition instruments by which to assess *any* infancy population – to say nothing of Down syndrome. Research that has been conducted has primarily been divided into two major approaches: psychometric and information-processing. The psychometric approach has been mainly characterized by comparing the intelligence test profiles of children with Down syndrome and other normal and mentally retarded groups. Both the Normalcy and Uniqueness questions have been addressed. Gibson (1978) provides an excellent review of these findings as well as those inspired by information-processing models. A variety of studies have suggested that children with Down syndrome may have particular cognitive deficits with respect to short-term memory and certain rehearsal strategies (see Gibson, 1978).

Although the psychometric and information-processing approaches have given us valuable insights into the cognitive architecture of adolescents and adults with Down syndrome, they have not provided much of a developmental account of the cognitive mechanisms they have isolated nor have they conveyed an understanding of the abilities and deficits of *infants* with Down syndrome. One reason for this resides in the lack of valid, standardized infancy tests with long-term predictive power (see Fagan & Singer, 1983; Kopp, 1983; and Kopp & McCall, 1982, for representative reviews). Absence of long-term predictability has made it possible for researchers to identify specific abilities that shape or underlie cognitive development.

It has recently been suggested by several investigators of infant perceptual and cognitive development that the failure in predicting later outcomes stems from fundamental flaws in the infant tests themselves (Caron & Caron, 1981; Caron, Caron, & Glass, 1983; Fagan, 1985; Fagan & McGrath, 1981; Fagan & Singer, 1983;

Rose, 1981; Rose, Gottfried, & Bridger, 1978; Rose & Wallace, 1985a, 1985b). These investigators have argued that the principal confound in these tests lies in their reliance on sensorimotor competence for the passing of these items rather than on the discrimination and memorial competence required for success on later intelligence tests. To be able to predict intelligence, it is necessary to tap the same processes and behaviors known to be related to later intelligence.

Consequently, in studies that have compared the performance of infants with Down syndrome and normally developing infants on psychometric tests, there is no way to know whether differences obtained were due to inherent differences in the populations or to the imprecisions of the instruments themselves. In this review we first describe alternative methods of assessment that have demonstrated long-term predictive power, and then turn to studies that have used such methods to characterize the attention, memory, and perceptual abilities of infants and children with Down syndrome.

The infant paradigms

There has literally been a revolution in the past 10 years in our understanding and appreciation of the abilities of human infants. Studies have shown that young infants have many impressive skills, including the ability (1) to form abstract concepts after only limited exposure to categorical exemplars (Cohen, 1979); (2) to discriminate numerosities in collections of up to three or four items (Starkey & Cooper, 1980); (3) to recognize objects that they have felt but never seen (Gottfried, Rose, & Bridger, 1977; (4) to understand ''metaphors'' (Wagner, Winner, Cicchetti, & Gardner, 1980); and, (5) to recognize emotional expressions in abstracted forms (Caron, Caron, & Myers, 1982).

A good part of the revolution in the study of infant perceptual and cognitive abilities has come about through the application of four fundamental paradigms. These paradigms or procedures are generally simple and designed such that passive attention – visual, auditory, or tactual – is all that is required. Because of this they are ideally suited for use with populations of infants who have trouble moving or speaking or are otherwise developmentally disabled. Therefore, they hold great promise for use in situations where traditional assessment batteries are either not applicable or not available (Cicchetti & Wagner, in press).

Preferential looking paradigm

Perhaps the simplest of the infant techniques consists of presenting the infant with two visual targets that differ on some experimentally controlled feature. To the extent that attention is differentially directed to one of the targets, we can conclude that the infant has discriminated one of the features that distinguishes the two targets. Of course, obvious confounding variables such as right–left positioning of the targets must be controlled. Note that we are less interested in discovering the actual preferences of the infants than in establishing their discrimination thresholds. Such a simple procedure as preferential looking has been used by Dobson and Teller (1978) to determine very precise estimates of the development of visual acuity in infants over the first year of life. The basis of the procedure consists in presenting gratings of differing stripe-width (spatial frequencies) corresponding to different Snellen acuity values (e.g., 20/100) paired with a homogenous gray target. Because infants prefer patterned stimuli to nonpatterned stimuli, when they no longer prefer the grating of the pure gray card, we can estimate their acuity. This technique is appropriate for any population where verbal responses cannot be gathered and where visual evoked potential studies are not practical.

It should be stressed that preferential looking is not limited to establishing psychophysical thresholds. Differences between stimuli can be made arbitrarily complex. Wagner and colleagues have previously adapted preferential looking to a situation where they have shown that infants of 6 to 12 months can associate dotted lines with pulsed tones and straight lines with pure tones, and rising and falling sweep tones with arrows that are pointed up or down. These abilities could be called "metaphorical mappings" because the events are related only in abstract ways (i.e., dotted lines and pulsed tones have nothing "physical" in common – Wagner et al., 1980).

Habituation paradigm

The habituation paradigm depends on the well-documented fact that infants (and other humans) get bored. It would be hyperbole to say that boredom is the sine qua non of intelligence and cognition because to be bored means that one recognizes the present as an instance of the past. Infants shown a visual target repeatedly will eventually reduce their average looking per exposure trial. If a new target that differs on some experimentally important feature is introduced (usually when the infant's attention has declined to 50% of what it initially was), the infant occasionally increases attention to the new target. If this occurs, it is likely that the infant has detected a change in the targets. If, on the other hand, attention does not increase, we cannot conclude necessarily that the infant has not discriminated the experimentally manipulated change. In such circumstances, the change may simply not be interesting enough to elicit an increase in attention. The continued inattention could also be due to fatigue. This is a very important point. Absence of evidence is not evidence of absence.

An increase in attention, however, is relatively umambiguous. The habituation procedure is extremely simple, but it is also extremely powerful because the differences between the habituation and test targets can be *conceptual* as well as *perceptual*. Such manipulations were the basis of the conclusion that 4-month-old infants can recognize numerosities (Starkey & Cooper, 1980).

It is important to note that habituation is "subject-controlled" (i.e., the subject controls the flow of information through the percentage of time spent in looking at a target). Habituation offers enormous promise to the assessment not only of normal infants but also of those infants with motoric difficulties as well as those who are nonverbal and developmentally delayed. The only behavioral requirement of the paradigm is that the subject be able to fixate visually. Visual acuity per se is not really a limiting factor, as the sizes of the objects and the distances of the subject can be controlled experimentally. Indeed, the procedure is so sensitive that it can even be used to assess visual acuity itself.

While the great majority of studies employing the habituation paradigm have depended on the visual modality, there is an important variant of the technique called the High Amplitude Sucking Procedure (HASP) that can be modified to establish discriminations in auditory and linguistic domains. In the HASP procedure, the infant is given a pacifier that contains a pressure transducer. A procedure is set up whereby the infant is presented an auditory (or visual) event as long as he or she sucks above a certain rate. If the rate declines below a prescribed level, the presentation is attenuated. At a prearranged point (e.g., when the rate is a certain value of the initial one), the experimenter introduces some change in the stimulus. If the sucking rate increases after the change, we can conclude that the infant has discriminated the change.

This procedure, although somewhat technically complicated to set up, has been used with great profit in a variety of contexts. Eimas (1975) was able to discover that young infants have the same categorical boundaries for identification of phonemes as do adults. Entus (1975) was able to determine that 4-month-olds process musical tones in the right hemisphere and linguistic stimuli (phonemes) in the left hemisphere.

A variety of this technique was used by DeCasper and his students (e.g., De-Casper & Fifer, 1980) to reveal newborns' recognition of their mothers' voices at 3 days of age, as well as their recognition of stories and songs they had heard repeatedly during the third trimester of pregnancy. Siqueland (1981) using the HASP procedure, found negative correlations between recognition of novelty and frequency of maternal birth complications. Obviously, it is only the imagination of the experimenter that places limits on this assessment technique.

Familiarization–novelty paradigm

The habituation paradigm depends on the natural tendency of humans to attend to changes in their environment. The familiarization–novelty paradigm (F–N) is designed around this fact. In this method, the infant is presented with a target for a certain preset number of "familiarization" trials, followed by a test trial in which the familiarization stimulus is paired with a novel stimulus. The important difference from the habituation paradigm is that the F–N procedure does not wait for the infant to reach his or her own level of reduced attention (the total exposure is controlled by the experimenter, not the child) and there are two target stimuli during the test phase (not just the one).

The F–N procedure (sometimes called the "paired-comparison technique") is generally more efficient than habituation in that it is quicker to administer and is more useful for making group comparisons. It is extremely general because the differences between the novel and familiar stimulus can be made arbitrarily complex by the experimenter. This procedure is probably the most frequently used of the infant perceptual discrimination paradigms.

The F–N procedure has provided researchers with an opportunity to document enormously sophisticated information-processing capacities on the part of infants. One such capacity that potentially has great clinical importance is cross-modal object recognition. For example, if we were allowed to explore an object haptically without visual feedback, and then were subsequently shown the object paired with a novel object, we would generally have little trouble distinguishing the two. This seemingly trivial capacity is in reality quite complex for it requires that we have requisite cortical centers for the initial sensory processing, and sufficient capacity to translate and compare the visual and tactual information. Verbal language affords older children and adults this ability. For infants to be capable of solving such problems, however, they must possess a preverbal means of coding sensory events from one modality into the terms of another. Using the F–N procedure, researchers have demonstrated such complex cross-modal discriminations in infants from birth to 1 year (Bushnell, 1986; Gottfried, Rose, & Bridger, 1977; Meltzoff & Borton, 1979; Rose, 1983; Wagner & Sakovits, 1986). Furthermore, Rose (1983) showed that cross-modal identification abilities were correlated with severity of prematurity and perinatal medical complications.

Another cognitive ability of young infants that was not suspected until recently has to do with abstract concept formation: categorization. Categorization is fundamental to thought and is defined as response equivalence to perceptually discriminable exemplars. It is our categorical ability that allows us to consider a whale as more similar to a mouse than to a shark. Although infants have not demonstrated this particular ability, they have shown the capacity to form perceptual categories that are adultlike in nature based on limited exposure to selected exemplars (see Cohen, 1979, for a review).

Conditioning

Conditioning is one of the oldest methods in the psychologist's arsenal. It is by far the most "demanding" of the infant paradigms in terms of cost, complexity, hardware requirements, and subject loss (i.e., due to time requirements, active compliance may decrease). It is, however, one of the most sensitive and powerful techniques available to the infancy research. The single greatest discriminating feature of the three other paradigms is that they are directed principally to the investigation of *group* differences. Their findings come from the comparison of preference scores to novel versus familial objects, yet no *individual* infant's preference can be compared to some statistical standard (i.e., chance) because not enough trials are completed by any one subject.

Conditioning, on the other hand, offers an opportunity to examine the abilities of *individual* infants and toddlers. It offers substantial control and predictive validity possibilities. It is especially suited to intervention strategies, and it is used routinely in institutions around the world. At present, however, there are no standardized problems to which one could compare different populations. Although conditioning represents a powerful treatment tool, it is not an effective assessment technique.

Applications of the infant paradigms

Together these four paradigms have opened up new vistas of research into the perceptual and cognitive development of infants. They have facilitated the discovery of new abilities in infants and revisions in our theories of development. They also open up new possibilities for formalized assessment of infants, including those with developmental disabilities. Nonetheless, we still must demonstrate that the abilities on which these methods depend (attention and preference for novel objects) have some clinical relevance. The question to be addressed is whether a young child who looks more quickly or for longer durations of time at a previously unseen or unexplored object will be more or less likely to develop greater competence later in life.

Fagan (1985) catalogued 15 studies that employed the novelty preference paradigm in the assessment of primarily premature infants, ranging in age from 3 to 12 months, and tested subsequently from 2 to 7.5 years of age. The 15 samples (total $N = 423$, $M = 28.2$, SD = 12.8) yielded an average predictive validity correlation of .44 (median = .42; range = .33 to .66; SD = .09), and the correlations are much higher if one limits them to at-risk populations or infants who are "failing to thrive." In these latter cases (three separate samples), the average correlation is .66 with a standard deviation of .06.

Rose and Wallace (1985a, 1985b) extend the conclusions reached by Fagan and others. In their studies, premature infants were assessed on the Bayley Scales at 6, 12, and 24 months; on a novelty preference measure at 6, 12, and 24 months; and on a measure of IQ (the Stanford–Binet and WISC-R) at 3, 4, and 6 years. Two findings are of note. First, the correlations of novelty preference with 6-year-old IQ average .54 and .64, compared with the Bayley MDI that correlates with IQ -0.27 and $-.14$. Second, and more significantly, novelty preference measures predict IQ *independently* of socioeconomic status. Each variable alone contributes equally to the variance in IQ when the other is partialed out (the semipartial correlations of infant novelty to 6-year IQ is .5), while novelty preference level and socioeconomic status (i.e., mother's education) are not intercorrelated. This has been independently demonstrated by Fagan and Singer (1983).

If one assumes that the novelty preference paradigm (in significant contrast to the Bayley Scales and other conventional infancy instruments) is tapping the same *kinds* of cognitive processes that are assessed by conventional IQ tests (i.e., perceptual integration, visual recognition memory, similarity recognition, etc.), these are not surprising results. Clearly, many infants who are born prematurely or who sustain significant birth complications demonstrate cognitive difficulties later in childhood. It has been hard, however, to identify, *in infancy,* those particular babies who are going to exhibit such deficits. It is reasonable to suggest that visual attention measures may achieve some success in this regard.

Many other studies have confirmed both the predictive and concurrent validity of attention and recognition memory scores (see Bornstein & Sigman, 1986, for a review). Fagan, Singer, Montie, & Shepherd (1986) administered a standardized F–N test to infants suspected to be at risk for later mental retardation. The sample included children born prematurely (birth weight < 1,500 g), or those with intra-uterine growth retardation, hypothyroidism, failure to thrive, or a history of mater-nal diabetes. The recognition memory test was administered four times between 3 and 7 months of age. Using a preestablished "risk-criterion," Fagan's test gener-ated hits (predict risk, outcome risk), false alarms (predict risk, outcome no risk), misses (predict no risk, outcome risk), and correct rejections (predict no risk, out-come no risk) of .90, .19, .10 (complement of .9), and .81 (complement of .19) respectively. These compared to .45 sensitivity and .38 specificity for the Bayley Scales. (In fact, a flip of a coin would have yielded higher sensitivity and specificity coefficients than did the Bayley Scales!) Several other studies have reported differ-ences between preterm infants and normal controls on both cross-modal recognition and visual recognition tests (Cohen, 1981; Rose, 1981; Rose, Gottfried, & Bridger, 1978; Rose & Wallace, 1985a, 1985b).

All of these investigations have centered on recognition memory for objects that vary in shape. One could argue that these tests are screening devices for significant delay because the perceptual function of shape recognition is so fundamental to later conceptual abilities. That is, if a child has trouble differentiating a circle from a square, then she or he is very likely to experience later delays – or so the argument would go. Some investigators have tried to extend these paradigms to tasks that go beyond the simple recognition of geometric shape. Caron and Caron (1981) ex-plored whether more sophisticated cognitive processes such as the ability to process invariant information (in particular the ability to extract invariant relational infor-mation) might also differentiate high risk from normal populations. Employing the F–N paradigm (presenting problems that tested for recognition of face–non-face, above–below, same–different face, and smiling–neutral face), they found that pre-terms (27–36 weeks) performed less well than term infants on all four problems. McDonough and Cohen (1982) employed the habituation paradigm, using a prob-lem requiring the infants to extract the concept of a "stuffed animal" from a series of six exemplars, to study a group of 16-month-old infants with cerebral palsy. These disabled infants were less able to extract the concept than age-matched nor-mal controls, although the difference was not found for 22-month-olds.

In summary, the validity of the novelty preference paradigm to predict cognitive delay has been established. Recognition memory is more valid both concurrently and predictively than conventional assessment instruments (at least when one limits the analyses to the level of *group* differences). In addition, it has the rare virtue of being uncontaminated by social class.

The fact that recognition memory scores predict group differences based on some metric of developmental disability, however, does not mean they have all the ad-vantages of a *standardized* score, such as the Bayley MDI. A Bayley score tells us exactly where a particular infant lies relative to his or her age peers. This is not yet the case for the results of recognition memory with recognition memory storage type tests, although some steps are being made in that direction. Fagan et al. (1986), for example, have devised a standardized battery of objects for infant assessment, with norms computed for individual trial times and ages. This protocol is based on the F–N paradigm and consists of a set of individual "problems" that are administered to the infants. An average novelty score is computed for each child based on his or her scores on three to four single problems. That score can be considered a "novelty preference coefficient."

A slightly different approach has been taken by Wagner and Sakovits (1986). The approach is based on a model of infant visual attention that is potentially well suited to predicting long-term developmental outcomes. The model stems from a dissatisfaction with the general attentional model underlying the standard novelty preference paradigm discussed above. Basically, the model posits that the novelty preference that is measured in the standard paradigm is the end point in a four-stage sequence whereby infants move from random (R) to familiarity (F) to random (R) to novelty (N) preference as the amount of exposure to the familiarizing stimulus is varied. Familiarity preference is not normally observed because, in general, the amount of time given for infants to explore the familiarization stimulus in the different experiments is sufficient to explore the object exhaustively and thus results in the infant's preferring the novel object. The RFRN model, as it is called, assumes there is a direct relationship between duration of processing and preference. Prior research on the RFRN model has demonstrated its validity in both intra-modal and cross-modal conditions, with object pairs of systematically varied complexity, with systematically varied exposure times to the familiarization stimuli, and with 6-, 9-, and 12-month-old infants (see Wagner & Sakovits, 1986, for a fuller elaboration).

If the RFRN model is a more complete characterization of infant attention and recognition memory, then it is natural to expect that it is better suited to predicting later developmental delay in at-risk infants. Other studies have centered on raw novelty preference averaged over a maximum of three trials per session, which results in low reliability between individual trials, and thus statistically limits the maximum predictive correlation. Familiarity preference (scores less than 50% novelty preference) would tend to depress correlations. Furthermore, infants with no preference (i.e., around 50% looking to the novel object) cannot be grouped with infants who show familiarity preference. What is needed is a way to compare an infant's individual profile with norms from all four phases of RFRN.

This raises a critical issue regarding the validity of attention measures. Virtually all studies have used group designs, and therefore it is not possible to use the data to predict how well a *particular* infant will perform as a 6-year-old. Because of this unfortunate design feature of the traditional novelty preference paradigm, an individual's particular score on a novelty test *cannot* be separated from his or her preference for that object *independently* of its novelty. That is why the small number of trials per session in the previous studies is unfortunate. This can only inflate the miss rate of the instrument. The RFRN model suggests a design that allows us to chart the flow of attention over time for each infant. This individual profile can then be compared to the normalized one for that infant's age-group, thus minimizing variations in looking related to the relative salience of individual objects and due to the temporal parameter.

In summary, the infant perceptual–cognitive paradigms hold significant promise for both the detection and the prediction of cognitive delay in groups of infants 9 months and older. Although there remain significant problems in extending these tasks to the prediction of outcome in individual clinical subjects, there is reason to be optimistic about the long-term standardization potential of some of the visual recognition memory tasks (e.g., Fagan et al., 1986).

Extending the paradigms to the study of Down syndrome

Given the enormous potential of the new paradigms, it is surprising that so few studies have exploited their promise with respect to either the Normalcy or the Uniqueness Question in infants with Down syndrome. The promise lies both in the fact that we can now meaningfully "match" infants on cognitive level (which the Bayley MDI does not do) as well as present the infants with problems that we know to be related to later IQ performance. Consequently, these paradigms should afford us the opportunity to examine properly the nature of the differences between, and the equivalences within, normal and retarded children's attentional and memory capacities.

The first studies to address explicitly the Normalcy Question were conducted by Miranda and Fantz (1973, 1974). In the 1974 study, three tasks based on the paired-comparison paradigm believed to reflect ordered levels of difficulty were presented to three age groups of infants with Down syndrome and normal infants (2 to 4 months, 5 to 7 months, and 8 to 10 months, respectively). The groups were thus CA- and not MA-matched. In every problem the normal infants showed a preference for the novel stimuli several weeks earlier than the group with Down syndrome. In addition, the most "complex problem" presented to the infants (discriminating a circular from a rectangular pattern) was not "solved" by the two younger groups with Down syndrome. However, the results did confirm that infants with Down syndrome have the capacity to acquire, store, and retrieve information at early ages and that the differences between Down syndrome and normal groups lay more in the speed of retrieval and encoding of visual stimuli than in basic cognitive differences.

In a follow-up longitudinal study, employing the preferential looking paradigm, Fantz, Fagan, and Miranda (1975) found that visual preferences for certain forms (e.g., bull's-eye vs. stripes, photographs vs. schematic faces, etc.) were delayed by 2 weeks to 4 months depending on the patterns presented. However, both the Down syndrome and the normal groups looked selectively more at patterns with more elements, angles, and contours than at simpler ones. The one major difference obtained was in the continued preference (up to the age of 33 weeks) of schematic face over the photograph by infants with Down syndrome (an effect that is reversed by 5 months of age in normal infants). This led Fantz and his colleagues to speculate that the Down syndrome group was delayed in their utilization of experience and social recognition. While the study did not demonstrate the existence of photograph over schematic face preference (at least up to 33 weeks), it is probable that it would have emerged eventually.

Fantz et al. (1975) also report data showing congruence between the Down syndrome and the normal groups.

The lack of retardation in Down syndrome infants in the development of patterns with more elements and angles and contour supports the interpretation that changes with age in preference for a number of elements in a pattern were likely related to the maturational and experiential perfection of elementary optical, oculomotor and neural mechanisms for pattern reception and visual-motor response – developments not retarded in Down syndrome infants – and not to increasing information-processing capacity or cognitive development that would be expected to be retarded in Down syndrome infants. (p. 321)

The fourth study to address explicitly the Normalcy issue with the infant paradigms was conducted by Cohen (1981). He used an habituation technique with a small group of infants with Down syndrome aged 19, 23, and 28 weeks. They were matched to a normally developing group of equal chronological age, sex, and socioeconomic status (SES). The number of testing sessions was also controlled. The habituation stimulus consisted of a 24 in. × 24 in. black-and-white checkerboard pattern and the posthabituation stimulus was a display of multicolored shapes. The main results of Cohen's study were that the number of habituation trials (the number of trials it took the infants to reach a criterion of 50% fixation to the habituation stimulus) was the same for both the Down syndrome group and the normal group at all ages; in contrast, the duration of looking during each trial was longer for the Down syndrome group at all ages. Moreover, the recovery of attention necessary for dishabituation was clearly present in only the older Down syndrome group (28 weeks).

These results indicate that infants with Down syndrome do habituate to visual displays and that they engage in longer fixations. In addition, these findings demonstrate that infants with Down syndrome do not clearly differentiate what they have habituated to compared to another pattern until they are somewhat older. At that time (7 months) they appear to behave like their CA-matched controls. This finding of longer fixations in infants with Down syndrome has been reported elsewhere (Hoffman, Salapatek, Kuskowski, & Cicchetti, 1979; Loveland, 1987).

In another study employing the habituation paradigm, Lewis and Brooks-Gunn (1984) were interested in determining whether habituation could be used as an index of central nervous system (CNS) integrity. Their study is significant for including other handicapped comparison groups. The sample was made up of infants with Down syndrome and cerebral palsy (CP), in addition to developmentally delayed (DD) and multiply handicapped (MH) infants. Four broad age ranges were investigated: 3 to 7 months, 8 to 16 months, 17 to 27 months, and 28 to 36 months. In addition to CA groupings, Lewis and Brooks-Gunn also computed MA scores based on the Bayley MDI.

Although such broad age ranges diminish somewhat the impact of the study, nonetheless several aspects of the results remain noteworthy. The youngest age group (3–7 months) did not show evidence of habituation–dishabituation. All other age groups (8–36 months) did. Although there was no normal control group, the habituation–dishabituation performance of the Down syndrome group was equal to the other handicapped groups (CP, DD, and other multiply handicapped). Furthermore, habituation scores were significantly correlated with MA (MDI) and CA for all infant groups.

In addition to global mean fixation scores (i.e., how long the infants looked at the particular targets), Lewis and Brooks-Gunn performed cluster analyses on the looking times, generating three patterns of responses that they then compared across groups. No differences in the proportion of infants exhibiting each looking pattern were found, thus motivating the conclusion that there were no differences between the infants with Down syndrome and the other comparison groups of handicapped infants on the habituation–dishabituation measure. We believe that this analysis ploy is particularly interesting and advocate that it be incorporated in future habituation studies.

The studies we have just discussed have all been concerned with visual recognition memory. The tasks have all involved visual *encoding* and visual *decoding*. A much more complex cognitive process is implicated in cross-modality encoding–decoding tasks. Such a problem requires the comparison of information that is stored in "different units." To recognize an object cross-modally requires, for example, that we translate the tactual information that we receive and the visual information that we receive and compare them in common "terms." There is only one study in the literature that has explicitly examined this question with infants with Down syndrome.

Lewis and Bryant (1982) employed a familiarization–novelty (paired-comparison) technique to investigate intramodality and cross-modality object identification in infants with Down syndrome and normal infants of equal developmental age (MA–MDI matched). Developmental-age groups of 12 and 17 months were targeted in a study that investigated whether the infants would visually recognize a shape that they had previously touched but not seen (cross-modal condition) and whether they would recognize a shape that they had previously seen (intramodal condition). There were two problems in each condition. As such, every child was presented with four tasks.

Lewis and Bryant were interested in this problem because of the well-established finding that tactual perception of adults with Down syndrome is particularly weak in comparison with other mentally retarded adults. Neither group of infants with Down syndrome showed evidence of cross-modal identification in either problem. The older developmental-age group of infants with Down syndrome showed intramodal identification on one of the visual–visual tasks. The younger and older groups of normal infants succeeded on both visual–visual tasks. The older normal group succceeded on both tactual–visual tasks, while the younger normal group succeeded on one of the tactual–visual tasks.

In a follow-up study, Lewis and Bryant examined the effect of touch on visual behavior. The infants looked at pairs of shapes, presented in a counterbalanced order, that could sometimes be touched and sometimes not. The infants with Down syndrome touched less and were less "coordinated" in their tactual exploration than the normal infants; however, both groups of infants made fewer and longer looks when they were allowed to explore the objects tactually. Lewis and Bryant interpret these findings as consistent with the hypothesis that infants with Down syndrome have a deficient sense of touch that is present early in life.

It is, of course, unclear whether the tactual deficit displayed by the infants with Down syndrome is due to an encoding problem in the tactual modality, to a difficulty in the translation of tactual information into units that are comparable to the visual units, or to generalized hypotonia. Would they, for instance, have failed the tasks if they had been given more time to explore the objects tactually during the encoding phase? Common sense tells us that it cannot be the case that infants with Down syndrome are incapable of *any* cross-modal identification tasks. However, the evidence that exists suggests that they do not do so with the facility of normal infants. It would be important to learn whether this difficulty is due to a tactual discrimination difficulty per se or to a "translation problem." Furthermore, it must be noted that the findings are in the form of "group-means." Variability in cross-modal performance must also be taken into account. It is likely that there exists significant overlap between the two distributions of Down syndrome and normal scores such that some infants with Down syndrome performed better than some normally developing infants.

While the Lewis and Bryant study is an interesting one, it should be noted that it is again a "main effect" finding in that infants with Down syndrome performed uniformly less well than normal infants. We cannot attribute this delay to any specific cognitive factor because there was no observed interaction between any manipulated variable and retardation group. It is worth noting, however, that Lewis and Bryant attempted to isolate the source of the difficulty observed in the first experiment by conducting the second experiment.

In general, the studies we have discussed suggest that the basic developmental processes of shape and pattern recognition are the same for infants with Down syndrome and for normal infants; however, the "pace" of development is slightly slowed in the case of Down syndrome. This is borne out by the studies employing the preferential looking technique that do not invoke the mechanisms of storage and retrieval memory since both stimuli are continuously present. These memory mechanisms are necessarily invoked by the habituation paradigm because each stimulus presentation has to be compared with the last one. In these situations the infants with Down syndrome again show some delay in long-term developmental "pace" but not in the nature of the representations that are formed. That is, infants with Down syndrome habituate to criterion in the same number of trials, although they process the stimuli for longer "bouts." This suggests that the basic encoding processes of shape perception are intact with Down syndrome.

However, since infants with Down syndrome do not dishabituate equivalently to

CA-matched controls until 7 months, infants with Down syndrome may store a more diffuse representation of basic patterns and shapes, or they may have difficulty retrieving the shape they have encoded and therefore not recognize a new shape as new. Both possibilities could account for their failure to dishabituate. By 7 months, these differences disappear and they perform equally to their CA matched normal peers. This is probably because the tasks are tapping fundamental and automatic cognitive processes that are themselves highly genetically determined (Fishbein, 1976). As such, they do not reveal differences that might otherwise emerge in higher-level processing.

The picture emerging from the cross-modal studies of Lewis and Bryant (1982) is one suggesting continuity with the known deficiency that adults with Down syndrome have on tactual recognition tasks. We do not yet know the source of this difficulty in infancy. It could be due to generalized hypotonia (Gibson, 1978) or to a cross-modality deficit.

We next consider two additional studies, which, although they do not explicitly incorporate the infant paradigms, nonetheless are germane to the concerns raised in our earlier discussions about the attention and recognition capacities of infants with Down syndrome. Specifically, these investigations provide insight into whether or not the problems noted in infants with Down syndrome are due to difficulties in *disengaging* from a significant visual display or to delays in processing the features of the displays.

A recent study by Loveland (1987) examined the behavior of infants with Down syndrome and normal infants matched for mental age (16–32 months) on tasks where they had to find objects that were reflected in a mirror. The tasks differed in complexity and included finding a rouge mark on the face, finding the mother, finding a toy, and free play in front of the mirror. This study was motivated by an interest in the effect of developmental disorders on the discovery of affordances (Gibson, 1979). Mirror behavior of infants with Down syndrome has been studied before within the context of its relationship to visual self-recognition and the self-concept (Mans, Cicchetti, & Sroufe, 1978). Mans and collaborators found that infants with Down syndrome could solve self-recognition tasks at the same developmental level at which normal children could solve them. The Loveland study basically confirmed these findings. The two groups were equally likely to solve the tasks. Whereas youngsters with Down syndrome were more attentive during some tasks, the normal toddlers displayed more positive affect during the mother-finding task than the youngsters with Down syndrome.

Loveland interprets these findings as demonstrating strong overall congruence between the developmental progress of children with and without Down syndrome in learning to use the mirror. The differences in affect are attributed to biological differences in the regulation of arousal (Cicchetti & Sroufe, 1978; Serafica & Cicchetti, 1976). Furthermore, Loveland attributes the differences in attentiveness to the failure of youngsters with Down syndrome to habituate to the mirror as normal children do.

The idea that individuals with Down syndrome manifest problems in the mechanisms of habituation had been suggested previously by Schafer and Peeke (1982). This is an extremely strong conclusion that merits some review. Schafer and Peeke addressed the issue of whether adults with Down syndrome were different from normal individuals on a cognitive parameter as fundamental as habituation. This research is in line with a series of studies showing that individuals with Down syndrome have increased amplitude in cortical evoked potentials, which has led to suggestions that individuals with Down syndrome are deficient with respect to the inhibitory capacity of their brains. That is, they do not decrease the magnitude of their responses to repetitive events (cf. Courchesne, 1989; Cicchetti & Sroufe, 1978; Ganiban, Wagner, & Cicchetti, Chapter 3, this volume).

The Schafer and Peeke study consisted in the presentation of fifty 60 db clicks every 2 seconds to 10 adults with Down syndrome and 10 normal adults. The auditory evoked cortical potentials were then analyzed. For the normal adults the amplitude of the evoked potential decreased significantly, whereas for the adults with Down syndrome it did not. It is worth noting that the *shape* of the auditory evoked potentials for both groups are remarkably similar in that they have the same negative and positive components – that is, they are time-locked together. They differ in amplitude, not frequency.

Schafer and Peeke apparently believe that if individuals with Down syndrome do not habituate to auditorily presented stimuli, this might suggest a possible neuro-biological substrate of mental deficiency. However, although it may well be true that the evoked potentials of individuals with Down syndrome are different from those of normal individuals, it is unlikely that individuals with Down syndrome *cannot* or *do not* habituate. As argued in earlier sections, habituation is a fundamental cognitive mechanism that can give overt evidence for the creation of a mental model of the world. In our view, habituation is the sine qua non of intelligence because without it, mental life would be impossible. There is ample behavioral evidence of individuals with Down syndrome being able to habituate to stimuli much more complicated than 60 db clicks. How can we reconcile these findings with the Schafer and Peeke study? One possibility, which is discounted by Schafer and Peeke but which we find compelling, is that the two groups probably differed on arousal level. If the repetitive auditory clicks were more aversive to the Down syndrome sample than to the normal sample (who were certainly told in advance that they would be hearing a series of clicks), this might have accounted for the failure to habituate. This is another example of how a main effect (as opposed to an interaction) for a retardation group is fairly uninterpretable, since the differences in means cannot be unambiguously attributed to the independent variable (i.e., retardation) as opposed to another confounded variable (e.g., arousal, hypotonia, etc.).

These concerns notwithstanding, the suggestion that one of the specific cognitive effects of Down syndrome has to do with inhibitory capacities is a compelling one and should be explored further. We would like to make a distinction between processing load differences and disengagement. Subjects might require more time to process a stimulus and thus appear to not habituate, or they might have processed the stimulus but be unable to "disengage" from it. This would be analogous to newborn visual behavior, which is occasionally characterized by "obligatory perception" in which the infant is "riveted" on a visual target and cannot easily "break off" (Stechler & Latz, 1966).

The studies just discussed have been concerned with perception and recognition memory – cognitive processes that are crucial to survival in virtually all higher organisms. We turn now to a uniquely human ability: language. In an innovative variant of the preferential looking technique, Glenn, Cunningham, and Joyce (1981), presented infants with Down syndrome and MA-matched normal infants (mean MA, 9 months) with an automated device that enabled them to choose to listen to one of a pair of auditory events. The subjects had to push a switch on one of two boxes to activate a sound track. The auditory discriminations consisted of a nursery rhyme sung by a female voice versus the same rhyme played on a flute, guitar, or trumpet, and a spoken nursery rhyme versus a repetitive piano tone. The impetus for this research was an interest in receptive language abilities in handicapped populations, because it is well known that children with Down syndrome evidence significant delay in expressive language (see Beeghly, Weiss-Perry, & Cicchetti, Chapter 10, this volume; Fowler, Chapter 9, this volume). Glenn and colleagues wanted to determine whether this deficit could be traced to an underlying comprehension deficit, because language comprehension generally is in advance of language production.

Overall, both groups showed a preference for the human voice. This led Glenn and collaborators to conclude there is no evidence for the hypothesis that it is lack of saliency of speech stimuli per se that accounts for the production deficit of infants and toddlers with Down syndrome. The strongest result of the study, however, concerned the interaction found between mental handicap and stimulus complexity. The infants with Down syndrome responded more to the spoken nursery rhyme than did the normal infants, whereas their responses to the tones were the same. Apparently the difference between tone and voice is more salient for infants with Down syndrome than for the normal infants – at least as measured by response duration and response frequency.

In a follow-up study Glenn and Cunningham (1983) extended their paradigm to an examination of whether infants with Down syndrome and normal infants discriminate between "motherese" and normal adult speech. Motherese is inflected speech characteristic of the speech patterns of adults to babies (and pets). It has recently been a subject of significant research activity in psycholinguistics – being seen as an important environmental vehicle for the child's learning of syntax (see Beeghly,Weiss-Perry, & Cicchetti, Chapter 10, this volume). They modified their apparatus to pose a choice of "baby talk" versus "adult talk." In addition they included a longitudinal component to the design by testing the infants both at MA 9 months and MA 18 months.

Both the infants with Down syndrome and normal infants showed preferences for baby talk over adult talk at both ages. There were, however, several interactions, the most important being that infants with Down syndrome significantly reduced their preference for baby talk over time while normal infants significantly increased their preference for baby talk. Glenn and Cunningham interpret this decline as implying that sometime between 12 and 24 months infants with Down syndrome "lose ground" in their receptive language abilities. The implication is that the older normal infants understand the baby talk better and thus are more motivated to produce it. During the second year the stimulus of the mother talking to the infant with Down syndrome loses some of its ability to maintain responses in the Down syndrome group because they have greater difficulty understanding language.

The studies by Glenn and colleagues (Glenn & Cunningham, 1983; Glenn et al., 1981) are noteworthy and raise several interesting issues. First, they illustrate the usefulness of preferential paradigms to address issues of consequence in cognitive development. Second, the designs of the studies are to be commended for being multifactorial. The existence of significant interaction effects lends further credence to the results being related to stimulus conditions rather than uncontrolled confounds of retardation.

However, some caveats should be kept in mind. First, the relationship between production and comprehension in language is a confusing one, and there is significant controversy among psycholinguists about how independent they are. There is evidence both of a clinical nature (i.e., the aphasias) and of an experimental nature that the two processes are fundamentally independent. Even anecdotal evidence confirms this. Any number of people can understand a language but cannot speak it. This is in fact the normal pattern of children of immigrant parents (the reverse pattern probably does not occur except in Wernicke's aphasia). In modern cognitive science parlance, comprehension is considered "bottom-up" while production is considered to be "top-down"; that is, speaking (production) requires the prior computation of syntax, semantics, and phonetics before the utterance is made, whereas understanding proceeds necessarily from phonetics to semantics. The phonemes have to be processed and the output of these computations passed on to the other language systems before we can understand an utterance.

It is certainly plausible to expect infants with Down syndrome to be delayed in top-down processing. Likewise, it is no surprise that they are not delayed in bottom-up processing. This, of course, does not mean that the decline in comprehension *could not* impact future production; however, it is hard to see why the younger infants with Down syndrome should prefer baby talk over adult talk more than they do at 18 months because they understand baby talk *less* at 18 months than the normal 18-month-olds. If poor comprehension did not hinder them at 9 months, why does it hinder them at 18 months?

Although the designs of these two studies are generally sound, they do contain significant methodological problems, the foremost being that the trials were administered by the infants' mothers (who, of course, were not blind to the group condition variable). We have no way of evaluating to what effect unconscious prompting on the part of the mothers could have affected the preference choices of the infants. Perhaps mothers of infants with Down syndrome are more concerned than mothers of normal infants that their 2-year-olds *not* prefer baby talk to adult talk.

The studies reviewed in the last section are useful examples of the power of the infant paradigms to address issues of concern to the researcher interested in Down syndrome. However, because none of the studies included other mentally retarded comparison groups, only the Normalcy Question has been addressed. It should be noted that the impetus for many of these studies came not from an interest in the cognitive specifics of Down syndrome per se, but rather from an attempt to find discriminative validity for the paradigms themselves. The assumption was that if a known mentally handicapped sample of infants performed less well on a habituation measure, that would validate the habituation measure. Now that the infancy paradigm has been validated, it is time to turn our efforts to designing new studies that address the Uniqueness Question as well as the Normalcy Question. In addition, we must start investigating the mechanisms underlying these differences, such as encoding versus decoding problems or difficulties with the auditory–visual integration of information. This can be accomplished by manipulating variables that are more specific than simply gross shape discrimination or pattern recognition. The studies by Glenn and her colleagues are good exemplars of the type of investigations that must be conducted.

Naturalistic studies of attention and memory

Although our primary goal in this chapter is to lobby for the new paradigms, we must also consider other studies of infants and toddlers with Down syndrome that have examined significant issues in attention, perception, and memory. A few noteworthy additional studies have been conducted on the development of attention in infants with Down syndrome. None employs one of the paradigms just described, yet each provides useful information about the similarities and differences in attentional patterns in infants with Down syndrome. They differ from the previous studies in being more "open-ended" in nature and more "natural" in their administration.

The first study we will consider was conducted by Vietze, McCarthy, McQuiston, MacTurk, and Yarrow (1983), who investigated three age-groups of infants with Down syndrome (6-, 8-, and 12-month-olds). Although there were no control groups of normal infants, Vietze and his colleagues present normative data from other studies to which they compare their Down syndrome sample. The study consisted of presenting infants with objects and containers and observing their reactions to them in three situations ranging from free manipulation of the objects through placing and removing the objects from the containers to overcoming a barrier to get a desired object. Vietze and his collaborators posited a developmental sequence to the exploratory activities progressing from mouthing and banging the objects through "mastery behavior."

The basic findings were that visual inspection alone of the objects decreased with age, while the amount of manipulation of the toys increased with age. The major dependent measure was relative preference of visual exploration versus manual exploration of objects. The pattern of data for the infants with Down syndrome was similar to that previously obtained with normals over developmental time in that older infants manipulated more and looked less. However, the infants with Down syndrome looked significantly more (and manipulated less) than nonhandicapped infants at all ages. Again, this is a main effect that is difficult to interpret. We do not know to which variable to attribute the difference. In such a case, retardation is reduced to delayed or "younger" but not "different."

In a follow-up study MacTurk, Vietze, McCarthy, McQuiston, & Yarrow (1985) extended the findings of the study conducted by Vietze and his colleagues. They examined the exploratory and "mastery" behaviors of a sample of 11 infants with Down syndrome and 11 normal infants matched on Bayley MDI. The infants were presented with 12 tasks that involved primarily the manipulation of popular commercially available toys. The mastery behaviors that MacTurk and associates were interested in varied from simply looking at the toys, manipulating them, persisting in solving the implicit problem of how they "worked," solving the problem (e.g., making a bell chime), socially sharing their activities with their mother or the experimenter, and off-task behaviors.

Rather than focus on the absolute levels of behaviors, they were interested in the patterns of how the two samples distributed their behaviors. This was done by computing transitional probabilities of the six basic mastery behaviors. Transitional probability analysis summarizes the probability of any one event's following another event. Two groups of subjects might display equal occurrences of different behaviors but might do so in different orders of sequences. This is basically what MacTurk and colleagues found. The infants with Down syndrome and the normal infants did not differ in the total amounts of behavior but did vary considerably in the distribution of behavior. Second, the analysis of transitional probabilities revealed similarities and differences. There was a striking similarity in most transitional patterns except for those involving looking. For the infants with Down syndrome, the "hub of behavior" was looking, in that they seemed to return to it after engaging in one of the other target behaviors. For the normal infants, the hub seemed to be "social behavior." MacTurk and collaborators hypothesize that infants with Down syndrome may have required more visual processing time to organize their response repertoire.

This finding is reminiscent of the report by Miranda and Fantz (1973), discussed in an earlier section, that infants with Down syndrome engage in longer fixations. What needs to be determined in interpreting these findings is the extent to which the longer fixations alone could have accounted for the patterned differences and, second, what effect the motor competence differences between the groups had on the results. MacTurk and colleagues matched their samples on mental indices but not motor indices. Because it is known that motor scores on the Bayley lag behind those of mental scores (Schneider & Brannen, 1981), the two groups of infants were not matched on motor level. This is particularly unfortunate because the tasks in this study require significant motor skills. However, the transitional probability analysis they employed can be genuinely sensitive to qualitative differences among groups and should be retained in future studies in this area.

A more naturalistic study was conducted by Gunn, Berry, and Andrews (1981).

They looked at two age groups of infants with Down syndrome (9 and 20 months). The dependent measure was degree of affective response to the repetition of an interesting visual event – a squeaky doll. The primary finding was that the degree of positive or negative affect was significantly correlated with cognitive development, assessed through the Bayley MDI. Although the study of Gunn and his collaborators did not include any normal comparison groups, the findings are consistent with the close association between cognitive and affective development that has been observed both in studies of normal infants (Sroufe & Wunsch, 1972) and in studies of infants with Down syndrome (Cicchetti & Sroufe, 1976, 1978).

A second study by Gunn, Berry, and Andrews (1982) examined the looking behavior of two groups of infants with Down syndrome and CA-matched normal infants (at 6 and 9 months of age) in a situation where they were with their mothers without toys. No maternal differences were found in vocalizations and holding behaviors, but the infants with Down syndrome looked almost twice as long at their mothers than did the normal infants. Gunn and colleagues interpret this finding as reflecting impoverished exploration competence on the part of the infants with Down syndrome. It is easy to incorporate this finding into that of the study by Vietze and his collaborators just discussed.

In another naturalistic study, Landry and Chapieski (1989) examined the joint attentional abilities of 12-month-old infants with Down syndrome during play interactions with their mothers. In this study the Uniqueness Question was addressed: Premature infants known to be at an elevated risk for developmental delay were compared to infants with Down syndrome. Unlike other studies, attempts were made to match infants for developmental level (mean developmental level for infants with Down syndrome = 10.50 months, SD = 1.02 months; mean developmental level for premature infants = 11.25, SD 1.09), and motoric ability (mean motor age for infants with Down syndrome = 9.25 months, SD = 1.12 months; mean motor age for premature infants = 9.25 months, SD = 1.38 months).

Within each group, infants' attentional capacity appeared to be easily taxed when they were required to attend jointly to their mothers and objects. However, the infants with Down syndrome seemed to have more difficulty than the premature infants. For example, when mothers attempted to direct their children's attention, the infants with Down syndrome were more likely than the premature infants to respond by looking at their mothers and not engaging in toy manipulation.

Additionally, the mothers within each group differed in the nonverbal strategies they used to direct their infants' attention. Mothers of children with Down syndrome tended to physically orient their children to toys and to introduce their children to new toys more than mothers of premature infants. Conversely, infants with Down syndrome also tended to be more passive in their play interactions and manipulated toys less than the premature infants.

These latter findings are consistent with previous studies that have compared infants with Down syndrome to normally developing infants (e.g., MacTurk et al., 1985; Vietze et al., 1983). However, these data also address the Uniqueness Question by comparing the attentional capacities of infants with Down syndrome with those of other infants known to be at risk for developmental delay. These data suggest that, again, infants with Down syndrome may have attentional difficulties unique to the Down syndrome genotype. However, further studies with other groups of children at risk for mental retardation are still needed to evaluate this possibility fully.

The next study of this group, carried out by Krakow and Kopp (1983), was perhaps the most extensive of the naturalistic studies conducted to date (see Kopp, Chapter 7, this volume, for an elaboration). This study is significant because it included a mentally retarded control group, thereby allowing the investigators to address the Uniqueness Question. It attempted to examine qualitative versus quantitative differences among infants with Down syndrome, mentally retarded infants of unknown etiology, and normal infants. Krakow and Kopp tried to show that qualitative differences can occur within the general pattern of coherent but delayed development (see Cicchetti & Beeghly, Chapter 2, this volume; Cicchetti & Pogge-Hesse, 1982; Hodapp & Zigler, Chapter 1, this volume). Krakow and Kopp videotaped a free-play situation where attention deployment to age-appropriate toys was monitored in both a structured and a nonstructured setting.

They found that there were differences between the normal and the two groups of handicapped infants in the duration of sustained attention, in the pattern of behavior during nonengagement with toys (i.e., normals never engaged in nonactivity), in the presence of throwing behavior in the infant's play repertoire, in the degree of object orientation and in the amount of glances that signal monitoring of the surround.

In one sense these results confirm the basic developmental thesis of Zigler and others. The two groups of handicapped infants showed patterns of play that are outwardly similar to MA-matched controls. If one considers, however, their "style" of play, more subtle differences emerge. There were major underlying differences found in attention deployment between the handicapped and normal groups, with some important distinctions noted between the infants with Down syndrome and those of unknown etiology. Compared to other mentally retarded infants, infants with Down syndrome were more like normal infants with respect to "engagement" with toys. On the other hand, the infants with Down syndrome tended to "ignore" the social surround more than the handicapped infants of unknown etiology. The infants with Down syndrome focused all their attention on the toys as opposed to the people around them. On this variable, the normal and unknown etiology groups of infants were more alike.

The Krakow and Kopp study is interesting in that it addresses both the Normalcy Question and the Uniqueness Question. When the unit of analysis is confined to *patterns* of behavior between infants with Down syndrome and normally developing infants, then differences evaporate. However, comparing infants with Down syndrome to other retarded infants of heterogeneous etiology (Uniqueness issue), qualitative differences emerge.

Methodological commentary on attention and memory studies

It is important to be cautious in interpreting the findings that have been reviewed. Although it is always difficult to compare results across studies, in the case of comparisons between infants with Down syndrome and normal infants, the problems are particularly acute. Three important points are worth making.

First, several of the studies that we reviewed underscored the fact that their outcome measures were correlated with the MDI of the Bayley Scales (1969) (i.e., the Lewis and Brooks-Gunn, 1984; the Gunn et al., 1981; and the Lewis and Bryant, 1982, studies). However, it is unclear what validation is involved given that the *infant* Bayley measure is itself uncorrelated with any meaningful cognitive measure in childhood. This critique would not apply to studies with toddlers where meaningful correlations can be obtained.

The second point concerns the issue of MA-matching. In the past, researchers who have examined infants with Down syndrome have employed CA-matched and MA-matched controls. In most studies, MA-matching is based upon Bayley MDI scores. Recently, however, researchers have started to question whether this infant measure taps the same processes and behaviors known to be related to later intelligence (Fagan, 1985; Fagan & McGrath, 1981; Fagan & Singer, 1983; Rose, 1981; Rose, Gottfried, & Bridger, 1978; Rose & Wallace, 1985a, 1985b). Consequently, it is questionable whether young infants with similar scores on the Bayley MDI have the same level of cognitive competence.

In addition, scores on the Bayley MDI may be affected by noncognitive abilities such as motor skills that could be confounded with the independent variable being manipulated (e.g., object exploration). For example, Schneider and Brannen (1981) have shown that infants with equivalent MDI scores may not have equivalent motor skills (as measured by the Bayley PDI, or "psychomotor index"). Although the Bayley MDI (1969) is affected by motor skills, the PDI is more sensitive to these abilities. Accordingly, infants with Down syndrome, who tend to be more motorically retarded than mentally retarded, also tend to have lower PDIs than MDIs in the first year of life (Cicchetti & Sroufe, 1976; Cowie, 1970). This means that MA-matched samples are not very well equated on motor abilities *or* mental abilities. Consequently, on tasks involving object manipulation or active exploration of the environment, infants and children with Down syndrome may be at a motoric disadvantage. Thus, differences obtained may be related to immature motor skills, rather than to other deficits. We suggest that researchers interested in cognitive and attention skills match their samples on recognition memory and attention performance rather than on the Bayley MDI. However, even if this is done, the designs of the studies must be improved.

Third, and most importantly, in any study of the differences between infants with Down syndrome and any mentally retarded or normal group, the claim that *different* cognitive processes are involved requires the demonstration of more than a main effect for retardation (or kind of retardation in the case of a Down syndrome–other mental retardation group study). Often, main effects for mental retardation on task performance indicate that performance and mental retardation are related. However, such relationships do not indicate whether mental retardation is the cause of poor task performance. For example, a number of non-task specific factors such as motivation, fatigue, familiarity with the stimuli, and the like, might produce uniformly lower performances on the part of the retarded.

Thus, if individuals with Down syndrome are uniformly "slower" than other mentally retarded subjects, or if they get uniformly lower means than normal persons, this does not support a "Difference" claim (Zigler, 1969). Rather, to support the "Difference" claim, individuals must perform differentially better or worse as a function of some manipulated variable (e.g., auditory vs. visual presentation, stimulus complexity, etc.). In other words, to postulate that a specific factor such as mental retardation or Down syndrome affects task performance, one must first demonstrate that an interaction between the factor and the stimulus condition exists. Consequently, future research should endeavor to manipulate retardation type and psychological operations in a multifactorial model.

To illustrate, consider the following study. Varnhagen, Das, and Varnhagen (1987) were able to show that adults with Down syndrome (compared to trainable mentally retarded adults without Down syndrome) were especially poor at long-term memory access for stimulus identification and at short-term storage and processing of auditory information. Subsequently, Varnhagen et al. were then able to isolate a specific memorial mechanism that could have accounted for the differences (i.e., the "articulatory loop," where one says the word to oneself before pronouncing it). The adults with Down syndrome did not show any difference in their performance in conditions where the words to be memorized were phonetically similar compared to a condition where the words did not sound the same. In contrast, the normal group had improved performance in the non-sound-alike condition. The study thus demonstrates an *interaction* between retardation group and condition and is an example of careful stimulus control and one that enhances our understanding of the specific cognitive deficits that characterize individuals with Down syndrome as opposed to other mentally retarded persons. Among the infancy studies we have reviewed, only the investigations by Glenn and colleagues (Glenn & Cunningham, 1983; Glenn et al., 1981) meet this criterion.

Interpretation of differences and equivalences

The "open-ended" naturalistic attention studies confirm the overall thrust of those using more controlled experimental situations. Infants with Down syndrome show consistent delays relative to normal infants with some differences emerging between Down syndrome and other mentally retarded groups.

Are there common threads that link the deficits we observe with infants with Down syndrome? First, as regards the Uniqueness Question, it is clear from the childhood and adult literature that persons with Down syndrome can be distinguished from other mentally retarded populations on certain psychological dimensions.

Let us first consider the Uniqueness Question. What very little evidence we have comes from the Krakow and Kopp (1983) study and suggests that infants with Down syndrome are slightly less disposed than other retarded infants to attend to important social features of their surround (e.g., their mothers) in a situation in which they are free to explore novel objects. On the other hand, infants with Down syndrome are in a sense "more riveted" and less affected by social demands than other infants. The mentally retarded infants, curiously, seek to reduce stimulation and spend a greater proportion of their time in "no activity."

Regarding the Normalcy Question, there is somewhat more to say. We have considered several studies that have reported differences in the performance of infants with Down syndrome and normal infants, either MA-matched or CA-matched. As we have stated, we do not regard MA-matched as very meaningful because we cannot be sure what is being matched. It is clear, however, that there exist both real differences and real similarities in the attention and memory behavior of infants with Down syndrome and normal infants. This state of affairs is, of course, not unlike that found with older children and adults with Down syndrome. We see no reason to expect that there *should* be a difference between infant performance in memory and attention because we believe in the fundamental continuity of mental operations from infancy to childhood (Bornstein & Sigman, 1986).

Basically, when the variables under investigation are perceptual or involve recognition memory, the differences are simply quantitative in nature. The Lewis and Bryant (1982) study did not show evidence of cross-modal recognition on the part of the infants with Down syndrome; however, we believe this would have been obtained had longer familiarization times been employed. Important differences do emerge in language preference tasks. These differences could be of significant consequence to language development, but we have yet to see a study that implicates a qualitative difference in specifically cognitive mechanisms on the part of the infant with Down syndrome.

In an important review of information processing in mentally retarded children and adults, some of whom had Down syndrome, Stanovitch (1978) provides a useful framework for examining the underlying mechanisms of information processing. Summarizing the information-processing approach of several investigators, he provides a general model of information processing that consists of four sequential stages of representing and processing steps during which the proximal stimulus is progressively transformed. The initial stage of processing is a short-term sensory storage system that preserves an intact visual representation of the stimulus for around 200 milliseconds. In Stage 2, this representation is then encoded into a more permanent representation (such as a name code), which is held in short-term memory. Stage 3 is presumed to be a central-processing stage in which manipulation of the stimuli are carried out. Manipulations include assessing association of the stimulus representation from long-term memory, accessing response codes or comparing to other stimuli in short-term memory. In Stage 4, a response program is selected based on the analyses completed in the previous stages. Below, we provide a brief summary of Stanovitch's review.

The four stages of processing (sensory storage, perceptual encoding, central processing, and response selection mechanisms) have all been extensively studied in mentally retarded persons. It seems clear that in terms of Stage 1 (sensory storage) there are no important differences between mentally retarded and normal children. Mentally retarded children are able to preserve in iconic memory an absolute representation of stimulus arrays for about 250 milliseconds. Their decay function is isomorphic to that of normal children. Differences obtained between mentally retarded and normal children in "whole-report" paradigms can be traced to unfamiliarity with the stimuli. When familiarity is controlled, mentally retarded and normal children perform equivalently in CA-matched designs.

Stage 2 of this model (perceptual encoding) has also been examined in mentally retarded persons. Studies have generally concentrated on the *rate* of information flow from sensory storage to longer-term storage. Again, mentally retarded and normal individuals of equal CA perform equivalently so long as stimulus familiarity is controlled and verbal response behaviors are minimized.

Stage 3 processes such as visual search, memory scanning, redundancy effects, and same–different judgments have been investigated. Mentally retarded persons have been shown to be subject to the same "laws" of cognition that CA-matched normal individuals are. For example, they are aided by redundancy in the stimulus sets in recall experiments and they obey Sternberg's (1966) serial-exhaustive search strategy in Sternberg-type tasks, and thus carefully evaluate each piece of information before responding to a task. Their behavior mirrors MA-matched controls in rate of processing but preserves isomorphism in response profiles with normal persons.

It is only in Stage 4 processes (response *selection* strategies) that there is evidence of significant deviations from the normal pattern. Mentally retarded persons appear to be *more* disturbed by such issues as stimulus response incompatibilities and they show greater interference on Stroop tests. These findings are the result of interactions between retardation and the independent variables being manipulated and implicate as much specific cognitive mechanisms as the causes of the effects.

How can we reconcile or characterize the patterns of differences and similarities that we find among groups of Down syndrome, other mentally retarded, and normal infants and children? One possible metaphor is that of hardware–software. In this metaphor, mental retardation is primarily, if not solely, a software problem. The computational hardware is all there (e.g., sensory information store, subitization, short-term memory, etc.) and the processing laws are obeyed (e.g., redundant information is processed more rapidly than nonredundant information; rehearsal in memory helps recall; lexical access occurs before semantic access; memory comparison in the Sternberg Paradigm (Sternberg, 1966) can be characterized as "serial-exhaustive"; etc.); however, the activation of cognitive subroutines (such as rehearsal) either are not present or are not initiated. The metacognitive execution of strategies is the source of observed deficits. Broadly speaking, this approach would characterize the work of Brown and Campione (1977) and Butterfield and Belmont (1977). In this approach the difference between Down syndrome and mentally retarded groups is not theoretically important and represents sample variance.

Conclusions and future directions

What, then, can we draw from our survey of research on cognition and attention in Down syndrome? We see several major directions in which future research would profitably be pursued.

First, we think it is imperative that researchers investigating the cognitive and attentional correlates of Down syndrome adapt their paradigms and experimental questions so as to take advantage of the novelty preference or habituation paradigms. Indeed, they should also endeavor to match their samples on recognition memory and attention measure scores before carrying out their experimental manipulations. Studies that do not do so are invariably constrained to "main effects" results.

Second, whenever possible, investigators should assess multiple domains of development concurrently. We take it as a basic assumption that assessments of only one domain are intrinsically incomplete because the infant and child do not engage the world with single competencies with all other variables controlled (Cicchetti & Wagner, in press). Rather, the child's response and subsequent interaction with the world are dependent upon the child's abilities across several domains and modalities as well as his or her inherent biological or genetic makeup. The innate capacities of children will determine their ability to perceive, understand, and engage the world effectively and appropriately given the expectations and stimulation provided by culture, parents, and peers. Thus, comprehensive assessments of development must examine the inherent capacities of infants and children, how these capacities affect their ability to engage the world, and the extent to which children meet and appropriately express the expectations established for them (see Berger, Chapter 4, this volume; Ganiban, Wagner, & Cicchetti, Chapter 3, this volume). Additionally, research must also assess the environment in which these children are expected to develop and to function (Bronfenbrenner & Crouter, 1983).

Third, cross-fostering of abnormal and normal developmental theory should be attempted. Understanding psychological development requires that we investigate deviations from the normal pattern (Cicchetti, 1984, in press; Rutter & Garmezy, 1983). Sternberg's triarchic theory of mental retardation (Sternberg & Spear, 1985) is a good example of this cross-fostering. Sternberg's theory of intelligence originally contained only one "axis." When he tried to extend it to mental retardation, he was obliged to consider and posit other axes as well. While he may have eventually reached these conclusions by an avenue other than that of mental retardation, the fact that his theory can accommodate mental retardation is one of its strengths.

Fourth, we believe it is important to investigate the pattern of individual differences in Down syndrome explicitly. Down syndrome has a range of effects across a vast array of psychological domains. There is significant variability *within* the population of Down syndrome. This variability is a significant source of important information about developmental mechanisms. We must endeavor to obtain a better sense of the individual variations in their performance across developmental domains.

Finally, future studies must break away from an emphasis on uncovering "main effects" and endeavor to examine multifactorially crucial psychological mechanisms. Although it is difficult and costly to do so, nonetheless it is possible.

An example we can offer of such a study (which, unfortunately, only targets cognitive processes) could be modeled on a study conducted by Strauss and Cohen (1978) that investigated the nature of their representations in a concept formation task. In this study, Strauss and Cohen were interested in whether 10-month-old infants could form a prototypical representation of serially presented schematic faces that varied along five dimensions (e.g., nose width, eye separation, nose length, etc.), with values on these dimensions varying from very small to very large (five values: 1–5). Even though the infants were rarely or never presented with "average" values on the dimensions (values of 3), they nonetheless formed a mental representation that was equivalent to a 3-3-3-3. That is, they ignored the extreme variations they were presented and created an internal schema that was not representative of what they had seen but was representative of a prototypical exemplar of the stimulus class they had been shown.

In another study, Strauss and Cohen tried to manipulate the nature of the prototype formed. It is known from the adult cognitive literature that we can form two kinds of prototypes, "modal" prototypes and "average" prototypes, depending on the nature of the category or concept and the discriminability of the values of the dimensions making up the category (e.g., how different a 3 value is from a 4 value) (Mervis, Chapter 8, this volume; Rosch & Mervis, 1975). Strauss and Cohen (1978) presented infants with a situation where the babies could form either a modal or an average prototype. Infants chose an average rather than a modal prototype, suggesting that they were more sensitive to the overall configuration of the face rather than to the specific features making up the faces.

It would be easy to extend such a design to address both the Normalcy and Uniqueness questions addressed in this chapter. We can only hope that future investigators will capitalize on the availability of these infant paradigms to extend the exciting and informative work that has been accomplished with adult mentally retarded populations (e.g., McDade & Adler, 1980; Marcell & Armstrong, 1982; Varnhagen, et al., 1987) to infants.

Finally, we think an important unresolved issue is the nature of the habituation–dishabituation deficit posited by many of the investigators whose research we have just reviewed. As we noted there are persistent reports that infants with Down syndrome are more "riveted" and visually attentive than normal infants. Does this stem from a failure of basic neurological inhibitory capacity, or does it simply reflect a "developmental" difference of longer processing or "schema construction" time?

References

Bayley, N. (1969). *The Bayley Scales of Infant Development*. New York: Psychological Corporation.
Bornstein, M., & Sigman, M. (1986). Continuity in mental development from infancy. *Child Development, 57*, 251–274.

Bronfenbrenner, U., & Crouter, A. C. (1983). The evolution of environmental models in developmental research. In P. Mussen (Ed.), *Handbook of child psychology* (pp. 357–414). New York: Wiley.

Brown, A. L., & Campione, J. C. (1977). Training strategic study time appointment in educable retarded children. *Intelligence, 1,* 94–107.

Bushnell, E. (1986). The basis of infant visual–tactual functioning – amodal dimensions of multimodal compounds? In L. Lipsitt & C. Rovee-Collier (Eds.), *Advances in infancy research* (Vol. 4, pp. 182–194). Norwood, NJ: Ablex.

Butterfield, E. C., & Belmont, J. M. (1977). Assessing and improving the executive cognitive functions of mentally retarded people. In I. Bialer & M. Sternlicht (Eds.), *Psychological issues in mental retardation* (pp. 277–318). New York: Psychological Dimensions.

Caron, A. J., & Caron, R. F. (1981). Processing of relational information as an index of infant risk. In S. L. Friedman and M. Sigman (Eds.), *Preterm birth and psychological development* (pp. 219–240). New York: Academic Press.

Caron, A. J., Caron, R. F., & Glass, P. (1983). Responsiveness to relational information as a measure of cognitive functioning in non-suspect infants. In T. Field & A. Sostek (Eds.), *Infants born at risk: Psychological, perceptual and cognitive processes* (pp. 181–209). New York: Grune & Stratton.

Caron, R., Caron, A., & Myers, R. (1982). Abstraction of invariant face expression in infancy. *Child Development, 53,* 1008–1015.

Cicchetti, D. (1984). The emergence of developmental psychopathology. *Child Development, 55,* 1–7.

Cicchetti, D. (in press). An historical perspective on the discipline of developmental psychopathology. In J. Rolf, A. Masten, D. Cicchetti, K. Neuchterlein, & S. Weintraub (Eds.), *Risk and protective factors in the development of psychopathology.* New York: Cambridge University Press.

Cicchetti, D., & Ganiban, J. (in press). The organization of coherence of developmental processes in infants and children with Down syndrome. In R. M. Hodap, J. A. Burack, and E. Zigler (Eds.), *Issues in the developmental approach to mental retardation.* New York: Cambridge University Press.

Cicchetti, D., & Pogge-Hesse, P. (1982). Possible contributions of the study of organically retarded persons to developmental theory. In E. Zigler & D. Balla (Eds.), *Mental retardation: The developmental–difference controversy* (pp. 277–318). Hillsdale, NJ: Erlbaum.

Cicchetti, D., & Sroufe, L. A. (1976). The relationship between affective and cognitive development in Down syndrome infants. *Child Development, 47,* 920–929.

Cicchetti, D., & Sroufe, L. A. (1978). An organizational view of affect: Illustration from the study of Down's syndrome infants. In M. Lewis & L. Rosenblum (Eds.), *The development of affect* (pp. 309–351). New York: Plenum.

Cicchetti, D., & Wagner, S. (in press). Alternative assessment strategies for the evaluation of infants and toddlers: An organizational perspective. In S. Meisels & J. Shonkoff (Eds.), *Handbook of early intervention.* New York: Cambridge University Press.

Cohen, L. B. (1979). Our developing knowledge of infant perception and cognition. *American Psychologist, 34,* 894–899.

Cohen, L. B. (1981). Examination of habituation as a measure of aberrant infant development. In S. L. Friedman & M. Sigman (Eds.), *Preterm birth and psychological development.* (pp. 241–253). New York: Academic Press.

Cohen, L. B., Sigman, M., Parmalee. A. H., and Beckwith, L. (1982). Perinatal risk and developmental outcome in preterm infants. *Seminars in Perinatology, 6*(4), 334–339.

Cohen, L. B., & Strauss, M. S. (1979). Concept acquisition in the human infant. *Child Development, 50,* 419–424.

Courchesne, E. (1988). Physioanatomical considerations in Down syndrome. In L. Nadel (Ed.), *The psychobiology of Down syndrome* (pp. 291–314). Cambridge, MA: MIT Press.

Cowie, V. (1970). *A study of the early development of mongols.* Oxford: Pergamon Press.

DeCasper, A. J., & Fifer, A. P. (1980). Of human bonding: Newborns prefer their mothers' voices. *Science, 208,* 1174–1176.

Dobson, V., & Teller, D. (1978). Visual acuity in human infants: A review and comparison of behavioral and electrophysiological studies. *Vision Research, 18,* 1469–1483.

Eimas, P. D. (1975). Speech perception in early infancy. In L. B. Cohen & P. Slapatek (Eds.), *Infants' perception: From sensation to cognition* (Vol. 2, pp. 193–231). New York: Academic Press.

Entus, A. K. (1975). *Hemispheric asymmetry in processing dichotically presented speech and nonspeech stimuli to infants.* Paper presented at meeting of the Society for Research in Child Development, Denver.

Fagan, J. (1985) *Early novelty preference and later intelligence.* Paper presented at meeting of the Society for Research in Child Development, Toronto.

Fagan, J. F., & McGrath, S. K. (1981). Infant recognition memory and later intelligence. *Intelligence, 5,* 121–130.

Fagan, J. F., & Singer, L. T. (1983). Infant recognition memory as a measure of intelligence. In L. P. Lipsitt (Ed.), *Advances in infancy research* (Vol. 2, pp. 31–78). Norwalk, NJ: Ablex.

Fagan, J., Singer, L., Montie, J., & Shepherd, P. (1986). Selective screening device for the early detection of normal or delayed cognitive development in infants at risk for later mental retardation. *Pediatrics, 78*(6), 1021–1026.

Fantz, R. L., Fagan, J. F., & Miranda, S. B. (1975). Early visual selectivity. In L. B. Cohen & P. Salapatek (Eds.), *Infant perception: From sensation to cognition,* Vol. 1: *Basic visual processes* (pp. 249–346). New York: Academic Press.

Fishbein, H. D. (1976). *Evolution, development and children's learning.* Pacific Palisades, CA: Goodyear Publishing.

Gibson, D. (1975). Chromosomal psychology and Down's syndrome. *Canadian Journal of Behavioural Science, 7,* 167–191.

Gibson, D. (1978). *Down's syndrome: The psychology of mongolism.* Cambridge: Cambridge University Press.

Gibson, J. J. (1979). *The ecological approach to visual perception.* Boston: Houghton Mifflin.

Glenn, S. M., & Cunningham, C. C. (1983). What do babies listen to most? A developmental study of auditory preferences in nonhandicapped infants and infants with Down's syndrome. *Developmental Psychology, 19*(3), 332–337.

Glenn, S. M., Cunningham, C. C., & Joyce, P. F. (1981). A study of auditory preferences in nonhandicapped infants and infants with Down's syndrome. *Child Development, 52,* 1303–1307.

Gottesman, I. I. (1963). Genetic aspects of intelligent behavior. In N. Ellis (Eds.), *Handbook of mental deficiency* (pp. 253–296). New York: McGraw-Hill.

Gottfried, A., Rose, S., & Bridger, W. (1977). Cross-modal transfer in human infants. *Child Development, 48,* 118–123.

Gottfried, A., Rose, S., & Bridger, W. (1978). Effects of visual, haptic, and manipulatory experiences on infants' visual recognition memory of objects. *Developmental Psychology, 14,* 305–312.

Gunn, P., Berry, P., & Andrews, R. J. (1981). The affective response of Down's syndrome infants to a repeated event. *Child Development, 52,* 745–748.

Gunn, P., Berry, P., & Andrews, R. J. (1982). Looking behavior of Down syndrome infants. *American Journal of Mental Deficiency, 87*(3), 344–347.

Hoffman, M., Salapatek, P., Kuskowski, M., & Cicchetti, D. (1979). *Evidence for visual memory in the evoked potential of human infants.* Presented at the Society for Research in Child Development Meeting, San Francisco, April.

Kopp, C. (1983). Risk factors in development. In P. H. Mussen (Ed.), *Handbook of child psychology* (4th ed., Vol. 1, pp. 1081–1188). New York: Wiley.

Kopp, C., & McCall, R. (1982). Predicting later mental performance for normal, at-risk, and handicapped infants. In P. B. Baltes & O. G. Brim (Eds.), *Life-span development and behavior* (Vol. 4). New York: Academic Press.

Krakow, J. B., & Kopp, C. (1983). The effects of developmental delay on sustained attention in young children. *Child Development, 54,* 1143–1155.

Landry, S. H., & Chapieski, M. L. (1989). Joint attention and infant toy exploration: Effects of Down syndrome and prematurity. *Child Development, 60,* 103–118.

Lewis, M., & Brooks-Gunn, J. (1984). Age and handicapped group differences in infants' visual attention. *Child Development, 55,* 858–868.

Lewis, V., & Bryant, P. E. (1982). Touch and vision in normal and Down's syndrome babies. *Perception, 11,* 691–701.

Loveland, K. (1987). Behavior of young children with Down syndrome before the mirror: Finding things reflected. *Child Development, 58,* 928–936.

MacTurk, R., Vietze, P., McCarthy, M., McQuiston, S., & Yarrow, L. (1985). The organization of exploratory behavior in Down syndrome and non-delayed infants. *Child Development, 56,* 573–585.

Mans, L., Cicchetti, D., & Sroufe, L. A. (1978). Mirror reactions of Down's syndrome infants and toddlers: Cognitive underpinnings of self-recognition. *Child Development, 49,* 1247–1250.

Marcell, M. M., & Armstrong, V. (1982). Auditory and visual sequential memory of Down syndrome and nonretarded children. *American Journal of Mental Deficiency, 87*(1), 86–95.

McCall, R. B. (1981a). Early predictions of later IQ: The search continues. *Intelligence, 5,* 141–147.

McCall, R. B. (1981b). Predicting developmental outcome: Résumé and redirection. In C. C. Brown (Ed.), *Infants at risk: Assessment and intervention* (pp. 57–70). New York: Johnson & Johnson.

McDade, H., & Adler, S. (1980). Down syndrome and short-term memory impairment: A storage or retrieval deficit? *American Journal of Mental Deficiency, 84*(6), 561–567.

McDonough, S. C., & Cohen, L. B. (1982). *Use of habituation to investigate concept acquisition on cerebral palsified infants.* Paper presented at meeting of the International Conference for Infant Studies, Austin, TX.

Meltzoff, A. N., & Borton, R. W. (1979). Intermodal matching by human neonates. *Nature, 282,* 403–404.

Miranda, S. B., & Fantz, R. L. (1973). Visual preferences of Down syndrome and normal infants. *Child Development, 45,* 651–660.

Miranda, S. B., & Fantz, R. L. (1974). Recognition memory in Down's syndrome and normal infants. *Child Development, 54,* 1168–1175.

Rosch, E., & Mervis, C. (1975). Family resemblances: Studies in the internal structure of categories. *Cognitive Psychology, 7,* 573–603.

Rose, S. A. (1981). Lags in the cognitive competence of prematurely born infants. In S. L. Friedman & M. Sigman (Eds.), *Preterm birth and psychological development* (pp. 255–269). New York: Academic Press.

Rose, S. A. (1983). Differential rates of visual information processing in full-term and pre-term infants. *Child Development, 54,* 1189–1198.

Rose, S. A., Gottfried, A. W., & Bridger, W. H. (1978). Cross-modal transfer in infants: Relationship to prematurity and socioeconomic background. *Developmental Psychology, 14*(6), 643–652.

Rose, S. A., & Wallace, I. (1985a). Visual recognition memory: A predictor of later cognitive development in preterms. *Child Development, 56,* 843–852.

Rose, S. A., & Wallace, I. (1985b). Cross-modal and intramodal transfer as predictors of mental development in full-term and preterm infants. *Developmental Psychology, 21,* 949–962.

Rutter, M., & Garmezy, N. (1983). Developmental psychopathology. In P. Mussen (Ed.), *Handbook of child psychology* (Vol. 4, pp. 775–911). New York: Wiley.

Sameroff, A., & Chandler, M. (1975). Reproductive risk and the continuum of caretaking casualty. In F. Horowitz (Ed.), *Review of Child Development Research* (Vol. 4). Chicago: University of Chicago Press.

Schafer, E., & Peeke, H. (1982). Down syndrome individuals fail to habituate to cortical evoked potentials. *American Journal of Mental Deficiency, 87,* 332–337.

Schneider, J., & Brannen, E. (1981). A comparison of two evaluation tools used to assess children with Down's syndrome. *Physical and Occupational Therapy in Pediatrics, 1,*(1), 19–29.

Serafica, F., & Cicchetti, D. (1976). Down syndrome children in a strange situation: Attachment and exploration behaviors. *Merrill-Palmer Quarterly, 22,* 137–150.

Siqueland, E. R. (1981). Studies of visual recognition memory in preterm infants: Differences in development as a function of perinatal morbidity. In S. L. Friedman & M. Sigman (Eds.), *Preterm birth and physiological development* (pp. 271–288). New York: Academic Press.

Sroufe, L. A., & Wunsch, J. (1972). The development of laughter in the first year of life. *Child Development, 43*, 1326–1344.

Stanovitch, K. (1978). Information processing in mentally retarded individuals. *International Review of Research in Mental Retardation, 9*, 29–60.

Starkey, P., & Cooper, R. G. (1980). Numerosity perception in human infants. *Science, 210*, 1033.

Stechler, G., & Latz, E. (1966). Some observations on attention and arousal in the human infant. *Journal of the American Academy of Child Psychiatry, 5*, 517–525.

Sternberg, S. (1966). High-speed scanning in human memory. *Science, 153*, 652–654.

Sternberg, R., & Spear, L. (1985). A triarchic theory of mental retardation. *International Review of Research in Mental Retardation, 13*, 301–326.

Strauss, M., & Cohen, L. (1978). *Infant immediate and delayed memory for perceptual dimensions.* Unpublished manuscript. University of Illinois.

Varnhagen, C., Das, J. P., & Varnhagen, S. (1987). Auditory and visual memory span: Cognitive processing by TMR individuals with Down syndrome or other etiologies. *American Journal of Mental Deficiency, 91*(94), 398–405.

Vietze, P., McCarthy, M., McQuiston, S., MacTurk, R., & Yarrow, L. (1983). Attention and exploratory behavior in infants with Down syndrome. In T. Field & A. Sostek (Eds.), *Infants born at risk: Perceptual and physical processes* (pp. 251–268). New York: Grune & Stratton.

Wagner, S., & Sakovits, L. (1986). A process analysis of infant visual and cross-modal recognition memory: Implication for an amodal code. In L. Lipsitt & C. Rovee-Collier (Eds.), *Advances in infancy research* (Vol. 4, pp. 196–217). Norwood, NJ: Ablex.

Wagner, S., Winner, E., Cicchetti, D., & Gardner, H. (1980). Metaphorical mapping in human infants. *Child Development, 52*, 728–731.

Weisz, J., & Yeates, K. (1981). Cognitive development in retarded and nonretarded persons: Piagetian tests of the similar structure hypothesis. *Psychological Bulletin, 90*, 153–178.

Weisz, J., & Zigler, E. (1979). Cognitive development in retarded and nonretarded persons: Piagetian tests of the similar sequence hypothesis. *Psychological Bulletin, 86*, 831–851.

Zigler, E. (1969). Developmental versus difference theories of mental retardation and the problem of motivation. *American Journal of Mental Deficiency, 73*, 536–556.

Zigler, E., & Balla, D. (Eds.), *Mental retardation*. Hillsdale, NJ: Erlbaum.

6   Sensorimotor development of infants with Down syndrome

Carl J. Dunst

The purpose of this chapter is to review and synthesize available data regarding the sensorimotor development of infants with Down syndrome. The term *sensorimotor development* refers to qualitative changes in the psychological functioning of infants occurring during the period from birth to the beginnings of symbolic and representational thought. Qualitative changes in psychological functioning reflect the infant's capacity to acquire, store, and use information about the social and nonsocial world. The study of the sensorimotor capabilities of infants has its roots in Baldwin's (1895, 1897) psychobiological model of child development; reached the forefront of psychology with Piaget's (1936/1952, 1937/1954, 1945/1951) publication of his trilogy on infant intelligence; and has more recently been the focus of attention, most notably reflected in the work of McCall (1979) and Uzgiris (1983).

The notions of sequence, stage, and structure are central to the study of psychological (cognitive) functioning in general (Flavell, 1982a, 1982b) and sensorimotor development in particular (Uzgiris, 1987). The term *sequence* refers to the constant and invariant order of acquisition of progressively more complex cognitive competencies. The term *stage* refers to the distinct forms of behavior that are manifested at different ages or periods of development. The term *structure* refers to the manner in which different manifestations of behavior bear some developmental (stagelike) relationship to one another, and share some sort of common mediator or denominator.

The sensorimotor period is generally considered to consist of six progressively more complex types of psychological sets of competencies (Piaget, 1952). Each level in this sequence is defined by classes of behavior that exemplify distinct stages of development. Piaget (1952) describes these stages in terms of the various types of adaptations the infant is capable of making in response to different environmental demands. At each stage of development, cognitive adaptations are manifested in

Appreciation is extended to Peggy Mankinen, Sherra Vance, Johnna Clontz, Carol Trivette, and Pat Condrey for assistance in preparation of this chapter. Work reported in this chapter was supported, in part, by a grant from the N.C. Department of Human Resources, Division of Mental Health, Mental Retardation and Substance Abuse, Research Section (#82A22).

180

different domains of performance: problem solving, object permanence, spatial relationships, causality, time, vocal imitation, gestural imitation, and play (Piaget, 1951, 1952, 1954). The manner in which these different sensorimotor capabilities are interrelated defines the structure of sensorimotor intelligence.

This chapter examines sensorimotor development from a neo-Piagetian perspective with a particular focus on explicating developmental processes in infants with Down syndrome (Cicchetti & Pogge-Hesse, 1982; Dunst, 1984). Three aspects of sensorimotor development are examined: stage-related properties, factors that influence the acquisition of sensorimotor competencies, and interdependencies with other developmental domains. The stage-related properties that are examined include stage sequencing, stage transitioning, and stage structuring. The influential bases of sensorimotor development are examined in terms of factors that affect the acquisition of sensorimotor competencies. The relationships between affect, motivation, temperament, and sensorimotor development are examined in terms of interdependencies among developments in these different behavior domains. The manner in which sensorimotor development is related to the acquisition of other behavior competencies is the focus of a number of other chapters in this volume (e.g., Beeghly, Weiss-Perry, & Cicchetti, Chapter 10).

As part of the review, synthesis, and critical examination of different aspects of sensorimotor development, contrasts between infants with Down syndrome and both nonretarded and retarded infants are made to discern similarities and differences in the processes of acquisition of sensorimotor competencies. These types of comparisons bear directly on the developmental–difference controversy (see Zigler & Balla, 1982). To the extent that infants with Down syndrome (and other retarded children) show similarities in their processes of acquisition of sensorimotor behaviors relative to nonretarded infants, we would have evidence regarding the universality of developmental processes. To the extent that processes of acquisition differ, the nature of the disparities in development would be established, and suggest the manner in which etiology influences various aspects of cognitive development.

Studies that have utilized Piagetian and neo-Piagetian frameworks for investigating the developmental characteristics of sensorimotor development have proliferated in recent years. These various studies constitute the primary source of material for this chapter.[1] Another source of data comes from a study completed by the author specifically for this chapter. This investigation is hereafter referred to as the Down Syndrome Study. The subjects were 85 infants with Down syndrome who participated in an early intervention program (Dunst, 1982, 1985). As part of their participation in this program, the subjects were administered both the Piagetian-based Uzgiris and Hunt (1975) scales and the Bayley (1969) infant scales (Mental Scale and Infant Behavior Record) at regular intervals in order to discern changes in cognitive development over time. The Uzgiris–Hunt scales measure sensorimotor development in seven domains: object permanence, means–ends abilities, vocal imitation, gestural imitation, operational causality, spatial relationships, and schemes for relating to sensorimotor intelligence as explicated by Piaget (1951, 1952, 1954).

The Uzgiris–Hunt scales were administered, on the average, four times per subject. A total of 310 complete protocols of the scales were available for the total sample. A subsample of the subjects ($N = 31$) were administered the scales longitudinally on 5 to 9 occasions ($M = 6.40$, $SD = 1.31$). Thus, the data are partly cross-sectional and partly longitudinal. Analyses were performed separately for the entire sample and the longitudinal subsample in order to determine if the two sets of data produced similar or different findings. Unless otherwise indicated, the results for the full sample and longitudinal subsample were identical for the particular results reported.

Results from the analyses of the Down Syndrome Study data relevant to the foci of this chapter will be described in a number of sections to fill in gaps, shed light on certain developmental questions, and support or refute the contentions of other investigations regarding sensorimotor development. Methodologically, this investigation examined several different aspects of sensorimotor functioning at different developmental junctures from birth to the age of attainment of the highest-level achievements on the Uzgiris–Hunt scales. Sensorimotor functioning was examined at successive 4-month age ranges (0–4, 4–8, 8–12, etc.), periods of time that either roughly demarcate the outer bounds of different stages of the sensorimotor period (Piaget, 1952) or time periods that are considered important transitional points in the genesis of sensorimotor competence (e.g., McCall, 1979; Uzgiris, 1983).

Stage-related properties of sensorimotor development

Piaget (1960, 1973) as well as others (Flavell, 1971, 1972, 1982b; Wohlwill, 1973) have proposed certain stage-related properties of cognitive development. These include stage sequencing, stage transitioning, and stage structuring. These different stage criteria provide a basis for describing and explaining processes of cognitive-developmental change and stability.

Stage sequencing is examined in terms of two different aspects of sensorimotor development: age-related changes and ordinality in development. Age-related changes refer to the extent to which higher levels of achievement are attained at progressively older ages. Developmental level regressed on chronological age (CA) provides a basis for establishing the developmental function of a behavior construct (McCall, 1979; Wohlwill, 1973). Ordinality refers to the extent to which Stage 1 behaviors always precede the appearance of the Stage 2 behaviors, Stage 2 behaviors always precede those of Stage 3, and so on. Both stage sequencing characteristics are important with regard to the establishment of the constant and invariant order in the acquisition of sensorimotor behaviors.

The term *stage transitioning* refers to both the relationships between successive stages, levels, or landmarks in development (Campbell & Richie, 1983; Flavell, 1972; Uzgiris, 1987) and stabilization in the mastery of cognitive competencies (Inhelder, 1966, 1968). The study of between stage relationships concerns itself with the establishment of causal–functional links between successive achievements in development. Stabilization in development has generally been studied with regard to (1) regressions in development and (2) the relative amount of time necessary for movement from one level of development to the next. Both stage transitioning characteristics provide a basis for disentangling the processes of acquisition of sensorimotor capabilities.

Stage structuring is examined in terms of both between-domain interrelationships and continuity in the structural organization of sensorimotor capabilities across time. Between-domain relationships refers to the extent to which different domains of sensorimotor performance are interrelated, and thus form a structural totality or *structure d'ensemble* (Piaget, 1973). Structural continuity refers to the extent to which the "form" of the organizational aspects of different sensorimotor domains are similar at different developmental junctures. Both stage structuring characteristics provide a basis for discerning the nature of organization and continuity in development.

Cicchetti and Pogge-Hesse (1982) and Dunst (1984) describe the manner in which the study of the stage-related properties of cognitive development among retarded persons can contribute to developmental theory building. Most notably, these investigations stress the contributions that the study of retarded children can make to our understanding of developmental *processes,* particularly with regard to factors that affect behavior organization and behavior change. Cicchetti and Pogge-Hess (1982) point out that because retarded children's pace of development is slower, it provides a better vantage point from which to separate coincidental synchronies in development from convergences and discontinuities in development that have mediational bases. Dunst (1984) argues for a broader-based perspective from which to view early cognitive growth, and the mechanisms that directly and indirectly affect processes involved in the acquisition of sensorimotor competencies.

It would appear that the study of the sensorimotor development of children with Down syndrome and other retarded children can contribute to developmental theory in a number of important ways. First, we may learn about the manner in which development proceeds in atypical populations and how etiology, as an independent variable, affects the course of development. Second, it may be possible to isolate factors affecting development because the slower pace of development of retarded infants permits a better vantage point from which to identify causal and mediational variables affecting change. Third, additional light may be shed on the developmental–difference controversy through the systematic examination of developmental processes among different groups of infants. With these major aims in mind, a systematic examination of the sensorimotor development of nonretarded infants, infants with Down syndrome, and other retarded infants was undertaken.

Stage sequencing

Age-related changes, or the *developmental function* of the relationship between CA and some behavioral construct (e.g., sensorimotor intelligence), provide an indication of order in the acquisition of different levels of a developmental construct. Developmental level regressed on age depicts sequential order with respect to the age-variable but not the invariant order based on the hypothesized relationships between successive levels of a developmental construct (e.g., object permanence). This difference is fundamentally important with regard to the stage sequencing notion. Order based on a postulated sequence of achievements requires that ordinality be determined not with respect to age but with respect to the relationship between items or landmarks chosen to represent points along a developmental continuum. Each type of scaling provides a different perspective from which to determine the sequential order of sensorimotor development.

Age-related changes

The extent to which stagelike progressions in different sensorimotor domains (object permanence, means–ends abilities, vocal imitation, etc.) are correlated with CA and mental age (MA) of nonretarded infants, infants with Down syndrome, and other retarded individuals has been examined in a number of studies. Table 6.1 shows data from 14 investigations, organized into three categories of studies: nonretarded, infants with Down syndrome, and heterogeneously formed groups of retarded individuals. As can be seen, strong age-related changes have been found in the majority of studies. These data indicate that higher level of sensorimotor development can be expected to be manifested at higher age levels.

Several things are worth noting about these age-related data. First, and not unexpectedly, the correlations between CA and sensorimotor level are substantial and highly significant in studies of nonretarded infants. Second, in all the studies of infants with Down syndrome, the magnitude of the correlation coefficients are moderate to substantial except for vocal imitation, indicating that the age-related changes for this sensorimotor construct are not as great as those for the other sensorimotor domains. Third, in those studies of older retarded persons (Barnes & Dunst, 1984; Rogers, 1977), level of sensorimotor development is not at all correlated with CA. This finding is consistent with results from other studies of older children and adults functioning at the sensorimotor level (see Uzgiris, 1987), and indicates that for older severely to profoundly retarded individuals, covariation between CA and sensorimotor level becomes minimal with increasing age. Taken together, however, the data shown in Table 6.1 provides considerable evidence that there is generally substantial covariation between both MA and CA (except for the exceptions noted above) and level of sensorimotor performance among nonretarded infants, infants with Down syndrome, and other retarded persons.

Further examination of Table 6.1 shows that for those studies that calculated correlations between sensorimotor level and both CA and MA, the correlations with MA are higher than those with CA. In order to determine if covariation was greater for MA compared to CA, intrastudy tests of significance were performed between the average correlations obtained in the different investigations. Correlation coefficients were converted to Fisher z scores; the mean of the scores computed; the average z_s converted back to average r_s; and the differences between the r_s for CA and MA tested using the Hotelling formula. This method takes into consideration, and corrects for, the correlation between CA and MA. The majority (70%) of the

Table 6.1. Correlations among chronological age (CA), mental (MA), and sensorimotor development reported in 14 investigations

Study	N	CA (months)			Correlation with CA							Correlation with MA						
		Mean	SD	Range	OP	ME	VI	GI	OC	SR	SO	OP	ME	VI	GI	OC	SR	SO
Nonretarded:																		
Uzgiris & Hunt (1974)	84	10.00	—	1–23	.94**	.94**	.88**	.91**	.86**	.91**	.89**	—	—	—	—	—	—	—
Decarie (1965)	90	11.00	—	3–20	.86**	—	—	—	—	—	—	.92**	—	—	—	—	—	—
Corman & Escalona (1969)	247	—	—	1–27	.83**	—	—	—	—	.84**	—	—	—	—	—	—	—	—
Watson & Fischer (1977)	36	19.00	—	13–26	—	—	—	—	—	—	.59*	—	—	—	—	—	—	—
Down syndrome:																		
Dunst (1981a)	7	11.14	4.08	7–18	.80*	.83**	.49	.78*	.79*	.94**	.93**	.94**	.98**	.69	.92**	.86**	.97**	.86**
Dunst & Rheingrover (1983)	21	13.07	5.19	3–23	.86**	.70**	.54**	.70**	.62**	.88**	.87**	.84**	.83**	.72**	.82**	.82**	.89**	.91**
Dunst & Rheingrover (1983)	30	15.39	8.96	3–32	.74**	.68**	.19	.67**	.55**	.71**	.84**	.86**	.87**	.63**	.84**	.72**	.86**	.76**
Down Syndrome Study	85	20.48	11.14	1–55	.76**	.68**	.51**	.68**	.72**	.72**	.69**	.84**	.77**	.68**	.77**	.77**	.82**	.78**
Hill & McCune-Nicolich (1981)	30	33.20	8.61	20–53	—	—	—	—	—	—	.44**	—	—	—	—	—	—	.75**
Mentally retarded:																		
Dunst (1980a)[a]	36	14.42	7.36	3–27	.89**	.82**	.67**	.75**	.86**	.89**	.90**	.91**	.87**	.83**	.88**	.91**	.88**	.94**
Dunst (1978a)[b]	28	16.80	8.47	6–30	.81**	.41*	.49**	.55**	.22	.59**	.61**	.83**	.84**	.61**	.79**	.69**	.87**	.91**
Dunst et al. (1981)[c]	143	19.07	10.55	3–66	.55**	.51**	.22*	.35**	.41**	.47**	.49**	.73**	.75**	.61**	.69**	.71**	.78**	.77**
Barnes & Dunst (1984)[d]	28	129.93	60.60	48–120	.12	.01	-.12	.20	.13	.03	.01	.90**	.85**	.57**	.83**	.90**	.85**	.75**
Rogers (1977)[e]	40	152.00	—	106–179	ns[f]	ns	ns	ns	—	ns	—	.40**	.48**	—	[.46**][g]	.73**	.73**	—

Note: OP = object permanence; ME = means–ends/problem solving; VI = vocal imitation; GI = gestural imitation; OC = operational causality; SR = spatial relationships; SO = Schemes for relating to objects/symbolic play. *$p < .05$; **$p < .01$. Dash means statistic not reported.

[a] The sample included 12 Down syndrome, 6 brain damaged, 5 spina bifida, 5 at-risk, 4 cerebral palsied, and 4 mentally retarded infants with unknown etiology.

[b] The sample included 13 Down syndrome, 6 brain damaged, 5 cerebral palsied, 2 hydrocephalic, 1 microcephalic, and 2 mentally retarded children with unknown etiology.

[c] The sample included 29 Down syndrome, 29 cerebral palsied, 33 at-risk, 17 mentally retarded infants with cranial anomalies, and 35 mentally retarded infants with unknown etiology.

[d] Unspecified heterogeneous group of mentally retarded and physically impaired persons.

[e] The sample included 13 encephalic, 4 chromosomal, 4 mentally retarded due to cultural factors, and 19 mentally retarded children with unknown causes.

[f] Correlation coefficients not reported (ns = nonsignificant).

[g] The correlation was between a combined measure of both gestural and vocal imitation and mental age.

Table 6.2. *Comparisons of the differences between the correlations of chronological age (CA) and mental age (MA) with sensorimotor development*

Study	N	CA			MA			t
		Mean	SD	Range	Mean	SD	Range	
Nonretarded:								
Decarie (1965)	90[a]	.86[b]	—	—	.92[b]	—	—	2.87**
Down syndrome:								
Dunst (1981a)	7	.83	.15	.49–.94	.90	.09	.69–.98	0.55
Dunst & Rheingrover (1983)	21	.76	.13	.54–.88	.84	.06	.72–.91	1.28
Dunst & Rheingrover (1983)	30	.66	.07	.19–.84	.80	.09	.63–.86	1.59
Down Syndrome Study	85	.69	.06	.57–.76	.78	.05	.68–.84	2.48**
Hill & McCune-Nicolich (1981)	30	.44	—	—	.75	—	—	2.69*
Mentally retarded:								
Dunst (1980a)	36	.84	.09	.67–.90	.91	.03	.83–.94	2.29*
Dunst (1978a)	28	.55	.18	.41–.81	.81	.11	.61–.91	2.73*
Dunst et al. (1981)	143	.43	.11	.22–.55	.72	.06	.61–.78	4.69**
Barnes & Dunst (1984)	28	.06	.07	−.12–.20	.83	.11	.57–.90	5.12**

Note: $*p < .05$; $**p < .01$. Dash means statistic not available.
[a] See Table 6.1 for a description of the characteristics of the subjects in the studies.
[b] The mean r_s were determined using Fischer Z transformations.

CA–MA differences were statistically significant (see Table 6.2). These findings indicate that MA rather than CA is the better covariate of sensorimotor level. The only analyses that did not produce significant differences were studies of infants with Down syndrome. In the Dunst (1981b) study this is probably due to the small sample size ($N = 7$). The results for the two samples of infants with Down syndrome in the Dunst and Rheingrover (1983) study suggest similar covariation between both CA and MA and sensorimotor level, and indeed the magnitude of the differences between the CA–MA contrasts are, in all but one instance, smaller for the infants with Down syndrome compared to the other samples of subjects.

In order to determine whether or not the degree of covariation between sensorimotor level and both CA and MA was similar or different for nonretarded infants, infants with Down syndrome, and other retarded children, between diagnostic group comparisons were made among the average r_s in studies that employed the seven Uzgiris and Hunt (1975) scales. Analyses were restricted to studies with subjects who were chronologically, on the average, less than 2 years of age. Data were aggregated from three studies of infants with Down syndrome (Dunst, 1981a; Dunst & Rheingrover, 1983; Down Syndrome Study) and three studies of nonadult retarded individuals (Dunst, 1978a, 1980a; Dunst, Brassell, & Rheingrover, 1981), and compared with the data reported by Uzgiris and Hunt (1975). The correlation coefficients were converted to Fisher z scores; the average of the scores computed;

Table 6.3. *Comparisons of the average correlations in studies of nonretarded, Down syndrome, and mentally retarded infants*

Subjects	N	CA			MA		
		Mean	SD	Range	Mean	SD	Range
Nonretarded[a]	84	.91	.03	.86–.94	—	—	—
Down syndrome[b]	143	.74	.16	.19–.94	.84	.09	.63–.98
Mentally retarded[c]	207	.65	.21	.22–.90	.83	.10	.61–.94
Comparison of mean r's:							
Nonretarded vs. Down syndrome		$Z = 4.14, p < .001$			$Z = 2.27, p < .01$		
Nonretarded vs. mentally retarded		$Z = 5.72, p < .001$			$Z = 2.47, p < .01$		
Down syndrome vs. mentally retarded		$Z = 1.58$, ns			$Z = .06$, ns		
Comparison of variances:							
Nonretarded vs. Down syndrome		$F(83, 142) = 28.44, p < .001$			$F(83, 142) = 9.00, p < .001$		
Nonretarded vs. mentally retarded		$F(83, 206) = 49.00, p < .001$			$F(83, 206) = 11.11, p < .001$		
Down syndrome vs. mentally retarded		$F(142, 206) = 1.71, p < .01$			$F(142, 206) = 1.23$, ns		

Note: ns = nonsignificant; dash means data not available for analysis.
[a] Uzgiris and Hunt (1975)
[b] Dunst (1981a); Dunst and Rheingrover (1983); Down Syndrome Study.
[c] Dunst (1978a, 1980); Dunst et al. (1981)

and comparisons made between groups. Table 6.3 shows the results for these analyses. There were significant differences between the mean r_s for the nonretarded infants and subjects with Down syndrome, and the nonretarded and retarded subjects, for both the CA and MA comparisons. Likewise, there were significant differences for the same comparisons in terms of variability around the mean r_s. The former set of findings indicates that degree of covariation between age and sensorimotor level is greater among nonretarded infants compared to infants with Down syndrome and other retarded infants. The latter set of findings indicates that intercorrelation variance is greater among children with Down syndrome and other retarded children. These sets of findings may be taken as evidence of greater heterogeneity in the sensorimotor development of children with Down syndrome and other retarded children.

The data regarding the covariation between CA and MA with level of sensorimotor performance among nonretarded infants, infants with Down syndrome, and other retarded persons may be taken as an indication that higher levels of achievement can be expected to be attained with increasing age of the child. However, the analytic approach upon which these data are based assumes a linear relationship between the independent and dependent measures, an assumption that may not be

Table 6.4. *Means and standard deviations for chronological age (CA), mental age (MA), developmental quotient (DQ), and sensorimotor domain at 10 age levels (Down Syndrome Study)*

| | Chronological age range (months) | | | | | | | | | | | | | | | | | | | |
| | 0–4: (N=9) | | 4–8: (N=28) | | 8–12: (N=47) | | 12–16: (N=41) | | 16–20: (N=45) | | 20–24: (N=29) | | 24–28: (N=32) | | 28–32: (N=25) | | 32–36: (N=22) | | F<8.274 |
	M	SD	M	SD	M	SD	M	SD	M	SD	M	SD	M	SD	M	SD	M	SD	
Chronological age	2.89	0.82	6.08	1.19	10.10	1.16	14.00	1.25	17.73	1.20	21.82	1.21	26.25	1.25	29.84	0.97	33.75	.98	1960.57[c]
Mental age[a]	2.81	1.02	4.34	1.30	6.54	1.56	8.96	2.32	11.43	2.06	14.15	2.71	16.47	7.26	15.92	4.37	18.46	2.27	67.37
Developmental quotient[a]	84.76	13.81	69.98	22.27	61.34	13.31	62.37	16.18	60.69	11.13	59.63	9.44	55.91	10.82	52.10	13.62	54.63	6.89	7.43
Object permanence (14)[b]	1.86	1.07	2.30	1.10	4.09	1.32	5.73	2.23	7.57	1.83	9.60	2.24	10.28	2.76	10.80	3.25	12.90	1.48	85.54
Means–ends (13)	1.83	1.17	2.96	1.43	5.92	2.10	7.15	2.55	8.96	1.41	9.99	1.16	10.03	1.94	10.55	2.31	11.49	.96	68.69
Vocal imitation (9)	1.89	.93	2.28	.94	2.55	1.32	3.53	1.45	4.27	.99	4.71	1.34	5.27	1.63	4.89	1.77	5.62	1.29	26.04
Gestural imitation (9)	1.68	.83	1.64	.75	2.01	1.15	3.27	1.59	4.62	1.63	5.84	2.19	6.76	2.16	6.61	2.79	8.45	.99	54.62
Operational causality (7)	1.50	.55	1.96	.92	2.82	.75	3.27	.81	3.82	.96	4.45	1.12	5.13	1.36	5.51	1.44	6.32	.64	56.78
Spatial relationships (11)	2.11	1.45	3.53	1.26	5.31	.97	6.37	1.53	7.78	1.57	9.32	1.70	9.59	1.77	9.73	1.86	10.82	.40	92.36
Schemes (10)	1.33	.52	2.56	1.11	4.33	1.09	6.28	1.41	7.11	1.32	7.79	.76	8.00	1.50	8.20	1.08	8.82	.91	100.60

[a] Bayley scales of infant development. DQ was computed as MA/CA × 100.
[b] The number in parentheses indicates the number of scale steps (ordinal score) on the Uzgiris–Hunt scales.
[c] All between-age contrasts significant beyond the .0001 level.

entirely tenable for children with Down syndrome and other retarded children. It is widely thought that the mental development of infants with Down syndrome is not linear but, rather, curvilinear; that is, changes in MA per unit change in CA become progressively smaller at older age levels (e.g., Dicks-Mireaux, 1972). It is therefore reasonable to expect that the sensorimotor development of infants with Down syndrome may show similar relationships.

The extent to which the sensorimotor development of infants with Down syndrome was linear or curvilinear was examined among the infants in the Down Syndrome Study. The independent variables were CA and domain of sensorimotor performance (the seven Uzgiris–Hunt scales). Patterns of sensorimotor development were examined at 9 age levels (0–4, 4–8, 8–12, etc.) between birth and 36 months of age. The dependent measures were the ordinal, stage placement, and developmental age equivalent scores of the scale steps (Dunst, 1980b). Ordinal scores are those equal to the highest item passed (achieved) in each sensorimotor domain. Stage placement scores and developmental ages were used because the number of items (steps) on each of the Uzgiris–Hunt scales is different, and therefore between-domain contrasts are not possible using ordinal scores. Stage placement scores and developmental age levels, however, permit between-scale comparisons because the unit of measure is the same for the different scales.

Table 6.4 shows the means and standard deviations at each of the nine age groupings for CA, MA, and DQ (Developmental Quotient), and the ordinal scores for the seven Uzgiris–Hunt scales. As expected, there were significant differences on each of the measures for between age-level comparisons. Figure 6.1 graphically depicts the relationship between CA and both MA and the total sensorimotor scores (sum of the seven separate ordinal scores) on the Uzgiris–Hunt scales. MA regressed on CA shows the typical curvilinear pattern characteristic of infants with Down syndrome. The pattern of development for sensorimotor performance is also curvilinear.

The specific nature of the developmental functions of the subjects in the Down Syndrome Study were tested by regressing MA, the ordinal scores for the separate Uzgiris–Hunt domains, and the total Uzgiris–Hunt scores on CA at three separate age ranges (0–12, 12–24, 24–36), and testing the differences between the regression coefficients. These contrasts determine whether the slopes of the regression lines at the different age ranges differ significantly from one another, and thus provide evidence for a progressive slowing down in development. The results are shown in Table 6.5. As can be seen, the third-year regression coefficients are in all instances smaller than those for the first and second year, and the majority are statistically significant. A progressive slowing down in development is evident between both the first and third (B_1 vs. B_3) and second and third (B_2 vs. B_3) years. Of particular note is the fact that MA and sensorimotor development, with the exception of object permanence and operational causality, show very similar patterns of changes over time. This may be taken as evidence that the developmental functions of mental and sensorimotor development are much alike with respect to the "slowing down" phenomenon.

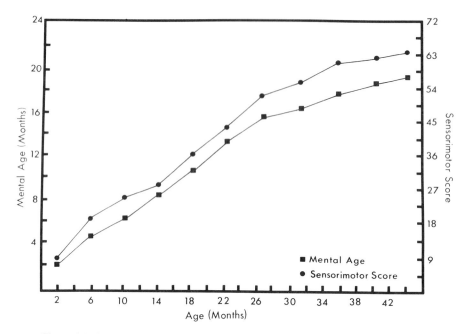

Figure 6.1. Patterns of mental and sensorimotor development for infants with Down syndrome. (*Note:* The total sensorimotor score was computed as the sum of the ordinal scores for the seven Uzgiris–Hunt scales.)

Table 6.5. *Regression coefficients at three age ranges for mental age and sensorimotor development (Down Syndrome Study)*

	Regression coefficients			t tests		
	B_1: 0–12 months	B_2: 12–24 months	B_3: 24–36 months	B_1 vs. B_2	B_1 vs. B_3	B_2 vs. B_3
Mental age[a]	.517	.641	.304	.91	1.66*	2.59**
Object permanence	.396	.477	.334	.70	.43	1.11
Means–ends	.681	.333	.169	2.78**	4.45***	2.10*
Vocal imitation	—[b]	.173	.051	—	—	1.94*
Gestural imitation	—[b]	.346	.196	—	—	1.72*
Operational causality	.194	.159	.135	.65	.89	.49
Spatial relationships	.441	.386	.139	.61	3.25***	2.94**
Schemes	.413	.213	.101	2.56**	3.59***	2.07*
Total sensorimotor score[c]	2.272	2.084	1.125	.39	1.89*	3.18***

Note: * $= p < .05$; ** $p < .01$; *** $p < .001$. Dash means data not available for analysis.
[a] Bayley mental scale.
[b] Insufficient data/variability to compute regression coefficient.
[c] Sum of the ordinal ranks on the seven Uzgiris–Hunt scales.

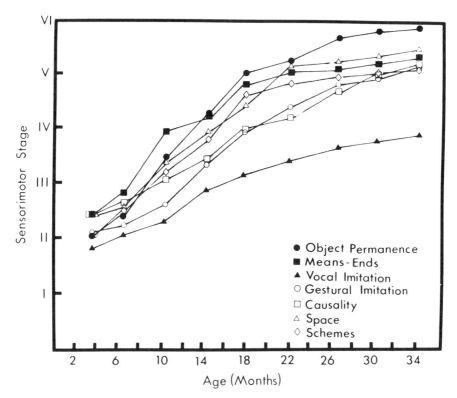

Figure 6.2. Patterns of development (stage levels) in separate sensorimotor domains for infants with Down syndrome.

The patterns of development for the infants with Down syndrome in terms of both stage placement scores and developmental ages are shown in Figures 6.2 and 6.3, respectively. The extent to which the developmental functions for the separate sensorimotor domains were similar was determined through a 9 Groups (Age Level) × 7 Domains (Object Permanence, Vocal Imitation, Causality, etc.) repeated measures Analysis of Variance (ANOVA) for both the stage placement and developmental age scores. The analyses yielded the expected main age effects for both Piagetian stage, $F(8, 295) = 89.91$, $p < .0001$, and developmental level, $F(8, 295) = 82.07$, $p < .0001$. There were also significant main effects for between sensorimotor domain comparisons for both Piagetian stage, $F(6, 1770) = 150.24$, $p < .0001$, and developmental level, $F(6, 1770) = 73.26$, $p < .0001$. Both sets of main effects were qualified by age × domain interactions for both Piagetian stage, $F(48, 1770) = 6.02$, $p < .0001$, and developmental level, $F(48, 1770) = 4.63$, $p < .0001$. Examination of Figures 6.2 and 6.3 shows that these interactions are manifested most notably in the slowing down of vocal imitation with increasing age. Thus, the only domain of sensorimotor performance with a developmental function that is clearly different is vocal imitation.

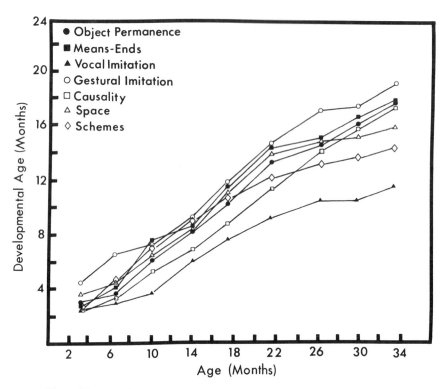

Figure 6.3. Age of acquisition of levels of sensorimotor development in separate domains for infants with Down syndrome. (*Note:* Developmental ages taken from Dunst, 1980b)

Ordinality in development

The principal method used to determine the extent to which infants acquire sensorimotor behaviors in an invariant stagelike progression has been Green's (1956) version of Guttman's (1950) method of scaling patterns of response. The procedure, termed *scalogram analysis,* discerns whether subjects, in response to a series of items rank-ordered by difficulty, succeed to a certain point and fail all subsequent items. For a group of infants administered the same series of items (either cross-sectionally or longitudinally), the procedure yields an Index of Consistency (I), where any value between .50 and 1.00 is considered an ordinal scale. The closer the I value is to 1.00, the more invariant the ordinal sequence.

Scalogram analysis has been widely used to determine ordinality in the achievement of sensorimotor progressions. As Uzgiris (1987) points out, this method permits a test of whether or not an individual's pattern of acquisition of sensorimotor behavior conforms to a hypothesized sequence of attainments (e.g., as posited by Piaget) where the different steps in the sequence may be taken as indications of progressively more complex levels of competence. Thus, in contrast to order in sensorimotor performance anchored on age, ordinality provides a measure of order grounded in theory regarding the types of progressions one would expect in development.

Table 6.6 shows the Indices of Consistency obtained in nine studies. Taken together, the data from these investigations provide converging evidence to support the fact that nonretarded infants, infants with Down syndrome, and other retarded children acquire sensorimotor behaviors in stagelike progressions. In those instances where $I < .50$, the findings should be interpreted with caution and not be taken as evidence disconfirming the stage sequencing criterion. These particular studies (Kopp, Sigman, & Parmelee, 1973; Rogers, 1977; Silverstein, Brownlee, Hubbell, & McLain, 1975) attempted to establish ordinality for within-stage as well as for between-stage sequences. Piaget claimed ordinality for between-stages of development only. Consequently, when Rogers (1977) scaled stage placements instead of both within- and between-stage items ($I = .30$), she found that her sample manifested sensorimotor behavior in a stagelike progression ($I = .79$). With regard to the major focus of this chapter, it is particularly interesting to note that patterns of ordinality among infants with Down syndrome are very much like those of nonretarded infants. This indicates that at least for these particular infants with Down syndrome, they manifested sensorimotor behavior in the same stage-level sequence as do nonretarded youngsters.

The fact that the Indices of Consistency reported in most studies are less than unity indicates there were some deviations from the hypothesized patterns of acquisition of sensorimotor attainments. The manner in which inversions or reversals occur in the acquisition of sensorimotor sequences has recently been examined in detail by Uzgiris (1987) for a group of 12 nonretarded infants followed longitudinally from 1 to 25 months of age. Deviations from the expected sequence of attainments were highest for the means–ends and schemes for relating to objects scales and lowest for the operational causality scale. Of all the deviations, the majority (all but two) involved adjacent within-stage items. As Uzgiris (1987) points out, the inversions do not invalidate the stage sequencing criterion but rather indicate the need to reconsider the conceptual ordering of several of the scale steps on the Uzgiris–Hunt test.

Comparisons of the inversions reported by Uzgiris (1987) for nonretarded infants with those found by Dunst (1981a) for infants with Down syndrome show remarkable similarities. The same inversion reported by Uzgiris for object permanence was found by Dunst. Subjects demonstrated reversal in searching for an object disappearing outside the visual field (Step 4) before they manually searched for a partially hidden object (Step 3). The dominant inversion found by Dunst on the means–ends scale was the same as reported by Uzgiris. The subjects demonstrated the use of a string to obtain a desired object (Step 9) before demonstrating an understanding of the support relationship by inhibiting the use of the support when an object was held above it (Step 8).

Dunst found two major inversions on the vocal imitation scale. Vocalizing in response to babbling sounds (Step 4) was more likely to occur before vocalizing in

Table 6.6. *Green's Index of Consistency obtained in nine separate investigations*

Study	N	CA (months)			Green's Index (I) of Consistency						
		M	SD	Range	OP	ME	VI	GI	OC	SR	SO
Nonretarded:											
Uzgiris & Hunt (1975)	84	10.00	—	1–23	.97	.81	.89	.95	.99	.91	.80
Corman & Escalona (1969)	247	—	—	1–27	1.00	—	—	—	—	.98	—
Kopp et al. (1973)	24	—	—	7–18	.75–1.00	.49–1.00	—	—	—	—	—
Watson & Fischer (1977)	36	19.00	—	13–26	—	—	—	—	—	—	.58
Down syndrome:											
Dunst (1981a)[a]	7	11.14	4.08	7–18	.89	.82	.82	.81	.88	.96	.67
Hill & McCune-Nicolich (1981)	30	33.20	8.61	20–53	—	—	—	—	—	—	.88
Mentally retarded:											
Kahn (1976)	63	66.63	—	42–126	.97	.98	1.00	1.00	.92	.81	—
Rogers (1977)	40	152	—	106–179	.77	.57	[.76][b]		—	.33–.79	—
Silverstein et al. (1975)	64	168	41.76	—	.58–.70	—	—	—	—	.30–.46	—

Note: OP = object permanence; ME = means–ends; VI = vocal imitation; GI = gestural imitation; OC = operational causality; SR = spatial relationships; SO = schemes for relating to objects. Dash means statistic not reported.

[a] Ordinality determined from longitudinal data for seven subjects administered the Uzgiris–Hunt scales an average of 5 or 6 times (total N = 36).
[b] Ordinality determined for both vocal and gestural imitation combined.

response to cooing sounds (Step 3), and vocalizing in response to unfamiliar sound patterns (Step 6) was more likely to occur before imitation of babbling sounds or familiar words (Step 5). The latter inversion was also reported by Uzgiris. Both Uzgiris and Dunst found the identical inversion on the gestural imitation scale. Attempting to imitate unfamiliar, invisible gestures (Step 7) was attained before imitation of unfamiliar, visible gestures (Step 6). Only one subject demonstrated an inversion on the space scale in the Dunst study, but it was the dominant deviation reported by Uzgiris. Visually directed reaching (Step 4) was achieved before sound localization (Step 3).

Two dominant inversions were found by Dunst on the scheme scale. The subjects were more likely to demonstrate complex actions with objects (Step 6) before visually examining objects in an exploratory manner (Step 5), and subjects were more likely to demonstrate dropping or throwing objects (Step 7) before demonstrating complex actions with objects (Step 6). Neither of these two instances of inversions were reported by Uzgiris.

Despite the few minor differences found in the Uzgiris and Dunst studies, the results are remarkably similar, and provide encouraging evidence that not only do infants with Down syndrome attain sensorimotor competencies in the same order as do nonretarded infants, but that deviations are nearly identical for both populations of subjects. These deviations appear to be due more to task difficulties and measurement considerations (see Uzgiris, 1987) than to theoretical problems with the stage sequencing criterion. Again, this cannot be taken as support against the proposition that sensorimotor development is ordinal in nature. Kopp et al. (1973), as well, reported that characteristics of sensorimotor tasks rather than theoretical problems with Piaget's theory accounted for inversions in development.

Summary

The studies examined in this section showed considerable similarities in the manner in which infants with Down syndrome and nonretarded infants manifest stagelike progressions in sensorimotor development. Both the age-related and ordinality data showed, respectively, that infants with Down syndrome manifest progressively more complex sensorimotor competencies at higher age levels and that the order of acquisition is invariant. The only major difference found between infants with Down syndrome and nonretarded infants was the degree of covariation between age and sensorimotor level. Infants with Down syndrome were found to show more heterogeneity in sensorimotor performance as measured by patterns of correlation between CA, MA, and sensorimotor level. The same was found for heterogeneously formed groups of retarded infants. Taken together, however, the conclusion can be made that infants with Down syndrome and other retarded infants (but not mentally retarded adults) acquire sensorimotor competencies in a stagelike manner that is more similar than different compared to nonretarded infants.

The analyses of the Down Syndrome Study data showed that patterns of acquisition of sensorimotor competencies are curvilinear and reflect a ''slowing down'' phenomenon. Moreover, the developmental functions of all but vocal imitation were much alike with respect to the slowing-down process. The rate of acquisition of vocal imitation relative to the other six Uzgiris–Hunt scale domains was much slower. This datum, together with the findings from the correlational analyses (see Table 6.1), shows that vocal imitation is the only sensorimotor domain for which patterns of development are clearly different among infants with Down syndrome.

Stage transitioning

Between-stage relationships

Establishing the fact that a progression of developmental attainments forms an invariant sequence does not demonstrate a functional relationship between the behaviors in the progression. As noted by Flavell (1970):

The empirical demonstration that some *A* reliability precedes some *B* in the ontogenesis ought to be regarded as only the beginning of the developmentalist's task. The next step would obviously be trying to hypothesize an other-than-temporal connection between *A* and *B*, which could account for, or at least make plausible, the observed temporal one. (p. 1035)

Flavell (1972) proposed that there are at least five major types of categories of causal–functional relationships that might explain temporal sequences in development. These are *addition, substitution, modification, inclusion,* and *mediation.*

Addition refers to developmental sequences where *A* and *B* are acquired in succession, but *B* does not replace *A;* it is simply added to the child's repertoire of behaviors. *Substitution* refers to developmental sequences where *B* more or less replaces or substitutes for *A* once *B* is fully acquired. *Modification* refers to developmental sequences where *A* and *B* are acquired in succession, but *A* undergoes changes due to the acquisition of *B,* and subsequently becomes part of *B. Inclusion* refers to developmental sequences where A_1 and A_2 become integrated or coordinated to form a new behavior *B. Mediation* refers to developmental sequences where *A* facilitates or mediates the acquisition of *B,* but once *B* is acquired, *A* can function independently.

Indirect tests of the possible causal linkages between behaviors in a developmental progression come from studies that have examined the correlations between level of achievement at one point in time with level of achievement at a subsequent measurement occasion (King & Seegmiller, 1973; Uzgiris, 1973). These types of analyses are predicated on the assumption that attainment of a certain level of competence at Time 1 will correlate with level of competence at Time 2, and reflect some sort of facilitating or mediating relationship between the different achievements. These types of analyses have been carried out only in terms of correlations between performances for the same domain of sensorimotor development (e.g., object permanence). The findings have not been particularly revealing. Neither the correlations between achievements at different age levels (King & Seegmiller, 1973) nor correlations between infants' age of acquisition of achievements of progressively more complex sensorimotor competencies (Uzgiris, 1973) have proved useful for discerning possible relationships between different stages or levels of performance.

Uzgiris (1987) provides an extensive discussion of the manner in which Flavell's (1972) proposed types of causal–functional relationships might be operating during the genesis of sensorimotor competence. Dunst (1984), as well, offers several suggestions regarding how one might go about empirically testing between stage relationships. He illustrated this with data gathered in a study examining the stagelike characteristics of infant communication development (Dunst, 1978b, 1979, 1980c; Holdgrafer & Dunst 1986). This communication model includes seven levels (stages) of development, the first six of which parallel the achievements of the sensorimotor period (Piaget, 1952). The seventh corresponds to the entry into the preoperational period. The model analyzes communicative behavior according to its component parts (gestural, visual, vocal, and verbal behaviors), which permits determination of level of communication competence as well as the mechanisms that permit isolation of factors that contribute to acquisition of communicative competencies.

As part of a study (Dunst, 1979, 1980c) designed to test hypotheses generated from this neo-Piagetian model of communicative development, data were gathered that suggest the types of developmental relationships that may be operating in the genesis of communicative development. The subjects were 12 nonretarded infants and 12 infants with Down syndrome and their mothers. Each sample was divided into two subgroups of six subjects each – those functioning primarily at Piagetian sensorimotor Stage 4 and those functioning at Stage 5. Subjects at these two particular developmental levels were studied because it has been suggested that these stages represent a major transitional point in the genesis of communicative competence (Bates, 1976; Sugarman-Bell, 1978).

Each mother–infant dyad was observed in a free-play situation where the types of gestures, visual behaviors, and vocal behaviors manifested by the infants were recorded. Gestures were coded according to one of three types: *Stage 3* (e.g., touches mother); *Stage 4* (e.g., extends arms out to be picked up); and *Stage 5* (e.g., giving and showing objects). Visual and vocal behaviors were coded in terms of the frequency at which the infants looked at or vocalized to their mothers, and the proportion and frequency at which there were concomitant (interpatterned) *looks at mother–vocalized to mother* (LV), *gesture-looks at mother* (GL), and *gesture-looks at mother–vocalizes to mother* (GLV) behaviors.

A Groups (Down syndrome vs. Nonretarded) × Levels (Stage 4 vs. Stage 5) × Gestural Type (3 vs. 4 vs. 5) repeated measures ANOVA for the nonverbal communication data yielded a main effects for levels, $F(1, 20) = 15.65$, $p < .01$, and a levels × gestural type interaction, $F(3, 60) = 16.08$, $p < .001$. There were no significant differences between groups nor any interactions involving the grouping factor. Thus, the patterns of development for the infants with Down syndrome and nonretarded infants were identical, and may be taken as evidence that the two groups of infants manifested early communication behaviors in a similar manner for these particular developmental (stage) levels.

With regard to the possible relationships between stages of development, the results suggested a *substitution* relationship. As the Stage 5 infants manifested progressively more complex types of gestures, less complex (i.e., Stage 3) gestures were more or less dropped from their repertoires or at least were less likely to be used as communicative acts.

Preliminary analyses of the subjects' looking and vocalizing data indicated that the infants with Down syndrome and nonretarded infants spontaneously *looked at their mothers* at the same frequency, but that Stage 5 infants manifested the criterion behavior more frequently than the Stage 4 infants, $F(1, 20) = 5.53$, $p < .05$. Similarly, the Stage 5 infants *vocalized to mother* more frequently than did the Stage 4 infants, $F(1, 20) = 28.38$, $p < .001$. All infants, however, did look at and vocalize to their mothers during the play episodes. The average number of *looks at mother* behaviors were, respectively, 12.33 ($SD = 6.28$) and 15.67 ($SD = 6.31$) for the Stages 4 and 5 nonretarded infants, and respectively, 5.83 ($SD = 3.19$) and 20.67 ($SD = 13.11$) for the Stages 4 and 5 infants with Down syndrome. The average number of *vocalizes to mother* behaviors were, respectively, 2.67 ($SD = 2.42$) and 8.00 ($SD = 6.23$) for the Stages 4 and 5 nonretarded infants, and, respectively, 1.17 ($SD = 1.16$) and 15.16 ($SD = 7.11$) for the Stages 4 and 5 infants with Down syndrome.

A series of Groups × Levels ANOVAs for each of the interpatterned behaviors (LV, GL, GLV) as the dependent measures produced no significant group differences for either the frequency or proportion of behaviors for groups, but significant main effects for levels on all six criterion behaviors. That is, the Stage 5 infants manifested both higher frequencies and proportions of LV, GL, and GLV behavior sequences. No significant groups × levels interactions were found for any of the analyses. The latter indicates that infants with Down syndrome and nonretarded infants showed identical patterns of behavior interpatterning (Dunst, 1979).

With regard to possible functional relationships among behaviors, the data suggested an *inclusion* relationship between gestural, visual, and vocal behaviors inasmuch as all the subjects *gestured toward, looked at,* and *vocalized to* their mothers, but that only Stage 5 infants were able to *interpattern* the behaviors in a functional way. That is, the Stage 5 infants integrated behaviors already in the repertoire in a manner that resulted in the coordination of separate behaviors to form a new behavior totality or schemata.

By no means are the Dunst (1979, 1980c) data conclusive regarding between stage relationships. The data are, however, noteworthy for several reasons. First, with regard to patterns of acquisition of sensorimotor behavior, the findings indicate that infants with Down syndrome and nonretarded infants acquire communicative behaviors as well as demonstrate the ability to interpattern behavior in a very similar manner. Second, with regard to the stage transitioning criterion, the strategy employed by Dunst illustrates that when sensorimotor competencies are examined in terms of their component parts, it is possible to discern the manner in which behavior organization occurs as part of developmental change (see also Beeghly, Weiss-Perry, & Cicchetti, Chapter 10, this volume).

Stage stabilization

Stabilization in the acquisition of sensorimotor competencies has generally been studied in terms of regressions in development (*oscillations,* in Inhelder's 1966, 1968, terminology) and the amount of time necessary to progress from one level of development to the next. Regressions in development refer to the manifestation of a certain level of functioning at one point in time but the failure to demonstrate the same competency at a subsequent measurement occasion (Uzgiris, 1987). Regressions are generally taken as indications of reorganizations (instability) in development where assimilation of environmental events has not fully occurred. The amount of time needed to move from one level of development to the next is considered a means whereby the ''relative'' degree of difficulty of between stage transitions can be determined (Mervis & Cardoso-Martins, 1984).

Regressions in development. Uzgiris (1987) provides an extensive review of available data regarding regressions in development found in studies of nonretarded infants. Declines in performance have been found to occur between 2% and 20% of the time, with the highest declines occurring between 15 and 18 months, and the lowest declines occurring between 5 and 12 months. In her own work with nonretarded infants followed longitudinally during the first and second years, Uzgiris (1987) found the overall level of regression to be 7%, with the lowest occurring in the means–ends domain (5%) and the highest in the vocal imitation domain (12%). Examination of the amount of regressions occurring at different age levels found the lowest occurring between 5 and 12 months of age (range = 1% to 8%) and the highest occurring between 15 and 17 months (range = 13% to 20%).

The extent to which regressions in sensorimotor development occur among infants with Down syndrome was discerned from a set of data collected by Dunst (1981a). In this investigation, the Uzgiris–Hunt scales were administered to seven subjects on five or six occasions at 3- to 5-week intervals ($M = 29.34$ days). The subjects' mean CA and MA were, respectively, 11.14 ($SD = 4.08$) and 7.67 ($SD = 3.10$) months at the beginning of the study.

Regressions were first determined for individual sensorimotor domains for all assessments combined, and comparisons made with the percentages of regressions reported for nonretarded infants (Uzgiris, 1987). Chi-square analyses between the percentage of regression for the nonretarded infants versus infants with Down syndrome were performed using the percentage of regression for the nonretarded infants as the expected value. Table 6.7 presents these data and their accompanying analyses. The mean percentage of regression for the subjects with Down syndrome was 17.56 (range = 8.57 to 25.71). In every case, the percentages of regressions were greater for the subjects with Down syndrome and statistically significant. On the average, there were more than twice as many instances of regressions among the infants with Down syndrome.

Uzgiris (1987) also reported the percentage of regressions that occurred at different age levels in order to assess the developmental junctures at which regressions

Table 6.7. *Percentages of regression for the highest level of achievement across assessment sessions*

	Group			
Scale	Nonretarded	Down syndrome	Ratio	Chi square
Object permanence	6.70	10.81	1:1.6	5.04*
Means–ends	4.60	16.22	1:3.5	58.70**
Vocal imitation	11.70	25.71	1:2.2	33.55**
Gestural imitation	9.90	25.71	1:2.6	50.49**
Operational causality	7.00	14.28	1:2.0	15.14**
Spatial relationships	4.70	8.57	1:1.8	6.37*
Schemes	4.70	21.62	1:4.6	121.82**
Average	7.04	17.56	1:2.5	31.30**

Note: *$p < .05$; **$p < .001$.
Sources: Data for the nonretarded group are from Uzgiris (1987); those for the Down syndrome group are from Dunst (1981a).

Table 6.8. *Mean percentages of regression for the highest level of achievement at five age levels*

	Group			
Age level (months)	Nonretarded	Down syndrome	Ratio	Chi square
5–6.9	4.10	12.98	1:3.2	38.46**
7–8.9	6.60	19.23	1:2.9	48.34**
9–10.9	5.20	7.14	1:1.4	1.15
11–12.9	2.85	11.90	1:4.2	57.47**
13–14.9	8.20	30.95	1:3.8	126.23**

Note: **$p < .001$.
Sources: Data for the nonretarded group are from Uzgiris (1987). Those for the Down syndrome group are from Dunst (1981a).

were lowest and highest. The same was done with the Dunst (1981a) data and contrasts made with the data reported by Uzgiris. The results are shown in Table 6.8. With the exception of the 9- to 10.9-month age level, the percentage of regressions among the infants with Down syndrome were significantly greater than among the nonretarded subjects.

Morss (1983), in a longitudinal study of object permanence development among nonretarded infants and infants with Down syndrome, examined the extent to which successes at one testing were likely to be repeated at subsequent measurement occasions. The percentage of repeated successes were 77% and 61% for the nonretarded and Down syndrome samples, respectively. The differences were statistically significant, indicating that the infants with Down syndrome were less likely to demonstrate repeated successes across measurement occasions. Stated differently, the infants with Down syndrome were more likely to show regressions in development across measurement occasions.

The higher levels of regressions in development among infants with Down syndrome have been interpreted by Morss (1983) as evidence indicating that the sensorimotor development of retarded infants is different from that of nonretarded infants. On the surface, available data would appear to offer evidence for this contention. However, upon reflection, the larger degrees of regressions may be an artifact of the slower pace of development of infants with Down syndrome. It may be the case that nonretarded infants' rate of development, relatively speaking, is so much more rapid that the possibility of discerning regressions is lessened. In contrast, because the rate of development of infants with Down syndrome is slower, the possibility of finding regressions may be increased.

This probability was tested with data from the Dunst (1981a) study by taking into consideration the slower pace of development of the infants with Down syndrome in determining percentage of regressions. The subjects in this investigation were also administered the Griffiths (1954) mental development scales. Their mean General Developmental Quotient (GDQ) at the times of regressions was 70. The percentage of regressions for the individual sensorimotor domains was reduced by this ratio (.70) and compared to the percentages reported by Uzgiris (1987). The analyses produced significant differences for four of the seven Uzgiris–Hunt scales: means–ends, $\chi^2 = 19.80$, $p < .001$; vocal imitation, $\chi^2 = 6.76$, $p < .05$; gestural imitation, $\chi^2 = 13.22$, $p < .001$; and schemes for relating to objects, $\chi^2 = 46.26$, $p < 001$. The overall percentage of regression was also significant: $\chi^2 = 7.83$, $p < .05$. Thus, regressions were generally still greater among the infants with Down syndrome even after their slower pace of development was taken into consideration.

Transitional timing. It has been suggested, based on psychometric test data, that infants with Down syndrome have a more difficult time making the transition from sensorimotor to symbolic functioning (Gibson, 1978). According to Gibson (1978), this "developmental wall" is most evident in the transition from sensorimotor Stage 5 to sensorimotor Stage 6 functioning.

Mervis and Cardoso-Martins (1984) recently tested Gibson's contention in a study that examined the amount of time it required infants with Down syndrome and nonretarded infants to move from Stage 5 to Stage 6 functioning in the object permanence and means–ends domains (Uzgiris & Hunt, 1975). Six infants with Down syndrome and six nonretarded infants were tested every 6 to 12 weeks and the ages at which the landmarks representing Stage 5 and Stage 6 functioning determined. Using the age of acquisition of the Stage 5 behaviors as anchor points, the amount of time it required to manifest Stage 6 behaviors was determined for individual subjects. The index used as the measure of stage transitioning was the age of attainment of the Stage 6 landmark minus ($-$) the age of acquisition of the Stage 5 landmark divided ($\div$) by the age of acquisition of the Stage 5 attainment. These ratios were summed across subjects within groups as a basis for discerning relative difficulty for the two groups of infants. The ratios for infants with Down syndrome and nonretarded infants were nearly identical for both the object permanence and means–ends domains. The investigators interpreted these findings as evidence that infants with Down syndrome have no more difficulty making the transition to Stage 6 functioning than do nonretarded infants.

The type of study conducted by Mervis and Cardoso-Martins (1984) is sorely needed in order to determine how stage transitioning occurs. However, a number of problems with this study make the investigation questionable as an empirical test of stage transitioning. First, the fact that the subjects were tested every 6 to 12 weeks calls into question the accuracy of the attainment ages for the Stage 5 and Stage 6 landmarks. For the nonretarded subjects, the difference between attainment of the Stage 5 and Stage 6 object permanence tasks was, on the average, 12.33 days (for four infants the difference were zero). Uzgiris (1987), who tested her subjects monthly, reported an average difference of 44.1 days between the same landmarks. Thus, the Mervis and Cardoso-Martins (1984) findings would appear, in part, to be due to an artifact of the testing schedule they employed. Second, for the particular landmarks used to assess means–ends performance, Uzgiris (1987) found that 11 out of her 12 subjects attained these scale steps in reverse order. She attributed this to the motor demands and measurement problems involving the Stage 5 scale step. Thus, it is questionable whether the means–ends landmarks used by Mervis and Cardoso-Martins provide a basis for assessing transitional timing. Third, it is questionable whether age of attainment of the Stage 5 landmark is the most appropriate benchmark against which the slower pace of development of infants with Down syndrome should be taken into consideration. A better index would be the ratio of developmental level divided by CA since this index is a more direct measure of developmental pace. Therefore, it must be concluded that whereas the approach taken by Mervis and Cardoso-Martins (1984) is conceptually sound, the method used to assess stage transitioning is questionable.

The amount of time necessary to move from stage to stage was examined for the longitudinal subsample ($N = 31$) in the Down Syndrome Study (Dunst, 1988) taking into consideration the problems just noted with the Mervis and Cardoso-Martins (1984) investigation. This was accomplished in the following manner. First, the ages of attainment of the landmarks on the Uzgiris–Hunt scales were determined for each subject by considering the child's CA at the test occasion as a reasonable estimate of the acquisition age of the highest item passed in each domain. Second, in the event that no age was assigned to a landmark used as a measure of a certain stage of performance (see Table 6.9), the age of attainment was estimated using a procedure described by Hunt, Paraskevopolous, Schickendanz, & Uzgiris (1975). This was done by dividing the age difference between items on either side of the landmark by two (2) and adding the result to the age of acquisition of the lower-level item to obtain an estimate of the age at which the infant achieved the landmark. Third, the amount of time necessary to move from one stage to another was determined for each subject by subtracting the age of acquisition of the higher-level achievement from the age of acquisition of the lower-level achievement. Fourth, the result obtained in Step 3 was adjusted by multiplying the difference by the child's DQ at the time of the assessment of the lower level achievement. Fifth, the average time necessary to move from stage to stage was determined for both the unadjusted and adjusted differences, and comparisons made with data reported by Uzgiris (1987) for nonretarded infants. These results are shown in Table 6.9.

The analyses of the unadjusted differences produced significant findings for 20 out of the 25 comparisons. Seventeen of the 20 differences showed that the nonretarded infants took less time to move from one stage of development to the next. In three instances (gestural imitation, causality, space), the infants with Down syndrome took less time to move from one stage to the next, although in every case the nonretarded infants attained the scale steps used as indices of the different stages of performance at earlier ages than did the infants with Down syndrome. Close inspection of the transitioning data showed that in those instances where the differences favored the infants with Down syndrome, the more rapid "bridging" of between stages of development was almost entirely because prior stage transitioning took so much longer. This increased the "basal" age used as the benchmark for determining the amount of time required to move from one stage to the next. In other words, in instances where it took the infants with Down syndrome longer to move from one stage to the next, subsequent stage transitioning often occurred more rapidly.

Examination of the adjusted differences taking into consideration the slower pace of development of the infants with Down syndrome showed that it still generally took longer for these subjects to move from one stage to the next. Significant differences favoring the nonretarded infants were found in 10 separate instances, most of which involved transitioning from Stages 3 to 4 and Stages 4 to 5. Of particular interest are the findings pertaining to the transitioning from Stages 5 to 6. In two instances, the differences favored the nonretarded infants while in two other instances they favored the infants with Down syndrome. These particular sets of findings call into question Gibson's (1978) contention that infants with Down syndrome face a "developmental wall" in the transition from Stage 5 to Stage 6 functioning.

Summary

With the exception of the evidence indicating that infants with Down syndrome and nonretarded infants show very similar patterns of behavior interpatterning for between-stage transitions, the data examined in this section indicated that stage stabilization was different for the two groups of infants. Infants with Down syndrome showed a larger percentage of regressions in development as well as generally took much longer to move from stage to stage. Both sets of results were found even after the slower pace of development of the infants with Down syndrome was taken into consideration. It is therefore reasonable to conclude that the manner in which stage

Table 6.9. *Average number of days necessary to move from stage to stage for nonretarded and Down syndrome infants*

	Unadjusted								Adjusted							
	Stage 2–3		Stage 3–4		Stage 4–5		Stage 5–6		Stage 2–3		Stage 3–4		Stage 4–5		Stage 5–6	
	M	SD	M	SD	M	SD	M	SD	M	SD	M	SD	M	SD	M	SD
Object permanence																
Nonretarded[a]	74.7	25.0	44.5	19.0	26.8	23.5	200.7	51.0	—		76.4	69.7	123.9	75.6	190.3	84.3
Down syndrome[b]	70.2	43.8	113.4	86.1	139.2	78.0	200.3	76.1	41.4	31.2						
	$t=-.32$		$t=2.65*$		$t=4.72*$		$t=-.07$		$t=3.07*$		$t=1.50$		$t=4.20*$		$t=-.37$	
Means–ends																
Nonretarded	—		39.8	18.5	166.4	29.5	252.5	61.5	—		93.1	89.1	201.8	115.2	343.2	148.8
Down syndrome	—		108.3	79.5	236.4	115.5	393.0	145.8	—							
			$t=2.85*$		$t=1.99*$		$t=3.09*$				$t=1.98*$		$t=1.01$		$t=1.96*$	
Vocal imitation																
Nonretarded	10.3	12.5	184.7	37.0	—		—		—		154.6	76.8	—		—	
Down syndrome	140.2	88.2	219.4	122.7	—		—		94.8	77.0						
	$t=4.92*$		$t=.94*$						$t=3.66*$		$t=1.27*$					
Gestural imitation																
Nonretarded	39.2	24.5	76.4	47.5	45.8	54.0	276.7	57.0	—		152.5	76.8	156.6	93.1	67.2	36.9
Down syndrome	108.3	69.9	238.7	100.3	229.8	112.1	114.0	63.0	65.2	55.7						
	$t=3.23*$		$t=5.15*$		$t=5.08*$		$t=3.35*$		$t=1.50$		$t=3.04*$		$t=3.58*$		$t=9.54*$	
Operational causality																
Nonretarded	37.5	19.0	85.3	22.5	252.1	39.5	225.4	61.0	—		92.1	54.5	140.5	98.7	240.2	104.2
Down syndrome	185.6	66.8	147.7	70.4	154.8	70.4	326.5	126.6	134.4	50.3						
	$t=7.33*$		$t=2.93*$		$t=4.38*$		$t=2.53*$		$t=6.29*$		$t=.41*$		$t=3.69*$		$t=.43$	
Spatial relationships																
Nonretarded	45.6	18.5	55.0	23.0	147.9	35.5	134.6	65.5	—		51.1	89.1	249.6	101.7	74.0	34.7
Down syndrome	63.2	42.7	74.1	92.1	330.0	133.5	103.0	33.6	36.4	35.0						
	$t=1.30*$		$t=.69*$		$t=4.54*$		$t=1.86*$		$t=-.88$		$t=.14$		$t=3.29*$		$t=3.57*$	
Schemes																
Nonretarded	74.1	18.0	57.5	31.0	121.5	38.5	218.7	65.0	—		100.7	59.8	153.0	76.3	286.8	124.0
Down syndrome	115.3	43.9	140.74	74.8	167.5	67.1	346.1	147.9	76.6	36.4						
	$t=2.79*$		$t=3.53*$		$t=2.12*$		$t=2.65*$		$t=.05$		$t=2.25*$		$t=1.31$		$t=1.72*$	

Notes: The adjusted scores are the average number of days reduced by the childrens' DQ at the age of attainment of the lower stage level item (see text). Comparisons of both the unadjusted and adjusted scores for the Down syndrome infants are against the unadjusted scores for the nonretarded infants. $*p < .05$. Dash means data not available for analysis.

[a] Uzgiris (1987).

[b] Down Syndrome Study (longitudinal sample).

transitioning occurs among infants with Down syndrome is generally different than that for nonretarded infants. The data provide evidence to suggest that stabilization in the both attainment and assimilation of sensorimotor capabilities occurs much slower among infants with Down syndrome compared to nonretarded infants.

Stage structuring

The term *stage structuring* is used here in a restricted sense that deserves both definition and comment. Stage structuring is used to refer to two aspects of cognitive functioning: (1) the extent to which performances in different sensorimotor domains are interrelated and form some structural totality; and (2) the extent to which the structural organization of sensorimotor development remains constant or similar over time.

Stage structuring has generally been studied in terms of either stage congruence or the correlations among the achievements of the various domains of sensorimotor development. Stage congruence is a measure of the extent to which an infant's stage of performance in one sensorimotor domain corresponds to stage of performance in another domain. For example, for a sample of subjects administered the seven Uzgiris–Hunt scales, there are 21 pairwise stage congruence indices. Correlational analyses provide a measure of the extent to which the rank ordering of scores for subjects in one domain corresponds to the rank orderings of scores in other sensorimotor domains.

Stage congruence and interdomain correlations have often been implicitly treated as analogous measures despite evidence to the contrary. Although complete stage congruence between the performance in separate domains would result in a high correlation between the achievements in the different branches of development, it does not necessarily follow that lack of stage congruence would yield a low correlation. In fact, it would be possible to have complete lack of stage congruence but a substantial correlation between the achievements in two domains. In this case, each child's development on one scale would be relatively advanced compared to performance on another scale, but the infants making up the sample would nonetheless show one-to-one correspondence in terms of their rank orderings in the respective branches of development. Correlational analyses yield information regarding covariation among variables that are independent of actual levels of performance; and stage congruence analyses yield information regarding developmental synchronies (i.e., same stage performances) but tell us nothing about the degree of covariation where stage congruence is not found. Thus, each type of data provides different information regarding the structural aspects of cognitive development.

Methodologically, three separate approaches have been employed for discerning the structural aspects of sensorimotor development. Stage congruence and correlational analyses have been performed in studies where the ages of the subjects have (1) varied across the entire sensorimotor period (Dunst & Rheingrover, 1983; Kahn, 1976; Rogers, 1977; Silverstein et al., 1975; Woodward, 1959); (2) been the same (Corman & Escalona, 1969; King & Seegmiller, 1973; Kopp et al., 1973; Uzgiris,

1973; Wachs & Hubert, 1981); or (3) covered narrowly constrained age ranges (Dunst, 1981; Dunst, Gallagher, & Vance, 1982). In a number of instances, CA or MA has been partialed from the correlation matrix of sensorimotor performance in order to obtain an estimate of covariation if all the subjects had been the same age (Dunst & Rheingrover, 1983; Uzgiris & Hunt, 1975). Still further, studies have differed in terms of the age variable used to group subjects. Some investigators have used CA (e.g., Wachs & Hubert, 1981) while others have used MA (e.g., Dunst et al., 1982).

The differing approaches used to examine the structural features of sensorimotor development would be expected to influence the nature of the findings. In terms of correlational analyses, one would expect spuriously high correlations between the achievements in different domains of sensorimotor performance where the subjects' ages were permitted to cover the entire sensorimotor period. This is the case because sensorimotor functioning levels would be expected to vary concomitantly with the age of the child, as was shown from data presented in Table 6.1. Where the subjects are all the same age or age has been statistically controlled, one would expect spuriously low correlations because of the restricted range of possible scores in the dependent variables and the statistical removal of age as a moderating variable affecting the magnitude of the correlation coefficients. Where the subjects' ages covered a narrowly constrained age range, one would expect degrees of covariation that reflect the fact that parallel attainments from different domains would not be expected to be mastered at exactly the same time but within a time period that would provide ample opportunity for different forms of the same stage competency to manifest themselves. Dunst et al. (1982) have argued that the strategy of studying stage structuring at different, narrowly constrained age ranges is most consistent with Piaget's (1952) contentions that same stage attainments would be expected to emerge within a specified period of time.

Another major difference in studies that have examined stage structuring has been the instruments used to measure sensorimotor performance. This, as well, would be expected to influence the nature of the findings. A number of investigators have employed the Casati-Lezine scales (Bovet, Dasen, & Inhelder, 1974; Dasen, Inhelder, Lavallee, & Retschitzki, 1978; Lezine, Stambak, & Casati, 1969); others, the Uzgiris–Hunt scales (Dunst & Rheingrover, 1983; Dunst et al., 1982; King & Seegmiller, 1973; Uzgiris, 1973); while other investigators have used either other Piagetian-based scales or have employed measurement procedures that the investigators themselves developed (e.g., Rogers, 1977; Watson & Fisher, 1977). The use of different measurement procedures would be expected to produce somewhat different findings depending upon the particular sensorimotor competencies that were assessed. This is especially likely in studies that have employed measures of limited types of sensorimotor behaviors (e.g., Casati–Lezine scale) compared to studies that have used broad-based measures (e.g., Uzgiris–Hunt scales).

The above differences in studies that have investigated stage structuring make direct comparisons between investigations somewhat difficult. In the discussions that follow, comparisons will be made to the extent possible, but with an explicit

Table 6.10. *Percentages of stage congruence reported in 10 investigations*

Study	Scale	Domains	Stage congruence Mean	SD	Range
Nonretarded:					
Lezine et al. (1976)	Casati-Lezine	OP, ME, ME/SR	71	—	58–87
Bovet et al. (1974)	Casati-Lezine	OP, ME, ME/SR	65	—	30–85
Dasen et al. (1978)	Casati-Lezine	OP, ME, ME/SR	79	—	59–96
Watson & Fischer (1977)	Uzgiris-Hunt, IDS[a]	OP, SO/PP	53	—	—
Down syndrome					
Dunst & Rheingrover (1983)	Uzgiris-Hunt	OP, ME, VI, GI, OC, SR, SO	34	15	2–56
Cicchetti & Mans-Wagener (1987)	Uzgiris-Hunt	OP, ME, OC, SR	64	12	50–79
Down Syndrome Study	Uzgiris-Hunt	OP, ME, VI, GI, OC, SR, SO	41	14	17–60
Down Syndrome Study	Uzgiris-Hunt	OP, ME, OC, SR	53	6	42–58
Mentally retarded:					
Dunst et al. (1981)	Uzgiris-Hunt	OP, ME, VI, GI, OC, SR, SO	33	16	6–56
Rogers (1977)	IDS[a]	OP, ME, SR, VI/GI	29	17	10–57
Woodward (1959)	IDS[a]	OP, ME/SO, CR	65	—	43–87

Notes: Notations for domains are as follows: OP – object permanence; ME – means–ends; VI – vocal imitation; GI – gestural imitation; OC – operational causality; SR – spatial relationships; SO – schemes for relating to objects; PP – pretend play; and CR – type of circular reaction. Two domains that are separated by a slash (/) indicates that the scale used to measure sensorimotor performance assessed both types of competencies. Dash means statistic not reported.
[a] IDS = investigator developed scale.

attempt to point out methodological differences that might account for differing sets of findings. Also, where possible, methodological differences will be taken into consideration through reanalysis of the data in order to produce results that are directly comparable.

Stage congruence

Table 6.10 shows the overall percentage of stage congruence reported in 10 separate investigations. The studies are organized according to diagnostic group and the domains of sensorimotor development for which stage congruence was determined. Substantial levels of stage congruence have been found in studies of nonretarded infants that have employed the Casati–Lezine scales as measures of sensorimotor performance. Somewhat lower levels of stage congruence have been reported in studies of infants with Down syndrome, although the lower levels are, in part, due to the particular sensorimotor domains for which stage congruence was determined. In the Down Syndrome Study, for example, the overall percentage of stage congruence was 41% when all seven Uzgiris–Hunt scales were used, but rose to 53% when only the same scales (object permanence, means–ends, causality, space) used

Table 6.11. *Percentage of stage congruence reported for individual pairwise scale comparisons in studies of Down syndrome and mentally retarded infants (according to sensorimotor domains)*

	OP			ME			VI		
	DS	DS	MR	DS	DS	MR	DS	DS	MR
Object permanence (OP)	—	—	—	37	56	56	29	29	14
Means–ends (ME)				—	—	—	2	17	7
Vocal imitation (VI)							—	—	—
Gestural imitation (GI)									
Operational causality (OC)									
Spatial relationships (SR)									
Schemes (SO)									

by Cicchetti and Mans-Wagener (1987) were analyzed. Likewise, when only the Uzgiris–Hunt scales (object permanence, means-ends, space) that are analogous to the Casati–Lezine scales were analyzed, the percentage of stage congruence was 55%. Taking into consideration these methodological differences, the percentage of stage congruence for nonretarded infants averages about 70%, whereas the overall percentage of stage congruence for infants with Down syndrome is around 60%. A somewhat lower (47%) level of stage congruence was found in the Dunst et al. (1981) study of retarded children when the same methodological differences were considered.

With the above differences and recalculations of the data in mind, the percentage of stage congruence for infants with Down syndrome is about 10% lower than for nonretarded infants and about 10% higher than for mentally retarded children. More specifically, the percentage of stage congruence for nonretarded infants, infants with Down syndrome, and mentally retarded infants was 71%, 64%, 55%, and 47% for the Casati–Lezine (Bovet et al., 1974; Dasen et al., 1978; Lezine et al., 1969), Cicchetti and Mans-Wagener (1987), Down Syndrome Study, and Dunst et al. (1981) studies, respectively, when only corresponding sensorimotor scales are analyzed. These data may be taken as evidence for somewhat greater heterogeneity (Flavell, 1982a) in the organization of sensorimotor development among infants with Down syndrome and other mentally retarded infants.

This heterogeneity is especially reflected in the range of the percentage of stage congruence for individual pairwise sensorimotor domain contrasts. Table 6.11 shows the percentage of stage congruence for individual pairwise comparisons for the three studies (Dunst & Rheingrover, 1983; Dunst et al., 1981; Down Syndrome Study) that used the seven Uzgiris–Hunt scales. The highest percentage of congruence was found for [OP, ME], [SR, SO], and [OC, SO].[2] The lowest percentage of stage

GI			OC			SR			SO		
DS	DS	MR	DS	DS	MR	DS	DS	MR	DS	DS	MR
21	35	19	28	37	32	34	51	41	33	42	31
7	25	21	33	54	39	46	58	45	38	53	41
52	36	31	29	30	21	19	20	14	28	26	23
—	—	—	39	39	35	41	38	38	40	40	39
			—	—	—	45	57	38	56	59	48
						—	—	—	56	60	54
									—	—	—

Sources: Dunst and Rheingover (1983) for first DS; Down Syndrome Study for second DS; Dunst et al. (1981) for MR.

congruence was found for [ME, VI], [VI, SR], and [ME, GI]. The average percentage of congruence for the two sets were, respectively, 51% ($SD = 9$) and 15% ($SD = 8$). There is a difference of 36% between the stage congruence percentages, which is quite substantial and statistically significant, $\chi^2 = 19.63$ $p < .001$. This particular finding indicates that degree of congruence varies considerably as a function of the particular sensorimotor domains examined, and may be taken as evidence that same stage performance for pairwise comparisons is generally much lower than Piaget's theory would suggest.

The extent to which overall levels of stage congruence varied according to age level has been examined in four separate studies (Cicchetti & Mans-Wagener 1987; Down Syndrome Study; Dunst et al., 1981; Lezine et al., 1969). Bearing in mind the differences already noted that account for variability in the absolute levels of stage congruence for different studies, a *U-function trend* emerged in percentage of stage congruence at the different age levels. Percentage of congruence was highest between 2 and 6 months and 18 and 22 months, and lowest in the 10- to 18-month range. This may be taken as evidence for greater heterogeneity during the middle portion of the sensorimotor period, with heterogeneity being defined in terms of the lack of stage congruence for all pairwise comparisons taken together.

When stage congruence for individual pairwise comparisons were examined at different age levels in the Down Syndrome Study, a *U*-function trend was found for 15 out of the 21 contrasts. The *U*-function findings showed same stage performance lowest in the 10- to 18-month range. A trend toward a linear function was found for six pairwise comparisons [OP, ME], [GI, OP], [GI, SO], [GI, SR], [GI, SO], [GI, ME]. The linear trend was most evident for pairwise contrasts involving gestural imitation.

Overall, the percentage of stage congruence found in studies with nonretarded infants, infants with Down syndrome, and other retarded persons is much lower than Piaget's theory would suggest. The data examined here revealed an age-related effect in terms of percentage of stage congruence, with concordance highest at the lower and upper bounds of the sensorimotor period and lowest in the 10- to 18-month range. This may be taken as evidence for reorganization in sensorimotor development during this time period. Although somewhat lower compared to non-retarded infants, the patterns of stage congruence manifested by infants with Down syndrome was very similar and suggests that patterns of reorganization parallel one another for the two samples of infants.

Correlational analyses

The structional characteristics of sensorimotor development based on correlational data have been examined using either hierarchical cluster analysis or factor analysis. Cluster analysis is a procedure designed to partition a set of variables into optimally homogeneous groups (Johnson, 1967). This analytic strategy has been used in a number of studies that have employed the seven Uzgiris–Hunt scales as the measures of sensorimotor performance. For the 21 pairwise comparisons, the procedure begins by forming a cluster among the two most highly correlated domains, and proceeds in a stepwise manner combining scales until all the domains that are substantially correlated are optimally connected.

Principal components factor analysis using varimax rotation (Nunnally, 1967) has been used in all the available studies that have examined the organizational aspects of sensorimotor development. This particular type of factor analysis produces a set of optimally related (correlated) solutions where the scales constituting the content of the different factors are orthogonal (i.e., uncorrelated with one another), so that multiple factor solutions may be taken as evidence of multidimensionality in behavior organization.

Factor analysis differs from cluster analysis primarily in terms of how "group membership" is determined. Factor analysis produces groupings based on an optimal, linear combination of variables taken together, whereas cluster analysis produces groupings based on the magnitude of the correlations taken in pairs. Consequently, cluster analysis will almost always produce a greater number of "groupings" than will factor analysis.

Cluster analyses. Cluster analysis has been used in several studies of nonretarded infants (Silverstein, McLain, Brownlee, & Hubbell, 1976), infants with Down syndrome (Dunst et al., 1982; Dunst & Rheingrover, 1983), and other retarded infants (Dunst et al., 1981). All four of these investigations examined stage structuring at different age levels between 4 and 24 months (CA for the nonretarded infants and MA for both infants with Down syndrome and other retarded infants).

Several major trends emerged from the different analyses. First, multiple sets of solutions were obtained in all the studies. This suggests that sensorimotor intelligence is not a unitary construct *(structure d'ensemble)* but rather is made up of varied components and sets of competencies. Second, the sets of solutions for the nonretarded infants, infants with Down syndrome, and other retarded infants were very similar between 4 and 12 months, although the similarities were not necessarily manifested at the same developmental junctures. Third, for the 12 sets of solutions obtained in the four separate studies, vocal imitation formed a separate cluster in half of the cases or combined to form a cluster including gestural imitation in five other instances. Imitation would appear to constitute a separate form of sensorimotor ability that bears little developmental relationship (correlation) with the other sensorimotor domains. Fourth, the sets of findings obtained for the Dunst et al. (1982) sample of infants with Down syndrome showed that there were considerable shifts in the patterns of organization of sensorimotor development during the period from 4 to 24 months. Of the five sets of solutions, [VI, GI], [OP, SO], and [ME, SR] were the only pairwise scales that repeated themselves in three out of five clustering networks. This finding may be taken as evidence that there is little structural continuity in sensorimotor development.

The aggregate of the findings from the different cluster analyses show a number of similarities in patterns of organization of sensorimotor behaviors among nonretarded infants, infants with Down syndrome, and other retarded infants. This was most evident with regard to clusters involving [VI, GI] and to a lesser extent [OP, ME] and [SR, SO]. Perhaps most notable were the considerable shifts in patterns of organization at different age levels. This may be taken as evidence for reorganizations in development. Indeed, if any firm conclusion can be made about stage structuring, it is that changes in patterns of organization are the rule in the genesis of sensorimotor competence.

Factor analyses. The most extensive data base on the structural features of sensorimotor development come from studies of the factor analysis of the performances on the Uzgiris–Hunt scales. Some factor analyses were independently performed by other investigators (Down Syndrome Study; Dunst et al., 1981; Dunst & Rheingrover, 1983; Silverstein et al., 1975; Wachs & Hubert, 1981), while other analyses were done specifically for this chapter from correlational data presented in original reports (King & Seegmiller, 1973; Uzgiris, 1973). The seven available studies have produced some 54 sets of solutions at six different age levels, which makes the data messy and interpretation somewhat difficult. In order to make sense out of the different sets of data, the results from the Down Syndrome Study are presented first as the benchmark against which the other sets of analyses are compared to discern similarities and differences in patterns of organization.

The structural organization of sensorimotor development was examined in the Down Syndrome Study at mental age levels of 0–4, 4–8, 8–12, 12–16, 16–20, and 20–24 months. The matrices of correlations among the seven Uzgiris–Hunt scales were subjected to principal components analyses using varimax rotation. The analyses were performed with unities in the diagonals, and factors with eigenvalues exceeding 1.0 were retained for rotation. A factor loading of .40 or greater was used to define factor membership. The extent to which the solutions at the six age

Table 6.12. *Factor analysis solutions and coefficients of congruence for the Down Syndrome Study sample (by mental age group in months)*

Sensorimotor domain	0–4			4–8	8–12	12–16		16–20			20–24		
	I	II	III	I	I	I	II	I	II	III	I	II	III
Object permanence	−13	91	17	89	66	65	16	45	56	11	−08	84	05
Means–ends	94	11	20	80	77	76	12	30	80	−16	−03	−06	94
Vocal imitation	13	72	−45	60	67	12	82	−13	02	85	65	55	−04
Gestural imitation	−77	28	32	68	73	13	88	36	13	76	17	89	−12
Operational causality	92	11	23	77	73	62	47	84	05	06	58	02	65
Spatial relationships	73	−24	51	86	77	86	00	78	23	02	83	−20	11
Schemes	19	01	86	76	75	52	36	−07	81	25	86	23	05
Individual factor variance:	42	22	20	60	53	35	26	25	24	20	32	27	19
Total Variance:			84	60	53	61			69				78

Age level (months)		Coefficients of congruence												
0–4	I	—	—	—	48	47	69	01	55	42	−26	15	03	83
	II	—	—	—	56	54	35	63	22	38	63	17	86	09
	III	—	—	—	63	61	69	24	54	72	06	58	16	31
4–8	I				—	99	93	71	76	79	52	73	59	56
8–12	I					—	90	77	73	77	58	76	59	86
12–16	I						—		83	81	18	67	30	69
	II						—	—	38	36	92	62	78	19
16–20	I								—	—	—	51	25	58
	II								—	—	—	46	39	57
	III								—	—	—	53	80	−16

Notes: Decimal points have been omitted. Factor loadings exceeding .40 have been underlined to emphasize factor membership. Coefficients of Congruence equal to or exceeding .80 have been underlined to identify congruent factor solutions.

groups were similar or different was determined using a measure of congruence developed by Tucker (1951; Harman, 1976). This procedure determines whether the weights (factor loadings) for the same set of variables at the different age levels are sufficiently congruent to conclude that the patterns of factor loadings reflect similar organization among the variables. The method yields a Coefficient of Congruence where a value of .80 or greater is taken as evidence of congruent structure among the variables.

Table 6.12 presents the factor analysis findings and the Coefficients of Congruence for all pairwise, between-age comparisons. Three factors were obtained at the 0–4 month level, one each at the 4–8 and 8–12 month levels, two at the 12–16 month level, and three each at the 16–20 and 20–24 month levels. This pattern of findings represents a *U*-function between the number of factors and the different age levels. The number of factors are smallest at the middle age-groups (4–8, 8–

12, 12–16) and greatest at the lower and upper bounds of the sensorimotor period. This may be taken as evidence of greater organization (covariation) in behavior during the period from 4 to 16 months. Thus, although it was found that stage congruence tends to be lowest during this particular age span, interdomain covariation in performance is greatest.

The bottom portion of Table 6.12 shows the extent to which the factor solutions obtained at the different age levels were congruent. Of the 68 pairwise comparisons, only 10 (15%) of the factors were sufficiently similar. This may be taken as evidence that there are considerable shifts in the patterns of organization of behavior at the different age levels. In those instances where congruence was established, 7 out of the 10 acceptable Coefficients of Congruence were along the diagonal of the coefficient matrix, indicating that when congruence was found, it tended to be between adjacent age levels. This suggests that shifts in patterns of organization are gradual rather than abrupt.

Examination of the specific patterns of factor loadings shows, with the exception of the 4–8 and 8–12 month levels where single, unitary solutions were obtained, that only 4 out of 21 pairwise scales ([ME, OC], [OC, SR], [SR, SO], [VI, GI]) factored together on 3 out of the 4 remaining solutions. Only three scales factored together more than once on the multiple factor solutions: [OP, OC, SR].

Comparison of the factor solutions from the Down Syndrome Study with those from other investigations (Dunst et al., 1981; Dunst & Rheingrover, 1983; King & Seegmiller, 1973; Silverstein et al., 1975; Uzgiris, 1973; Wachs & Hubert, 1981) finds both similarities and differences in the organizational features of sensorimotor development. Comparisons were made at six age levels (0–4, 4–8, 8–12, 12–16, 16–20, 20–24 months) between the three major groups of infants (nonretarded, Down syndrome, mentally retarded).

A number of major findings emerged from inspection of the factor analyses in the various studies. First, with the exception of the 4–8 month age level, multiple solutions were generally found, indicating multidimensionality in the patterns of sensorimotor organization. Second, some noticeable trends were evident in the data. [OP, ME], [OP, SO], [ME, SR], [ME, SO] [OC, SR], [OC, SO], and [SR, SO] loaded substantially on 50% of the solutions. Likewise, [VI, GI] factored together on 50% of the solutions. Each of these pairwise comparisons may be taken as evidence that the performance on the different scales have some common structure that is likely to manifest itself at almost all the developmental junctures at which patterns of organization have been examined. Third, interstudy comparisons find certain similarities in patterns of organization. Contrasts of the solutions for the Dunst et al. (1981) study of retarded subjects with the findings for the Down syndrome at the 4–8, 8–12, and 12–16 month levels shows almost identical factor solutions. This suggests that homogeneously and heterogeneously constituted groups of retarded infants show quite similar patterns of sensorimotor organization. At the 16–20 month level, the solutions involving vocal and gestural imitation in King and Seegmiller (1973), Wachs and Hubert (1981), and Down Syndrome Study were identical, which suggests that at least in terms of imitation abilities at this age level, nonretarded infants and infants with Down syndrome show similar patterns of organization.

The extent to which there was congruence in the factor solutions obtained in the various studies was also examined. The Coefficients of Congruence for the Down Syndrome Study solutions were compared with those solutions obtained in all other studies. Of 300 pairwise comparisons, only 39, or 13% of the solutions, were substantially congruent. These findings indicate very little similarity in overall patterns of organization. When examined for separate diagnostic groups, the percentage of congruent solutions were 11%, 8%, and 23% respectively for the nonretarded, Down syndrome, and retarded samples. The differences were statistically significant, $\chi^2 = 8.99$, $df = 3$, $p < .05$. When the analyses were limited only to the data for pairwise comparisons for the identical age levels, the percentage of sufficiently congruent structures were 8%, 16%, and 42% for the nonretarded, Down syndrome, and mentally retarded samples. The differences were again statistically significant, $\chi^2 = 27.82$, $df = 3$, $p < 001$. Both sets of data suggest that the patterns of organization of the Down Syndrome Study subjects are most similar to the retarded subjects in the Dunst et al. (1981) study. However, inasmuch as these were the only investigations that employed the same strategy of examining patterns of organization at narrowly constructed mental-age ranges, it may be that the similarities are related more to methodology than the influences of etiology or mental retardation.

Summary

The data examined in this section indicate that the sensorimotor competence of infants with Down syndrome comprises different subsets of behavior (i.e., is multidimensional) and that there are considerable shifts in the overall patterns of organization at different age levels. Both nonretarded and mentally retarded infants were found to show similar shifts in patterns of organization although the "make-up" of the different sets of competencies were generally different for the three groups of infants. The only consistent results for two different samples of infants were found for the Down Syndrome Study infants and Dunst et al. (1981) sample of mentally retarded infants, although it was noted that the parallel sets of findings may have been due more to methodological than subject similarities.

Although it is tempting, based on the data reviewed in this section, to conclude that the stage structuring of infants with Down syndrome and nonretarded infants is different, such a conclusion may not be warranted. Comparative analyses of the structural characteristics of sensorimotor development among different groups of nonretarded infants performed by Wachs and Hubert (1981) found very few congruent factor solutions among the different samples. Therefore, the fact that infants with Down syndrome manifested different patterns of organization is not inconsistent with findings of other investigations. Indeed, if anything, the results from the analyses performed in this section show higher degrees of congruence than even Wachs and Hubert (1981) reported.

Two major conclusions may be made based on the data just examined. First, different sensorimotor competencies do not form a structure totality or *structure d'ensemble*. Rather, sensorimotor intelligence is comprised of subsets of competencies. Second, there is very little structural continuity in the genesis of sensorimotor intelligence. Rather, there are changing networks of competencies over the course of the first 2 years of life.

Influential bases of sensorimotor development

The purpose of this section is to examine (1) factors that affect the acquisition of sensorimotor behaviors and (2) the relationship between sensorimotor competencies and developments in other behavior domains.

The treatment of sensorimotor development as a dependent variable seeks to discern the manner in which the development (acquisition, learning, etc.) of sensorimotor capabilities is influenced by other factors, including heredity, etiology, the environment, and other present and past organism–environment transactions (Baltes, Reese, & Nesselroade, 1977). The study of the relationship between sensorimotor competence and developments in other behavior areas seeks to discern the manner in which there are interdependencies which reflect some common developmental process. Both types of relationships are embodied in the paradigm

$$B = f(X),$$

where B is related to, varies as a function of, or otherwise is influenced or affected by X.

Although the $B = f(X)$ paradigm does not necessarily imply that B *causes X*, but only that a discernible relationship can be explicated between the two variables, the nature of the relationship is such that cause–effect inferences are likely to be drawn from data that conform to this relationship. (A detailed discussion of causation is beyond the scope of this chapter – see, e.g., Cohen & Cohen, 1983, chap. 9; Cook & Campbell, 1979, chap. 1; Kenny, 1979; for further discussion of this issue.) Although it is the ultimate goal of the science of developmental psychology to establish the nature of cause–effect relationships (Baltes et al., 1977), our state-of-the-art knowledge concerning sensorimotor development is such that we would be stepping on soft ground if other than conditional statements regarding the relationships among variables were to be made at this time.

Environmental influences on sensorimotor development

The extent to which the acquisition of sensorimotor competencies is influenced by environmental events has been examined in two types of studies. The first has examined how different conditions of rearing affect the age of attainment of different levels of sensorimotor competence. The second has examined how the use of "curricula" and other training procedures have positive influences on the development of sensorimotor behaviors. Both types of studies are concerned with the degree to which sensorimotor development, the dependent variable, is affected by different environmental events and manipulations, the independent variables.

Conditions of rearing

Hunt and his colleagues (Hunt, 1976, 1980; Hunt et al., 1975, 1976; Paraskevopoulos & Hunt, 1971) have amassed a considerable body of evidence indicating that different conditions of rearing affect the rate of acquisition of sensorimotor competencies. The approach Hunt has taken is to treat rearing condition as the independent variable and age of acquisition of different sensorimotor landmarks as the dependent variable, and to compare groups of infants varying in terms of rearing condition in order to determine the degree to which the environment, broadly conceived, has facilitating or retarding effects on sensorimotor development.[3]

The rearing conditions that Hunt has studied have varied along a continuum ranging from home-reared infants participating in an early intervention program to institutionally reared infants for whom no special provisions of enrichment or stimulation were provided. The results, presented in the following paragraphs, demonstrate the influence of rearing condition on sensorimotor development. The attainment of the highest level, Stage 6 achievements on the Uzgiris–Hunt scales, have differed as much as 38 weeks among infants reared under favorable versus unfavorable conditions. Hunt (1980) described this substantial variability as the "range of reaction" of the environment, and interpreted the findings as evidence for a high degree of plasticity in the rate of acquisition of sensorimotor competencies resulting from environmental variations.

A number of studies have compared the effects of home versus institutional placements upon rates of development among children with Down syndrome (e.g., Bayley, Rhodes, Gooch, & Marcus, 1971; Francis, 1971; Stedman & Eichorn, 1964). It has generally been found that home-reared children manifest higher levels of mental and language development, suggesting that rearing condition influenced the development of children with Down syndrome. Stedman and Eichorn (1964) found debilitating effects of institutional placement even for a group of infants who participated in a special enrichment program within an institution. Bayley et al. (1971), who followed the same subjects in the Stedman and Eichorn (1964) study until the children were 8 years of age, found that the home-reared children functioned at higher levels of mental, motor, and social development on nearly all outcome measures at 2, 5, 6, and 8 years of age. However, when the institutionalized sample was involved in an intensive language-training program beginning when the children were between 5 and 6 years of age, a number of the differences between groups dissipated. The latter finding illustrates the potent influence of the environment on development, and indicates that even some of the debilitating effects of institutional rearing can be overcome as late as 6 years of age.

The degree to which the sensorimotor development of children with Down syndrome and other retarded children is influenced by rearing condition was examined for the present chapter through a systematic comparison of the age of acquisition of different sensorimotor landmarks by various groups of infants differing in both etiology and rearing condition (Badger, 1971, 1972; Down Syndrome Study, Dunst, 1978a; Escalona & Corman, 1969; Hunt, Mohandessi, Ghodesi, & Akiyama, 1976; Paraskevopoulos & Hunt, 1971; Uzgiris, 1987; Wohlhueter & Sindberg, 1975). The Uzgiris (1987), Badger (1971, 1972), Escalona and Corman (1969), Paraskevopoulos and Hunt (1971), and Hunt et al. (1976) studies included infants with no identifiable pathology. The Uzgiris (1987) sample was from lower- to upper-middle socioeconomic status (SES) backgrounds; children of nonworking mothers; and all home-reared. The Badger (1971, 1972) sample included infants from low SES backgrounds who participated in a center-based early intervention program designed to optimize learning opportunities for the children. The Escalona and Corman (1969) sample was from lower- to middle-class backgrounds; and all were home-reared.

The Paraskevopoulos and Hunt (1971) study included three samples of subjects of lower SES backgrounds from Athens, Greece. One sample was a home-reared group of infants of working mothers whose children attended a day-care program. The other two groups were infants placed in orphanages awaiting adoption with caregiver–child ratios of 3 to 1 and 10 to 1 respectively. The Hunt et al. (1976) study included five samples of infants living in a Tehran, Iran, orphanage. Each differed in terms of the types of enrichment they received. The infants were all "foundlings" without known parents or relatives. The Iran infants were more "advantaged" than the institutionalized Greek infants in the sense that even without the special forms of interventions provided by Hunt et al. (1976), the infants were generally provided as much stimulation and enrichment as possible.

The Down Syndrome Study included home-reared infants from predominately lower to middle SES backgrounds who participated in a home-based early intervention program. The sample was divided into two groups: one was followed longitudinally, and the other was assessed cross-sectionally. The Dunst (1978a) study included a heterogeneously formed group of handicapped infants from lower to upper SES backgrounds who participated in a center-based early intervention program. The subjects in the Wohlhueter and Sindberg (1975) study were a heterogeneous group of mentally retarded children with different etiologies living in a state institution for the retarded.

In order to determine the effects of rearing condition on acquisition of sensorimotor competencies, the mean age of attainment of the landmarks on the seven Uzgiris–Hunt scales were ascertained in as many instances as possible, to determine whether or not rearing condition influenced sensorimotor development. Because the number of possible pairwise comparisons (105) among the 15 samples of subjects would produce a staggering number of contrasts for the 72 Uzgiris–Hunt scale items, only 5 items per scale corresponding to Stages 2 through 6 of the sensorimotor period were selected for analysis.[4]

A series of *t* tests were performed between the ages of attainment of the landmarks for the longitudinal sample in the Down Syndrome Study and the ages of attainment in all the other studies to determine the influence of rearing condition and etiology on acquisition of sensorimotor competencies. Only pairwise contrasts with the Down Syndrome Study are reported since these analyses are most germane to the purpose of the present chapter. (The interested reader should see Hunt et al., 1976, for a description of the effects of condition of rearing for the various samples of nonretarded subjects.)

The comparisons of the Down Syndrome Study versus home-reared, nonretarded samples (Badger, 1971, 1972; Escalona & Corman, 1969; Uzgiris, 1987) showed, not unexpectedly, that the nonretarded infants attained the various landmarks at an earlier age in nearly every instance except for gestural imitation. The results of the analyses for the infants with Down syndrome versus Badger sample indicated that both groups of subjects acquired the Stage 3 and Stage 6 gestural imitation landmarks at about the same age.

The comparisons of the Down Syndrome Study versus the three Paraskevopoulos and Hunt (1971) samples of Greek infants produced 13 significant findings. In the majority of instances (69%), the differences favored the infants with Down syndrome. The majority of advantages favoring the infants with Down syndrome were found for comparisons involving the two institutionalized samples. However, in only 3 of 13 instances (23%) did the home-reared Greek sample attain the landmarks at earlier ages compared to the infants with Down syndrome. Thus, the home-reared infants with Down syndrome participating in an early intervention generally acquired sensorimotor competencies at the same or at a faster rate than did infants who were without pathology but were disadvantaged in terms of rearing condition (i.e., institutionalized) or SES status (home-reared).

The types of experiences provided the five waves of subjects in the Hunt et al. (1976) study varied on a continuum from no active attempts to influence development (Wave 1) to nonspecific enrichment (Wave 3) to active attempts to affect development through provision of nonsocial and social learning experiences (Wave 5). The results of the analyses involving the Waves 1, 2, and 3 infants showed that the Down Syndrome Study sample often acquired the Stage 2 and 3 landmarks before the institutionalized samples, but that the highest level achievements were generally acquired earlier by the samples without pathology. However, in only 22% of the cases did the Iran samples in Waves 1, 2, and 3 attain the landmarks at earlier ages compared to the infants with Down syndrome. In contrast, comparisons with the Waves 4 and 5 infants showed that in the 23 instances where significant differences were found, 21, or 91%, favored the Iran samples. Thus, although the rate of development of the infants with Down syndrome was generally similar to that of the "untutored" Waves 1, 2, and 3 infants, their rates of development were much slower compared to the Waves 4 and 5 infants who received structured intervention.

There were no significant differences between the longitudinal and cross-sectional samples of infants in the Down Syndrome Study for any of the 45 comparisons. The comparisons of the Down Syndrome Study versus the Dunst (1978a) sample showed that the infants with Down syndrome attained seven landmarks at an earlier age than did the heterogeneously formed group of retarded subjects. Inasmuch as these two groups of infants differed both in terms of etiology and type of early intervention (home vs. center), it is difficult to separate out the differential influences, if any, of these two factors. The differences between the Down Syndrome Study and institutionalized mentally retarded samples (Wohlhueter & Sindberg, 1975) were highly significant, and in all instances favored the infants with Down syndrome. Again, inasmuch as the infants differed in terms of etiology, how much the delays in the acquisition of sensorimotor competencies are attributable to institutionalization cannot be adequately determined.

In summary, the infants in the Down Syndrome Study acquired sensorimotor competencies at a slower rate compared to both home-reared, advantaged nonretarded infants and institutionalized but "tutored" nonretarded infants; at about the same rate compared to both home-reared, disadvantaged nonretarded infants and other retarded infants who participated in an early intervention program; but at a faster rate compared to both nonretarded and retarded institutionalized children. Rearing condition would therefore seem to contribute to the rate of acquisition of sensorimotor competencies among infants with Down syndrome and other retarded children. However, evidence from a number of sources suggests that it is not rearing condition per se but, rather, specific components of the home environment that positively influence sensorimotor functioning (Piper & Ramsey, 1980; Smith & Hagen, 1984). These include both environmental arrangements (e.g., organization of the physical and temporal environment) and caregiver behaviors (e.g., maternal responsiveness).

Training studies

A number of investigations have sought to determine whether the use of curricula and other forms of training affect the acquisition of sensorimotor competencies among infants with Down syndrome and other mentally retarded children. The major efforts in this area have involved the use of procedures designed to enhance the acquisition of object permanence (Brassell & Dunst, 1978; Kahn, 1978; Morss, 1984). The subjects in the Brassell and Dunst (1978) study were mentally retarded, physically impaired, and developmentally at-risk infants, including infants with Down syndrome. The Kahn (1978) study included eight subjects, six of whom were children with Down syndrome. All of the subjects in the Morss (1984) study were infants with Down syndrome. Each study included a control group for which no object permanence training was provided. The method of training was relatively similar in all three investigations. Repeated presentations and restructuring of standard object permanence tasks (e.g., Uzgiris and Hunt, 1975) constituted the method of enhancing acquisition of the construct. Typically, targeted behaviors were broken down into smaller learning steps, or task-analyzed according to their component parts, and systematic efforts were implemented to foster the acquisition of the behaviors necessary to demonstrate different levels of the object permanence construct. The results of all three studies showed that the children participating in the training program acquired progressively more complex object permanence competencies, and that the amount of progress demonstrated by the experimental subjects was significantly greater than for control subjects.

Two studies have examined the extent to which training procedures influenced acquisition of sensorimotor competencies in developmental areas in addition to object permanence. Dunst (1974) conducted a single-subject study in which a set of curricula procedures (Dunst, 1981b) was used to facilitate means–ends, object permanence, vocal imitation, gestural imitation, and play behaviors in a 3-month-old infant with Down syndrome. The seven Uzgiris–Hunt scales were the dependent measures of sensorimotor performance. A multiple baseline design across sensorimotor domains established the efficacy of the intervention procedures. The design consisted of three separate intervention periods, where one, three, and one sensorimotor domains were targeted, respectively, and intervention procedures implemented to foster acquisition of the types of competencies within each target area. The results showed that the gains in the intervention areas were significantly greater than progress in the nonintervention areas.

Kahn (1981) reported results from a study designed to assess the impact of different types of sensorimotor training on the acquisition of cognitive skills. Four groups of mentally retarded subjects were included in the study. The first received training in object permanence, the second in means–ends skills, and the third in language acquisition. The fourth served as a control group. Differential influences of training were found in all instances. Although the subjects all demonstrated gains across an 18-month period of time, progress was generally greater in the particular areas in which training was provided. These findings support the results from other training studies that have demonstrated specificity with regard to the effects of training (see Dunst, 1981b).

Summary

The evidence examined in this section strongly suggests that rearing condition as well as learning opportunities have positive influences on the sensorimotor development of infants with Down syndrome. Although home-reared, nonretarded infants' rate of development was generally much more rapid than for home-reared infants with Down syndrome, the latter often demonstrated more advanced levels of sensorimotor competence relative to infants without pathology but reared under less favorable conditions. Moreover, the results from the training studies indicated that rate of acquisition of sensorimotor competencies was much greater compared to infants not receiving training (see Dunst, Snyder, & Mankinen, 1989, and Hanson, 1981, for reviews of additional studies documenting the impact of early intervention with infants with Down syndrome). Taken together, both sets of findings suggest that the range of reaction (Hunt, 1980) of the environment is much alike for both infants with Down syndrome and nonretarded infants, and that the sensorimotor development of infants with Down syndrome can be influenced positively by rearing condition and provision of learning opportunities.

Relationship between affect, motivation, temperament and sensorimotor development

The organizational view of development so lucidly advanced by Cicchetti and his colleagues (e.g., Cicchetti & Pogge-Hesse, 1981; 1982; Cicchetti & Sroufe, 1976, 1978) stresses the interdependencies among developments in different behavior domains. According to these investigators, developmental organization is reflected in patterns of interdependencies, and the manner in which these interdependencies represent evolving systems of how the infant adapts to different environmental demands. Evidence regarding the relationships between sensorimotor development and other behavioral competencies is examined in this section.

Sensorimotor development and affect

The study of the relationship between affective and cognitive development is one area of investigation for which data substantiate the organizational view. Because data from these studies are reviewed elsewhere in this volume (see Cicchetti & Beeghly, Chapter 2), the discussion here is restricted only to findings specifically examining how sensorimotor development and affect are related among infants with Down syndrome. The pertinent evidence comes from a study by Cicchetti and Sroufe (1976). The subjects in this study were 14 infants with Down syndrome followed longitudinally from 4 to 24 months of age. The infants were tested monthly on a series of standardized items designed to elicit smiling and laughter. At 13 months of age, the Uzgiris–Hunt object permanence and causality scales were administered to the subjects. Age of first smile and first laughter as well as the total amount of smiling and laughter were correlated with sensorimotor performance. The mean correlations for the 11 indices of affective expression and object permanence and causality were, respectively, .76 ($SD = .06$) and .78 ($SD = .08$). All 22 correlations were statistically significant. Cicchetti and Sroufe (1976) interpreted these findings as evidence for strong affective–cognitive ties in development that supported an integrated view of behavior organization.

Sensorimotor development and motivation

A version of the organizational view of development has been advanced by Hunt (1965, 1971) with regard to the relationship between sensorimotor and motivational development. Hunt's theory of motivation stresses the extent to which optimally incongruent tasks challenge and motivate the infant, whereas tasks that have already been mastered tend to elicit boredom and those beyond the cognitive capabilities of the infant fail to engage his or her attention and interest. A fundamental tenet of Hunt's theory is the pleasure derived from cognitive mastery. Equally fundamental is the hypothesized inverted-U relationship between the degree of cognitive challenge and the amount of gratification experienced. Tasks that are optimally challenging elicit little or no signs of gratification. Both smiling and laughter have been found to be particularly reliable indices of cognitive mastery among nonretarded infants (see McCall & McGhee, 1977), and patterns of affective responding have generally conformed to the hypothesized inverted-U function.

The optimal stimulation hypothesis was examined by Dunst (1981c) in a study that assessed the extent to which infants with Down syndrome smiled and laughed in response to successful and unsuccessful completion of the items on the Uzgiris–Hunt scales. The subjects were administered the scales in their own homes on five or six occasions over a 4-month period. During each assessment, the subject's affective behavior was recorded to the successful and unsuccessful completion of each item administered.

To test the hypothesis that the manifestation of affective behavior would be curvilinearly related to level of sensorimotor performance, the subjects' sensorimotor capabilities were divided into three performance levels: easy (successful); optimal (successful); and unsuccessful. Optimally successful was defined as the highest two levels of performance attained on each scale. The easy level was defined as the two items below optimal performance. The difficult level was defined as the two items above the highest item passed in each domain. The hypothesis that sense of pleasure would be greatest to successfully completed items was supported. Subjects demonstrated positive affect to successfully completed tasks ($M = 14.63$) at a rate of nearly four times that manifest in response to unsuccessful tasks ($M = 4.21$). The hypothesis that solutions to optimally challenging tasks would produce a greater sense of pleasure than solutions to easy tasks was supported only for vocal imitation. On the other scales, positive affect occurred as frequently to both the easy and optimal performance level tasks.

Sensorimotor development and temperament

The relationship between infant temperament and learning has been established in a number of studies (Dunst & Lingerfelt, 1985; Krafchuk, Sameroff, & Bakow, 1976; Matheney, Dolan, & Wilson, 1974; Peters-Martin & Wachs, 1981; Stevenson & Lamb, 1979; Wachs & Gandour, 1983). Wachs and Gandour (1983) found that Piagetian level of sensorimotor development at 6 months of age was significantly correlated with the temperament dimensions of approach and intensity at this same age level. Peters-Martin and Wachs (1981) found that several dimensions of temperament (threshold, persistence, and adaptability, respectively) measured at 6 months of age were significantly correlated with vocal imitation ($r = .66$), causality ($r = .38$), and space ($r. = .46$) performance at 12 months of age. Likewise, Stevenson and Lamb (1979) found that several sociability dimensions of temperament were highly correlated with Uzgiris–Hunt scale performance among 1-year-old infants.

The extent to which temperament was related to sensorimotor development among infants with Down syndrome was examined in the Down Syndrome Study. The dependent measures were the seven Uzgiris–Hunt scales. The independent measures of temperament were the Bayley Scales Infant Behavior Record (IBR) items. The 10 IBR items included in the analyses were: social orientation, cooperativeness, fearfulness, emotional tone, object orientation, goal directedness, attention span, endurance, activity level, and reactivity.

Canonical correlation analysis was used to identify which IBR items were significantly related to which sensorimotor competencies. The analyses were performed at four mental-age levels (4–8, 8–12, 12–16, 16–20) in order to determine whether the patterns of relationships were similar at the different age levels. (Insufficient data were available at the 0–4 and 20–24 month levels to perform the canonical correlation analyses.) The canonical correlations between the IBR and sensorimotor scores were, respectively, .79 ($p < .01$), .81 ($p < .05$), .73 ($p < .08$), and .79 ($p < .001$) at the four age levels. On the average, 61% ($SD = 5.60$) of the variance in sensorimotor performance was accounted for by the IBR dimensions of temperament. This set of findings provides evidence for strong interdependencies between temperament and sensorimotor functioning.

Examination of the sensorimotor scales/IBR items that had canonical variable loadings exceeding .35 yielded the following patterns: 4 to 8 months [SO/Emotional Tone], 8 to 12 months [OP, ME, VI, GI, OC, SR Fearfulness, Emotional Tone, Activity Level, Reactivity], 12 to 16 months [GI, SR, SO/Cooperativeness, Attention Span, Activity Level, Reactivity], and 18 to 20 months [OP, GI, SR, SO/ Activity Level, Reactivity]. Gestural imitation loaded substantially on all four canonical solutions, while both spatial relationships and schemes for relating to objects did so on three out of the four solutions. The three IBR items that were consistently related to sensorimotor performance were emotional tone, activity level, and reactivity. Thus, although there were strong relationships between sensorimotor functioning and temperament, there was considerable specificity in the nature of the relationships.

Summary

Taken together, the data reviewed in this section provide considerable evidence in support of an organizational view of development between sensorimotor functioning and affect, motivation, and temperament among infants with Down syndrome. In studies where correlations were calculated between sensorimotor and social functioning, 60% of the variance was accounted for by the relationship between the two developmental domains (Cicchetti & Sroufe, 1976; Down Syndrome Study). This is twice as high as generally found in studies of nonretarded infants (see Lamb, 1982), although methodological differences may account for a portion of this variability. Nonetheless, the available evidence indicates, as Cicchetti and his colleagues (Cicchetti & Pogge-Hesse, 1981, 1982; Cicchetti & Sroufe, 1976, 1978) have repeatedly demonstrated, that there are strong ties between the acquisition of cognitive and social competencies, and that the manifestation of these relationships are much alike for nonretarded infants and infants with Down syndrome.

Conclusion

The following were the major findings from this review and analysis of the literature of the sensorimotor development of infants with Down syndrome:

· Both age-related changes and ordinality in the acquisition of sensorimotor competencies among infants with Down syndrome were very similar to that of nonretarded infants.
· Infants with Down syndrome showed a progressive slowing down in the acquisition of sensorimotor competencies with increasing age; where the slowing down phenomenon was most pronounced for vocal imitation.
· Available evidence regarding the manner in which infants with Down syndrome and nonretarded infants integrate behaviors in the transition from lower to higher levels of functioning was much like for both groups of children.
· Infants with Down syndrome showed a greater incidence of regressions in development and took longer to move from stage to stage compared with nonretarded infants, even after the slower pace of development of the infants with Down syndrome was taken into consideration.
· Available evidence concerning the structural aspects of sensorimotor intelligence among infants with Down syndrome showed that their infant cognitive abilities comprised subsets of competencies and that there was little structural continuity in the patterns of organization at different age levels.
· Comparisons of the stage functioning characteristics of infants with Down syndrome and nonretarded infants showed both similarities and differences in patterns of organization, although methodological differences in the various studies made direct comparative analyses difficult at best.
· Evidence regarding the extent to which the acquisition of sensorimotor competencies among infants with Down syndrome were affected by the environment showed that rearing condition, specific aspects of home environments, and training efforts enhanced the attainment of progressively more complex types of sensorimotor behaviors.
· Available evidence showed that there were strong relationships between sensorimotor functioning and affective, motivation, and temperament development among infants with Down syndrome, although the specific nature of these relationships is unclear at this time.

The aggregate of all the findings, albeit the differences in stage stabilization, provide evidence to support the developmental position (Zigler & Balla, 1982) that the sensorimotor development of infants with Down syndrome and nonretarded infants is more similar than different. Despite their slower pace of development, infants with Down syndrome showed remarkably similar changes in their acquisition and organization of sensorimotor competencies.

Since the translation of Piaget's (1951, 1952, 1954) trilogy on sensorimotor intelligence into English, we have witnessed a burgeoning number of studies examining the early cognitive development of nonretarded infants, infants with Down syndrome, and other retarded infants. According to Baltes et al. (1977), the task of developmental psychology is *"the description, explanation, and modification (optimization) of intraindividual change in behavior and interindividual differences in such changes"* (p. 84). With regard to the sensorimotor development of infants with Down syndrome, the focus of most research efforts has been the description of developmental change and stability. We now have a substantial body of evidence describing the characteristics of sensorimotor development among infants with Down syndrome and other retarded infants. Also, a burgeoning body of evidence documents the role that early experiences (intervention) play in enhancing the acquisition of sensorimotor competencies (see especially Dunst, 1986; Dunst et al., 1989). What we do not have is much evidence regarding the explication of factors affecting the acquisition and organization of sensorimotor capabilities. Further advances are likely to be made only when investigators begin to examine and isolate the causal and mediational factors affecting change and stability in sensorimotor development.

Establishment of relationships among variables is only one of the developmentalist's tasks. Another is explaining these relationships. What are the factors that affect the manner in which stage sequencing occurs? What are the conditions that influence the organization of sensorimotor abilities and the ways in which shifts occur in patterns of organization? Are these shifts a result of organismic factors or the way in which the environment shapes the course of developmental change? What are the specific aspects of the environment that affect change? Does sensorimotor functioning affect social development, or vice versa? Is there a transactional relationship between these developmental domains? Are both affected by a third, moderating variable? These as well as other questions must be addressed if we are to further our knowledge and understanding of the processes of acquisition of sensorimotor development. In summarizing the data on the relationship between infant cognitive and social functioning, Lamb (1982) concluded that "the evidence regarding the relationship between sociability and cognitive performance in infancy remains frustratingly inconclusive" (p. 236). This statement could easily be expanded to say "despite more than a 25-year history of the study of sensorimotor development, the evidence regarding the relationships between heredity, etiology, the environment, sensorimotor functioning, and social development remains frustratingly inconclusive." Further advances are likely to be made only when explanatory models are applied to the study of sensorimotor functioning as both a dependent and an independent variable. A shift toward the application of such models is clearly indicated.

Notes

1 In a number of instances, data presented in the published reports were reanalyzed for purposes of this chapter. In several other cases, unpublished data from the studies were analyzed in order to shed light on various aspects of sensorimotor functioning among infants with Down syndrome.

2 This notation system will be used to represent those particular sensorimotor domains that show strong interdependencies with one another. (*note:* OP = object permanence; ME = means–ends; VI = vocal imitation; GI = gestural imitation; OC = operational causality; SR = spatial relationships; SO = schemes for relating to objects.)

3 As noted by Paraskevopoulos and Hunt (1971); "While it is easy to specify the conditions of rearing that influence development, rearing condition as an independent variable is highly limited insofar as specifying the characteristics of the infant–environment interaction" (p. 304).

4 The specific scale steps were as follows: OP (2,3,5,9,14), ME (1,4,6,9,13), VI (2,4,5,8,9), GI (1,2,4,7,9), OC (1,3,4,5,7), SR (3,4,6,9,11), and SO (2,5,6,9,10). The reader should consult Uzgiris and Hunt (1975) or Dunst (1980b) for a description of these landmarks.

References

Badger, E. (1971). A mother's training program – the road to a purposeful existence. *Children, 18,* 168–173.

Badger, E. (1972). A mother's training program – A sequel article. *Children Today, 1*(13), 7–12.

Baldwin, J. M. (1895). *Mental development in the child and the race: Methods and processes.* New York: Macmillan.

Baldwin, J. M. (1897). *Social and ethical interpretations in mental development.* New York: Macmillan.

Baltes, P., Reese, H., & Nesselroade, J. (1977). *Life-span developmental psychology: Introduction to research methods.* Monterey, CA: Brooks/Cole.

Barnes, C., & Dunst, C. J. (1984). *Sensorimotor development of mentally retarded children.* Unpublished study, Western Carolina Center, Morganton, NC.

Bates, E. (1976). *Language and context: The acquisition of pragmatics.* New York: Academic Press.

Bayley, N. (1969). *The Bayley Scales of Infant Development.* New York: Psychological Corporation.

Bayley, N., Rhodes, L., Gooch, B., & Marcus, M. (1971). Environmental factors in the development of institutionalized children. In S. Hellmuth (Ed.), *Exceptional Infant,* Vol. 2: *Studies in subnormalities* (pp. 450–472). New York: Brunner/Mazel.

Bovet, M. C., Dasen, P. R., & Inhelder, B. (1974). Etapes de l'intelligence sensorimotrice chez l'enfant Baoule. *Archives de Psychologie, 41,* 363.

Brassell, W. R., & Dunst, C. J., (1978). Fostering the object construct: Large-scale intervention with handicapped infants. *American Journal of Mental Deficiency, 82,* 507–510.

Campbell, R. L., & Richie, D. M. (1983). Problems in the theory of developmental sequences: Prerequisites and precursors. *Human Development, 26,* 156–172.

Cicchetti, D., & Mans-Wagener, L. (1987). Stages, sequences, and structures in the organization of cognitive development in Down syndrome infants. In I. C. Uzgiris & J. McV. Hunt (Eds.), *Infant performance and experience* (pp. 281–310). Urbana–Champaign: University of Illinois.

Cicchetti, D., & Pogge-Hesse, P. (1981). The relation between emotion and cognition in infant development: Past, present, and future perspectives. In M. Lamb & L. Sherrod (Eds.), *Infant social cognition* (pp. 205–272). Hillsdale, NJ: Erlbaum.

Cicchetti, D., & Pogge-Hesse, P. (1982). Possible contributions of the study of organically retarded persons to developmental theory. In E. Zigler & D. Balla (Eds.), *Mental retardation: The developmental difference controversy* (pp. 277–318). Hillsdale, NJ: Erlbaum.

Cicchetti, D., & Sroufe, L. A. (1976). The relationship between affective and cognitive development in Down's syndrome infants. *Child Development, 47,* 920–929.

Cicchetti, D., & Sroufe, L. A. (1978). An organizational view of affect: Illustration from the study of Down syndrome infants. In M. Lewis & L. Rosenblum (Eds.), *The development of affect* (pp. 309–350). New York: Plenum.

Cohen, J., & Cohen, P. (1983). *Applied multiple regression/correlation analysis for the behavioral sciences* (2nd ed.). Hillsdale, NJ: Erlbaum.

Cook, T. D., & Campbell, D. T. (1979). *Quasi-experimentation: Design and analysis issues for field settings.* Chicago: Rand McNally.

Corman, H. H., & Escalona, S. K. (1969). Stages of sensorimotor development: A replication study. *Merrill-Palmer Quarterly, 15,* 351–361.

Dasen, P., Inhelder, B., Lavallee, M., & Retschitzki, J. (1978). *Naissance de l'intelligence chez l'enfant Bauole de Côte d'Ivoire.* Berne: Hans Huber.

Decarie, T. G. (1965). *Intelligence and affectivity in early childhood.* New York: International Universities Press.

Dicks-Mireaux, M. J. (1972). Mental development of infants with Down's syndrome. *American Journal of Mental Deficiency, 77,* 26–32.

Dunst, C. J. (1974). *Patterns of cognitive skills acquisitions among developmentally delayed infants.* Paper presented at the annual meeting of the American Association on Mental Deficiency, Toronto, June.

Dunst, C. J. (1978a). *Patterns of sensorimotor development among children in the Kennedy Center Experimental School Infant Unit.* Unpublished manuscript, George Peabody College of Vanderbilt University, Nashville, TN.

Dunst, C. J. (1978b). A cognitive–social approach for assessment of early nonverbal communicative behavior. *Journal of Childhood Communication Disorders, 2,* 110–123.

Dunst, C. J. (1979). *Cognitive-social aspects of communicative exchanges between mothers and their Down's syndrome infants and mothers and their nonretarded infants.* Unpublished doctoral dissertation, George Peabody College of Vanderbilt University, Nashville, TN.

Dunst, C. J. (1980a). *Sensorimotor development of mentally retarded and handicapped infants.* Unpublished study, George Peabody College of Vanderbilt University, Nashville, TN.

Dunst, C. J. (1980b). *A clinical and educational manual for use with the Uzgiris–Hunt scales.* Baltimore: University Park Press.

Dunst, C. J. (1980c). *Developmental characteristics of communicative acts among Down's syndrome infants and nonretarded infants.* Paper presented at the biennial meeting of the Southeastern Conference on Human Development, Alexandria, VA, April.

Dunst, C. J. (1981a). Test settings and the sensorimotor performance of Down syndrome infants. *Perceptual and Motor Skills, 53,* 575–578.

Dunst, C. J. (1981b). *Infant learning.* Hingham, MA: Teaching Resources.

Dunst, C. J. (1981c). Social concomitants of cognitive mastery in Down's syndrome infants. *Infant Mental Health Journal, 2,* 144–154.

Dunst, C. J. (1982). *Early intervention, social support, and institutional avoidance.* Paper presented at the annual meeting of the Southeastern American Association on Mental Deficiency, Louisville, KY, November.

Dunst, C. J. (1984). Toward a social–ecological perspective of sensorimotor development among the mentally retarded. In P. Brooks, R. Sperber, & C. McCauley (Eds.), *Learning and cognition in the mentally retarded* (pp. 359–387). Hillsdale, NJ: Erlbaum.

Dunst, C. J. (1985). Rethinking early intervention. *Analysis and Intervention in Developmental Disabilities, 5,* 115–201.

Dunst, C. J. (1986). Overview of the efficacy of early intervention programs: Methodological and conceptual considerations. In L. Bickman & D. Weatherford (Eds.), *Evaluating early intervention programs for severely handicapped children and their families* (pp. 79–147). Austin, TX: PRO-ED.

Dunst, C. J. (1988). Stage transitioning in the sensorimotor development of Down syndrome infants. *Journal of Mental Deficiency Research, 32,* 405–410.

Dunst, C. J., Brassell, W. R., & Rheingrover, R. M. (1981). Structural and organisational features of sensorimotor intelligence among retarded infants and toddlers. *British Journal of Educational Psychology, 51,* 133–143.

Dunst, C. J., Gallagher, J., & Vance, S. (1982). *Developmental characteristics of sensorimotor intelligence among mentally retarded infants: Preliminary findings.* Paper presented at the Gatlinburg Conference on Research in Mental Retardation/Developmental Disabilities, Gatlinburg, TN, April.

Dunst, C. J., & Lingerfelt, B. (1985). Maternal ratings of temperament and operant learning in two-to-three-month-old infants. *Child Development, 56,* 555–563.

Dunst, C. J., & Rheingrover, R. M. (1983). Structural characteristics of sensorimotor development among Down's syndrome infants. *Journal of Mental Deficiency Research, 27,* 11–22.

Dunst, C. J., Snyder, S. W., & Mankinen, M. (1989). Efficacy of early intervention. In M. Wang, M. Reynolds & H. Walberg, (Eds.), *Handbook of special education* (Vol. 3, pp. 259–294). Oxford: Pergamon.

Escalona, S., & Corman, H. (1969). *Albert Einstein scales of sensorimotor development.* Unpublished manuscript, Albert Einstein College of Medicine, Department of Psychiatry, New York.

Flavell, J. (1970). Concept development. In P. Mussen (Ed.), *Carmichael's manual of child psychology* (3rd ed., pp. 983–1059). New York: Wiley.

Flavell, J. H. (1971). Stage-related properties of cognitive development. *Cognitive Psychology, 2,* 421–453.

Flavell, J. H. (1972). An analysis of cognitive developmental sequences. *Genetic Psychology Monographs, 86,* 279–350.

Flavell, J. H. (1982a). On cognitive development. *Child Development, 53,* 1–10.

Flavell, J. H. (1982b). Structures, stages, and sequences in cognitive development. In W. A. Collins (Ed.), *The concept of development: The Minnesota symposia on child psychology* (Vol. 15, pp. 1–28). Hillsdale, NJ: Erlbaum.

Francis, S. H. (1971). Effects of own-home and institution-rearing on the behavioral development of normal and mongol children. *Journal of Child Psychology and Psychiatry and Allied Disciplines, 12,* 173–190.

Gibson, D. (1978). *Down syndrome: The psychology of mongolism.* New York: Cambridge University Press.

Green B. (1956). A method of scalogram analysis using summary statistics. *Psychometrika, 21,* 79–88.

Griffiths, R. (1954). *The abilities of babies.* London: University of London Press.

Guttman, L. (1950). The basis for scalogram analysis. In S. Stouffer (Ed.), *Measurement and predictions* (pp. 60–90). Princeton, NJ: Princeton University Press.

Hanson, M. J. (1981). Down's syndrome children: Characteristics and intervention research. In M. Lewis & L. Rosenblum (Eds.), *The uncommon child* (pp. 83–114). New York: Plenum.

Harman, H. (1960). *Modern factor analysis.* Chicago: University of Chicago Press.

Hill, P., & McCune, Nicolich, L. (1981). Patterned play and patterns of cognition in Down's syndrome children. *Child Development, 52,* 611–614.

Holdgrafer, G. & Dunst, C. J., (1986). Communicative competence: From research to practice. *Topics in Early Childhood Special Education, 6*(3), 1–22.

Hunt, J. McV. (1965). Intrinsic motivation and its role in psychological development. In D. Levine (Ed.), *Nebraska symposium on motivation* (Vol. 13, pp. 189–282). Lincoln: University of Nebraska Press.

Hunt, J. McV. (1971). Intrinsic motivation and psychological development. In H. M. Schroder & P. Suedfeld (Eds.), *Personality, theory, and information processing* (pp. 131–177). New York: Ronald Press.

Hunt, J. McV. (1976). The utility of ordinal scales inspired by Piaget's observations. *Merrill-Palmer Quarterly, 22,* 31–45.

Hunt, J. McV. (1980). Implications of plasticity and hierarchical achievements for the assessment of development and risk of mental retardation. In D. Swain, R. Hawkins, L. Walker, & J. Penticuff (Eds.), *Exceptional infant,* Vol. 4: *Psychosocial risks in infant-environment transactions* (pp. 3–54). New York: Brunner/Mazel.

Hunt, J. McV., Mohandessi, K., Ghodesi, M., & Akiyama, M. (1976). The psychological development of orphanage-reared infants: Intervention with outcomes (Tehran). *Genetic Psychology Monographs, 94,* 177–226.

Hunt, J. McV., Paraskevopoulos, J., Schickendanz, D., & Uzgiris, I. (1975). Variations in the mean ages of achieving object permanence under diverse conditions of rearing. In B. Friedlander, G. Sterritt, & G. Kirk (Eds.), *The exceptional infant,* Vol. 3: *Assessment and intervention* (pp. 247–262). New York: Brunner/Mazel.

Inhelder, B. (1966). Cognitive development and its contribution to the diagnosis of some phenomena of mental deficiency. *Merrill-Palmer Quarterly, 11,* 299–319.

Inhelder, B. (1968). *The diagnosis of reasoning in the mentally retarded.* New York: Day. (Originally published 1943.)

Johnson, S. C. (1967). Hierarchical clustering schemes. *Psychometrika, 32,* 241–254.

Kahn, J. V. (1976). Utility of the Uzgiris and Hunt scales of sensorimotor development with severely and profoundly retarded children. *American Journal of Mental Deficiency, 80,* 663–665.

Kahn, J. V. (1978). Acceleration of object permanence with severely and profoundly retarded children. *AAESPH Review, 3,* 15–22.

Kahn, J. V. (1981). *Training sensorimotor period and language skills with severely retarded children.* Paper presented at the meeting of the Council for Exceptional Children, New York, April.

Kenny, D. A. (1979). *Correlation and causality.* New York: Wiley.

King, W., & Seegmiller, B. (1973). Performance of 14- to 22-month-old Black, firstborn male infants on two tests of cognitive development: The Bayley Scales and the Infant Psychological Development Scale. *Developmental Psychology, 8,* 317–326.

Kopp, C. B., Sigman, M., & Parmelee, A. H. (1973). Longitudinal study of sensorimotor development. *Developmental Psychology, 10,* 687–695.

Krafchuk, E., Sameroff, A., & Bakow, H. (1976). *Newborn temperament and operant head turning.* Paper presented at the Southeast regional meeting of the Society for Research in Child Development, Nashville, TN.

Lamb, M. E. (1982). In H. Reese & L. Lipsett (Eds.), *Advances in child development and behavior* (Vol. 16), New York: Academic Press.

Lezine, I., Stambak, M., Casati, I. (1969). Les estapes de l'intelligence sensorimotrice. *Montographie de Centre de Psychologie Appliquée,* no. 1. Paris: Les Editions de Centre de Psychologie Appliquée.

Matheny, A., Dolan, B., & Wilson, R. (1974). Bayley's Infant Behavior Record: Relations between behaviors and mental test scores. *Developmental Psychology, 10,* 696.

McCall, R. B. (1979). Qualitative transitions in behavioral development in the first two years of life. In M. Bornstein & W. Kessen (Eds.), *Psychological development from infancy: Image to intention* (pp. 183–224). Hillsdale, NJ: Erlbaum.

McCall, R. B., & McGhee, P. E. (1977). The discrepancy hypothesis of attention and affect in human infants. In I. C. Uzgiris & F. Weizmann (Eds.), *The structuring of experience* (pp. 179–210). New York: Plenum.

Mervis, C. B., & Cardoso-Martins, C. (1984). Transition from sensorimotor Stage 5 to Stage 6 by Down syndrome children: A response to Gibson. *American Journal of Mental Deficiency, 89,* 99–102.

Morss, J. R. (1983). Cognitive development in the Down's syndrome infant: Slow or different? *British Journal of Educational Psychology, 53,* 40–47.

Morss, J. R. (1984). Enhancement of object-permanence performance in the Down's syndrome infant. *Child: Care, Health, and Development, 10,* 39–47.

Nunnally, J. C. (1967). *Psychometric theory.* New York: McGraw-Hill.

Paraskevopoulos, J., & Hunt, J. McV. (1971). Object construction and imitation under differing conditions of rearing. *Journal of Genetic Psychology, 119,* 301–321.

Peters-Martin, P., & Wachs, T. (1981). *A longitudinal study of temperament and its correlates in the first year of life.* Paper presented at the meeting of the Society for Research in Child Development, Boston.

Piaget, J. (1951). *Play, dreams, and imitation in childhood.* (C. Gattegno & F. Hodgson, Trans.). New York: Norton. (Originally published 1945).

Piaget, J. (1952). *The origins of intelligence in children.* (M. Cook, Trans.). New York: International Universities Press. (Originally published 1936).

Piaget, J. (1954). *The construction of reality in the child.* (M. Cook, Trans.). New York: Basic Books. (Originally published 1937).

Piaget, J. (1960). The general problems of the psychobiological development of the child. In J. Tanner & B. Inhelder (Eds.), *Discussions in Child Development* (Vol. 4, pp. 3–27). New York: International Universities Press.

Piaget, J. (1973). *The child and reality.* New York: Grossman.

Piper, M., & Ramsey, M. (1980). Effects of early home environment on the mental development of Down syndrome infants. *American Journal of Mental Deficiency, 85,* 39–44.

Rogers, S. (1977). Characteristics of the cognitive development of profoundly retarded children. *Child Development, 48,* 837–843.

Silverstein, A., Brownlee, L., Hubbell, M., & McLain, R. (1975). Comparison of two sets of Piagetian scales with severely and profoundly retarded children. *American Journal of Mental Deficiency, 80,* 292–297.

Silverstein, A., McLain, R., Brownlee, L., & Hubbell, M. (1976). Structure of ordinal scales of psychological development in infancy. *Educational and Psychological Measurement, 36,* 355–359.

Smith, L., & Hagen, V. (1984). Relationship between the home environment and sensorimotor development of Down syndrome and nonretarded infants. *American Journal of Mental Deficiency, 89,* 124–132.

Stedman, D. J., & Eichorn, D. H. (1964). A comparison of the growth and development of institutionalized and home-reared mongoloids during infancy and early childhood. *American Journal of Mental Deficiency, 69,* 391–401.

Stevenson, M. B., & Lamb, M. E. (1979). Effects of infant sociability and the caretaking environment of infant cognitive performance. *Child Development, 50,* 340–349.

Sugarman-Bell, S. (1978). Some organizational aspects of preverbal communication. In I. Markova (Ed.), *The social context of language* (pp. 49–66). New York: Wiley.

Tucker, L. R. (1951). *A method for synthesis of factor analysis studies* (Personnel Research Section Report No. 984). Washington, D.C.: Department of the Army.

Uzgiris, I. C. (1973). Patterns of cognitive development in infancy. *Merrill-Palmer Quarterly, 19,* 181–204.

Uzgiris, I. C. (1983). Organization of sensorimotor intelligence. In M. Lewis (Ed.), *Origins of intelligence* (2nd ed., pp. 135–189). New York: Plenum.

Uzgiris, I. C. (1987). The study of sequential order in cognitive development. In I. C. Uzgiris & J. McV. Hunt (Eds.), Infant performance and experience (pp. 129–167). Urbana–Champaign: University of Illinois Press.

Uzgiris, I. C., & Hunt, J. McV. (1975). *Assessment in infancy: Ordinal scales of psychological development.* Urbana: University of Illinois Press.

Wachs, T., & Gandour, M. (1983). The relationship of temperament and environment to cognitive development at six months: A test of the organismic specificity hypothesis. *International Journal of Behavior Development, 6,* 135–152.

Wachs, T., & Hubert, N. (1981). Changes in the structure of cognitive-intellectual performance during the second year of life. *Infant Behavior and Development, 4,* 151–161.

Watson, M. W., & Fisher, K. W. (1977). A developmental sequence of agent use in late infancy. *Child Development, 48,* 828–830.

Wohlhueter, M. J., & Sindberg, R. (1975). Longitudinal development of object permanence in mentally retarded children: An exploratory study. *American Journal of Mental Deficiency, 79,* 513–518.

Wohlwill, J. F. (1973). *The study of behavioral development.* New York: Academic Press.

Woodward, M. (1959). The behavior in idiots interpreted by Piaget's theory of sensorimotor development. *British Journal of Educational Psychology, 29,* 60–71.

Zigler, E., & Balla, D. (1982). *Mental retardation: The developmental difference controversy.* Hillsdale, NJ: Erlbaum.

7 The growth of self-monitoring among young children with Down syndrome

Claire B. Kopp

Introduction

At some point during the early years, parents begin to impose limits on their child's behaviors. Restrictions are placed on where and when the child may crawl and toddle, on the objects that may be touched and explored, and the degree that caregiver and family routines may accommodate child whims. At about the same time, the child is informed about expectations for standards for conduct. Messages are given about cleanliness, respect for others and their possessions, and what constitutes acceptable behavior in one or another situation.

Despite the earnestness of parent intentions, few of their messages are initially understood by the child. Gradually, though, using gestures, declaratives, commands, affective cues, regularity, and repetition, parents make their wishes clear. In time, children start to discern the implications of requests and prohibitions, and begin to accede to their parents' demands. But more than this, children eventually internalize their parents' standards for conduct, and act upon them even when they are alone. They are able to regulate their own behavior. These achievements also suggest that a degree of predictability has become part of the child's day-to-day behavior. Increasingly, children will be asked to respond to additional standards for conduct, and to do so on their own.

This evolving scenario is not easily orchestrated. It requires parents who are responsive to, and feel a sense of responsibility for, their children. It involves children who are attentive, who try to understand, and who want to go along with parent wishes. And it demands fine tuning of parent expectations with child abilities along with the ability to adapt to unexpected situations and events. Although it is the parent who initially takes on the primary role and tailors it to the child, without

Appreciation is extended to Susan Markowitz, Diane Parham, and Sara Rushbrook for their help in various aspects of the research with the children with Down syndrome, and to Joanne B. Krakow, Brian E. Vaughn, and Kim L. Johnson for their overall contribution to the self-control studies. This research was supported by contract #300-77-0306, Bureau of Education for the Handicapped, U.S. Office of Education, 1977-1982, B. K. Keogh & C. B. Kopp, Co-Principal Investigators.

231

question both parent and child have to go along with each other in order for self-regulation to evolve.

Although developmentalists do not fully understand the specifics of caregiver input and the processes involved in the child's adherence to and internalization of caregiver standards, advances are being made. Research involving topics associated with self-regulation, particularly with young normally developing children, continues.

In marked contrast, there has been a dearth of studies about young handicapped children and their development of self-regulation. This is troublesome because the clinical literature provides numerous examples of dysfunctional self-regulation among older handicapped children in both educational and social settings. Disturbances in cognitive processing are often implicated (e.g., Douglas, 1980; Harris, 1978), but how these problems come about and interface with self-regulatory abilities is poorly understood. Similarly not known are the role and the influences provided by the child's parents. Thus, from an educational and rearing standpoint, there is strong impetus to determine how young handicapped children develop self-regulation, and when and where problems might arise. From a developmental and theoretical perspective, it would be useful to know how closely the ontogeny of self-regulation among handicapped children parallels that of normally developing ones, and the specific cognitive abilities and processes that are associated with successful versus problematic self-regulation.

Children with Down syndrome were the handicapped group chosen to explore these issues. The selection was based on the following: First, these children represent a sizable proportion of the mentally retarded. Thus, it could be helpful to parents, teachers, and the children themselves to illuminate further their course of development. Second, various types of cognitively oriented interventions have been offered to these children and their parents, but relatively few social interventions have been implemented. Nonetheless, parents report the existence of social problems, and there is indication that children with Down syndrome are overly impulsive (Gibson, 1978). Research might be able to specify some of the factors involved, and ultimately findings could be applied to intervention efforts. Finally, a large data base exists about children with Down syndrome. These data have potential value when attempts are made to infer relationships and linkages.

This chapter focuses on both child and caregiver issues, although greater emphasis is given to developmental questions vis-à-vis the child. The first section deals with conceptual and developmental perspectives. The second is data-based and summarizes results obtained with both young normally developing and Down syndrome children and their mothers.

The literature on caregivers and children

Caregivers

Human beings are exposed to social conventions from the first days and months of life, but "becoming socialized" takes years. One of the more demanding aspects of the process requires children to become aware of and to conform to standards of socially appropriate behavior, and to begin to assume responsibility for their own acts, particularly in the absence of external monitors (Bandura, 1977; Block & Block, 1980; Luria, 1961; Mischel, 1983; Vygotsky, 1962). The emergence of these abilities, often labeled self-regulation, is a major developmental achievement with implications that extend throughout life (Harter, 1983; Kendall & Braswell, 1985; Lidz, 1978; Markus & Nurius, 1984; Mischel, 1983).

Self-regulation probably has both social and cognitive origins. Some of these surely arise from caregiver belief systems and practices which are transmitted to the child during the socialization process. Caregivers define standards, convey them to the child, and work toward getting the child to adapt to them particularly around issues of social conventions and expectations for behavior within the family and society at large.

Not surprisingly, the role of caregivers has been highlighted in the self-regulation literature and often deals with characteristics of caregivers perceived to be *vital* in the transmission of standards. One group of investigators suggests caregiver attributes such as sensitivity and responsivity are critically important for facilitating child compliance and other forms of self-regulation (e.g., Ainsworth, Blehar, Waters, & Wall, 1978; Arend, Gove, & Sroufe, 1979; Stayton, Hogan, & Ainsworth, 1971). Parental sensitivity, or *tolerance,* as it is also termed, is considered essential when dealing with toddlers whose rapid maturation of motor and language skills makes them especially tuned to the environment and particularly vulnerable to repressive restrictions (Rexford, 1978).

Another perspective holds that the critical aspect of transmission turns on the role of caregiver structure and organization of child activities that are inherent in communication patterns (Luria, 1960; Vygotsky, 1979; Wertsch, 1984). Briefly stated, this perspective argues that the process of thinking evolves from shared social activities. Recent research using Vygotskian theory has emphasized "the zone of proximal development." This refers to a situation where a child has partially mastered a task, but with caregiver participation can see the task to its successful completion. Findings indicate that caregivers tailor their speech and actions both to a child's level of functioning and also to a perceived next step (Wertsch, 1979). Irrespective of task, caregivers appear to provide a structured agenda for the child taking into account age and level of self-monitoring behavior that is displayed (Rogoff, Malkin, & Gilbride, 1984).

A third perspective holds that the child's self-regulatory abilities grow out of specific types of control techniques used by caregivers (Lytton, 1979; Minton, Kagan, & Levine, 1971; Schaffer, 1984). This research provides valuable descriptions of mothers' behaviors in compliance situations involving 2- and 3-year-old children. For example, "attention getting," use of indirect commands, task structuring, and concomitant verbal and nonverbal messages are common strategies employed by mothers of children in the second year (summarized in Schaffer, 1984). Maternal behaviors specifically associated with child compliance include suggestive verbal controls enhanced by nonverbal signals that are timed appropriately (Lytton, 1979, 1980; McLaughlin, 1983; Schaffer & Crook, 1978, 1980).

In sum, a synthesis of the caregiver literature suggests that sensitive parents, tuned to their children's characteristics, who use a variety of attention-getting mechanisms, and who organize the child's milieu, will have the most chance of conveying standards to the child. That these variables are important is given credence by findings reported in both the research and clinical literatures about dysfunctional mothering. Mothers who are depressed, anxious, abusive, poorly educated, or preoccupied for one or another reason (e.g., maternal illness, family disruptions, etc.) are less able to provide appropriate external controls for the child that, in turn, are associated with out-of-control behaviors on the part of the child (see Hetherington, Cox, & Cox, 1979, 1982; Lidz, 1978; Malone, 1978).

The child

Without doubt, the caregiver makes a critical contribution to the child's growth of self-regulation. But also without doubt, the caregiver cannot make the child adopt standards and values. The child must want to do so, must understand something about the nature of requests or expectations, and must have a way of responding as required. In other words, developmental cognitive and motivational factors appear to be implicated.

Surprisingly, child-related developmental issues are barely touched upon in the aforementioned studies related to caregivers and young children. Nonetheless, the complexities of self-regulation argue for a child-oriented developmental perspective that is integrated with themes about caregivers. This need was the catalyst for Kopp's (1982) attempt to formulate a description of the emergence and growth of early forms of self-regulation. Questions that formed the conceptual foundation included when the child might be expected to understand caregiver expectations, how this might occur, and what form it might take.

Kopp (1982) suggested that the development of self-regulation is probably highly dependent upon the child's developing cognitive system. Because intelligent, adaptive behavior first appears around the end of the first year, it is most probable that nascent aspects of self-regulation make their initial appearance around the second year. In order to provide support for these ideas, Kopp reviewed the literature on cognitive changes and suggested how they could interface with early forms of self-regulation. The ideas originally discussed in Kopp (1982) have been modified slightly. The developmental perspective briefly summarized in the next section reflects a portion of her revised version.

A developmental perspective

In Kopp's view, there are forms of behavioral modulation that occur long before the child becomes responsive to standards for conduct. Whether such forms of modulation are later associated with awareness and acceptance of standards is not known. All are discussed, however, primarily to provide a longitudinal perspective on the evolution of control behaviors in general.

The first phase is referred to as *neurophysiological modulation*. This is a form of modulation in which arousal states are modulated, and reflex behaviors are exhibited as organized patterns of functional behaviors. The infant can respond to incoming stimuli, self-soothe, and "shut out" stimuli that are too intrusive by drifting into sleep or crying. This form of modulation appears during the initial months of life.

A second phase, *sensorimotor modulation,* signifies the infant's ability to engage in voluntary motor acts and modify them in response to situational factors that come into play. This antecedent phase of self-regulation is presumed to occur from about 3 to 12 months of age.

Because the infant of this age has a relatively primitive level of perceptual–cognitive capabilities, it is highly likely that sensorimotor modulation is nonintentional, does not involve consciousness or awareness of the meaning of a situation, and does not involve preconsidered volitional restraints. There is, nonetheless, a limited form of appraisal of the environment. Most often this is seen in infant responsiveness to strange individuals, novel objects, or unusual situations. Typically, the response is to hold back motorically and psychologically until the situation is looked over. Sometimes the infant references the caregiver, possibly as a means to reduce uncertainty (Campos & Stenberg, 1981).

Another form of behavioral inhibition occurring toward the end of this phase involves the cessation of an activity as the result of a loud voice and negative affect displayed by the caregiver. This marks the emergence of the caregiver's systematic and ongoing use of phrases such as *"NO!" "DON'T TOUCH!" "STOP THAT!"* that are directed to the crawling or walking infant who is seemingly and suddenly into everything. The fact that the infant holds back and inhibits, albeit due to surprise or fear, may be the first indication of the ability to respond in some way to caregiver standards.

A third phase labeled *control* is characterized by signs of the emerging ability of infants to demonstrate actual awareness of social and task demands around standards for conduct (e.g., protection of caregiver possessions, adherence to "rules" for safety, etc.), and to initiate, maintain, or cease behaviors accordingly. This competence is probably a derivative of the dramatic qualitative and quantitative changes in comprehension and in cognitive processing skills that occur during the last part of the first year and the beginning of the second. Control is considered to occur from about 12 to 24 months.

Control is initially observed in the form of compliance to simple caregiver requests such as "no shoes on the table." Shortly thereafter, a form of *self-initiated compliance* is observed, in which the child approaches and then retreats from a previously prohibited object on his or her own. This represents an impressive growth because in order to show self-initiated compliance the child has to integrate caregiver expectations with the production of an appropriate response without external assistance.

Whatever the child's capability in terms of exercising control, it is likely tied to the presence of certain signals and cues that help the child remember expectations. Because of this, control is likely to be highly situation specific.

Self-control is the term used to designate the fourth phase. It emerges sometime during or after the emergence of comprehension, representational thinking, and recall memory, and is thus linked to these cognitive advances. Self-control involves compliance, the ability to delay (at least for a short while), the ability to modulate behaviors on demand (e.g., talk softly), and the ability to comply with expectations for standards in the absence of external monitors. Self-control is associated with the child's beginning understanding that he or she has a continuing, independent identity; this "identity" (self) can make things happen, which in turn affects others.

In addition, self-control implies that the child begins to remember (without the presence of cues) caregiver dictums and expectations about acceptable and unacceptable behavior. Presumably, the child who has self-control can rely more on his or her own memory than on specific cues that arise in specific situations. Thus, behavior ought to show some consistency across contexts. Nonetheless, at times the child in the self-control phase becomes locked in nonproductive patterns of behavior because there is little flexibility of thought.

A final phase is labeled *self-regulation*. Getting under way sometime during or after the third year of life (and extending into childhood and later), self-regulation represents a distinctly mature and maturing form of control. It subsumes all of the components just mentioned, and in general is variable and pliant to diverse demands for standards for conduct. Similar to other phases, self-regulation is associated with certain cognitive competencies. In this instance these are presumed to include reflection, use of strategies that involve introspection and evaluation, and the ability to apply contingency rules to behavior. These cognitive processes are probably crucial facilitators of flexible thinking and the ability to modify behavior quickly, as appropriate.

Although this framework requires empirical study and validation, its cognitive emphasis does have some support from the clinical literature. As has been noted, dysfunctional forms of self-regulation are often described among children who have impairments in cognitive functioning, including the mentally retarded, learning disabled, and hyperactive (e.g., Douglas, 1980).

An integration

Taken together, the ideas discussed above suggest that the emergence and development of self-regulation among normally developing children are very dependent upon the ability of caregivers to impart information about standards to their children, and the ability of children to understand and to act upon their caregivers' expectations. An implicit assumption is that with normal development and with caregivers who are relatively sensitive and sensible, the components of self-regulation will develop without major, long-term perturbations. This implies neither that the course will invariably be smooth, nor that situational factors will be unimportant.

But what can be expected about the development of self-regulation in instances where children have significant developmental delays and subsequent major cognitive impairments? Might caregivers have to carry the socialization burden longer and more forcefully? Can the handicapped child learn self-regulation equivalent to his or her normally developing peers but over a longer period of time? Can the level of self-regulation ultimately attained be linked directly to the child's level of cognitive functioning? These questions have direct bearing on children with Down syndrome.

The next section briefly sets the stage for research by summarizing some of the characteristics of parents of young children with Down syndrome and of the children themselves. This information is helpful in formulating expectations and hypotheses about trends in self-regulation.

Down syndrome

Young children

In terms of self-regulation, the most salient attributes that ought to be considered about the child include the following: Down syndrome is associated with moderate to severe mental retardation. There are some suggestions that the mental age attained may approximate the level of preoperational thought, or in some cases be slightly higher (e.g., see Gibson, 1978). Abilities that most often show dysfunction are abstract reasoning, problem solving, and language competencies (see summaries Beeghly, Weiss-Perry, & Cicchetti, Chapter 10, this volume; Fowler, Chapter 9, this volume; Gibson, 1978; Kopp & Parmelee, 1979). The sequence and organization of behaviors of infants and young children with Down syndrome are similar to those of normally developing children of similar developmental age (e.g., Cicchetti & Pogge-Hesse, 1982; Cicchetti & Sroufe, 1976; Kopp, 1983; Krakow & Kopp, 1983; Markowitz, 1980; Serafica & Cicchetti, 1976; Thompson, Cicchetti, Lamb, & Malkin, 1985). Taken together, these findings suggest that the antecedents and the early phases of control behaviors ought to be grossly similar among Down syndrome and normally developing children. In terms of emergence of specific components, some form of behavioral inhibition should emerge first, then compliance and self-initiated compliance, and so on.

Going beyond developmental trends, recent research on infants and children with Down syndrome indicates that even though many forms of behavior are similar, variations do occur. It has been noted, for example, that young Down syndrome children differ in the intensity of the responses that they display and the degree to which they use components of their behavioral competencies (e.g., Buckhalt, Rutherford, & Goldberg, 1978; Cicchetti & Sroufe, 1976, 1978; Cytryn, 1975; Emde, Katz, & Thorpe, 1978; Jones, 1977, 1980; Krakow & Kopp, 1983; Markowitz, 1980; Stone & Chesney, 1978; Thompson et al., 1985). Emotional expressiveness is often dampened, vocalizations are few, signaling behaviors are frequently inappropriate, nonreciprocal, or asynchronous. The ability to respond to nuances in the environment is often variable.

The fact that "reading" the milieu is problematic leads to speculation that manifestations of self-regulation might also be affected. In particular, this could occur in situations where cues are not always salient but demands for certain kinds of behavior are unvarying. Many caregivers, for example, are quite explicit and unyielding about appropriate child behaviors related to safety. Yet constant reminders for the child, such as a highly visible roadway sign signifying danger, are not always available.

In sum, a reasonable expectation is that the development of self-regulation among children with Down syndrome will approximate that shown by normally developing children of similar developmental age. Differences may be anticipated in the degree of effectiveness of self-regulating attempts.

Caregivers

The rich and diverse literature on self-regulation vis-à-vis parents of normally developing children does not have a counterpart in the literature on Down syndrome. Nonetheless, inferences can be made, on the basis of existing studies, about how caregivers socialize their Down syndrome children toward standards.

By way of background, the literature suggests that parents of children with Down syndrome demonstrate interactions that signify their awareness of their child's "normality" and "abnormality". Described by Roskies (1972), this duality is a function of parental realization (possibly intuitive) that certain facets of child development and child behaviors are manifested irrespective of a child's condition. Alternatively, caregiver responses are also predicated upon the knowledge that the child differs from others in observable and significant ways.

Findings from studies of parents of young Down syndrome children support this theme of duality. Caregivers do show depression and frustration and occasional nonappropriate responses (e.g., Emde & Brown, 1976). Yet caregivers are resilient and, like parents of normally developing children, learn to adapt their responses to the level of the child (e.g., DeLoache, 1984; Rogoff et al., 1984). As examples, they modify the speed and complexity of their nonverbal and verbal signals to child capability (e.g., Buckhalt et al., 1978; Markowitz, 1980). Caregivers can also be quite directive and exhibit assertive patterns over interactions (Jones, 1980). Presumably these are adaptive responses that occur when the child is not sufficiently tuned in to the environment or to the caregiver.

When transmission of standards is involved, parents of children with Down syndrome probably use techniques similar to those displayed by parents of normally developing children. The former might be more directive in situations that they view as especially important and where the child seems less responsive than seems acceptable. By and large, then, more comparability than difference ought to be expected in attempts to move the child toward self-regulation.

Research

The child's development of self-control

Normally developing sample. Our initial research studies focused upon normally developing children presumed to be in the phase of self-control. The basic questions that were posed centered on the developmental course of self-control and mediators that might be associated with its growth.

Self-control was operationalized in two ways, both taking into account the relatively limited language ability of most children in the second and third years of life. One was a measure of compliance to a maternal request, and the other was a measure of the child's ability to delay touching a desirable object. Both situations are analogous to everyday experiences of young children.

The compliance task involved interaction of child and mother in a toy clean-up task. The child had been playing for 10 minutes with a group of toys when, at a specified signal, the child's mother asked him or her to put all of the toys on a nearby shelf. The mother was encouraged to use whatever procedures she felt comfortable with. Child actions were coded for time to first cleanup act, categories of behavior demonstrated by the child during the 6 minute cleanup period (e.g., positive response – picks up toy and puts away, ignores mother, argues with mother), and an overall rating of compliance for the entire period (see Vaughn, Kopp, & Krakow, 1984, for details).

Two different tasks were used to assess the child's ability to inhibit and delay. One involved going along with E's request not to touch a bright red plastic old-fashioned telephone. (This was a toy that almost called out Touch me!) In this situation, child and mother were seated at the same side of a table, with mother ostensibly reading a magazine. An experimenter came to the opposite side of the table and placed the telephone before the child. Explaining its features, the experimenter then mentioned that he or she had to leave in order to get more toys. The child was admonished not to touch the telephone until the person returned. The experimenter left and waited for 150 seconds, or sooner if the child touched the telephone before the end of the period. The variable of interest was duration of waiting time.

The second delay measure involved a two-segment find-the-raisin game. Child and mother sat on the same side of the table (mother was not reading) and the experimenter sat across from the child. Using three plastic cups, the experimenter hid a raisin under one of the cups. The child was asked to wait, and then was told to find the raisin. The first task segment consisted of six short trials of 20 seconds in which the variable of interest was the number of trials the raisin was not picked up. The second segment consisted of a final trial of 120 seconds with duration of waiting the variable of interest.

A total of 72 normally developing children and their mothers (maternal data are reported later) were seen at ages of 18, 24, and 30 months. Stability, reliability, and consistency of the child measures were evaluated and found to be satisfactory (see details in Vaughn et al., 1984). Using data reduction techniques, four standardized and composited delay scores and three compliance factors – Compliance, Noncompliance–Avoid, and Noncompliance–Argue – were examined for developmental trends (for details see Vaughn et al., 1984).

Findings revealed significant age-related increases for the delay tasks and for the Compliance factor. On the telephone task, for example, 18-month-olds waited an average of 10 seconds, whereas 30-month-olds waited 113 seconds. Within-age comparisons for the delay tasks indicated that coherence across tasks increased with age. That is, the child who waited on the telephone task would be likely to wait also on the raisin task or vice versa.

In terms of Compliance, findings showed a significant age related increase. The factor labeled Noncompliance–Argue showed a nonsignificant increase with age, whereas the factor Noncompliance–Avoid was highest for the 24-month-olds. Coherence in performance across compliance and the two delay tasks showed a positive relationship only among the oldest children. This meant that children who were likely to delay were also likely to comply. Finally, correlational analyses revealed modest, although significant, positive relationships with developmental test data for the older children.

The most important practical information that came out of this study was the finding related to consolidation of behavior. Most apparent with older children, the data indicated that by 2½ years children begin to show a degree of stability and predictability in their self-control behaviors despite variations in context. Once children of this age show signs of adhering to standards, they can be trusted within limits to do so.

With this study as background, we proceeded to explore self-control among young children with Down syndrome. Primary goals were to determine similarities and differences in the development of delay and compliance among children of equivalent developmental ages, and to also examine maternal behaviors.

The sample of children with Down syndrome. If optimal research conditions had prevailed, a comparable number of subjects who were normally developing and who had Down syndrome would have been recruited for all of the studies that were conducted. As it was, approximately 25 children with Down syndrome were involved in the research. These children's performance was analyzed. When a sufficient number of them demonstrated developmental ages similar to those of the normally developing sample, they became the sample of interest.

Fifteen children (9 males) had measured developmental ages between 24 and 40 months with a mean developmental age of 29 months. This sample had a mean Gesell developmental quotient of 63.9, with one score at 45 and others ranging between 55 and 77. Chronological ages varied from 31 to 60 months. The children were generally in good health, albeit close to half had visual problems that had been corrected. Parents were in their early thirties; only a small number of mothers had college degrees, whereas half of the fathers had graduated from 4-year programs.

In order to be able to make group comparisons, the normally developing child subject file was scanned in order to select a subsample who were of equivalent developmental age and gender to the children with Down syndrome. Seventeen normally developing children met the criteria and were placed in this group. Their mean developmental quotient was 115, developmental ages ranged from 23 to 40 months, and chronological ages from 18 to 30 months. All of the children were healthy. Their parents were in their early thirties, and a majority were college graduates.

Results pertaining to delay performance are discussed first. Findings showed that the children with Down syndrome performed appreciably poorer on both the telephone and raisin measures than the comparison subsample of normally developing children. For example, the mean delay score for the telephone task was 23.3 (SD 30.9) seconds for the children with Down syndrome and 71.5 (SD 61.6) seconds for the normally developing group. On the raisin task (long trial) where the variable of interest was the time taken to touch the cup (which hid the raisin), the Down syndrome sample waited an average of 43.8 (SD 54.6) seconds, whereas the normally developing sample waited 57.5 (SD 53.3) seconds.

In general then, these mean scores suggested that the children with Down syndrome responded more quickly than their age-matched normally developing peers. However, it should be noted that the Down syndrome group did considerably better in the raisin task. In this situation two adults were present and one of them interacted with the child; further, the task was segmented into short time periods, and it involved a food reward. Of interest, these situational factors had less effect on the performance of the normally developing group. In fact, these children did slightly poorer; they waited less on the raisin task than on the telephone task.

However different the mean scores of the groups were, they do not reveal the entire picture of performance. As seen in the preceding paragraphs, standard deviations within both groups of children were sizable. In order to determine if the attributes of a few children were masking the capability of others, the data was reanalyzed. Using a cut-point of 10 seconds (the score obtained with normally developing 18-month-olds; see Vaughn et al., 1984), responses were tabulated for the number of children whose scores fell at or below this level, or above. Ten children in the Down syndrome sample had scores of 7 seconds or less (66%), and five others waited for 27, 44, 62, 78, and 93 seconds. Using the same cut-point, three children in the normally developing sample waited less than 10 seconds (18%), five children waited from between 21 and 34 seconds, and the rest were spread between 35 and 150 seconds.

Clearly, a degree of very fast responsivity was found for some of the children in both samples, but a greater proportion was found among the group of Down syndrome children. Was this a stable child characteristic? In order to determine if delay on the telephone task was related to delay on the raisin task, correlational analyses were performed on scores for both of the tasks. The correlation coefficient obtained for the children with Down syndrome was essentially zero, for the normally developing children $r = .71$, $p.0$. Stated another way, the children in the normally developing sample showed coherence in behavior in the delay tasks. Those that waited longer on one task tended to wait longest on the other; similarly, those that responded quickly on one were also likely to do so on the other. (Considering the findings from the group as a whole, this is not surprising). However, this accord was not found in the sample of Down syndrome children. Only five children showed coherence; one of the children who waited longest on the telephone task (78 seconds) waited for a long period on the raisin task (120 seconds), and four children waited very short periods on both tasks.

In sum, each group showed a great deal of variability on the telephone task, but the *key* group differences related to the high proportion of children with Down syndrome whose waiting time was very short, and the inability of any child with Down syndrome to wait the entire testing period for the telephone task. Further, it was difficult to find individual consistency in performance from one delay task to the other.

The delay situation, particularly the telephone task, had elicited many interesting child behaviors – some of which appeared to be used as self-distractors to avoid looking at or touching the telephone. In preliminary analyses with normally developing children, Johnson & Kopp (1981) found that production of nonverbal and verbal behaviors (which were not telephone-directed) was associated with proportionately longer waiting times. These nontelephone behaviors clearly possessed a strategic-like quality on the order of a diversionary tactic.

The question that arose was whether the child with Down syndrome had difficulty with delay that was related to limited production of diversionary behaviors. Subsequently in microanalyses of behaviors demonstrated during the telephone task, it was found that Down syndrome children rarely turned away from the telephone. They also produced few nontelephone distractors such as squirming around in their chairs, looking at their hands, or gazing at the ceiling (these types of responses were relatively common among the normally developing sample) but engaged in more general activity per minute than did the normally developing sample (see Kopp, Krakow, & Johnson, 1983). Thus, the Down syndrome child's ability to delay was hampered by inability to disengage from the attractive stimulus, which possibly was itself linked to levels of heightened movements that did not permit total responsibility to task demands.

Parenthetically, it may be that excess activity is a function of developmental immaturity or is related to the elevated levels of stereotypic behaviors often evidenced by the children with Down syndrome (e.g., see Krakow & Kopp, 1983). This characteristic is even demonstrated in relatively rich instances of pretend play. In one example observed in the laboratory, a boy with Down syndrome picked up a toy coffeepot and cups, simulated pouring a liquid into the cups, and then offered his mother "chocolate." She held the cups while he poured. The child made the same offer eight additional times, and did not vary the play scene at all. The issue of *activity* merits additional study.

Turning from the analysis of delay to the compliance task, in terms of overall compliance, both groups showed similarities in most behaviors. The only trend to emerge was a slight difference in noncompliance patterns. The children with Down syndrome tended to ignore their mothers slightly more than did the normally developing children.

Additional analyses indicated no discernible relationship between compliance or noncompliance patterns and the delay scores. This may have been a function of the small sample sizes and the attenuated scores for the compliance task. The finding goes against the data obtained with the large group of normally developing children (see Vaughn et al., 1984) where coherence was found across both delay and compliance for the oldest children.

In conjunction with the studies of compliance and delay, complementary analyses were run to explore developmental issues related to anticipated age trends. Recall in the studies of normally developing children, both compliance and delay showed significant increments in performance (18 to 30 months) as a function of both developmental and chronological ages. A similar trend was predicted for the sample of children with Down syndrome.

Because of the small size of the sample of children with Down syndrome (and the equivalent normally developing sample), nonparametric correlations were run between compliance and delay on the one hand and developmental age, chronological age, and developmental quotient on the other. As might be expected, the coefficients for the normally developing sample were either significant or showed a strong trend for both developmental and chronological ages and task performance. There was no relationship with developmental quotients, but this was anticipated because a very modest trend had been found in the large sample with only the oldest children (see Vaughn et al., 1984).

In contrast, the coefficients for the sample of children with Down syndrome were quite variable. Compliance was significantly related (positively) to developmental age, whereas performance on the telephone task showed a significant positive relationship to chronological age and a negative relationship to developmental quotient. There were no significant relationships for the raisin task. The finding for the telephone task is an enigma because it suggests that older, lower functioning children were the ones able to wait longest on the telephone task.

In sum, despite the difficulty encountered by the Down syndrome sample on waiting tasks, these children were able to function similarly to developmental age peers on a self-regulation task that tapped compliance to a toy-cleanup request. Surprisingly, developmental trends in performancce were variable.

Maternal responses to the child: compliance task

It would have been useful if our research paradigms had included an examination of maternal behaviors in both a delay and a compliance setting. However, the compliance situation was the only one where plans had been made to integrate systematically mother and child activities.

Bear in mind the compliance situation required mothers to ask their children to put toys away after a 10-minute play period. Mothers were free to organize this cleanup as they wished. In all, a total of 15 maternal behaviors were displayed. Each behavior was reviewed, operationally defined, coded, and subjected to interobserver reliability tests. The list of behaviors and their operational definitions can be found in Table 7.1. As can be seen, behaviors ranged from organizational ones to those that involved bribes or threats. A few composite scores were developed, and these are included as well.

Table 7.1. *Maternal behaviors*

Touches for attention: Mother (M) lightly touches Child (C) or gently moves him or her in an effort to direct his gaze toward her or toward task.

Other strategies for attention: M says "watch," "look," "see," or some other attention getting word, whistles, waves a hand in front of child's face, or calls child's name.

Points and pats: M points to or pats objects to facilitate child compliance. Examples include pointing to the basket of toys, patting the shelf on which the toys are to be placed, or pointing out toys to be picked up.

Moves toys to child: M picks up toy and places it near C.

Physical guidance: M directs C to task by touching and moving his body or an object he is holding. This category includes acts that are directive and task oriented; it excludes acts such as touching for attention.

Organizes and directs: M explains task, defines task situation, hands toy to C, tells C where toys should be put, or tells C to move in a way that will facilitate task: "Hold the basket," "Put the truck here," "Put it on the bottom shelf."

Models task: M demonstrates task to C and often accompanies demonstration with statements such as "Watch me," "I'll show you how," or a similar term.

Game: M structures task by turning it into a play activity. Examples include M telling C to put the baby to sleep on the shelf, to park the truck in the garage (on the shelf), or to count the toys into the bucket. Use of a toy as a diversionary strategy is not counted.

Shares: M verbally suggests task is a joint effort. Tells C she will help, or she needs him or her to help her, or they will do the cleanup together.

Asks for favor: M attempts to get C compliance by suggesting the C do the task particularly for her. M uses terms such as "Do it for me," "Put this away for Mommy," "I would appreciate it if you . . ."

Incentive: M suggests that a positive outcome will follow C's compliance in the cleanup task. Examples include telling child there will be more toys to play with later, or other games will follow the cleanup.

Warning: M tells C that some negative outcome will occur if C does not follow her directives. An example includes telling C that nothing else will occur until cleanup is accomplished.

Grabs: M firmly and abruptly takes hold of child to gain attention or to move toward task. This category denotes rough handling of C and has a punitive quality.

Gives up: M ceases to give task-oriented directives for the cleanup.

Non-task-oriented verbalizations: M makes comments that are not directly related to the task, and divert C's attention away from the task.

Composite scores: (see note below).

Physical closeness: A 6-point rating of M's actual proximity to C.

Task participation: A 6-point rating of percentage of toys M puts away herself.

Investment in C compliance: M's continued or sporadic involvement with C in order to see the task to completion.

Note: Details about composite scores can be obtained from the author.

Among mothers of normally developing children of any age (18, 24, 30 months) or any level of child compliance, the most common behaviors displayed were organize/direct, points/pats, and use of attention-getting strategies (Kopp, 1985, 1987). In order to present the data most economically, a principal components analysis was done. Three factors and a single variable accounted for almost half of the common variance.

The first factor, labeled Mother as Definer and Organizer, included behaviors of touch for attention, use of attention-getting strategies, points and pats, and organizes and directs. The second factor, labeled Mother as Helper, included *moves toy closer to child, models,* and *plays put-toy-away game with the child.* Factor three, labeled Mother as Partner, included participation and shares task with child. The single variable was active involvement with the child. The first factor was the only one to show significant age-related changes. Mothers of older children (or those children who were most compliant) showed reductions in organizational and attention-getting strategies.

That mothers were less active in organizing the task for the older normally developing children suggests that the behavioral coherence found for delay and compliance among the 30-month-olds was due to within-child capabilities and not to situational condition driven by specific maternal acts. That is, the mother did not make the child comply nor did she make the child delay. The children appeared to be responding to task demands on their own. Further evidence for this child competence came from informal reviews of videotapes. The differences among mothers of younger versus those of older children were striking. The former had ''to work'' to get responsivity from the child, the latter literally and figuratively sat back in their chairs once they had told the child what to do.

What about mothers of the Down syndrome sample and the mothers of the equivalent group of normally developing children? Group comparisons were made of maternal behaviors using the codes described in Table 7.1. Because the sample sizes were small and the number of variables relatively large, it was essential to reduce the number of variables. In order to have an appropriate subject–variable ratio, maternal behaviors were categorized into conceptual categories that exactly mirrored the factors obtained from the principal components analysis (described in an earlier section). Accordingly, one cluster was called Mother as Organizer and Director, a second was called Mother as Helper, and a third, Mother as Partner.

Findings revealed that the only significant difference that emerged between the two groups was that mothers of children with Down syndrome showed a greater amount of organizing and directing. A trend was found for mothers of normally developing children to show a greater amount of partnership in the task than did mothers of children with Down syndrome. The results are summarized in Table 7.2.

These findings are consonant with other reports that show mothers of children with Down syndrome are sometimes more active and directive than mothers of normally developing children (e.g., Field, 1977). This may be an adaptive response to inattentive children.

Table 7.2. *Comparison of number of maternal acts*

Behavioral categories (a priori, based on previous studies)	Maternal groups	
	DS	ND
Director: (touch for attention; other strategies for attention; points and pats; organizes and directs)	88.33 (37) ($t = 2.11, p$ .04)	58.81 (39)
Helper: (move toy closer; model; make task a game)	4.13 (6.8) ns	3.5 (6.3)
Partner: (share; overall task participation)	3.73 (3.1) ($t = 1.88, p$ .07)	6.0 (3.7)

Note: DS, mothers of children who had Down syndrome; ND, mothers of children who were normally developing (for this analysis, the number of DS mothers was 15; for ND mothers, 16).

Summing up

The conceptual themes and the data presented in this chapter are attempts to understand how young children begin to adopt the standards for behavior espoused by their caregivers. The ideas and the data ought to be viewed as beginnings because the issues are very complex. However, findings clearly reveal increments in compliance and delay performance among normally developing children in the second and third years of life. Along with this, coherence in performance becomes more solidified. The behavior of mothers also reveals developmental trends; when their children show more competent compliance, they reduce their organizational efforts.

These general findings served as a framework for the examination of the monitoring behaviors of children with Down syndrome. Demands for delay were very difficult for children with Down syndrome. Their most obvious stumbling block was encountered in the telephone task. They could not seem to generate tactics that would help them delay, particularly when few environmental supports were available to draw upon. The question that we cannot answer is whether performance would have been improved if mothers had been more directly involved in the task. Nonetheless, the data unequivocally implicate within child cognitive processes in delay. Even very young normally developing children can produce diversionary means that appear to facilitate waiting. Young children with Down syndrome of similar developmental age do not appear to be able to do so on their own.

This finding is all the more surprising because the children were equated for developmental ages. The equivalent groups were assembled on the bases of scores on subdomain portions of the Gesell developmental test (e.g., motor, adaptive) as well as with overall developmental scores. Although developmental tests are not perfect instruments, presumably similarity in a developmental age score for a particular subdomain represents some degree of similarity in actual knowledge or abilities.

One can only conclude, then, that the children with Down syndrome had a knowledge base similar to that of their normally developing peers. Why was the knowledge not used to advantage? One clue may come from studies of older children. Brown, Bransford, Ferrara, and Campione (1983) recently described differences in children's abilities to access their own knowledge. In one example, they report, academically unsuccessful school-age children had difficulty spontaneously organizing information they already knew in order to learn a new task. They did not ask themselves about the relevance of certain items of information or the meaning of certain facts. In contrast, academically successful children probed their own information base, asked themselves questions, and used self-generated prompts. The authors suggest that "superficial processing" demonstrated by the academically unsuccessful students could lead to further deficits. Unfortunately, the authors do not discuss possible origins of difficulties with accessing knowledge.

The theme of accessing and organizing knowledge makes sense and may partially explain why striking group differences can be obtained when children are equated on developmental age but differ in intellectual competencies revealed by developmental quotients. The brighter children in the sample we studied, when given a difficult task (i.e., telephone), somehow used their knowledge to generate ways to facilitate their delay. Granted, at this age this was probably done in a very primitive, nonintrospective way. Nonetheless, the children with Down syndrome could not do this; they did not seem able to use and apply information appropriately when they were on their own. They did appreciably better on the raisin delay task and in the compliance situation when external help was available.

As so often happens with research directed to exceptional children, as many questions as answers come out of the studies. This research has not been an exception. It is difficult, for example, to explain why a cohesive pattern of developmental age relationships and the self-control tasks was not obtained. Whether this is due to the restricted sample size, or to some other factor, is not known. But the finding does need to be explored with other samples.

Similarly, questions arise around the results obtained with the mothers. To be sure, findings go along with previous reports suggesting that mothers of children with Down syndrome are more directive and less playful than mothers of normally developing children. Yet one of the questions that comes to mind is whether child compliance for both groups was in fact similar because the mothers of the children with Down syndrome worked to get good performance from their children. Or, it could be argued, the children were similarly competent in this task, but the mothers were utilizing an interactive style that had become part of their repertoire. This, too, is an issue that ought to be studied further.

Finally, there is the question of identifying which within-child factors and which caregiver factors interface to facilitate the growth of self-regulation skills. This research has only been able to hint at answers. But the question and its empirically derived answers are critical for understanding the growth of self-regulation and the nature of interventions that should be provided if dysfunction arises.

Future directions

Although the broad configurations of the antecedents and emergence of self-regulation have been outlined, additional research is necessary to amplify our understanding of developmental and individual difference trends. It will be advantageous to pinpoint specific mediators of problematic self-regulation. This may ultimately improve the social and educational functioning of handicapped children whose self-regulatory abilities are often erratic.

At the most basic level, it may be useful to conceptualize distortions in self-regulation as due to failures in interactive communications. By this is meant that the following could occur: Appropriate messages about expectations for standards for conduct are not conveyed to the child by caregivers, or, the child may have difficulty in attending to a message, realizing its implications for behavior, or modulating behavior sufficiently quickly to meet situational demands. The first situation may arise because caregivers themselves may have serious problems of their own (e.g., emotional stress, insensitivity to others) or they may have difficulty *reading* the child's behavioral *signals*. Caregivers, for example, often have implicit assumptions about children's development such that if a child seems *mature* in one domain of functioning, they believe that holds true for other domains. Or if a child seems responsive in one situation, they expect like behavior in other situations. But it takes perceptive caregivers to sort through the meanings of the varied behaviors young children display and to know how and when to ask for one or another response from the child.

From the standpoint of children, there are any number of conditions that potentially make them less receptive to caregiver expectations than they might otherwise be. Preoccupation with certain activities may be one condition, but more pervasive may be these children who generally are just not responsive. A mentally retarded child may get the message but not know how to tap his behavioral repertoire to bring out the appropriate response. A deaf child may *receive* most of her caregiver's message but misinterpret one crucial element. An overly active child may be so mesmerized with his own movements that his caregiver's expectation is received but quickly put aside. Or a child who is constantly testing her own or others' limits may test caregiver limits with respect to expectations for behavior. In all of these situations, the children are not producing behavioral communications anticipated by caregivers. A cycle is started that is difficult to terminate.

The point to the above is that numerous caregiver, child, and situational factors exist that alone or together contribute to adequate or poor self-regulation. Teasing out these factors will be a challenge but will be beneficial to children and caregivers, and to our own understanding.

References

Ainsworth, M.D.S., Blehar, M. C., Waters, E., & Wall, S. (1978). *Patterns of attachment*. Hillsdale, NJ; Erlbaum.

Arend, R. A., Gove, F. L., & Sroufe, L. A. (1979). Continuity of individual adaptation from infancy to kindergarten: A predictive study of ego-resiliency and curiosity in preschoolers. *Child Development, 50,* 950–959.

Bandura, A. (1977). *Social learning theory*. Englewood Cliffs, NJ: Prentice-Hall.

Block, J. H., & Block, J. (1980). The role of ego-control and ego-resiliency in the organization of behavior. In W. A. Collins (Ed.), *Minnesota Symposium of Child Psychology* (pp. 53–107). Hillsdale, NJ: Erlbaum.

Brown, A. L., Bransford, J. D., Ferrara, R. A., & Campione, J. C. (1983). Learning, remembering, understanding. In J. H. Flavell & E. M. Markman (Eds.), *Handbook of child psychology: Cognitive development* (Vol. 3). New York: Wiley.

Buckhalt, J., Rutherford, R. & Goldberg, R. (1978). Verbal and non-verbal interaction of mothers with their Down's Syndrome and nonretarded infant. *American Journal of Mental Deficiency, 82*(4), 337–343.

Campos, J. J., & Stenberg, C. (1981). Perception, appraisal, and emotion: The onset of social referencing. In M. E. Lamb & L. R. Sherrod (Eds.), *Infant social cognition: Empirical and theoretical considerations*. Hillsdale, NJ: Erlbaum.

Cicchetti, D., & Pogge-Hesse, P. (1982). Possible contributions of the study of organically retarded persons to developmental theory. In E. Zigler & D. Balla (Eds.), *Mental retardation: A developmental-difference controversy*. Hillsdale, NJ: Erlbaum.

Cicchetti, D., & Sroufe, L. A. (1976). The relationship between affective and cognitive development in Down's syndrome infants. *Child Development, 47,* 920–929.

Cicchetti, D., & Sroufe, L. A. (1978). An organizational view of affect: Illustration from the study of Down's syndrome infants. In M. Lewis & L. Rosenblum (Eds.), *The development of affect*. New York: Plenum.

Cytryn, L. (1975). Studies of behavior in children with Down's Syndrome. In E. J. Anthony (Ed.), *Explorations in child psychiatry* (pp. 271–285). New York: Plenum.

DeLoache, J. S. (1984). What's this? Maternal questions in joint picture book reading with toddlers. *Quarterly Newsletter of the Laboratory of Comparative Human Cognition, 6,* 87–95.

Douglas, V. I. (1980). Treatment and training approaches to hyperactivity: Establishing internal or external control. In C. K. Whalen & B. Henker (Eds.), *Hyperactive children: The social ecology of identification and treatment*. New York: Academic Press.

Emde, R. N., & Brown, C. (1978). Adaptation after the birth of a Down's syndrome infant: A study of six cases, illustrating differences in development and the countermovement between grieving and maternal attachment. *Journal of the American Academy of Child Psychiatry, 17,* 299–323.

Emde, R. N., Katz, E. L., Thorpe, J. K. (1978). Emotional expression in infancy: II. Early deviation in Down's Syndrome. In M. Lewis & L. A. Rosenblum (Eds.), *The development of affect*. New York: Plenum.

Field, T. (1977). Effects of early separation, interactive deficits and experimental manipulation on infant–mother face-to-face interaction. *Child Development, 48,* 763–771.

Gibson, D. (1978). *Down's syndrome: The psychology of mongolism*. Cambridge: Cambridge University Press.

Harris, R. I. (1978). Impulse control in deaf children: Research and clinical issues. In L. S. Liben (Ed.), *Deaf children: Developmental perspectives*. New York: Academic.

Hetherington, E. M., Cox, M., & Cox, R. (1982). Effects of divorce on parents and children. In M. Lamb (Ed.), *Non-traditional families*. Hillsdale, NJ: Erlbaum.

Johnson, K., & Kopp, C. (1981). The emergency of strategy production in a delay task. Presentation, American Psychological Association, Los Angeles, August.

Jones, O.H.M. (1977). Mother–child communication with prelinguistic Down's syndrome and normal infants. In R. Schaffer (Ed.), *Studies in mother–infant interaction*. New York: Academic Press.

Jones, O.H.M. (1980). Prelinguistic communication skills in Down's syndrome and normal infants. In T. M. Field (Ed.), *High risk infants and children*. New York: Academic Press.

Kendall, P. C., & Braswell, L. (1985). *Cognitive-behavioral therapy for impulsive children*. New York: Guilford.

Kopp, C. B. (1982). The antecedents of self-regulation. *Developmental Psychology, 18,* 199–214.

Kopp, C. B. (1983). Risk factors in development. In M. Haith & J. Campos (Eds.), *Infancy and psychobiology* (Vol. 2). (From P. Mussen (Ed.), *Manual of child psychology*). New York: Wiley.

Kopp, C. B. (1985). The maternal side of child compliance. Paper presented at the biennial meeting of the Society for Research in Child Development, Toronto.

Kopp, C. B. (1987). The growth of self-regulation: Caregivers and children. In N. Eisenberg (Ed.), *Contemporary issues in developmental psychology*. New York: Wiley.

Kopp, C. B., Krakow, J. B., & Johnson, K. L. (1983). Strategy production by young Down syndrome children. *American Journal of Mental Deficiency, 88,* 164–169.

Kopp, C. B., & Parmelee, A. H. (1979). Prenatal and perinatal influences on behavior. In J. Osofsky (Ed.), *Handbook of infant development*. New York: Wiley.

Krakow, J. B., & Kopp, C. B. (1983). The effects of developmental delay on sustained attention in young children. *Child Development, 54,* 1143–1155.

Lidz, T. (1978). Discussion. In E. N. Rexford (Ed.), *A developmental approach to problems of acting out* (rev. ed.). New York: International Universities Press.

Luria, A. R. (1960). Verbal regulation of behavior. In M.A.B. Brazier (Ed.), *Conference on central nervous system and behavior*. New York: Josiah Macy Foundation.

Luria, A. R. (1961). *The role of speech in the regulation of normal and abnormal behavior*. New York: Liveright.

Lytton, H. (1979). Disciplinary encounters between young boys and their mothers and fathers: Is there a contingency system? *Developmental Psychology, 15,* 256–268.

Lytton, H. (1980). *Parent–child interaction: The socialization process observed in twin and singleton families*. New York: Plenum.

Malone, C. A. (1978). Some observations on children of disorganized families and problems of acting out. In E. N. Rexford (Ed.), *A developmental approach to problems of acting out* (rev. ed.). New York: International Universities Press.

Markowitz, S. L. (1980). *Mother–infant interactions with normal and Down syndrome infants*. Unpublished doctoral dissertation, University of California, Los Angeles.

Markus, H. J., & Nurius, P. S. (1984). Self-understanding and self-regulation in middle childhood. In W. A. Collins (Ed.), *Development during middle childhood: The years from six to twelve*. Washington, DC: National Academy Press.

McLaughlin, B. (1983). Child compliance to parent control techniques. *Developmental Psychology, 19,* 667–673.

Minton, C., Kagan, J., & Levine, J. A. (1971). Maternal control and obedience in the two-year-old. *Child Development, 42,* 1873–1894.

Mischel, W. (1983). Delay of gratification as process and as person variable in development. In D. Magnusson & U. L. Allen (Eds.), *Human development: An interactional perspective*. New York: Academic Press.

Rexford, E. N. (1978). *A developmental approach to problems of acting out* (rev. ed.). New York: International Universities Press.

Rogoff, B., Malkin, C., & Gilbride, K. (1984). Interaction with babies as guidance in development. In B. Rogoff & J. V. Wertsch (eds.), *Children's learning in the "zone of proximal development"* (W. Damon [Ed.], *New directions for child development, No. 23*.) San Francisco: Jossey-Bass.

Roskies, E. (1972). *Abnormality and normality: The mothering of thalidomide children*. Ithaca, NY: Cornell University Press.

Schaffer, H. R. (1984). *The child's entry into a social world*. London: Academic Press.

Schaffer, H. R., & Crook, C. K. (1978). The role of the mother in early social development. In H. McGurk (Ed.), *Issues in childhood social development*. London: Methuen.

Schaffer, H. R., & Crook, C. (1980). Child compliance and maternal control techniques. *Developmental Psychology, 16,* 54–61.

Serafica, F., & Cicchetti, D. (1976). Down's syndrome children in a strange situation: Attachment and exploration behaviors. *Merrill-Palmer Quarterly, 22,* 137–150.

Stayton, D. J., Hogan, R., & Ainsworth, M.D.S. (1971). Infant obedience and maternal behavior: The origins of socialization reconsidered. *Child Development, 42,* 1057–1069.

Stone, N., & Chesney, B. (1978). Attachment behaviors in handicapped infants. *Mental Retardation, 16*(1).

Thompson, R., Cicchetti, D., Lamb, M., & Malkin, C. (1985). The emotional responses of Down syndrome and normal infants in the strange situation: The organization of affective behavior in infants. *Developmental Psychology, 21,* 828–841.

Vaughn, B. E., Kopp, C. B., & Krakow, J. B. (1984). The emergence and consolidation of self-control from eighteen to thirty months of age: Normative trends and individual differences. *Child Development, 55,* 990–1004.

Vygotsky, L. S. (1962). *Thought and language.* Cambridge, MA: MIT Press.

Vygotsky, L. S. (1978). *Mind in society,* M. Coles, V. John-Steiner, S. Scribner, & E. Souberman (Eds.). Cambridge, MA: Harvard University Press.

Wertsch, J. V. (1979). From social interaction to higher psychological processes: A clarification and application of Vygotsky's theory. *Human Development, 22,* 1–22.

Wertsch, J. V. (1984). The zone of proximal development: Some conceptual issues. In B. Rogoff and J. V. Wertsch (Eds.), Children's Learning in the "Zone of Proximal Development." *New directions for child develop, no. 23.* San Francisco: Jossey-Bass.

8   Early conceptual development of children with Down syndrome

Carolyn B. Mervis

Without the ability to categorize, a child's life would be chaotic, since his or her world contains an infinite number of discriminably different entities. Assigning objects or events or attributes to categories provides the child's world with stability: Each entity no longer must be treated as unique. Entities assigned to the same category are alike in important respects, and thus can be treated similarly. Categories also allow a child to go beyond the information perceptually available from observing an entity, to make inferences about that entity. Consider the case of an opaque object that is currently stationary. Once the category assignment of that object is known, a child can predict both the internal (invisible from the surface) attributes of the object and the functions or characteristic actions of the object (based largely on the correlated form attributes).

These points have been made repeatedly in the literature concerned with categorization by nonhandicapped human adults (e.g., Bruner, Goodnow, & Austin, 1956; C. B. Mervis & Rosch, 1981; E. E. Smith & Medin, 1981). Given the importance that has been ascribed to categorization, one would expect very young children to form categories spontaneously regardless of whether the children had Down syndrome or were developing normally. The purpose of this chapter is to consider the development of categorization by both children with Down syndrome and nonhandicapped children. Much of the chapter will focus on the results of a longitudinal study I recently conducted in collaboration with Claudia Cardoso-Martins and Cynthia Mervis (e.g., Cardoso-Martins, 1984; Cardoso-Martins & C. B. Mervis, 1984,

Several people have made important contributions to the longitudinal study reported in this chapter. . Claudia Cardoso-Martins and Cindy Mervis collaborated with me on all aspects of this study. Kimberlee Chamberlain, Patricia Christensen, and Julie Nakamura assisted us with data collection and reduction. We thank the mothers and children who were involved in the study for their enthusiastic participation. The theory presented in this chapter has been improved by numerous discussions with John Pani. Marjorie Beeghly and Dante Cicchetti provided constructive criticisms of previous versions of this chapter. The longitudinal study was supported by the Department of Education, grant #DEG 008002485, and by the National Science Foundation, grant #BNS 81-21169. Preparation of this chapter was supported by the National Science Foundation, grant #BNS 84-19036.

1988; Cardoso-Martins, C. B. Mervis, & C. A. Mervis, 1985; C. B. Mervis, 1982, 1984; C. B. Mervis & C. A. Mervis, 1984; C. B. Mervis, 1988). When available, other research also will be discussed.

Simultaneous consideration of the development of categorization by children with Down syndrome and nonhandicapped children provides a unique opportunity for expanding our knowledge concerning categorization, for several reasons. First, the comparative study of children with Down syndrome and nonhandicapped children is important from a theoretical perspective. As described in sections that follow, the linguistic input that middle-class prelinguistic children with Down syndrome receive concerning names for objects differs systematically from the input middle-class nonhandicapped children receive. Therefore, a comparison of the categories initially formed by the two groups of children provides a basis for addressing a crucial theoretical question: Are children's initial categories formed based on the labels that children hear in reference to objects, or are these categories formed based on the children's cognitive structures? At the same time, this comparison should provide evidence concerning universal aspects of categorization that transcend mental status. Given the fundamental nature of categorization, one would expect at least certain of its aspects to be independent of cognitive abilities, once a baseline level of cognitive development was attained.

Second, correlation of certain characteristics of maternal linguistic input to children with Down syndrome with rate of vocabulary acquisition by these children should provide insight into an additional theoretical question: Which aspects of linguistic input, if any, are important for enhancing vocabulary development? It appears that this insight cannot be gained from the correlation of maternal linguistic input and rate of vocabulary acquisition by nonhandicapped children, either because mothers of nonhandicapped children are relatively uniform in the linguistic input they provide (Eheart, 1982) or because the threshold amount of specific types of input required by nonhandicapped children is very low, and therefore is provided routinely by virtually all mothers (Newport, Gleitman, & Gleitman, 1977). At the same time, the correlational study of maternal linguistic input and rate of vocabulary acquisition by children with Down syndrome should have practical implications as well. Linguistic input features that are strongly related to rate of vocabulary acquisition can be incorporated profitably into intervention programs focusing on enhancing the cognitive and language development of both children with Down syndrome and children with other handicaps (see Spiker, Chapter 13, this volume).

Third, consideration of the methods used by mothers of nonhandicapped children to teach their children new vocabulary also has practical implications. As described in sections that follow, the category formation of nonhandicapped children is more advanced than that of children with Down syndrome even when the two groups are equated for cognitive level. Therefore, consideration of the methods that mothers use to teach vocabulary to nonhandicapped children should provide an excellent basis for intervention techniques designed to promote vocabulary acquisition by children with Down syndrome or other handicaps affecting cognitive development.

This chapter focuses on the development of concrete object categories. The labels for these categories constitute the largest class of words in children's early vocabularies (Nelson, 1973; see Gentner, 1982, for a discussion of why children acquire nouns before verbs). The chapter is organized as follows: First, I consider several possible methods of studying early conceptual development and the types of data available concerning conceptual development by children with Down syndrome. I explain why the primary measure to be used concerns the child's lexicon. I then discuss three aspects of early lexical development that are important from a theoretical perspective, with regard to the nature of the early words that children produce. First, do these words refer to whole objects or to parts of objects? Second, what types of objects do early words refer to? Is it possible to make predictions about the types of objects that will serve as the referents of children's early words? Third, do children's early words refer to concepts at a variety of taxonomic levels, or does one level predominate? Is it possible to predict what level this will be?

I then discuss our recent research program designed to address a variety of questions concerning early conceptual development by both children with Down syndrome and nonhandicapped children. I begin by describing the methodology used in our longitudinal study. I then present part of a new theory of lexical development that the research program was designed to test and extend. After that, I consider the data relevant to three aspects of the theory. First, the extension of children's early categories is considered. That is, is it possible to predict which objects children will include in a given category? Second, the basis for the extension of children's early categories is considered. Third, the basis for the evolution of children's early categories to conform to the corresponding adult categories is discussed. Integral to this topic is a consideration of methods mothers use for teaching new vocabulary. After these discussions, three additional types of data obtained in our longitudinal study are considered. These data address other issues concerning the course of early lexical development. First, the mental age and sensorimotor cognitive level of the children at the onset of referential language comprehension and the onset of referential language production is examined. Rate of vocabulary acquisition relative to rate of cognitive development also is discussed. Second, maternal linguistic style when talking with the child is considered. Are there systematic differences between the mothers of the children with Down syndrome and the mothers of the nonhandicapped children in the manner in which they talk with their children? Third, the potential effect of differences in maternal linguistic style on rate of vocabulary acquisition by children with Down syndrome is examined.

In the chapter's final substantive section, data concerning categorization by older children are discussed. These data are interpreted within the framework of the theory of categorization proposed by Rosch and C. B. Mervis (e.g., Rosch & C. B. Mervis, 1975; C. B. Mervis, 1980; C. B. Mervis & Pani, 1980). In the final section, some implications of the findings concerning conceptual development are discussed.

Methods of studying early conceptual development

A variety of methods has been used to study early conceptual development. This section briefly reviews these methods and the general results obtained. The choice of techniques to be considered in the remainder of the chapter is then explained.

The primary method that has been used to consider conceptual development in infancy is habituation (e.g., the papers reviewed in L. B. Cohen & Gelber, 1975); conditioning has been used occasionally (e.g., Husaim & L. B. Cohen, 1981). The results of these studies suggest that nonhandicapped 10-month-olds are able to form categories according to the same basic principles adults use; however, 7-month-olds rely on very different principles (L. B. Cohen & Younger, 1983). Although Kopp (1983), in her review of studies of the early development of children with Down syndrome, cites one study of habituation by infants with Down syndrome (L. B. Cohen, 1981), this study was not concerned with categorization. Thus, no data are available concerning the category formation principles used by infants with Down syndrome. The habituation technique is valuable for addressing the issue of the principles infants are capable of using when forming categories. However, the technique at present cannot be used to address issues concerning spontaneous category formation by infants. The problem is that when the habituation technique is used, it is impossible to determine whether the child had formed the category being studied prior to the experiment, or has learned the category during the course of the experiment, based on the "instruction" provided by the experimenter. Reznick and Kagan (1983) are attempting to develop methods to address this issue.

Recently, a new technique has been developed to study preexisting (i.e., nonexperimentally induced) categories. The extension of a child's category is measured based on a response the child has developed that is unique to members of that category. So far, this technique has been used only in case studies of individual nonhandicapped children. Golinkoff and Halperin (1983) used an affective response one infant consistently made when he saw an animal to determine the extension of his *animal* category. Benelli, D'Odorico, Levorato, and Simion (1977) used the functional response of attempting to suck to study one infant's *pacifier* category. C. B. Mervis (1985) used the functional response of attempting to blow to study one 9-month-old's *horn* category. In this study, a wide range of potential category members was included, and the infant was tested twice, 2 weeks apart. The results of this study indicated that the infant had formed a stable category and was relying on the same basic principle of category formation as adults use, although the extension of the infant's category was not identical to that of the corresponding adult category. The reasons for the differences will be discussed in a later section. No studies of infants or toddlers with Down syndrome have been carried out using this technique. The technique is excellent for studying certain types of spontaneously formed categories but is limited to categories for which a unique functional or affective response is available. The technique also is limited to the period prior to the onset of object substitution play (about age 16 months for nonhandicapped children). Once children deliberately substitute one object for another, the technique is no longer useful, because it is impossible to determine whether any overextensions the child makes are categorical or instead playful.

Other types of nonverbal techniques have been used with older infants and children. The infant studies have involved object-sorting tasks. These studies generally have required the infant to divide objects into two groups; within each group, the objects are usually identical or differ only minimally (e.g., Ricciuti, 1965; Sugarman, 1983). Thus, these studies do not address the issue of the basis for infant categorization. Results, based on measures of sequential touching of objects or physical division of the objects into groups, corroborate the results of studies using other techniques. Older infants are capable of forming categories. No studies of infants or toddlers with Down syndrome have been conducted using object-sorting techniques.

Studies with children of a variety of ages have been conducted using either object- or picture-sorting tasks or match-to-sample tasks. The results of the first studies of nonhandicapped children (e.g., Goldman & Levine, 1963; Olver & Hornsby, 1966; J. Thompson, 1941) suggested that nonhandicapped children younger than about 8 years did not form the same types of categories as adults. The results of more recent studies, however, indicate that even young nonhandicapped children form the same categories as adults, although the extensions of the categories are often not identical (e.g., Neimark, 1974; Rosch, C. B. Mervis, Gray, Johnson, & Boyes-Braem, 1976; Saltz, Soller, & Siegel, 1972). In the only study involving children with Down syndrome, Tager-Flusberg (1985a) found that 11-year-olds with Down syndrome also form the same categories as adults, although again the extensions are not identical. When a principled selection of objects is used, sorting techniques provide excellent insights into children's categorizations. The available studies employing this technique are reviewed in the final substantive section of this chapter, in the context of an important theoretical prediction concerning the relationship between child and adult categories.

The final method that has been used to study conceptual development involves determining the extension of a child's categories based on either language comprehension or language production. In the production task, the child is asked to label a variety of objects. In the comprehension task, the child may be asked to select a single object (from a choice of a few objects) that is named by the word the experimenter produces. Alternatively, the child may be asked to select all of the objects that are named by the word the experimenter produces, from a large set of objects. The former comprehension technique is most often used with older infants and young children, while the latter technique frequently is used with older children. In addition, researchers sometimes collect data concerning spontaneous comprehension or production. The results of studies with nonhandicapped toddlers indicate that, given the child has formed a particular category, the extension of that category will be similar, although often not identical, to the corresponding adult category (e.g., K. Chapman, 1983; C. B. Mervis, 1984; Rescorla, 1980, 1981; Thompson & R. S. Chapman, 1977). Parallel results are obtained, whether measured by comprehension or production (C. B. Mervis & Canada, 1983). The same results were obtained in a longitudinal study of toddlers who had Down syndrome (C. B. Mervis, 1982, 1984, 1988). C. B. Mervis (1982, 1984, 1988) has shown that the toddler categories are based on the same basic principle as adult categories. The results of studies with nonhandicapped children indicate that for certain types of categories, the children's extensions are the same as the adult extension, while for other types, the extensions are similar but not identical (Anglin, 1977; C. B. Mervis, 1987; Rosch et al., 1976). Tager-Flusberg (1985b, 1986) has found that 11-year-olds who had Down syndrome spontaneously formed categories that were similar, but not identical, to the corresponding adult categories. The deviations fit the developmental predictions made by C. B. Mervis (1980).

This chapter focuses on studies conducted using the comprehension and production methods of assessing conceptual development. The available studies concerning sorting and match-to-sample tasks also are considered. In part, this decision is forced by the available data; as indicated in the brief review above, no data concerning infants or children with Down syndrome have been collected using other methods. However, the comprehension–production method is important in its own right. The lexicon is critical for the child; it allows the child to communicate his or her categories to other people. At the same time, it allows the child to understand what other people are saying, and thereby to gain access to their categorization system. Almost all concrete nouns are labels for categories of objects. Thus, measures of word comprehension and production provide a direct indication of the extension of the category corresponding to the word, as well as a basis for inferences concerning the intension of the category. Therefore, the study of early lexical development provides insight into the child's category structures. From a research perspective, measurement of comprehension and production is probably the most direct method now available for studying spontaneously formed categories.

Nature of children's early words

Given the importance of categorization, and the importance of the lexicon for communicating about categorization, it is unfortunate that so little data on either early categorization or early lexical development of children with Down syndrome are available. Neither topic is discussed in the two major texts on Down syndrome (Benda, 1960; Gibson, 1978). A search of the literature yielded very few studies. One sorting study including children with Down syndrome as subjects has been reported (Tager-Flusberg, 1985a). One longitudinal study using lexical measures of categorization has been conducted (e.g., Cardoso-Martins, 1984; Cardoso-Martins, C. B. Mervis, & C. A. Mervis, 1985; C. B. Mervis, 1984). Tager-Flusberg (1985b; 1986) has conducted the single cross-sectional study of this type. In addition, one study of the words included in the early lexicons of toddlers with Down syndrome has been reported (Gillham, 1979), and one other study included a measure of vocabulary size at age 36 months (Strominger, Winkler, & L. T. Cohen, 1984). Thus, the only data available concerning the actual content of the early lexicons of children with Down syndrome are the data collected by Gillham. In this section, these data are used, along with data collected on the early lexical development of nonhandicapped children, to address three important theoretical issues concerning the words included in children's early lexicons.

Referents of early words: parts or wholes?

Wittgenstein (1958) has argued that pointing at an object at the same time as providing a label leads to an ambiguous situation, because pointing allows for an infinite number of referents (e.g., the whole object, parts of the object, attributes of the object, actions involving the object). To disambiguate the deictic utterance or gesture, there must be an agreed-upon convention concerning its referent. All theories of early lexical development have postulated the same convention. Thus, an important assumption underlying these theories is that children initially believe that when a person points at or otherwise indicates an object for which the child does not already know a name, the accompanying word refers to the whole object.

Despite the importance of this assumption, there are virtually no data available that address it directly. Because comprehension generally precedes production (e.g., Clark & Hecht, 1983; Huttenlocher, 1974; Keenan & MacWhinney, 1987), the most relevant data are comprehension data. The form–class comprehension errors reported in case studies of two nonhandicapped children support the assumption. Hoffman's son initially assumed that *hot* meant "stove" (Hoffman, 1968; cited in Macnamara, 1982). My son initially assumed that "hot" meant "cuplike object," "more" meant "juice-like beverage," and "night-night" meant "bedlike object" (C. B. Mervis, 1987). Velleman, Mangipudi, and Locke (in press) report similar examples for young children with Down syndrome. Further support for the assumption is provided by preliminary analyses of the early entries in a diary study of my son's early lexical development. These analyses indicated that when Ari learned a verb, it initially was comprehended and produced in reference to the action of an object whose name he already comprehended (C. B. Mervis, 1987).

To address experimentally the hypothesis concerning young children's initial beliefs regarding referents of novel words, Laurel Long and I have conducted a study using artificial stimuli (Mervis & Long, 1987). In this study, the experimenter pointed directly at a part of an object at the same time as she provided a nonsense syllable label. She then removed the original object and placed three additional objects in front of the child. One object had the same overall shape as the initial object but did not have the part that was labeled; one object had a different overall shape but did have the labeled part in the same position as in the original object; and one object had a different overall shape and did not have the part that was labeled. The child was asked to show the experimenter the [label]. The data obtained from nonhandicapped 18-month-olds strongly support the hypothesis that young children believe that a word used in reference to a novel type of object refers to the whole object, rather than a part of the object. The subjects almost always treated the word used to label the part as though the word referred instead to the whole object.

Production data, although less useful than comprehension data for testing the whole-object assumption, are still valuable. The results of two group studies, one of which included children with Down syndrome, can be considered in reference to this assumption. Only the whole-object-prior-to-object-part aspect of the hypothesis can be addressed by these data. Because the referents of the children's words were not given in the reports of these studies, it is impossible to determine whether the verbs or attribute words produced were used initially in reference to objects whose names were already known. Nelson (1973), in considering the first 10 words produced by the 18 nonhandicapped children in her study, found that most of these words were names for whole objects. None of the children produced any word for a part of an object as one of his or her first 10 words. However, by the time a 50-word vocabulary had been attained, many of the children were able to produce the names for a few body parts. Given the number of different people and animal words that the children knew prior to producing any body part words, it is likely that the latter initially were produced in reference to objects whose names already were known. No other part words appear to have been produced.

Gillham (1979), in a study of 4 children with Down syndrome and 14 nonhandicapped children, also found that the children's first 10 words consisted primarily of names for whole objects. The list of early words for the children with Down syndrome included three body parts (hair, eye, ear); the list for the nonhandicapped children included two body parts (nose, eye). Although the number of children who produced each of these words was not indicated, Gillham's lists of early words were arranged by number of children who produced each word. It is clear from the positions of the body part words that very few of the children produced them. On the other hand, almost all of the high-frequency words were labels for either people or animals. Thus, it is quite likely that the children who did produce body parts initially produced these words in reference to either people or animals whose category names were already known. Only one other part word was produced early. One of the nonhandicapped children produced "button." No item of clothing likely to include buttons was among the first 10 words learned; however, it is possible that the child who produced "button" initially produced the word in reference to a button on an object whose name the child already comprehended. It is also possible that this child learned "button" in reference to a button that was not attached to another object. Examination of the play session transcripts from our longitudinal study indicates that none of the children with Down syndrome ever produced any word for a part of an object. This was true even though the toys available included several animals, so referents for body part words were readily available.

Gillham provides two additional lists: a list of the words included by at least half of the children with Down syndrome in their first 50 words and a list of the words included by more than 20% of the nonhandicapped children in their first 100 words. No additional part words were included in the list for the children with Down syndrome. In addition to the part words included in the early words, the list for the nonhandicapped children included several additional body parts and also "drawer." No item of furniture that contains drawers was included in the list. Thus, "drawer," if it was used solely in reference to individual drawers rather than in reference to the object containing the drawers, would constitute an exception to the prediction. Note that this word was acquired relatively late, however; it was included in the first 100 words of fewer than a third of the children.

Adults appear usually to honor the whole-object convention in talking to their young children. For example, Ninio and Bruner (1978) and Ninio (1980) found that in a bookreading situation, approximately 95% of maternal deictic utterances referred to whole objects. For the few exceptions, the utterances usually were marked to indicate explicitly the relationship between the whole object and the singled-out part, attribute, and the like (e.g., "That's the kitty's ear," rather than "That's an ear.") Shipley, Kuhn, and Madden (1983) found that when mothers label both a whole object and a part of that object, the label for the object precedes the label for the part 98% of the time. This tendency of mothers to label whole objects is probably helpful to lexical acquisition. However, maternal labeling patterns do not form the entire basis for the children's acceptance of the whole-object principle. As the case study data just reported indicated, very young children sometimes decide that labels for attributes of objects are in fact labels for the objects themselves. In addition, Ninio (1980) found that when a mother asks her young child, "What's this?" the child almost invariably answers with an object label, even when the mother makes clear from an adult perspective (e.g., by touching or tapping a specific part) that she is asking about a part. Further, Gillham (1979) reported that early language-training programs often focused initially on color words, with the result that the children did not learn any words. When the focus was changed to object words, however, the children were more successful. Thus, the value of maternal adherence to the whole-object principle may derive primarily from its fit with the child's intrinsic belief in that principle.

In summary, the available data strongly support the whole-object hypothesis. Young children initially believe that when a person points at or otherwise indicates an object for which the child does not already have a name, the accompanying word refers to the whole object. This belief is held consistently by both nonhandicapped children and children with Down syndrome.

Children's object words: horizontal development

The acquisition of an object-word vocabulary involves two types of development: horizontal and vertical. Horizontal development refers to the acquisition of words at a single taxonomic level; for example, the acquisition of names for basic object categories. Vertical development refers to the acquisition of a set of taxonomically related terms to refer to a particular object; for example, the acquisition of coffee table, table, and furniture in reference to a single object. In this section, horizontal development is considered. Vertical development is considered in the next section.

When nonhandicapped children begin to talk, the words they produce are remarkably consistent. These words are not a random sample of the words used in child-addressed speech. Clark (1979), in reviewing a number of diary studies of the lexical development of nonhandicapped children, pointed out that initial nouns are concentrated on a limited subset of categories: types of food, clothing, animals, people, vehicles, toys, household items used in daily routines, and eventually body parts. These diary studies were conducted in the late 19th and early 20th centuries. The results of Nelson's (1973) and Gillham's (1979) more recent studies indicate that for nonhandicapped children, early vocabulary content at the present time is essentially the same as at the turn of the century.

The results of Gillham's (1979) study of the early lexicons of children with Down syndrome indicate that the initial nouns produced by these children are concentrated on the same subset of categories as for nonhandicapped children. Even within this subset, the particular exemplars chosen are remarkably consistent. For example, within the clothing category, both children with Down syndrome and nonhandicapped children produce such words as ''shoe'' and ''sockie'' early, while producing ''shirt'' and ''pants'' much later. In fact, 83% of the object words produced by at least half of the children with Down syndrome in their first 50 words were also produced by the nonhandicapped children within their first 50 words. Blind children's early words are very similar to those produced by sighted children (Bigelow, 1982; Landau & Gleitman, 1985; Mulford, 1988).

What is the basis for this impressively consistent choice of words? Several explanations were offered at the beginning of the century. Moore (1896) suggested that children first talk about things that have excited great interest. Guillaume (1927/1973) stated that children were most likely to name objects they could manipulate. Bohn (1914) argued that the ability of an object to change independent of the child was an important determinant of early vocabulary choice. More recently, two explanations that encompass these characteristics have been offered. Nelson (1973) argued that children become interested in objects that have ''salient properties of change'' (p. 33), that is, objects that either move independently or can be manipulated by the child. Nelson (1979), in a study of nonhandicapped 20-month-olds, has demonstrated that the more manipulable an object is, and the greater the number of specific action schemes evoked by the object, the more likely the child is to learn to name that object, when input labeling is controlled. Whitehurst, Kedesdy, and White (1982) have suggested that in addition to mobility, the novelty and salience of an object must be taken into account in order to explain individual differences in early vocabularies. The relative merits of the two proposals remain to be determined. However, it is clear that mobility, whether independent of the child or dependent on the child, is an important factor in determining if a word will be produced early.

Vertical development

An object can be categorized at each of several different levels. Psychologists usually consider three levels of abstraction. For example, a coffee table (subordinate) is a type of table (basic), which is a type of furniture (superordinate). Rosch et al. (1976) have argued that the basic level is more fundamental than the other levels.

The basic level is most fundamental because it is the most cognitively efficient level. It is the most general level at which category members have similar overall shapes and at which a person uses similar motor actions for interacting with category members. Although categories at all levels are based on correlated attribute clusters, the correlations are most apparent for basic level categories. Thus, basic level categories are the categories most differentiated from one another. In support of this claim, Tversky and Hemenway (1984) have demonstrated that members of a given basic level category are perceived to share the same parts, while members of other basic level categories within the same taxonomy tend to have different parts. In contrast, members of the various subordinate categories subsumed under a single basic level category are perceived as sharing parts; these categories differ on the basis of nonpart attributes. At the superordinate level, category members may be perceived to share no relevant part attributes at all. On the basis of the special characteristics of basic level categories, Rosch et al. (1976) have predicted that children will learn to categorize and to name objects at the basic level prior to other taxonomic levels.

There is considerable linguistic evidence in support of the primacy of the basic level for nonhandicapped children. Analyses of the diary records of the early vocabularies of 47 children (see the following paragraph for references) indicates that almost all of the words listed correspond to basic level categories. In addition, Stross (1973) and Dougherty (1978) have shown that the first botanical labels that children learn are names for basic level categories.

The relative priority of superordinate and subordinate labels can be examined based on the diary records just mentioned. These reports are generally of four types: lists of the first 50 words used; lists of the first 100 words used; lists of all words used at age 17–18 months (median number of words in the studies cited below = 156); and lists of words used at age 24 months (median number of words = 483). Examination of all studies of the first 50 words of 20 nonhandicapped children (Gruendel, 1977; Nelson, 1973) indicated that the range of superordinate words used was from 0 to 1 (median = 0). Studies of the first 100 words of 16 nonhandicapped children (Gillham, 1979; Gruendel, 1977) indicated that the range of superordinate words used was from 0 to 1 (median = 1); the range for subordinate words was the same (median = 0). Studies of the vocabulary of three nonhandicapped 17–18-month-olds (Bohn, 1914; Boyd, 1914; Nice, 1915) indicated that no superordinates or subordinates were used. Finally, studies of the vocabulary of nine nonhandicapped 24-month-olds (Bohn, 1914; Boyd, 1914; Grant, 1915; Holden, 1877; Jegi, 1901; Moore, 1896; Pelsma, 1910) indicated that the range of superordinate words used was 0 to 7 (median = 3); the range of subordinate words used was 0 to 8 (median = 1). Categories for which the basic level is likely to vary from child to child (e.g., the bird taxonomy; see Dougherty, 1978) were not included in these analyses, because it was impossible to determine the basic level for individual children. Thus, the actual number of superordinate and subordinate words produced may be slightly greater than those already indicated. In summary, analyses of the diary studies indicated that virtually all of the words that young children produce are names for basic level categories. Names for superordinate categories are slightly more prevalent than names for subordinate categories.

The results for the children with Down syndrome who participated in Gillham's (1979) study support the primacy of basic level names over names at other taxonomic levels. Examination of the vocabulary lists provided by Gillham indicate that other than proper names (which have not been considered in any of these analyses), every object word included was the name for a basic level category. No superordinate or subordinate names were listed. Analysis of the play session transcripts from our longitudinal study corroborate this finding. All object words used by the six children with Down syndrome during the play sessions were names for basic level categories. There was little evidence of comprehension of subordinate level names. (Superordinate level words were not tested.) These results obtained even though at the end of the study, the children were more than 3 years old. Even once children presumably know more than one name for a given object, the object's basic level name is consistently preferred by both children with Down syndrome and nonhandicapped children (Rosch et al., 1976; Tager-Flusberg, 1986).

There also is evidence that although mothers sometimes use subordinate level names when labeling objects for other adults, basic level names are almost always used in speech addressed to young children (Anglin, 1977; Blewitt, 1983; Brown, 1958). Blewitt (1983) also found that when subordinate names were used in speech addressed to young children, these names were often either directly preceded or directly followed by the relevant basic level name. These studies included only nonhandicapped children. However, informal examination of the transcripts from the play sessions in our longitudinal study suggest that the same constraints held for the mothers of the children with Down syndrome.

Thus, a variety of considerations supports the primacy of the basic level. The results of a categorization study using nonsense stimuli that were never named for the child (C. B. Mervis and Crisafi, 1982) indicate that category structure alone is sufficient to account for the primacy of the basic level. Other evidence that children's categorization decisions are often independent of linguistic input is presented in the next section. However, parental naming practices may facilitate the early acquisition of categories at the basic level.

Summary

Consideration of the evidence concerning three separate aspects of early lexical development important from a theoretical perspective indicates striking similarity between the qualitative aspects of the early vocabularies of children with Down syndrome and nonhandicapped children. Both groups of children initially accept the whole-object assumption concerning the meanings of novel words. The initial vocabularies of both groups of children are concentrated on the same limited subset of categories, and the particular words chosen from these categories are often identical. These words are names for objects either that move independently or that can be manipulated by the child. Finally, the initial vocabularies of both groups of children consist almost entirely of names for basic level categories.

A longitudinal study of early conceptual development: method

The next three sections examine a variety of issues regarding early conceptual development that have been addressed primarily by our longitudinal study of the early lexical development of both children with Down syndrome and nonhandicapped children. Because the emphasis in these sections will be on this study, it is important for the reader to be aware of the methodology used, which is described in this section.

Subjects

Six children with Down syndrome (three boys, three girls) and their mothers and six nonhandicapped children and their mothers participated in this study. The children with Down syndrome constituted the entire known surviving population of children with Down syndrome born in two small midwestern cities during a 3-month period in 1979. The nonhandicapped children were matched to the children with Down syndrome for sex and birth-order position. All children had hearing and vision within the normal range. All families were middle-class, and in all cases the mother was the primary caregiver. (The mothers of one child with Down syndrome and one nonhandicapped child worked part-time outside the home.) At the start of the study, the children with Down syndrome were between 17 and 19 months old. The nonhandicapped children were 9 months old. None of the children was able to comprehend or produce language referentially. The children were visited at home every 6 weeks for between 14 and 21 months.

Procedure

Each visit began with a 30-minute play period during which mother and child played together with a specially chosen set of toys. The play period was audiotaped. In addition, one observer recorded all the nouns and pronouns used by either mother or child, along with their referents. A second observer audiotaped a running commentary describing the nonverbal interaction (including, for the children with Down syndrome and their mothers, any manual signs produced and the context in which they were used).

After the play period, production testing and comprehension testing were carried out. First, the child was asked to name the toys, if there was any possibility that he or she could produce the names. Such a possibility was considered to exist if the child had produced any of the object names, either spontaneously or in imitation of the mother, during the play period, or if the mother thought her child could produce any of the object names. Next, the child's comprehension was tested. Four objects were placed in front of the child, and he or she was asked, "Is there an [*X*]?" The distractor objects were selected according to predetermined rules, to ensure that the objects most similar to members of the target category were used (see C. B. Mervis, 1984). If the child appeared tired or fussy, comprehension testing was discontinued and then completed within a few days.

In addition to the play period and the production and comprehension tests, some visits included assessments of cognitive development. Four measures were used: the object permanence and means–ends relations subscales of the Uzgiris and Hunt (1975) scales for sensorimotor development; the mental scale of the Bayley Scales of Infant Development (Bayley, 1969); and form L–M of the Stanford–Binet Intelligence Scale (Terman & Merrill, 1960).

The object permanence and means–ends relations subscales were administered at the first visit and at every second visit thereafter, until the child had passed all the items. These scales also were administered at the visit during which referential comprehension first was demonstrated and at the visit during which referential production first was demonstrated, even if these assessments originally had not been scheduled for those dates. The scales also were administered at the last visit, if the child had not yet passed all the items.

The mental scale of the Bayley test was administered at the end of the first visit (usually on the day following the first play session) and at regular intervals approximately 5 months apart throughout the remainder of the study. The Stanford–Binet test was administered to the nonhandicapped children at the visit closest to their second birthday and to the children with Down syndrome at either their last visit or their last two visits, depending on the child's performance on the Bayley test. One child with Down syndrome was not given the Stanford–Binet test because his family moved away before the test would have been appropriate.

Stimuli

The categories studied had to meet three criteria. First, the child's basic level category had to be expected to differ from the adult category labeled with the same name. Second, the labels for these categories had to be among children's earliest words (as determined by Gillham's [1979] and Nelson's [1973] lists). Third, a variety of exemplars expected to be included in the child-basic category but not the adult-basic category had to be available. Several categories met the first two criteria, but only three of these met the third: *kitty, car,* and *ball.* All three were included in the study. The toys used included true members of the category (by adult standards), related objects that I predicted to be members of the child-basic categories, and unrelated objects from the same superordinate categories, that were predicted not to be included in either the adult-basic or the child-basic categories.

To predict which items should be included in a child-basic category, I used the principle that basic level categories are the most general categories whose members share similar overall shapes and similar functions or characteristic actions. I began by observing the functions for nonhandicapped 13-month-olds of a prototypical exemplar (in toy form) of the adult-basic category labeled by each target word. I then predicted that any object that could fulfill these functions (whether or not these functions were appropriate for that object from an adult perspective) and that had a shape similar to the prototypical exemplar would be a member of the child-basic category. For example, I predicted that anything that could be thrown, could roll, and was approximately spherical would be included in the child-basic *ball* category.

Starting with the fifth visit, we included objects that were predicted to be members of the adult-basic categories but that might be excluded from the child-basic categories. The toys were varied occasionally, to keep the mothers and children from becoming bored. The toys used are listed in Table 8.1.

A new theory of early lexical development

This section describes part of a new theory of early lexical development. (For additional description, see C. B. Mervis, 1984; 1987; 1988.) Supporting data from the longitudinal study and other relevant studies are summarized at the end of each subsection. I argue that membership in young children's categories, including deviations from adult categories, can be predicted based on the same principles used to predict categorization by older children and adults. I further argue that, in many cases, children choose to attend to or emphasize different attributes from adults, because of limited experience or lack of knowledge of culturally appropriate functions and their correlated form attributes. In such cases, children will form categories that are not isomorphic to adult categories, even though young children's beliefs concerning the basis for initial category formation are based on the same principles as adults' beliefs. I claim that the evolution of children's early categories is dependent on the child realizing that, for particular objects, attributes that he or she had not attended to are important, and that a different categorization scheme is therefore equally or more plausible than the child's earlier scheme. The emphasis will be on the role of the child's own cognitive structures, including his or her beliefs concerning the basis for category formation, in the formation and evolution of his or her initial categories. However, I also consider the role played by adults in determining which categories the child could potentially form and how accurate these categories will be. Finally, I discuss the role of adults in the evolution of a child's categories: The manner in which the adult introduces new vocabulary often determines whether or not the new word will be comprehended, allowing category evolution to begin.

Child-basic categories: initial composition

As just mentioned, children's initial categories are basic level categories. However, these initial categories often will not correspond to the adult-basic category labeled by the same word. Such differences are to be expected; only the principles governing the determination of basic level categories were predicted to be universal (Dougherty, 1978; Rosch et al., 1976). The actual categories formed on the basis of these principles will vary because different groups notice or emphasize different

Table 8.1. *Toys used in the play sessions*

	Category		
	Ball	Car	Kitty
Predicted membership:			
Adult-basic and child-basic	rubber ball	sedan car	house cat
	whiffle ball	sports car	sachet cat[a]
	soccer ball	wooden car[a]	beanbag cat[a]
	football[a]	jeep[a]	potholder cat[a]
Child-basic only	multisided beads	van	panther
	Christmas ornament	bus	cougar
	round candle	moving truck	cheetah
	round owl bank	fire engine	leopard
	round bell	cement truck	tiger
		dump truck	lion
Neither	wooden blocks	airplane	dog
	Frisbee	helicopter	frog
	plastic keys	boat	parrot
			zebra
			squirrel
			rabbit
			walrus
			turtle
			elephant
			duck
			giraffe
			lobster
			camel
			dinosaur

Note: A subset of these toys was used in each of the play sessions. At the start of the study, five objects from each category were included: one predicted adult-basic and child-basic; three predicted child-basic-only; and one predicted neither. By the end of the study, nine objects from each category were included: two predicted adult-basic and child-basic; five predicted child-basic only; and two predicted neither. For many of the names listed, several different exemplars of the category labeled by that name were used over the course of the study.
[a] Potential undergeneralization object.

attributes of the same object as a function of different experiences or different degrees of expertise. Very young children often do not share adults' knowledge of culturally appropriate functions and their correlated form attributes, leading children to deemphasize attributes of an object that are important from an adult perspective. At the same time, children may notice a function (and its correlated form attributes) for that object which adults ignore. In such cases, children would emphasize attributes of the object that are unimportant to adults. Therefore, very young children's basic level categories will oftentimes differ from the corresponding adult-basic level categories.

When differences between child-basic and adult-basic categories occur, several relationships between the two types of categories may result. First, the child-basic category may be broader than the corresponding adult-basic category. These broad categories sometimes correspond to a more general level in the same taxonomy (see also Brown, 1958, 1978). For example, the child-basic *kitty* category might correspond to the adult *feline* category. In other cases, the child's broad category contains exemplars from several adult taxonomies. For example, the child-basic *ball* category might include round candles, round coin banks, and multisided beads, as well as objects adults would consider balls. Second, the child's category may be narrower than the corresponding adult category. For example, the child-basic *chair* category might not include beanbag chairs. Third, the child's category may overlap the adult's category; that is, the child's category may include objects that are excluded from the adult category while at the same time excluding objects that are included in the adult category. For example, the child-basic *car* category might include trucks but exclude dune buggies.

Previous theories of early lexical development have accounted for the differences between child and adult categories by postulating that children and adults attend to different numbers of attributes when making categorization decisions. Thus, Clark (1973) has claimed that the child attends to a proper subset of the attributes relevant to an adult. Consequently, the child's categories corresponding to his or her early words are broader than the adult categories labeled by the same words. Nelson (1974) has claimed that the child attends to a superset of the attributes relevant to an adult. Consequently, the child's categories are initially narrower than the corresponding adult categories. Development consists of either adding relevant attributes (Clark, 1973) or subtracting irrelevant attributes (Nelson, 1974) until the appropriate adult category is acquired. In contrast, I believe (see C. B. Mervis, 1982, 1984; C. B. Mervis & Canada, 1983; C. B. Mervis & C. A. Mervis, 1982) that although some differences between child and adult categories may be due to variations in the number of attributes attended to, this is not the major source of difference. Instead, one of the most important causes of the differences between child and adult categories is that children are attending to or emphasizing different attributes from adults (see also Carey, 1982).

For child-basic categories that are broader than the corresponding adult-basic category, there are three reasons why a child might attend to a different set of attributes or assign a different weight to an attribute. First, the child may not know about the cultural significance of certain attributes. For example, the child may not realize that a candle can be burned. Therefore, the wick of a round candle may be ignored, in favor of known attributes such as *round, rolls, can be thrown*. The round candle will accordingly be assigned to the child's *ball* category. Second, the child may be aware of the attributes that are important to the adult category assignment, but the salience of these attributes may sometimes be less for him or her than the salience of a different set of attributes. Thus, a child may consider a round candle to be both a candle and a ball. Third, the child may include false attributes in his or her decision process. For example, the mistaken belief that a zebra says "neigh" (as the child's mother may tell him or her; see C. B. Mervis & C. A. Mervis, 1982) may contribute to the child's decision to categorize it as a horse.

For child-basic categories that are narrower than the corresponding adult-basic category, the child often defines the acceptable range of values for a given attribute more narrowly, for attributes that both children and adults include in their decision processes. This situation often occurs because the child is not aware of cultural conventions concerning stylized representations. For example, both children and adults expect squirrels to have fur. However, very young children may require this fur to be plush and relatively plain. Thus, a toy squirrel made out of a polka-dot satin fabric may be excluded from a child's *squirrel* category but included in an adult's *squirrel* category.

In many cases for which the child-basic category overlaps the corresponding adult-basic category, the factors that contribute to overly broad and overly narrow categories operate simultaneously. For example, the child may include round banks and round candles in his or her *ball* category, because he or she is unaware of the cultural significance of the slot or the wick. At the same time, the child may exclude footballs from his or her *ball* category because the shape is too deviant from round. In other cases, the factor that is primarily responsible for overgeneralization may lead to overlap: The child emphasizes attributes that are irrelevant to the adult category, while ignoring an attribute that is crucial for the adult category. For example, Keil (1987) has argued that young children emphasize such attributes as being a friend of one's father and bringing one presents in determining membership in their *uncle* category. Young children ignore the kinship criteria that adults use. Thus, young children would be expected to include not only actual friendly adult uncles but also close male friends of the father in *uncle,* while excluding juveniles and unfriendly adults who are uncles by the kinship criterion.

As with adult-basic categories, child-basic categories are characterized by gradients of goodness-of-example. That is, some members of the category are more representative of the category than other members. The principles of family resemblance and contrast set (see Rosch & C. B. Mervis, 1975) govern the goodness-of-example of child-basic categories, just as for adult-basic categories. Thus, the most representative exemplars are those that share large numbers of attributes with many other exemplars of the category, while at the same time sharing few attributes with exemplars of related categories. However, the goodness-of-example structure of the child-basic category is not determined simply on the basis of the goodness-of-example structure of the corresponding adult-basic category. The two structures will sometimes differ, because children may attend to or emphasize different attributes from adults. For example, for an adult, a football is a ball, whereas a round bank is not. For a young child, a round bank may be a better example of *bank* than a football is; for some young children, the football may not even be a ball.

Which objects, then, should be included in an initial child-basic category? The principle that basic level categories are the most general categories whose members share similar overall shapes and similar functions or characteristic actions can be used to make predictions. An initial child-basic category should include those objects that, from a child's perspective, have similar overall shapes (or similar parts in particular configurations) and similar characteristic actions and/or can be used for similar functions.

One important factor that limits the predictability of the composition of child-basic categories concerns the initial exemplar or exemplars on which the child bases his or her category. As John Pani and I have shown (C. B. Mervis & Pani, 1980), when the initial exemplar is a good example of its category, a person (either child or adult) is likely to generalize appropriately to include other predicted members in his or her category. However, when the initial exemplar is a poor example of its category, the person is not likely to generalize appropriately at first. In many cases, he or she will form a category that is much narrower than the predicted category. Thus, the predictions made based on the basic level principle will be correct when children first form a category only if the initial exemplar is a good example of its category. The predictions eventually will hold even if the initial exemplar was a poor example. However, the child first will have to realize that the good examples are also members of the category.

In summary, very young children form basic level categories whose composition often differs from that of adult basic level categories. Children's categories may be broader than, narrower than, or may overlap, the corresponding adult categories. These differences occur because the child's limited knowledge of culturally appropriate functions of objects and their correlated form attributes leads him or her to emphasize different attributes or attribute values than adults do, for the same object. However, because child-basic categories and adult-basic categories are formed and structured according to the same principles, it is possible to predict the composition of child-basic categories.

Relevant results. The initial extension of the children's *ball, car,* and *kitty* categories was determined based on the data from the first comprehension test on which the category name was comprehended. For the children with Down syndrome, 14 of the 16 initial categories corresponded exactly to the predicted child-basic categories. In the two remaining cases, the football was excluded from the child's *ball* category. (One child with Down syndrome never comprehended "car" or "kitty.") For the nonhandicapped children, 17 of the 18 initial categories corresponded exactly to the predicted ones. One category was slightly overextended. Thus, for both groups of children, virtually all of the initial categories corresponded perfectly to the predicted child-basic categories.

Although these data indicate that children's initial categories took the predicted form, additional data are needed to determine if these categories are based on the children's cognitive structures (as predicted), or if the manner in which mothers label objects for their children also would provide the basis for forming the predicted child-basic categories. Results of previous studies (Cardoso-Martins & C. B. Mervis, 1985; C. B. Mervis & C. A. Mervis, 1982) indicate that mothers of nonhandicapped children often label objects with their child-basic names rather than their adult-basic names. Thus, for nonhandicapped children, one could argue that maternal labeling practices were a major contributor to the formation of the predicted child-basic categories. Cardoso-Martins and C. B. Mervis (1985) found, however, that mothers of children with Down syndrome almost never used child-basic, rather than adult-basic, names when speaking to their child with Down syndrome. Thus, if these children also formed the predicted child-basic categories, that would provide strong evidence in favor of the view that child cognitive structures were the major contributor to the formation of the predicted child-basic categories. Unfortunately, neither of these studies included measures of the child's categories.

These studies provided the impetus to the longitudinal study, the results of which replicated those of the previous ones with regard to maternal labeling patterns. The most relevant analysis involved whether or not mothers labeled at least one of the child-basic-only objects with its child-basic name during the play period on the day the child first demonstrated comprehension of that name. The mothers of the non-handicapped children used the child-basic name to label at least one of the child-basic-only objects in 67% of the test cases. In contrast, the mothers of the children with Down syndrome used the child-basic name to label at least one of the child-basic-only objects in 31% of the test cases. Thus, in most cases for the children with Down syndrome, and in several cases for the nonhandicapped children, maternal labeling patterns provided no inkling of the existence of a child-basic category that was not identical to the corresponding adult-basic category. Nevertheless, both groups of children consistently formed the predicted child-basic categories. These results strongly support the position that initial child-basic categories are formed on the basis of child cognitive structures rather than maternal labeling input.

The stimuli used in the longitudinal study were chosen primarily to allow us to consider cases of predicted overgeneralization. Although objects that might potentially be excluded by a child but included by an adult (leading to undergeneralization or overlap) were added in the fifth play session, by this time some of the children with Down syndrome and most of the nonhandicapped children already comprehended all three category names. Thus, if undergeneralization is most likely when children first begin to form a category, potential instances of undergeneralization may have been missed, due to the late introduction of relevant objects. The results of other studies (e.g., Anglin, 1977; C. B. Mervis, 1987; Nelson, Rescorla, Gruendel, & Benedict, 1978) indicate that undergeneralization, and also overlap, often occur during the period of early lexical development. For all three types of relationship, when data concerning adult labeling input are available, comparison of the adult input and the extension of the child's category strongly suggests that the reason the children's categories are not identical to the corresponding adult categories is that the children are attending to or emphasizing different attributes or attribute values from the adults, for the same objects.

The results of analyses of those categories that were underextended over the course of the study indicate that the internal structure of the children's categories was determined separately from the internal structure of the corresponding adult categories. Five of the six children with Down syndrome evidenced some undergeneralization, as did two of the nonhandicapped children. In all cases, the same pattern was followed. The child excluded the poorest exemplar of the adult-basic category (as determined by adult ratings) and included all of the predicted child-basic-only objects (which were excluded from the adult-basic category, as determined by adult ratings). For adults, the percentage of subjects who consider a given object not to be a member of a particular category is highly negatively correlated with the goodness-of-example ratings assigned that object by subjects who do consider it a category member. Thus, objects that are excluded by some children should be considered poorer exemplars of the category than objects included by all children. The obtained results indicate that the goodness-of-example structure of the child-basic category is not composed simply of the goodness-of-example structure of the adult-basic category, with the child-basic-only objects tacked on as the poorest exemplars. For the category exemplars used in this study, the same objects served as poor exemplars for both children and adults. However, the nonexemplars from the adults' perspective (the predicted child-basic-only objects) were actually good or moderate exemplars from the children's perspective. Such results would be expected, if children are attending to or emphasizing different attributes or attribute values from adults, for the same object.

The effects of the initial exemplar on initial category composition cannot be considered on the basis of the results of this study. However, the results of other studies are relevant. As discussed above, C. B. Mervis and Pani (1980), in a study using novel artificial stimuli, found that nonhandicapped 5-year-olds tended to form reasonably accurate (by adult standards) categories when the initial exemplar presented was a good example, but tended to undergeneralize or not generalize at all when the initial exemplar was a poor example. The data from the diary study of my son's early lexical development indicate that two of his earliest words were seriously undergeneralized. In both cases, Ari's initial category was based on a poor exemplar (C. B. Mervis, 1987). There are no relevant data available concerning children with Down syndrome. However, there are data concerning severely and profoundly handicapped children and adolescents, functioning at Stage 6 of the sensorimotor period. Hupp and C. B. Mervis (1982) found that these children were able to generalize a category name to novel exemplars if the initial exemplar or exemplars were all good examples of the category. However, if both good and poor exemplars were presented initially, the children performed at chance levels on the generalization tests. The results of these studies suggest that children with Down syndrome also would be most likely to generalize a category accurately if the initial exemplar was a good example of its category. Undergeneralization or no generalization would be expected if the initial exemplar was a poor example of its category.

Evolution of initial child-basic categories

Initiation of category evolution

Many initial child-basic categories will not be identical to the corresponding adult-basic categories. When an adult is conversing with a child, there are four circumstances under which the adult can use the adult-basic label for an object the child does not include in its adult-basic category, thus providing the child with an opportunity to learn this label and to change his or her categorization scheme. First, the child might notice important attributes on his or her own, and then call these attributes to an adult's attention. The adult would be likely to respond by acknowledging the attribute that the child had indicated and then labeling the object with its adult-basic name. For example, the child might point out a round bank's slot to the mother, in which case she probably would respond by commenting on the slot and then labeling the object "bank."

If the child has not noticed these important attributes on his or her own (or if the adult does not realize the child has), the adult may choose to point them out. This may be accomplished in two ways. First, the adult can show the child a critical form attribute(s) and/or demonstrate a critical function attribute(s) of an object, which serve to make it a member of its adult-basic category. Coincident with this highlighting of a critical attribute, the adult may label the object with its adult-basic name. These illustrations often are accompanied by verbal descriptions. For example, the adult might run a finger along the slot of a round bank, drop in a coin, and tell the child that this is a slot into which you put money. The adult would then label the object "bank." Alternatively, the adult might provide a verbal description, without a concrete illustration. Both these strategies could be used either spontaneously or in response to the child's use of a child-basic name to label the object in question.

Finally, the adult may label the object with its adult-basic name without either an implied request from the child (the first circumstance described) or some form of explanation (the second and third circumstances). The use of an adult-basic label alone constitutes an implicit statement of the existence of attributes that make the object a member of the named category. This strategy may also be used spontaneously or as a correction of the child's use of a child-basic name to label the object in question.

The four circumstances under which the adult labels an object with its adult-basic name should be differentially associated with success at leading the child to comprehend the new adult-basic label and to begin to form a new category, or to extend the category to include objects previously excluded from it. Success should be most likely to occur if either the child points out a relevant attribute or the adult provides a concrete illustration. In these cases, because the important attributes have been made explicit in a concrete manner, even the very young child often is able to see that they form the basis for a new category, or, in the case of an initially undergeneralized category, the basis for assignment of the object to its appropriate category. Success when the adult provides a verbal explanation without a concrete illustration is less likely. The child probably will not understand the explanation. The success of this method should increase as the child's vocabulary size increases. Success when the adult uses an adult-basic label without either a request from the child or an explanation is considerably less likely for young children. If this object is already included in a different child-basic category, then success is extremely unlikely. The metacognition required to realize that categories should be altered simply because a different label is used is relatively sophisticated. However, if the object has not yet been assigned to any category, and the child already has the appropriate category for this object, success is more likely. Indeed, children eventually believe that all objects should belong to some category, and therefore "look" for a category to which the unassigned object could be assigned. In some cases, the child may even ask, "What's that?" in reference to an unassigned object. Success in these cases is very likely.

Relevant results. To best evaluate the predictions concerning the relationship between method of introduction of the adult-basic label for an object previously included in a child-basic category labeled by a different name and child acquisition of the new name, controlled experiments are necessary. K. Chapman, Leonard, and C. B. Mervis (1986) have conducted a longitudinal experimental study involving two of the four methods: introduction of the adult-basic label with concrete illustration and introduction of the adult-basic label alone (in this case, accompanied by a statement indicating explicitly that the child-basic name was incorrect). These methods were used as feedback for the child's use of the child-basic level. For example, if a child called a round bank, "ball," in the illustration plus label condition, the adult would respond, "That's a bank. See, it has a slot you can put money in" (while running a finger along the slot). In the label alone condition, the adult would respond, "That's not a ball. That's a bank." As expected, the results indicated that, for both comprehension and production, acquisition of the adult-basic label was more likely following use of the label plus illustration method than following use of the label alone method. Only nonhandicapped children participated in this study.

The data from the present longitudinal study, although necessarily correlational, nevertheless can be used to provide a preliminary assessment of the relative efficacy of the various methods of adult-basic label introduction for leading the child to acquire this label in reference to an object previously included in a child-basic category labeled by a different name. To provide such an assessment, I have examined the transcripts from the longitudinal study play periods for mother–child interactions with members of the child-basic (but not adult-basic) *ball* category. These objects are listed in Table 8.1. Across the six children with Down syndrome, there were 16 cases in which a child eventually comprehended the adult-basic name for an object previously included in the child-basic *ball* category. In every case, the mother provided a concrete illustration of crucial form and/or function attributes during the play period immediately preceding the comprehension test on which the child first comprehended the word in question. In one case, the mother's use of the adult-basic label was also immediately preceded by the child's demonstration of a crucial form attribute of the object. In the preceding sessions, mothers had hardly ever provided concrete illustrations when the adult-basic labels were used.

Across the six nonhandicapped children, there were 20 relevant cases. In 16 of them, the mother provided a concrete illustration of crucial form and/or function attributes in the play session preceding the comprehension test on which the relevant word first was comprehended. In 2 of the 16 cases, the mother's use of the adult-basic label was also immediately preceded by the child's demonstration of a crucial function attribute of the object. Three of the remaining four cases involved maternal provision of only a verbal description of crucial form and/or function attributes of the object. In the preceding sessions, mothers had hardly ever provided concrete illustrations when the adult-basic labels were used. Thus, the results for both the children with Down syndrome and the nonhandicapped children provide preliminary support for the hypothesis that acquisition of the adult-basic label for an object previously included in a child-basic category labeled by a different name is most likely to occur when crucial form and/or function attributes are highlighted (by either the child or the mother) at the time the mother labels the object with its adult-basic name. Acquisition is less likely to occur following adult use of the adult-basic name accompanied by a verbal description alone, and is even less likely to occur following adult use of the adult-basic label by itself.

Course of category evolution

The child is most likely to notice or acknowledge important form and/or function differences for those objects that are least similar to the best example of the child-basic category. (In general, these objects also will be the ones least similar to the best examples of the adult-basic category labeled by the same word as the child-basic category.) Therefore, when an initially overgeneralized child-basic category (or the overgeneralized part of an overlapped category) begins to evolve, new categories that are represented by the atypical members of the original child-basic category should emerge before new categories represented by the more typical members of the original category. For example, when breaking down an initial child-basic *kitty* category, the child should form a *lion* category before forming a *panther* category. Similarly, if all eventual members of a new child-basic category are not assigned to that category simultaneously, the objects least similar to the other members of the initial child-basic category should be assigned to the new category first. (In general, these objects will be the better examples of the new category.) For example, if a child does not assign all trucks to his or her new *truck* category simultaneously, the child should assign cement trucks before pickup trucks, because cement trucks are less similar to other members of the initial child-basic *car* category than pickup trucks are.

Comprehension of the adult-basic name for an object previously included in an initial child-basic category is the first step in the evolution of that category to conform to the adult-basic category labeled by the same word. It often has been argued (e.g., Barrett, 1978, 1982; Clark, 1973, 1983) that upon learning a more appropriate name for an object, the child immediately discards the former name. That is, the old and the new categories immediately become disjunctive. This claim is based on data from either diary studies (which actually contain a few contradictions; see Lewis, 1936; Merriman, 1987) or observations of play rather than on systematic testing. In contrast, I would like to argue that the complete separation of the two categories is gradual. The child, in considering the object that is changing category membership, at first finds two sets of attributes salient: the set that makes the object a member of the initial category and the set that makes the object a member of the new category. Consequently, the child includes the object in both categories. That is, the very young child does not have a principle that precludes the simultaneous assignment of objects to two basic-level categories. (Older children and adults generally operate according to such a principle; see Tversky & Hemenway, 1984.) For a child to decide that an object should be excluded from its initial category, he or she must decide that only the set of attributes that makes the object a member of the new category is important, or in the case of previously included false attributes, that the two sets of attributes are contradictory (e.g., that a single animal does not say both "meow" and "grr"). At this point, the separation of the two categories will be complete. It is not clear what causes the child to make this decision. (For some possible influences, see C. B. Mervis, 1984; 1987.)

In summary, many child-basic categories initially are not identical to the corresponding adult-basic categories. Evolution occurs because the child realizes that the object(s) that is misassigned or unassigned has important attributes that make it a member of the adult-basic category. Successful initiation of evolution, as defined by child comprehension of the adult-basic label in reference to the relevant object, is most likely under two circumstances: Either the child has realized the importance of the relevant attributes on his or her own and points them out to the adult, who responds by providing the object's adult-basic name; or the adult provides a concrete illustration of these attributes, accompanied by the object's adult-basic name. Once category breakdown begins, the separation of the new category from the initial child-basic category is gradual. This separation is completed only when the child realizes that the attributes that led him or her to include the object in the initial child-basic category are either irrelevant for that object or not true of that object. In many cases in which the child-basic category becomes broader, the child must realize that the acceptable range of values for one or more important form and/or function attributes is larger than he or she previously had thought. In other cases, the child must realize that attributes he or she previously had considered irrelevant for the category in fact are relevant.

Relevant results. The course of evolution of the categories of both the children with Down syndrome and the nonhandicapped children correspond extremely well to the predicted course; see C. B. Mervis (1984) for detailed analyses. To illustrate this course, the evolution of the *ball* category of one child with Down syndrome will be described. The evolution of this category is presented in Table 8.2. At the end of the study, Myra's (a pseudonym) *ball* category had not yet completely evolved to correspond to the adult categorization scheme. This incomplete evolution was characteristic; across the two groups of children, complete evolution occurred for only 4 of the 34 initial child-basic categories.

Myra first comprehended "ball" when she was 20½ months old. Her initial *ball* category corresponded perfectly to the predicted child-basic category. The category

Table 8.2. *Evolution of Myra's initial* ball *category*

| | Category | | | |
	Ball	Football	Bell	Bank
Age[a]				
19 months	—			
20½ months	ball ornament bank bell			
23 months	ball bead[b] ornament bank bell			
24½ months	ball bead ornament bank bell		bell	
27½ months	ball football[c] bead ornament candle[c] bank bell		bell	
33 months	ball football bead ornament candle bank		bell	bank
34½ months[d]	ball football bead ornament candle	football	bell	bank

Note: This table is based on data from the comprehension tests.

[a] Age at which the category pattern first was obtained. (Note that throughout the study, all changes in categories represented progress toward the adult standard; no regressions occurred.)

[b] The bead was introduced at this visit.

[c] The football and the candle were introduced at this visit.

[d] This pattern was present until the end of the study, when Myra was 38½ months old.

began to evolve when Myra was 24½ months old. Two categories eventually emerged from *ball:* first *bell* and then *bank.* This order of emergence corresponds to the predicted order, based on adult judgments of how much each child-basic-only object was "like a ball." As predicted, *bell* and *bank* did not separate immediately from the *ball* category. That is, the categories at first were not considered mutually exclusive. The round bell was considered to be both a bell and a ball for several months; the round bank was considered to be both a bank and a ball for several weeks. This initial overlap was, as predicted, a general pattern for both groups of children. Overall, for categories emerging from any of the three initial child-basic categories, membership in the new and old categories initially was simultaneous in 93% of the tests cases for the children with Down syndrome and in 96% of the test cases for the nonhandicapped children. The predicted order of complete separation of categories from the initial child-basic *ball* category is identical to the predicted order of acquisition of the adult-basic categories. For Myra, the order of complete separation was the same as the order of initial acquisition. Thus, this order corresponded exactly to the predicted one.

Summary

Consideration of the evidence concerning early conceptual development, as measured by lexical methods, strongly supports the proposed theory of early lexical development, for both children with Down syndrome and nonhandicapped children. Furthermore, once again, as with the qualitative aspects of the vocabularies of the two groups of children, the similarity between qualitative aspects of conceptual development for the two groups of children is striking. Despite important differences in maternal labeling patterns, both the children with Down syndrome and the nonhandicapped children formed the predicted child-basic categories. This result suggests that the cognitive structures underlying early categorization are the same for both groups of children. The available evidence suggests that the internal structure of these categories is the same for the two groups of children, while differing from that for adults. The most effective method of introduction of a new label for an object already considered a member of a category labeled by a different name was the same for both groups of children. Finally, the course of evolution of an initial child-basic category was qualitatively the same for both groups.

Relationship between cognitive development and lexical development

The data from the longitudinal study are useful for investigating the relationship between cognitive development and vocabulary acquisition, for both comprehension and production, for a selected set of object words. As indicated in an earlier section, a comparison of Gillham's (1979) data concerning the early words of children with Down syndrome with the data obtained in studies of the early words of nonhandicapped children shows that the early productive vocabularies of the two groups of children are strikingly similar. At the same time, however, Gillham mentioned that rate of vocabulary acquisition was much slower for the children with Down syndrome than for the nonhandicapped children. This comment appears to have been based on a real-time comparison of rates of acquisition by the two groups of children. Differences in real-time rates might be expected, simply on the basis that rate of cognitive development is slower for the children with Down syndrome than for the nonhandicapped children. No studies of rate of productive vocabulary acquisition, adjusted for rate of cognitive development, have been conducted. There have been no studies of the early receptive vocabularies of children with Down syndrome. Thus, previous research does not provide insight into the relationship between rate of early vocabulary development and rate of cognitive development, for children with Down syndrome as compared to nonhandicapped children. The results of studies with older children and adults who had Down syndrome, however, indicate that the levels of language development (for both vocabulary and syntax) evidenced by these persons were less than would be expected based on their levels of cognitive development (e.g., Evans & Hampson, 1969; Lyle, 1959, 1960; Share, 1975; M. M. Thompson, 1963).

Based on the data from the longitudinal study, we were able to make two sets of comparison, each considering comprehension and production separately. First, we compared the levels of cognitive development of the children with Down syndrome and the nonhandicapped children, at the time referential acquisition of object names first was demonstrated. Second, we compared the vocabulary sizes of the two groups of children at comparable levels of cognitive development. The results of these analyses are summarized here; for a more detailed description, see Cardoso-Martins, C. B. Mervis, and C. A. Mervis (1985).

Cognitive level at the emergence of language

To determine the children's cognitive levels at the emergence of comprehension and production, two sets of measures were used. The first measure was the estimated mental age of the child, derived from a regression equation computed based on the child's Bayley (1969) test scores. Estimated mental age was determined separately for the first visit on which referential comprehension was demonstrated and the first visit on which referential production was demonstrated. The second measure was the child's level of sensorimotor cognitive development at these visits. This level was determined separately for object permanence and means–ends relations, based on the stage represented by the most advanced item passed on the relevant Uzgiris and Hunt (1975) subscale. Dunst's (1980) stage assignments were used.

At the time referential comprehension first was demonstrated, the mean mental age of the children with Down syndrome was 14.5 months (range: 13.3–15.2 months). The mean mental age of the nonhandicapped children was 13.8 months (range: 12.6–15.3 months). At the time referential production first was demonstrated, the mean mental age of the children with Down syndrome was 18.9 months (range:

16.6–21.5 months). The mean mental age of the nonhandicapped children was 19.5 months (range: 16.2–24.1 months). The mean mental ages and the range of mental ages for the two groups are strikingly similar. The mental age data for the children with Down syndrome are corroborated by the data Abrahamsen, Cavallo, and McCluer (1985) obtained in a training study concerned with the acquisition of manual signs. Four children with Down syndrome participated in this study. Three did not acquire referential use of any manual signs, despite training. The highest mental age for a child in this group was 15–16 months. The fourth child did acquire referential use of some manual signs; his mental age was 19 months.

At the time referential comprehension first was demonstrated, three of the children with Down syndrome were in Stage 5 of object permanence development; the remaining three were in Stage 6. Four of the nonhandicapped children were in Stage 5; the other two were in Stage 6. All the children in both groups were in Stage 5 of means–ends relations development. At the time referential production first was demonstrated, all of the children in both groups were in Stage 6 of object permanence development. For means–ends relations development, five children from each group were in Stage 5; the remaining child in each group was in Stage 6. Thus, the sensorimotor cognitive development of the two groups was virtually identical, at both the onset of comprehension and the onset of production. The sensorimotor stages of the children in the longitudinal study correspond to those previously reported for these language landmarks (e.g., R. S. Chapman, 1978; Corrigan, 1978; Folger & Leonard, 1978; Ingram, 1978; Ramsey, 1978).

Vocabulary sizes at different levels of cognitive development

To consider the children's rate of vocabulary development relative to their rate of cognitive development, we compared the vocabulary sizes of the children with Down syndrome and the nonhandicapped children at various mental ages and levels of sensorimotor development. We were able to consider four 2-month mental age ranges for which all children attained the requisite mental age during the course of the study: 13.0–14.9; 15.0–16.9; 17.0–18.9; 19.0–20.9. Within each of these ranges, we selected the visits at which the children with Down syndrome and their nonhandicapped matches had the most similar estimated mental ages. The differences between the estimated mental ages of the two children in a pair was never greater than .7 month. For each of these mental age ranges, the vocabulary sizes of the two groups of children were similar, whether measured by comprehension or by production.

However, a different pattern was obtained when sensorimotor cognitive development was considered. For object permanence, the children with Down syndrome comprehended fewer object names than the nonhandicapped children did, upon complete attainment of Stage 5, upon entry into Stage 6, and upon complete attainment of Stage 6. The differences for complete attainment of Stage 5 and complete attainment of Stage 6 were significant. Upon completion of Stage 6, the children with Down syndrome also produced significantly fewer object names than the non-handicapped children did. For means–ends relations, upon complete attainment of Stage 5, the children with Down syndrome comprehended and produced fewer words than the nonhandicapped children; the difference for comprehension was significant. Comparisons at the time of entry into Stage 6 and complete attainment of Stage 6 fit the same pattern, although too few children with Down syndrome reached these points during the course of the study to justify statistical analyses.

The results of a larger-scale study of eighty-one 36-month-olds with Down syndrome suggest that the differences found between the two groups in rate of vocabulary development as a function of rate of sensorimotor cognitive development also might have been obtained for mental age, had either more children been considered or the children's entire vocabularies, rather than just a subset of their vocabularies, been studied. Strominger et al. (1984) reported that the average vocabulary size of the children in their study was 18.5 words at age 36 months. The range of vocabulary sizes was from 0 to 85 words. The average vocabulary size of a nonhandicapped 36-month-old is 1,222 words (M. E. Smith, 1926). At 36 months chronological age, the average mental age of the children with Down syndrome in their study, as measured by performance on the Bayley test, was 20.6 months (Schnell, 1984). The average vocabulary size of a nonhandicapped 21-month-old is 118 (M. E. Smith, 1926). Thus, even when the children with Down syndrome and the nonhandicapped children are equated for mental age, the vocabularies of the children with Down syndrome are considerably smaller than those of the nonhandicapped children. Note, however, that the average vocabulary size for a nonhandicapped 18-month-old is 22 (M. E. Smith, 1926). This size is not much larger than that reported for the children with Down syndrome. The nonhandicapped children apparently have a spurt in vocabulary size between 18 and 21 months (see also Anisfeld, 1984). Thus, it appears that an important reason for the large discrepancy in vocabulary size between the two groups, even when they are on average equated for mental age, is that the nonhandicapped children are beginning their vocabulary spurt at a younger mental age than the children with Down syndrome.

The difference between the two groups of children in rate of vocabulary acquisition is probably due in part to specific cognitive deficits that children with Down syndrome may have. Deficits in both storage abilities (McDade & Adler, 1980) and retrieval abilities (Dodd, 1975; McDade & Adler, 1980) have been reported. In addition, Bilovsky and Share (1975) have found that children with Down syndrome have difficulty in encoding and decoding verbal stimuli. Because learning of vocabulary necessarily requires use of memory, problems in storing and retrieving information would be likely to hinder vocabulary acquisition. The difference in rate of vocabulary acquisition probably also is due to differences in maternal speech to the two groups of children. Several such differences are considered in the next section. An additional important potential difference concerns the likelihood that the mother will use the most effective strategies for teaching new vocabulary. In the previous section, it was shown that both children with Down syndrome and nonhandicapped children were most likely to learn new vocabulary when mothers provided concrete illustrations of critical attributes along with the new word. There is preliminary evidence from our longitudinal study that mothers of children with Down syndrome may be less likely to use this strategy than mothers of nonhandicapped children.

Summary

For the first time in the course of this chapter, a potentially important difference between the children with Down syndrome and the nonhandicapped children has been described. The children with Down syndrome acquired vocabulary at a rate significantly slower than would be expected, even when rate of cognitive development is taken into account. This result was obtained in our longitudinal study when measures of sensorimotor cognitive development were used. Further, a comparison of the results obtained by Strominger et al. (1984) with the vocabulary sizes reported by M. E. Smith (1926) yields the same finding for mental age. Note that McCarthy (1954) has suggested that M. E. Smith may have systematically underestimated the vocabulary sizes of the children in her study; thus, the actual differences between the children with Down syndrome and the nonhandicapped children may be even greater than reported above. The largest difference found in the comparisons involving sensorimotor cognitive development was obtained when vocabulary size upon complete attainment of Stage 6 of object permanence was considered. Corrigan (1978) has speculated that the vocabulary spurt for nonhandicapped children begins at about this time. The complete attainment of object permanence Stage 6 should occur at a mental age of about 21 months, which is about the chronological age at which the vocabulary spurt occurred for the children in M. E. Smith's study. Thus, these results combined suggest that a major reason for the large differences in size of vocabulary between children with Down syndrome and nonhandicapped children is that the vocabulary spurt for the children with Down syndrome does not begin at the mental age that would be expected, based on the findings concerning nonhandicapped children. Differences between the two groups of children in rate of vocabulary acquisition probably are due to both specific cognitive deficits that children with Down syndrome may have and linguistic input that is not optimal for vocabulary acquisition. Research with nonhandicapped children (e.g., Anisfeld, 1984) indicates that these children acquire a considerable number of words before syntactic acquisition begins. Thus, the problems that children with Down syndrome have with early vocabulary acquisition may lead to a further delay in the onset of syntax.

At the same time, it is important to note that the onset of referential language, whether measured by comprehension or production, occurred at the same level of cognitive development for the two groups of children. This was true both for measures of mental age and measures of sensorimotor development, as reflected in object permanence and means–ends relations development.

Maternal linguistic style and early lexical development

Maternal linguistic style

When mothers talk with their young nonhandicapped children, two different styles emerge (McDonald & Pien, 1982). Some mothers use a directive style, reflecting an intention to control the child's behavior. Other mothers use a conversational-eliciting style, reflecting an intention to elicit the child's participation in the conversation. McDonald and Pien have argued that there is a cluster of maternal language features associated with each style and that the two styles are incompatible. Thus, directive mothers seldom should engage in behaviors characteristic of the conversational-eliciting style. Mothers motivated by the intention to elicit conversation from the child seldom should attempt to control the child's behavior.

McDonald and Pien (1982) suggested that the directive style may be less adequate for fostering language development than the conversational-eliciting style. The results of studies investigating the impact of maternal language on language acquisition by nonhandicapped children suggest that certain features of the directive style (e.g., use of directives) may be detrimental for early language development (Nelson, 1973; Newport, Gleitman, & Gleitman, 1977). In contrast, certain features of the conversational-eliciting style (e.g., questions, comments on the child's activity or verbalization) correlate positively with measures of child language growth (Cross, 1978; Furrow, Benedict, & Nelson, 1979; Nelson, 1973; Newport et al., 1977).

Mothers of young children with Down syndrome use more commands than mothers of nonhandicapped children, whether the children are matched on chronological age, mental age, or language level (e.g., Buium, Rynders, & Turnure, 1974; Cardoso-Martins & C. B. Mervis, 1985; Weistuch, 1983). Relatively frequent use of commands clearly is associated with the directive style. It would seem likely, then, that mothers of children with Down syndrome also would use other language features characteristic of the directive style more frequently than mothers of nonhandicapped children. In addition, if, as McDonald and Pien (1982) argue, the two styles are incompatible, mothers of children with Down syndrome should be less likely than mothers of nonhandicapped children to use language features characteristic of the conversational-eliciting style.

Analysis of the transcripts of the play session tapes from our longitudinal study indicates that mothers of young children with Down syndrome are in fact more likely than mothers of young nonhandicapped children to use language features characteristic of the directive style of interaction and less likely to use language features characteristic of the conversational-eliciting style of interaction. The results of the analyses leading to this conclusion are summarized here; a more detailed description is presented in Cardoso-Martins and C. B. Mervis (1984, 1985). The language of the mothers was compared for each of five different play sessions during the study. At each of these sessions, the children with Down syndrome had similar estimated mental ages and similar receptive and productive vocabulary sizes to the nonhandicapped children.

The mothers of the children with Down syndrome were significantly more likely than the mothers of the nonhandicapped children to use the following language features characteristic of the directive style: requests for an action; prompts for an action; overall use of directives; and negative feedback for the child's vocalization. The mothers of the nonhandicapped children were significantly more likely to use one language feature characteristic of the directive style: test questions. The mothers of the nonhandicapped children were significantly more likely to use the following language features characteristic of the conversational eliciting style: real questions; action-reflective questions; verbalization-reflective questions; low constraint questions; positive feedback for the child's action; positive feedback for the child's verbalization; and overall positive feedback. The mothers of the children with Down syndrome were significantly more likely to use one characteristic of the conversational-eliciting style: vocalization-reflective questions.

The results of these analyses clearly point to a potentially important difference between mothers of children with Down syndrome and mothers of nonhandicapped children. Mothers of children with Down syndrome tend to use a directive style of interacting with their child, while mothers of nonhandicapped children tend to use a conversational-eliciting style of interaction. In the present context, this difference would be important if it were the case that the early acquisition of vocabulary was facilitated by maternal use of features associated with the conversational-eliciting style and/or hindered by maternal use of features associated with the directive style. The effect of certain maternal language features on early vocabulary acquisition is considered next. Afterward, some possible reasons for differences in maternal linguistic style between mothers of children with Down syndrome and mothers of nonhandicapped children are discussed.

Impact of maternal linguistic style on rate of lexical development

The results of the previous analyses indicated clearly that when talking with their children, mothers of children with Down syndrome used a different interaction style than mothers of nonhandicapped children did. Before considering the potential effects of these style differences on rate of lexical development by children with Down syndrome, however, a second variable concerning maternal linguistic behavior must be considered: semantic contingency of the child's linguistic or nonlinguistic behavior. It is quite possible that semantic contingency, rather than nondirectiveness per se, is the relevant maternal linguistic variable affecting early language acquisition (see Cross, 1978). The positive effects found for the conversational-eliciting style in previous research with nonhandicapped children have probably derived from the fact that most of the language features characteristic of this style of interaction refer to the child's behavior or focus of attention. On the other hand, the language features characteristic of the directive style of interaction do not, in general, refer to the child's behavior or focus of attention. It therefore makes sense that a high incidence of these language features would have a negative impact on language acquisition. However, directiveness does not co-occur automatically with lack of semantic contingency to the child's behavior. A few features characteristic of the directive style are semantically contingent on the child's behavior. In the present study, the mothers of the children with Down syndrome were significantly more likely than the mothers of the nonhandicapped children to use one such feature, negative feedback for the child's vocalization. Similarly, a few features characteristic of the conversational-eliciting style frequently do not refer to the child's behavior. In the present study, the mothers of the nonhandicapped children were significantly more likely to use one such feature, real questions. The pattern of results obtained in the analyses reported below can be used to address the question of whether any negative impact of maternal linguistic input on rate of vocabulary acquisition by children with Down syndrome is due to directiveness per se or to lack of semantic contingency on the child's behavior. Again, the results of these analyses are summarized here; a more complete account is provided in Cardoso-Martins and C. B. Mervis (1988).

The impact of maternal linguistic input on rate of vocabulary acquisition by children with Down syndrome was addressed through correlational analyses. Measures of maternal language taken from a visit occurring about halfway through the study were correlated with two measures of child language: cumulative number of different object names comprehended through the last visit in which all of the children with Down syndrome participated, and cumulative number of different object names produced through that visit. Third order partial correlations were used: child estimated mental age, receptive vocabulary size, and productive vocabulary size at the visit from which the maternal language measures were taken were partialed out of the correlations between measures of maternal language and the measures of child vocabulary acquisition.

Because we were interested in determining the impact of the style of interaction adopted by the mothers of the children with Down syndrome on vocabulary acquisition by these children, the maternal language features that differentiated between the two groups of mothers were chosen for inclusion in the correlational analyses. Because of the small number of subjects, the results should be considered suggestive. Nevertheless, a consistent pattern of results emerged. This pattern fit the semantic contingency explanation better than the directive style explanation. Two features were significantly negatively correlated with rate of child receptive or productive vocabulary acquisition: overall use of directives and real questions. The first of these features is associated with the directive style, but the second is associated with the conversational-eliciting style. Both features are associated with semantic noncontingency. Three features were significantly positively correlated with rate of vocabulary acquisition: positive feedback for the child's verbalization, overall positive feedback, and negative feedback for the child's vocalization. The first two of these features are associated with the conversational-eliciting style, but the third is associated with the directive style. All three are associated with semantic contingency on the child's behavior.

The basis for the positive impact of language features that generally are semantic contingent and the negative impact of language features that generally are semantically noncontingent is clear. The language features associated with semantic contingency include frequent references to the object of the child's attention. Therefore, these language features should make the relation between the object word and its referent particularly salient to the child, thus facilitating vocabulary acquisition. On the other hand, the language features associated with semantic noncontingency generally do not make the word-referent relation clear to the child, because these language features seldom include references to the focus of the child's attention. Roth's (1984) study of the relationship between maternal linguistic style and speed of maternal response to her nonhandicapped child's initiatives suggests that there are problems with a noncontingent style that extend beyond those just mentioned. Roth found a very strong positive correlation between the proportion of semantically contingent maternal utterances and the proportion of all maternal responses that occurred within one second of the child's initiative. Roth presents evidence that responses occurring more than one second after the child's initiative are likely to be much less valuable for the acquisition of vocabulary than are utterances occurring after a shorter delay. Rapid responses are particularly important because they maximize the probability that the response, assuming it is semantically contingent on the child's prior initiative, occurs while the child still is attending to the relevant object. Thus, mothers who adopt a semantically noncontingent style appear further to decrease the value of their input for vocabulary acquisition by taking too long to respond to their child, even when the response is semantically contingent.

Basis for differences in maternal linguistic style

Differences in maternal interactional intent probably in part explain the differences in linguistic style found between the mothers of the children with Down syndrome and the mothers of the nonhandicapped children. Bell (1964; Bell & Harper, 1977) and Jones (1977, 1979, 1980) have found that mothers of young nonhandicapped children tend to follow the child's initiatives when interacting with the child. Thus, these mothers would be expected to use a conversational-eliciting style of interaction. In contrast, Bell has found that mothers of children with handicaps are much less likely to follow their child's initiatives, and much more likely to expect the child to follow their initiatives. Jones has obtained the same result for mothers of children with Down syndrome. In addition, Jones (1980) has suggested that mothers of handicapped children may believe that their child needs more direction than nonhandicapped children do. These mothers may therefore feel more motivated than mothers of nonhandicapped children to direct their child's behavior.

Child factors also are important. The differences between the two groups of mothers probably reflect, in part, adaptive responses by the mothers of the children with Down syndrome to their children's handicaps. Children with Down syndrome often have been described as more passive and less socially responsive than nonhandicapped children (e.g., Buckhalt, Rutherford, & Goldberg, 1978; Jones, 1977, 1979,

1980). In addition, children with Down syndrome do not use language as often as nonhandicapped children do (Cardoso-Martins, 1984; Cardoso-Martins, C. B. Mervis, & C. A. Mervis, 1983; Gillham, 1979). It is possible, therefore, that mothers of children with Down syndrome feel less motivated than mothers of nonhandicapped children to try to elicit their child's participation in the conversation.

The results of a series of analyses we recently conducted support this possibility. When children first begin to talk, the only way that their mothers can elicit "conversation" from the child is to ask the child a "What's that?" type of question. The mothers of the children with Down syndrome asked (nonsignificantly) fewer of these questions than the mothers of the nonhandicapped children, even when only the play sessions beginning with the one in which the child first demonstrated referential production are considered. Moreover, those "What's that?" questions that the mothers of the children with Down syndrome did ask were significantly less likely than those asked by the mothers of the nonhandicapped children to refer to objects whose labels were included in the child's productive vocabulary. Of the "What's that?" questions addressed to the children with Down syndrome, 54% were asked in reference to an object for which the child could produce an appropriate label and 46% were asked in reference to an object for which the child could not. For the questions addressed to the nonhandicapped children, the corresponding figures were 69% and 31%. Interestingly, the percentage of "What's that?" questions that were answered correctly, given that the child could produce an appropriate label, was virtually identical for the two groups of children: 14% for the children with Down syndrome and 15% for the nonhandicapped children. Thus, when given the opportunity, the children with Down syndrome were as likely as the nonhandicapped children to hold up the child's end of the conversation.

Thus, both maternal factors and child factors probably are involved in the different styles adopted by the mothers of the two groups of children. At the same time, the mothers of the children with Down syndrome varied widely among themselves in how directive their speech to their child was. Corresponding variation was obtained in how semantically contingent on their child's behavior the speech of the mothers of the children with Down syndrome was. Ultimately, semantically contingent speech facilitated vocabulary acquisition by the children with Down syndrome. More research on the basis for use of the directive style in speech to children with Down syndrome clearly is needed. Individual differences analyses that address the question of why certain mothers are more likely than others to use semantically contingent speech to their child with Down syndrome would be particularly useful.

Category knowledge of older children

Virtually no research is available concerning the category knowledge of older children with Down syndrome. Tager-Flusberg (1985a, 1985b; 1986; results from the 1985b paper were described in a previous section) has conducted the only studies on this topic. Three groups of children participated in these studies: autistic children, mentally retarded nonautistic children, and nonhandicapped children. All groups were matched on scores on the Peabody Picture Vocabulary Test–Revised (Dunn & Dunn, 1981). Mean vocabulary ages were 5 years 2 months, 4 years 11 months, and 5 years 0 months for the three groups, respectively. Mean chronological ages were 10 years 5 months, 11 years 6 months, and 4 years 7 months. The mentally retarded group included children with a variety of etiologies. Five of these children had Down syndrome (Tager-Flusberg, personal communication, 1984). I was unable to obtain the data for the children with Down syndrome separately from the other children in the mentally retarded nonautistic group, but Tager-Flusberg has stated (personal communication, 1984) that the data for the children with Down syndrome were parallel to those for the mentally retarded group as a whole. Because data specifically on the children with Down syndrome are not available, the results of the studies are summarized here, rather than described in detail.

As mentioned in a previous section, categories are characterized by gradients of goodness-of-example: Some members of the category are more representative of that category than other members are. For example, a hammer is more representative of the category *tool* than a clamp is. Similarly, a dump truck is more representative of the category *truck* than a pickup truck is. Given the internal structure of categories, one would expect the probability that a child would include an object in a category to be a positive function of the goodness-of-example of that object in that category (C. B. Mervis, 1980). Children consistently should include good examples of the category in the category, because these exemplars are both the most representative of their own categories and the least similar (in general) to members of related categories. Thus, when children's categories are not identical to adult categories, the most frequent errors should be either undergeneralization involving exclusion of the peripheral members of the category, or overgeneralization involving inclusion of related nonmembers of the category. (Instances in which overlap would be more likely were discussed in a previous section; such instances should involve primarily younger children, as described in that section.) This pattern of results has been obtained in a large number of students of nonhandicapped children ranging in age from 2 years to 12 years (e.g., Anglin, 1977, for young children; results for children 5 years to 12 years are described in C. B. Mervis, 1980).

The data from Tager-Flusberg's studies provide a test of this prediction for 11-year-old children with Down syndrome. Tager-Flusberg conducted several studies relevant to this prediction, involving measures of both comprehension (1985b) and nonverbal categorization abilities (match-to-sample; 1985a). These studies involved basic level categories and superordinate categories; subordinate categories were not considered. The results indicated clearly that children with Down syndrome are able to form both basic and superordinate categories. Further, the categories of the children with Down syndrome are similar to those of the nonhandicapped children, as were the categories formed by the autistic children. The results of three separate studies confirmed the prediction based on category structure. In these studies, the children with Down syndrome were most likely to include as members pictures of objects that had been considered good examples of the category by adults. These children also were more likely to include peripheral members of the category than related nonmembers, and more likely to include related nonmembers than unrelated nonmembers. All these differences consistently were statistically significant. When errors of categorization were made, the two most frequent patterns were the expected ones: undergeneralization involving exclusion of peripheral examples, and overgeneralization involving inclusion of related nonmembers. Similar results were obtained for both the nonhandicapped children and the autistic children. Very few differences in the categories formed were found among the three groups of children.

These results pointed to another qualitative similarity between the conceptual development of children with Down syndrome and nonhandicapped children. In this case, the similarity is shared by autistic children as well. The categories evidenced by all three groups of children were structured according to prediction: Good examples by adult standards were more likely to be included in the children's categories than peripheral examples were. The pattern of overgeneralization and undergeneralization errors also correspond to the predicted one.

Conclusion

As the research reviewed in this chapter indicates, there is substantial overlap between the conceptual development of children with Down syndrome and that of nonhandicapped children. At the same time, important differences also have emerged. In this final section, I review these results in reference to three important questions. First, what have we learned about conceptual development, from a theoretical perspective, that we would not have known if data concerning children with Down syndrome had not been available? Second, what have we learned about the conceptual development of children with Down syndrome? Third, based on the answers to the first two questions, what suggestions can be made concerning the facilitation of conceptual development by children with Down syndrome?

Benefits of comparative research from a theoretical perspective

When considering the benefits of research on the conceptual development of children with Down syndrome from a theoretical perspective, two separate issues must be addressed. First, what have we learned about the universality of conceptual development, that transcends differences in intelligence? Second, what have we learned, beyond universality, that could not have been learned simply by the study of nonhandicapped children?

Universal aspects. Our knowledge of universal aspects of conceptual development has been enhanced greatly by consideration of the conceptual development of children with Down syndrome. Advances have been made concerning universal aspects of children's early vocabularies, early category development, and later category development. In all these cases, theoretical predictions concerning universality had been made, or universality had been assumed, but virtually no relevant data were available.

The research indicates three major similarities between children with Down syndrome and nonhandicapped children concerning qualitative aspects of early vocabularies. All three are strong candidates for universality. First, both young children with Down syndrome and young nonhandicapped children accept the whole-object hypothesis concerning the meaning of novel words. In particular, young children initially believe that when a person points at or otherwise indicates an object for which the child does not already have a name, the accompanying word refers to the whole object rather than to some attribute of that object. This finding is especially important because all theories of early lexical development have postulated this principle as the means of disambiguating deictic utterances or gestures. Second, the initial vocabularies of both groups of children are concentrated on the same limited subset of categories, and the particular words chosen from these categories often are identical. As predicted by several theorists, these words are labels for objects that either are capable of moving independently or that can be manipulated by the child. Finally, the initial set of concrete nouns acquired by both groups of children consists almost entirely of names for basic level categories. These categories are considered to be more fundamental than categories at other levels of abstraction, and therefore have been predicted to be acquired first. The input language provided by parents is concordant with many of the propensities shown by both groups of children. This concordance is undoubtedly helpful for vocabulary acquisition. However, the child is not responding simply to the input he or she receives. Instead, the young child selects from the available input those words that he or she decides refer to categories of interesting objects, and assigns those words accordingly. The sometimes dramatic errors that young children make concerning the referents of words (e.g., that "hot" is the label for cuplike objects) are testimony to the independent operation of the child's cognitive structures.

Several similarities, and potential universals, also have emerged from a comparative consideration of early categorization. The most important similarities are reiterated here. As noted, the early object words of both children with Down syndrome and nonhandicapped children are labels for basic level categories. However, these child-basic categories often are not isomorphic to the adult-basic categories labeled by the same name. The child-basic categories formed by the two groups of children are identical. As predicted, these categories are based on the shape–function principle of basic level category formation, applied from the young child's perspective. The internal structure of these child-basic categories is the same for both groups of children and, as predicted, is based on the child's application of category formation principles, rather than simply on linguistic input. For both groups of children, introduction of a new word as a name for an object that the child already includes in a category labeled by a different word is most successful if adult use of the word is accompanied by a concrete illustration of critical form and/or function attributes that make the object a member of the category labeled by the new word. The particular success of this method with young children was predicted; changes in categorization should occur when the child changes the attributes that he or she attends to or emphasizes, rather than simply because the child hears the object labeled with a different word. Such changes are most likely to occur when the relevant attributes are pointed out to the child explicitly, rather than when their existence only is implied.

A comparative consideration of category development by older children also yielded a major qualitative similarity, suggesting the universality of an important principle of category development. Both children with Down syndrome and nonhandicapped children are more likely to include good examples of a category in that category than to include poorer examples. This result was predicted based on the category structure principles of family resemblance and contrast set. In addition, the patterns of overgeneralization and undergeneralization that were predicted based on these principles were obtained for both groups of children.

Addressing other theoretical issues. Data concerning the conceptual development of children with Down syndrome are invaluable beyond addressing issues of universality. In certain cases, data relevant to particular theoretical claims cannot be obtained from nonhandicapped children. The research reviewed in this chapter can be used to address two such claims that I and my colleagues have made. First, I have argued that children's initial categories are determined by the children's cognitive structures rather than by the labeling patterns of their mothers. It is difficult to address this question based on data obtained from mother–nonhandicapped child dyads. This is because although the categories the children form differ in the predicted ways from the corresponding adult categories, the mothers often label objects with the name that is appropriate from the child's perspective rather than the adult perspective. This labeling pattern occurs even before the child demonstrates comprehension of the category name. Therefore, for nonhandicapped middle-class children, the child cognitive structures hypothesis and the maternal labels hypothesis both predict the same categories for the child. However, because the labeling patterns of mothers of children with Down syndrome in general differ systematically from those of mothers of nonhandicapped children, data from mother–child with Down syndrome dyads can be used to address the category-basis issue. Mothers of children with Down syndrome almost always label objects with the names that would be appropriate from an adult perspective. Therefore, examination of the initial categories formed by children with Down syndrome may provide a critical test. The results of this analysis indicated that the children with Down syndrome formed the categories predicted based on the child cognitive structures hypothesis, despite labeling input that corresponded to the adult categories rather than the child categories. This result provides strong support for the hypothesis that children's initial categories are determined by children's cognitive structures, rather than by the labels adults provide for objects.

Second, Cardoso-Martins and I have argued that rate of early vocabulary development is enhanced by maternal linguistic input that is semantically contingent on the child's linguistic or nonlinguistic behavior. Although occasional suggestive evidence, particularly for later linguistic development, has been obtained from data on mother–nonhandicapped child interaction, the results generally have been weak.

Indeed, correlational analyses based on maternal speech to the nonhandicapped children in the longitudinal study reported above indicated virtually no effects (Cardoso-Martins, 1984). Two explanations for these noneffects have been offered. First, there is not enough variability in the speech of mothers of nonhandicapped children to expect differential effects on vocabulary development. Second, the minimum threshold for input to nonhandicapped children is so low that all mothers provide it routinely, as evidenced by the rapid rate of vocabulary acquisition by nonhandicapped children. Given these explanations, research involving mothers and their children with Down syndrome is ideally suited to addressing the input effects issue. There is substantial variability among mothers of children with Down syndrome regarding linguistic input. In addition, the minimum threshold for input to children with Down syndrome is likely to be higher than for nonhandicapped children. The results of partial correlational analyses involving measures of maternal linguistic interaction features and child vocabulary size several months later are consistent with the position that there are strong positive effects of features associated with semantic contingency and negative effects of features associated with semantic noncontingency. Further, these analyses indicate that use of a directive style per se does not have a negative impact on early vocabulary development; the relevant variable instead is semantic contingency on the child's behavior.

Conceptual development of children with Down syndrome

In many important respects, the conceptual development of children with Down syndrome parallels that of nonhandicapped children, as just described. Thus, the concrete nouns included in the early vocabularies of children with Down syndrome are labels for specific types of basic level categories: those composed of objects that either can move independently or can be manipulated by the child. Children with Down syndrome use the whole-word hypothesis to help them determine the meanings of novel words. The children's initial basic level categories are determined according to the shape–function principle, the same principle that serves as the basis for adult-basic categories. However, because children apply this principle from a child perspective rather than an adult perspective, the child-basic categories often differ in predictable ways from the corresponding adult-basic categories. The basis for the categories of the children with Down syndrome derives from the child's cognitive structures, rather than from the labels the mother uses. Children with Down syndrome begin to comprehend language referentially at a mental age of approximately 13–15 months, during Stages 5 or 6 of object permanence development and Stage 5 of means–ends relations development. These children begin to produce language referentially at a mental age of approximately 17–21 months, during Stage 6 of object permanence development and Stages 5 or 6 of means–ends relations development. Rate of vocabulary development is positively correlated with the use of semantically contingent utterances by the mother. Older children with Down syndrome are most likely to include good examples of a category in the category and less likely to include more peripheral examples. Overextension is likely to involve inclusion of peripheral examples of related categories.

However, the conceptual development of children with Down syndrome differs from that of nonhandicapped children in at least one important way. Rate of vocabulary acquisition is significantly slower than for nonhandicapped children, even when the slower rate of cognitive development of the children with Down syndrome is taken into account. Children with Down syndrome appear to begin their vocabulary spurt at an older mental age than nonhandicapped children do. Thus, differences in rate of vocabulary development are especially apparent beyond mental ages of 20–21 months.

Both child factors and adult factors were proposed as potential explanations for the discrepancy in rate of vocabulary development. Children with Down syndrome appear to have specific memory deficits, involving both storage and retrieval, as well as difficulty encoding and decoding verbal stimuli. These problems are exacerbated by the relatively low level of semantic contingency contained in the speech addressed to them by their mothers (and probably by other adults). In addition, mothers of children with Down syndrome appear to be less likely than mothers of nonhandicapped children to introduce new vocabulary in an optimal manner. These characteristics of maternal speech to children with Down syndrome in turn are probably affected by child factors. Children with Down syndrome are more passive and less socially responsive than nonhandicapped children. In addition, children with Down syndrome use language less often than nonhandicapped children. Once again, the relative infrequency of language use is in part due to maternal factors; the mothers of children with Down syndrome are proportionally less likely than mothers of nonhandicapped children to ask the child questions whose answers are in the child's productive vocabularies. And again, child factors are probably partially responsible for this difference. Thus, the slower rate of vocabulary development of the children with Down syndrome appears to be due to a series of interrelated child and adult factors.

Suggestions for early intervention

The contents of previous sections of this chapter provide the basis for a large number of suggestions for facilitating the conceptual development of children with Down syndrome. These suggestions are based both on the commonalities observed in conceptual development by children with Down syndrome and nonhandicapped children and on the differences between the two groups of children and the two groups of mothers. An entire chapter could be devoted to the intervention question; here, I briefly discuss the most important of these implications. Only acquisition of concrete object categories and names for these categories are considered. However, once a variety of such categories and their names has been acquired, introduction of verb categories and attribute categories can begin, based on the same principles.

Intervention specifically related to conceptual development probably should begin at the end of Stage 4 or early in Stage 5 of the sensorimotor period. The child's mental age will probably be about 10 to 12 months at this time. During Stage 5 of the sensorimotor period, the child becomes sensitive to and interested in the properties of objects that are relevant to category assignment. For example, the child becomes interested in the roundness and rollability of a ball, where formerly he or she was interested only in more general properties of the ball, such as that it could be banged, batted at, or chewed on (Piaget, 1954; Uzgiris & Hunt, 1975). At this point, the child should become interested in categorization, and referential comprehension should follow within a few months of mental age.

The categories chosen for intervention should be categories of whole objects, so that they fit the child's whole-object hypothesis concerning the meaning of novel words. As Gillham (1979) has pointed out, programs that focus on attribute words are not successful. The object categories chosen should be basic level categories of objects that either can move independently or can be manipulated by the child. If possible, toys that the specific child is known to be interested in should be included. The objects available should include good (and possibly moderately good) examples of the categories.

The intervention should take the form of playing, rather than teaching. Thus, the adult should attempt to follow the child's initiatives, if the child is actively involved with a toy. If the child is not involved, the adult obviously must take the initiative; he or she should choose a toy the child is likely to find interesting and then show the child what is interesting about the object, for example, its special form features or its function. It is important to label the toy while the child is attending to it. Labels should be included in short phrases or short sentences. Young children are most likely to attend to the last word in an utterance. (This pattern would be expected as a derivative of Slobin's, 1973, operating principle, Pay attention to the ends of words.) Therefore, the object label generally should be the final word in the utterance. The object should be labeled frequently, rather than only once during each interaction with it. Very young children usually require many repetitions of a word, both within a single interaction and across several interactions with that object or other objects included in the category, before comprehending the word. Children with Down syndrome, because of their memory deficits, would be expected to require additional exposure to a word before comprehending it. Comprehension testing at first should be informal, involving asking the child to find the toy for the adult, in the context of playing. Once the child appears to comprehend a word, more formal comprehension testing can be conducted to determine if the child demonstrates referential comprehension and to determine the extension of the child's category. The procedure used in the longitudinal study can be followed. Errors that extend beyond the boundaries of the child-basic category (e.g., retrieving a set of keys when asked for a ball) should be corrected, but at this stage, errors that are within the boundaries of the child-basic category (e.g., retrieving a round bead when asked for a ball) should not be corrected. The latter pattern of response is expected and quite reasonable, given the attributes of the bead that the child is likely to notice. The suggested pattern of interaction, involving labeling objects that the child is attending to or interacting with, should be used not only as part of a formal intervention program, but also at home during everyday activities by the adults (or older children) who regularly interact with the child. Positive feedback for correct comprehension, whether comprehension occurs in an informal or a formal setting, is an important part of semantic contingency and as such is crucial to the success of the intervention.

Referential production can be expected to begin during late Stage 5 or Stage 6 of the sensorimotor period, at a mental age of about 16 to 20 months. As Gillham (1979) has pointed out, the most effective way to facilitate production is not to force the child to imitate words, but to ensure that comprehension of the word is well established. Cheseldine and McConkey (1979), in an intervention study involving parents of children with Down syndrome as the teachers, found that increasing semantic contingency led to improved language development, for children somewhat more advanced than the ones included in the longitudinal study. Thus, continuation of the same program should facilitate production as well as comprehension. Initially, errors should be corrected under the same circumstances as suggested for comprehension.

Eventually, adults should begin to teach the child the correct names for objects that the child is incorrectly (by adult standards) including in his or her child-base categories. The child is ready for this step at the time that he or she is able to appreciate the attributes that differentiate the object from other members of its initial child-basic category. The new labels should be introduced to the child according to the concrete illustration strategy described in a previous section. In addition, the adult should take advantage of situations that arise spontaneously, in which the child appears to have noticed one of these attributes on his or her own (e.g., the child is fingering the wick on a round candle that is included in his or her *ball* category). If the child is ready, these procedures should make it relatively easy to teach the child new names for objects previously included in categories that are incorrect from an adult perspective. However, the child will not automatically exclude the object from its previous category. Again, this is expected based on the normal development pattern, and should not be a source of concern.

Once comprehension of the correct (from an adult perspective) name of an object previously included in a different category is well established, the adult may want to begin correcting the child's production of the former name in reference to the object. Correction, if used, should follow the concrete illustration strategy. Correction should not be insisted on if the child indicates disagreement, for example, by playing with the object as if it were a member of the previous category, by repeating the name of the previous category, or by acting upset. Positive feedback for correct use of the new name is important.

There are three major goals for an intervention program concerned with early vocabulary acquisition. First, the child should learn, and learn correctly (from the child perspective at first, and later from the adult perspective), as many useful words as possible. Second, the child and the adults involved with the child should develop a pattern of interaction that is comfortable and productive for all of them.

Third, the child should be encouraged to use the words in his or her vocabulary spontaneously, for communication, both to express his or her ideas and to attempt to control the environment. The program outlined above should fulfill all three goals.

References

Abrahamsen, A., Cavallo, M. M., & McCluer, J. A. (1985). Is the sign advantage a robust phenomenon? From gesture to language in two modalities. *Merrill Palmer Quarterly.*

Anglin, J. M. (1977). *Word, object, and conceptual development.* New York: Norton.

Anisfeld, M. (1984). *Language development from birth to three.* Hillsdale, NJ: Erlbaum.

Barrett, M. D. (1978). Lexical development and overextension in child language. *Journal of Child Language, 5,* 205–219.

Barrett, M. D. (1982). Distinguishing between prototypes: The early acquisition of the meaning of object names. In S. A. Kuczaj II (Ed.), *Language development,* Vol. 1: *Syntax and semantics* (pp. 313–334). Hillsdale, NJ: Erlbaum.

Bayley, N. (1969). *Bayley Scales of Infant Development.* New York: Psychological Corporation.

Bell, R. Q. (1964). The effect on the family of a limitation in coping ability in the child: A research approach and a finding. *Merrill-Palmer Quarterly, 10,* 129–142.

Bell, R. Q., & Harper, L. V. (1977). *Child effects on adults.* Hillsdale, NJ: Erlbaum.

Benda, C. E. (1960). *The child with mongolism (congenital acromicria).* New York: Grune & Stratton.

Benelli, B., D'Odorico, L., Levorato, C., & Simion, F. (1977). Formation and extension of the concept of a prelinguistic child. *Italian Journal of Psychology, 3,* 429–448.

Bigelow, A. (1982) *Early words of blind children.* Paper presented at the International Conference on Infant Studies, Austin, TX, March.

Bilovsky, D., & Share, J. (1965). The ITPA and Down's syndrome: An exploratory study. *American Journal of Mental Deficiency, 70,* 78–82.

Blewitt, P. (1983). *Dog vs. collie:* Vocabulary in speech to young children. *Developmental Psychology, 19,* 602–609.

Bohn, W. E. (1914). First steps in verbal expression. *Pedagogical Seminary, 21,* 578–595.

Boyd, W. (1914). The development of a child's vocabulary. *Pedagogical Seminary, 21,* 95–124.

Brown, R. (1978). How shall a thing be called? *Psychological Review, 65,* 14–21.

Brown, R. (1978). A new paradigm of reference. In G. A. Miller & E. Lenneberg (eds.), *Psychology and biology of language and thought: Essays in honor of Eric Lenneberg* (pp. 151–166). New York: Academic Press.

Bruner, J. S., Goodnow, J. J., & Austin, J. G. (1956). *A study of thinking.* New York: Wiley.

Buckhalt, T. A., Rutherford, R. B., & Goldberg, K. E. (1978). Verbal and non-verbal interaction of mothers and their Down's syndrome and non-retarded infants. *American Journal of Mental Deficiency, 72,* 337–343.

Buium, N., Rynders, J., & Turnure, J. (1974). Early maternal linguistic environment of normal and Down's syndrome language-learning children. *American Journal of Mental Deficiency, 79,* 52–58.

Cardoso-Martins, C. (1984). *Early vocabulary acquisition by Down syndrome children: The roles of cognitive development and maternal language input.* Unpublished doctoral dissertation, University of Illinois, Urbana–Champaign.

Cardoso-Martins, C., & Mervis, C. B. (1984). *Maternal speech to Down syndrome and normal children: Interaction styles.* Paper presented at the Third International Congress for the Study of Child Language, Austin, TX, July.

Cardoso-Martins, C., & Mervis, C. B. (1985). Maternal speech to prelinguistic children with Down syndrome. *American Journal of Mental Deficiency, 89* 451–458.

Cardoso-Martins, C., & Mervis, C. B. (1988). *Maternal speech to young children with Down syndrome: Linguistic styles and its effects on early vocabulary acquisition.* Submitted for publication.

Cardoso-Martins, C., Mervis, C. B., & Mervis, C. A. (1983). *Early vocabulary acquisition by Down syndrome children: The relationship between language development and intellectual development.*

Paper presented at the Gatlinburg Conference on Research in Mental Retardation/Developmental Disabilities, Gatlinburg, TN, March.

Cardoso-Martins, C., Mervis, C. B., & Mervis, C. A. (1985). Early vocabulary acquisition by children with Down syndrome. *American Journal of Mental Deficiency, 90,* 177–184.

Carey, S. (1982). Semantic development: The state of the art. In E. Wanner & L. R. Gleitman (Eds.), *Language acquisition: The state of the art* (pp. 347–389). New York: Cambridge University Press.

Chapman, K. (1983). *Inappropriate word usage in young children: A longitudinal investigation.* Unpublished doctoral dissertation, Purdue University, West Lafayette, Indiana.

Chapman, K., Leonard, L. B., & Mervis, C. B. (1986). The effects of feedback on young children's inappropriate word usage. *Journal of Child Language, 13,* 101–117.

Chapman, R. S. (1978). Comprehension strategies in children. In J. Kavanaugh & W. Strange (Eds.), *Speech and language in the laboratory, school, and clinic* (pp. 308–327). Cambridge, MA: MIT Press.

Cheseldine, S., & McConkey, R. (1979). Parental speech to young Down's syndrome children: An intervention study. *American Journal of Mental Deficiency, 83,* 612–620.

Clark, E. V. (1973). What's in a word? On the child's acquisition of semantics in his first language. In T. E. Moore (Ed.), *Cognitive development and the acquisition of language.* New York: Academic Press.

Clark, E. V. (1979). Building a vocabulary: Words for objects, actions, and relations. In P. Fletcher & M. Garman (Eds.), *Language acquisition: Studies in first language development* (pp. 149–160). New York: Cambridge University Press.

Clark, E. V. (1983). Meaning and concepts. In P. H. Mussen (Ed.), *Carmichael's manual of child psychology,* Vol. III: *Cognitive development* (pp. 787–840). New York: Wiley.

Clark, E. V., & Hecht, B. F. (1983). Comprehension, production, and language acquisition. *Annual Review of Psychology, 34,* 325–349.

Cohen, L. B. (1981). Examination of habituation as a measure of aberrant infant development. In S. L. Friedman & M. Sigman (eds.), *Pre-term birth and psychological development.* New York: Academic Press.

Cohen, L. B., & Gelber, E. R. (1975). Infant visual memory. In L. B. Cohen & P. Salapatek (Eds.), *From sensation to cognition,* Vol. 1: *Basic visual processes* (pp. 347–403). New York: Academic Press.

Cohen, L. B., & Younger, B. (1983). Perceptual categorization in the infant. In E. Scholnick (Ed.), *New trends in conceptual representation: Challenges to Piaget's theory?* (pp. 197–220). Hillsdale, NJ: Erlbaum.

Corrigan, R. (1978). Language development as related to stage 6 object permanence development. *Journal of Child Language, 5,* 173–189.

Cross, T. G. (1978). Mothers' speech and its association with rate of linguistic development in young children. In N. Waterson & C. Snow (Eds.), *The development of communication* (pp. 199–216). New York: Wiley.

Dodd, B. J. (1975). Recognition and reproduction of words by Down's syndrome and non-Down's syndrome retarded children. *American Journal of Mental Deficiency, 80,* 306–311.

Dougherty, J.W.D. (1978). Relativity and salience in categorization. *American Ethnologist, 5,* 66–80.

Dunn, L. M., & Dunn, L. (1981). *Peabody Picture Vocabulary Test–Revised.* Circle Pines, MN: American Guidance Service.

Dunst, C. J. (1980). *A clinical and educational manual for use with the Uzgiris and Hunt scales of infant development.* Baltimore: University Park Press.

Eheart, B. K. (1982). Mother–child interactions with nonretarded and mentally retarded preschoolers. *American Journal of Mental Deficiency, 87,* 20–25.

Evans, D., & Hampson, M. (1969). The language of mongols. *British Journal of Disorders of Communication, 3,* 171–181.

Folger, M. K., & Leonard, L. B. (1978). Language and sensorimotor development during the early period of referential speech. *Journal of Speech and Hearing Research, 21,* 518–527.

Furrow, D., Nelson, K., & Benedict, H. (1979). Mothers' speech to children with syntactic development: Some simple relationships. *Journal of Child Language, 6,* 423–442.

Gentner, D. (1982). Why nouns are learned before verbs: Linguistic relativity versus natural partitioning. In S. J. Kuczaj II (Ed.), *Language development,* Vol. 2: *Language, thought, and culture* (pp. 301–334). Hillsdale, NJ: Erlbaum.

Gibson, D. (1978). *Down's syndrome: The psychology of monogolism.* London: Cambridge University Press.

Gillham, B. (1979). *The first words language programme.* London: George Allen & Unwin.

Goldman, A. E., & Levine, M. A. (1963). A developmental study of object sorting. *Child Development, 34,* 649–666.

Golinkoff, R. M., & Halperin, M. S. (1983). The concept of animal: One infant's view. *Infant Behavior and Development, 6,* 229–233.

Grant, J. R. (1915). The child's vocabulary and its growth. *Pedagogical Seminary, 22,* 183–203.

Gruendel, J. M. (1977). Referential extension in early language development. *Child Development, 48,* 1567–1576.

Guillaume, P. (1927/1973). Les debuts de la phrase dans le langage de l'enfant. *Journal de Psychologie, 24,* 1–25. Translated by E. V. Clark in C. A. Ferguson & D. I. Slobin (Eds.), *Studies of child language development* (pp. 522–541). New York: Holt, Rinehart & Winston.

Holden, E. S. (1877). On vocabularies of children under two years. *Transactions of the American Philological Association, 8,* 58–68.

Hupp, S. C., & Mervis, C. B. (1982). Acquisition of basic object categories by severely handicapped children. *Child Development, 53,* 760–767.

Husaim, J. S., & Cohen, L. B. (1981). Infant learning of ill-defined categories. *Merrill-Palmer Quarterly, 27,* 443–456.

Huttenlocher, J. (1974). The origins of language comprehension. In R. L. Solso (Ed.), *Theories in cognitive psychology: The Loyola symposium* (pp. 331–368). Potomac, MD: Erlbaum.

Ingram, D. (1978). Sensori-motor intelligence and language development. In A. Lock (Ed.), *Action, gesture, and symbol: The emergence of language.* New York: Academic Press.

Jegi, J. I. (1901). The vocabulary of a two-year-old child. *Child Study Monthly, 6,* 241–261.

Jones, O.H.M. (1977). Mother–child communication with prelinguistic Down's syndrome and normal infants. In H. R. Schaffer (Ed.), *Studies in mother–infant interaction* (pp. 379–401). New York: Academic Press.

Jones, O.H.M. (1979). A comparison study of mother–child communication with Down's syndrome and normal infants. In H. R. Schaffer & J. Dunn (Eds.), *The first year of life: Psychological and medical implications of early experience* (pp. 175–195). New York: Wiley.

Jones, O.H.M. (1980). Prelinguistic communication skills in Down's syndrome and normal infants. In T. M. Field (Ed.), *High-risk infants and children: Adult and peer interactions* (pp. 205–225). New York: Academic Press.

Keenan, J. M., & MacWhinney, B. (1987). Understanding the relationship between comprehension and production. In H. W. Dechert & M. Raupach (Eds.), *Psycholinguistic models of production.* Norwood, NJ: Ablex.

Keil, F. C. (1987). Conceptual development and category structure. In U. Neisser (Ed.), *Concepts reconsidered: Ecological and intellectual bases of categorization.* Cambridge: Cambridge University Press.

Kopp, C. B. (1983). Risk factors in development. In P. H. Mussen (Ed.), *Handbook of child psychology,* Vol. 2: *Infancy and developmental psychobiology* (pp. 1081–1188). New York: Wiley.

Landau, B., & Gleitman, L. R. (1985). *Language and experience: Evidence from the blind child.* Cambridge, MA: Harvard University Press.

Lewis, M. M. (1936). *Infant speech: A study of the beginnings of language.* London: Kegan Paul, Trench, Trubner & Co.

Lyle, J. G. (1959). The effect of an institution environment upon the verbal development of imbecile children. I. Verbal intelligence. *Journal of Mental Deficiency Research 3,* 122–128.

Lyle, J. G. (1960). The effect of an institution environment upon the verbal development of imbecile children. II. Speech and language. *Journal of Mental Deficiency Research, 4,* 1–13.

Macnamara, J. (1982). *Names for things: A study of human learning.* Cambridge, Mass.: MIT Press.

McCarthy, D. (1954). Language development in children. In L. Carmichael (Ed.), *Manual of child psychology* (2nd ed., pp. 429–630). New York: Wiley.

McDade, H. L., & Adler, S. (1980). Down syndrome and short-term memory impairment: A storage or retrieval deficit? *American Journal of Mental Deficiency, 84*, 561–567.

McDonald, L., & Pien, D. (1982). Mother conversational behavior as a function of interactional intent. *Journal of Child Language, 9*, 337–358.

Merriman, W. E. (1987). *Lexical contrast in toddlers: A reanalysis of the diary evidence.* Paper presented at the biennial meeting of the Society for Research in Child Development, Baltimore, MD, April.

Mervis, C. B. (1980). Category structure and the development of categorization. In R. J. Spiro, B. C. Bruce, & W. F. Brewer (Eds.), *Theoretical issues in the development of reading comprehension: Perspectives from cognitive psychology, linguistics, artificial intelligence, and education* (pp. 279–306). Hillsdale, NJ: Erlbaum.

Mervis, C. B. (1982). *Mother–child interaction and early lexical development.* Paper presented at the annual meeting of the Midwestern Psychological Association, Minneapolis, May.

Mervis, C. B. (1984). Early lexical development: The contributions of mother and child. In C. Sophian (Ed.), *Origins of cognitive skills* (pp. 339–370). Hillsdale, NJ: Erlbaum.

Mervis, C. B. (1985). On the existence of prelinguistic categories: A case study. *Infant Behavior and Development, 8*, 293–300.

Mervis, C. B. (1987). Child-basic object categories and early lexical development. In U. Neisser (Ed.), *Concepts reconsidered: The ecological and intellectual bases of categorization.* London: Cambridge University Press.

Mervis, C. B. (1988). Early lexical development: Theory and application. In L. Nadel (Ed.), *The psychology of Down syndrome.* Cambridge, MA: Bradford/MIT Press.

Mervis, C. B., & Canada, K. (1983). On the existence of competence errors in early comprehension: A reply to Fremgen & Fay and Chapman & Thomson. *Journal of Child Language, 10*, 431–440.

Mervis, C. B., & Crisafi, M. A. (1982). Order of acquisition of subordinate, basic, and superordinate level categories. *Child Development, 53*, 258–266.

Mervis, C. B., & Long, L. M. (1987). *Words refer to whole objects: Young children's interpretation of the referent of a novel word.* Paper presented at the biennial meeting of the Society for Research in Child Development, Baltimore, MD, April.

Mervis, C. B., & Mervis, C. A. (1982). Leopards are kitty-cats: Object labeling by mothers for their 13-month-olds. *Child Development, 53*, 267–273.

Mervis, C. B., & Mervis, C. A. (1984). *Reduction of lexical overextensions: The roles of maternal attribute illustrations and corrections.* Paper presented at the Third International Congress for the Study of Child Language, Austin, TX, July.

Mervis, C. B., & Pani, J. R. (1980). Acquisition of basic object categories. *Cognitive Psychology, 12*, 496–522.

Mervis, C. B., & Rosch, E. (1981). Categorization of natural objects. *Annual Review of Psychology, 32*, 89–115.

Moore, K. C. (1896). The mental development of a child. *Psychological Review, Monograph Supplement, 1*(3).

Mulford, R. (1988). First words of the blind child. In M. R. Smith & J. L. Locke (Eds.), *The emergent lexicon: The child's development of a linguistic vocabulary.* New York: Academic Press.

Neimark, E. (1974). Natural language concepts: Additional evidence. *Child Development, 45*, 508–511.

Nelson, K. (1973). Structure and strategy in learning to talk. *Monographs of the Society for Research in Child Development, 39* (1–2, Serial No. 149).

Nelson, K. (1974). Concept, word, and sentence: Interrelations in acquisition and development. *Psychological Review, 81*, 267–285.

Nelson, K. (1979). Explorations in the development of a functional semantic system. In W. A. Collins (Ed.), *Children's language and communication. The Minnesota Symposia on Child Development* (Vol. 12). Hillsdale, NJ: Erlbaum.

Nelson, K., Rescorla, L., Gruendel, J., & Benedict, H. (1978). Early lexicons: What do they mean? *Child Development, 49,* 960–968.

Newport, E. L., Gleitman, H., & Gleitman, L. R. (1977). Mother, I'd rather do it myself: Some effects and non-effects of maternal speech style. In C. E. Snow & C. A. Ferguson (Eds.), *Talking to children: Language input and acquisition* (pp. 109–149). London: Cambridge University Press.

Nice, M. M. (1915). The development of a child's vocabulary in relation to environment. *Pedagogical Seminary, 22,* 35–64.

Ninio, A. (1980). Ostensive definition in vocabulary teaching. *Journal of Child Language 7,* 565–573.

Ninio, A., & Bruner, J. (1978). The achievement and antecedents of labeling. *Journal of Child Language, 5,* 1–15.

Olver, R. R., & Hornsby, J. R. (1966). On equivalence. In J. S. Bruner, R. R. Olver, P. M. Greenfield et al., *Studies in cognitive growth* (pp. 68–85). New York: Wiley.

Pelsma, J. R. (1910). A child's vocabulary and its development. *Pedagogical Seminary, 17,* 328–369.

Piaget, J. (1954). *The construction of reality in the child.* New York: Basic Books.

Ramsey, D. (1978). Object word spurt, handedness and object permanence in the infant. (Doctoral dissertation, University of Denver, 1977). *Dissertation Abstracts International, 38,* 1147B.

Rescorla, L. A. (1980). Overextension in early language development. *Journal of Child Language, 7,* 321–335.

Rescorla, L. A. (1981). Category development in early language. *Journal of Child Language, 8,* 225–238.

Reznick, J. S., & Kagan, J. (1983). Category detection in infancy. In L. P. Lipsitt & C. K. Rovee-Collier (Eds.), *Advances in infant research* (Vol. 2). Norwood, NJ: Ablex.

Ricciuti, H. (1965). Object grouping and selective ordering behavior in infants 12 to 24 months old. *Merrill-Palmer Quarterly, 11,* 129–148.

Rosch, E., & Mervis, C. B. (1975). Family resemblances: Studies in the internal structure of categories. *Cognitive Psychology, 7* 573–605.

Rosch, E., Mervis, C. B., Gray, W. D., Johnson, D. M., & Boyes-Braem, P. (1976). Basic objects in natural categories. *Cognitive Psychology, 8,* 382–439.

Roth, P. L. (1984). *Temporal and discourse properties in different styles of maternal speech to infants.* Paper presented at the Third International Congress for the Study of Child Language, Austin, TX, July.

Saltz, E., Soller, E., & Siegel, I. E. (1972). The development of natural language concepts. *Child Development, 43,* 1191–1202.

Schnell, R. R. (1984). Psychomotor evaluation. In S. M. Pueschel (Ed.), *The young child with Down syndrome* (pp. 207–226). New York: Human Sciences Press.

Share, J. B. (1975). Developmental progress in Down's syndrome. In R. Koch & F. F. de la Cruz (Eds.), *Down's syndrome (mongolism): Research, prevention and management* (pp. 78–86). New York: Brunner/Mazel.

Shipley, E. F., Kuhn, I. F. & Madden, E. C. (1983). Mothers' use of superordinate terms. *Journal of Child Language, 10,* 571–588.

Slobin, D. I. (1973). Cognitive prerequisites for the development of grammar. In C. A. Ferguson & D. I. Slobin (eds.), *Studies of child language development.* New York: Holt, Rinehart & Winston.

Smith, E. E., & Medin, D. L. (1981). *Categories and concepts.* Cambridge, MA: Harvard University Press.

Smith, M. E. (1926). An investigation of the development of the sentence and the extent of vocabulary in young children. *University of Iowa Studies of Child Welfare, 3*(5).

Strominger, A. Z., Winkler, M. R., & Cohen, L. T. (1984). Speech and language evaluation. In S. M. Pueschel (Ed.), *The young child with Down syndrome* (pp. 253–261). New York: Human Sciences Press.

Stross, B. (1973). Acquisition of botanical terminology by Tzeltal children. In M. Edmonson (Ed.), *Meaning in Mayan languages* (pp. 107–142). The Hague: Mouton.

Sugarman, S. (1983). *Children's early thought: Developments in classification.* Cambridge: Cambridge University Press.

Tager-Flusberg, H. (1985a). Basic level and superordinate level categorization by autistic, mentally retarded, and normal children. *Journal of Experimental Child Psychology, 40,* 450–469.

Tager-Flusberg, H. (1985b). The conceptual basis for referential word meaning in children with autism. *Child Development, 56,* 1167–1178.

Tager-Flusberg, H. (1986). Constraints on the representation of word meaning: Evidence from autistic and mentally retarded children. In M. Barrett & S. A. Kucza II (Eds.), *The development of word meaning* (pp. 69–81). New York: Springer-Verlag.

Terman, L. M., & Merrill, M. A. (1960). *Measuring intelligence.* Boston: Houghton Mifflin.

Thompson, J. (1941). The ability of children of different grade levels to generalize on sorting tests. *Journal of Psychology, 11,* 119–126.

Thompson, M. M. (1963). Psychological characteristics relevant to the education of the pre-school mongoloid child. *Mental Retardation, 1,* 148–151.

Thompson, J. R., & Chapman, R. S. (1977). Who is "Daddy" revisited: The status of two-year-olds' overextended words in use and comprehension. *Journal of Child Language, 4,* 359–375.

Tversky, B., & Hemenway, K. (1984). Objects, parts, and categories. *Journal of Experimental Psychology: General, 113,* 169–193.

Uzgiris, I., & Hunt, J. McV. (1975). *Assessment in infancy: Ordinal scales of psychological development.* Urbana: University of Illinois Press.

Velleman, S. L., Mangipudi, L., & Locke, J. L. (in press). Prelinguistic phonetic contingency: Data from Down syndrome. *First Language.*

Weistuch, L. (1983). *The effects of maternal training on language use.* Paper presented at the Gatlinburg Conference on Research in Mental Retardation/Developmental Disabilities, Gatlinburg, TN, March.

Whitehurst, G. J., Kedesdy, J., & White, T. G. (1982). A functional analysis of meaning. In S. A. Kuczaj II (Ed.), *Language development,* Vol. 1: *Syntax and semantics* (pp. 397–427). Hillsdale, NJ: Erlbaum.

Wittgenstein, L. (1958). *The blue and brown books.* Oxford: Blackwell.

9 Language abilities in children with Down syndrome: evidence for a specific syntactic delay

Anne E. Fowler

It has been claimed that the development of language in children with Down syndrome is but a slow-motion replica of the normal course of acquisition, identical in all respects but rate of acquisition (Lenneberg, 1967). Despite delays in the onset and timing of language development, the language structures that are acquired by children with Down syndrome have consistently been described as normal and unremarkable in the order of their appearance. In the speech of children with Down syndrome, there has been no evidence of deviant forms or constructions not observed at some stage of normal development (Bloom & Lahey, 1978; Evans & Hampson, 1968; Rondal, 1975; Rosenberg, 1982; Ryan, 1975).

Our discussion does not challenge the standard view of Down syndrome language as "delayed without deviance." How it differs is by shifting attention away from the issue of deviance (or lack thereof) to focus upon substantial, unexplained delays in acquiring language structure. In particular, this chapter covers two robust features of Down syndrome language that have previously drawn little attention, but which call for an explanation. The first is that the ultimate syntactic and morphological levels achieved by most individuals with Down syndrome are consistently low across a number of studies, independent of assessment procedures. The second is that this limited language development cannot be explained as a simple function of general intellectual development, or as a function of more general verbal or communicative skill (see Beeghly, Weiss-Perry, & Cicchetti, Chapter 10, this volume). In making these points, the evidence for a specific syntactic deficit is examined, and it is asked whether particular areas within syntax or morphology pose special difficulties for the child with Down syndrome. Finally, to account for individual differences within the Down syndrome population, potential factors bearing on the rate and extent of the delay are introduced. Cognitive, maturational, and linguistic factors contributing to individual differences will be discussed.

This paper was supported by a grant from the March of Dimes Birth Defects Foundation (12-113) to L. Gleitman, R. Gelman & A. Fowler; and by an NICHD post-doctoral fellowship (1-F32-HD-06543). Lila Gleitman's contribution to this paper is gratefully acknowledged, as are helpful comments from Marjorie Beeghly, Susan Brady, and Rochel Gelman.

302

The issue in this chapter pertains to how children with Down syndrome acquire knowledge of the grammatical structures of English, including both syntax and morphology. Knowledge of grammatical structures include such things as the use of word order to express meaning (as in, *Fish ate Tom* versus *Tom ate fish*), compliance with constraints on how words can be combined and moved (e.g., subjects before verbs), and appropriate use of functors both within and across words (e.g., use of infinitive markers as in *I want to go* or of the grammatical marker *s* in *she wants ice cream*). Evidence for acquisition of this knowledge is sought through analyses of spontaneous production, through standardized language assessment batteries, and through experimental techniques contrived to demonstrate comprehension or elicit production of structures not otherwise apparent. Although our primary interest is in the acquisition of syntax, we seek to place its development within a broader context of verbal and communicative function, including lexical development (vocabulary), acquisition of communicative skill (conversational interactions, use of gesture), and general "verbal" ability (culturally transmitted knowledge about the world such as is assessed in standardized intelligence tests). Individual differences in phonology (the sound structure of the language) will not be addressed in this chapter.

A developmental approach to the study of language

Although research on language development in children with Down syndrome has proliferated for some time, only recently have studies begun to yield consistent and coherent conclusions regarding the course of language learning in these children. This has been accomplished by adherence to important methodological and developmental principles. Because these principles serve as guidelines in this chapter for the evaluation of research findings, they will be briefly discussed.

First, it is important to restrict the focus of study to *biologically well-defined subgroups,* ideally for comparison with other equally well-defined contrast groups. All the studies presented have focused on children with Down syndrome exclusively. Although published research on contrast groups is minimal as yet, ongoing language studies of children with Fragile-X (Paul, Cohen, Breg, Waxton, & Herman, 1984), autism (Tager-Flusberg, Calkins, Nolin, Baumberger, Anderson, & Chadwick-Dias, submitted), and Williams syndrome (Bellugi, in press) increase the likelihood of comparisons in the near future with children having Down syndrome (see Scarborough, Rescorla, Tager-Flusberg, Fowler & Sudhalter, unpublished ms.)

A second developmental principle derives from the *modularity* hypothesis of cognition: One cannot conduct language research without at least acknowledging the hypothesis that language is acquired, processed, and represented independently of other cognitive domains. (See Lenneberg, 1967, for an early statement of this hypothesis, supported, in part, by his findings from research on language learning in children with Down syndrome; see Fodor, 1983, for a more recent statement of the position and for a discussion of what constitutes relevant data; see Keil, 1981, for a discussion of modularity from a developmental perspective). There are several methodological points following from the modular point of view. First, it suggests that mental age (MA) may serve as no more than a rough guideline for typical behavior, since it usually averages over several distinct domains. Although it remains of interest to compare global measures of language, memory, perception, and the like with mental age expectations, one cannot make judgments of deviance in regard to a particular structure without reference to other progress in that whole domain. Thus, it becomes only sensible to rely upon a general measure from *within* the language domain for fine-grained comparisons of language structures across individuals or populations. Similarly, to make serious statements about the specificity of the language deficit in Down syndrome, it is essential to show growth in another well-defined nonlinguistic domain (e.g., see work by Cornwell, 1974, and Gelman & Cohen, 1988 for exploratory studies on number knowledge in children with Down syndrome). An important corollary of the modularity hypothesis is that one must in turn treat the subdomains of language and communication (phonology, morphology, syntax, lexicon, nonverbal communication, and discourse) as potentially separable and distinct domains (see Abrahamson, Cavallo, & McLuer,1985; Beeghly, Hanrahan, Weiss, & Cicchetti, 1985; Beeghly, Weiss-Perry, & Cicchetti, Chapter 10, this volume; and Mervis, Chapter 8, this volume, for relevant studies).

The third developmental principle governing this discussion is the possibility of distinct *stages* in the development of grammatical structures (e.g., Bowerman, 1982; Hyams, 1986; Karmiloff-Smith, 1979). Although Brown (1973) introduced language stages more as descriptive aids than as theoretical constructs, they have proven to be extremely useful heuristics in studies of language development over the years. Quite distinct grammatical systems are connoted by the prelinguistic stage and each of the five subsequent stages outlined by Brown (1973). A great deal of information would be sacrificed if performance of children at several stages of language development were collapsed into a single average score. One cannot, for example, average together the scores of two children at a one-word stage (Stage I) and one child with simple syntactic structures (Stage III) and claim that children with Down syndrome are on average in language Stage II (consistently combining words). Moreover, questions asked about language abilities in children with Down syndrome may have quite different answers depending on the language level under study.

Finally, one cannot overlook that *maturational factors* (e.g., as indexed by chronological age) may exert a unique effect on development in children with Down syndrome. Indeed, it is well known that IQ declines with age in this population (Zeaman & House, 1962). Relatively rapid mental age growth in the preschool years is interrupted by plateaus in growth that become both lengthier and more frequent in the school-age years, with an actual decline in MA scores apparent by adolescence (Gibson, 1966). More current work raises the possibility that early onset of Alzheimer's disease may explain the decline in IQ, at least in part (Gibson, 1978; Ross, Galaburda, & Kemper, 1984; see Wisniewski, Miezejeski, & Hill, 1988, for a critical discussion). It remains to be determined whether chronological age (CA) exerts a unique effect on language development in children with Down syndrome. One issue has concerned whether children with Down syndrome cease to acquire language after a critical period for language learning has passed. Lenneberg (1967) argued that at puberty language learning was no longer possible owing to a loss of brain plasticity. This claim was based, in part, on the language growth curves observed in his longitudinal study of 62 children with Down syndrome. Over a 3-year period, children with Down syndrome who had attained puberty failed to make any discernible progress in acquiring language structure; this was in contrast to younger children in whom some growth was observed (Lenneberg, Nichols, & Rosenberger, 1964). Although Lenneberg's critical period hypothesis and the data on which it was based have since been challenged on many important details (Best, Hoffman, & Glanville, 1982; Dennis & Whitaker, 1977; Molfese, 1977; St. James-Roberts, 1981), a critical period of language acquisition remains an important theoretical construct regarding the ability to learn language (spoken or signed) beyond the preschool years (Krashen, 1975; Newport & Supalla, 1980). Further research on the role of maturational factors in children with Down syndrome may prove an important empirical base for testing and refining the critical period hypothesis (see also Cicchetti & Beeghly, Chapter 2, this volume).

To summarize the research perspective adopted in this chapter, an attempt has been made to keep in mind sources of variability hypothesized to be important for normal language development. These include choosing a well-defined subgroup, identifying the particular component of language being studied, assessing the language level at which the child is functioning, and evaluating the significance of chronological age. It is hoped that this approach will provide us with a sharper descriptive picture of the language abilities of children with Down syndrome and bring us closer to an explanatory account of their difficulties.

Characterizing the delay: is there a pattern?

In an overview of studies conducted in the 1950s and 1960s, Evans and Hampson (1968) concluded that there was no problem of language acquisition unique to children with Down syndrome. They reported that first words could appear any time from 1 year to 6 years of CA, and first sentences any time from 1 year to 17 years CA. There appeared to be little correlation between IQ and language level, and except for a generally higher incidence of articulatory and voice defects, there was no consistent relationship between how children with Down syndrome compared with other groups of retarded children. On the basis of these findings, they argued that further research specifically directed to language in individuals with Down syndrome would be unrewarding. (See Bloom & Lahey, 1978, and Rosenberg, 1982, for similar views).

In fact, however, research focusing exclusively on children with Down syndrome consistently reports a large discrepancy between measured language skill and expectations based on mental age assessment. In the same paper quoted from above, Evans and Hampson (1968) noted that the "worst" area of development in individuals with Down syndrome is language and that they lag behind MA-matched controls in language by as much as 50%. Although the definitions of "verbal" and "nonverbal" are often quite general and vary from study to study, a large body of evidence points to a delay in speech relative to traditional motor, intellectual, and social indices (see Gibson, 1978, for a comprehensive review). To cite one example, Thompson (1963) tested 29 children with Down syndrome (CA 5;0 to 6;11) on the Stanford–Binet and Vineland Social Maturity Scale; not one child had language skills equivalent to his overall MA score and most children were more mature on the Vineland than on the Stanford–Binet. More recently and on a much broader scale, Wisniewski et al. (1988) report identical findings: In a clinical sample of 194 persons with Down syndrome, ranging in age from 2 to 70 years, and with IQs extending from profound up into the low normal range, only one individual had normal language; that individual suffered from a rare form of mosaic Down syndrome rather than the more typical trisomy 21. "Across all levels of cognitive function [they] observed language deficits disproportionate to those observed for nonverbal abilities" (p. 331). This relative deficit for language is apparent over time as well. In a large-scale longitudinal study of home-reared children followed from birth, Share (1975) reported that, throughout childhood, developmental performance on language measures was below motor and personal–social skills as assessed by the Gesell developmental norms. Recent studies of very young children suggest that the deficiencies in language and language-related skills may extend back to the very earliest stages of development (Dameron, 1963; Share, Koch, Webb, & Graliker, 1964; see also Greenwald & Leonard, 1979; Mahoney, Glover, & Finger, 1981; and Mervis, Chapter 8, this volume).

Further support for a specific language deficit in Down syndrome is provided by comparisons with other subgroups of the retarded population, matched for CA and IQ. On the basis of such studies, typically involving a heterogeneous contrast group of retarded individuals, it has often, though not always, been claimed that individuals with Down syndrome are "the most severely language handicapped" (Evans, 1977; see also Johnson & Abelson, 1969). One study claiming specific linguistic deficiencies in children with Down syndrome (Burr & Rohr, 1978) looked not at the development of grammatical or syntactic skills, per se, but focused instead on the pattern of processing and expressive skills suggested as underlying language ability and assessed in the Illinois Test of Psycholinguistic Abilities (ITPA, McCarthy & Kirk, 1961). On this test, children with Down syndrome showed a consistent disadvantage in the auditory tasks relative to comparable visual tasks; this auditory disadvantage was both more pervasive and greater in magnitude than that found for three groups of retarded children matched on IQ and CA, but whose retardation derived from perinatal, postnatal, environmental, or undiagnosed causes. (See Marcell & Armstrong, 1982, for additional evidence for a specific auditory deficit Down syndrome involving comparisons with normal IQ kindergarteners). Taking a different perspective, Wing (1975; cited in Gibson 1978) found that children with "organic brain damage" experienced even greater language problems than those found for children with Down syndrome matched for IQ and age. In sum, there is much evidence to suggest that Down syndrome is characterized by a specific impairment within the language domain; further details on the nature and scope of this deficit are developed in the section that follows.

Limits on language structure: differential delays within the communication/verbal domain

The evidence reviewed above suggests that children with Down syndrome experience difficulties with verbal measures that are incommensurate with their general developmental status. However, in the studies discussed, the language skills are usually not well defined or contained and the contrast skill or score is often a vague, all purpose measure. In this section, the argument is taken further. First, we review evidence that the sentence structures employed by children with Down syndrome are limited in absolute terms. Second, we argue that syntactic limitations extend beyond difficulties observed in other areas within the communication/verbal domain. A large number of studies point to a split between lexical and structural knowledge; a growing literature suggests that syntactic development may also lag behind other closely related abilities such as communicative function, sensorimotor development, and symbolic play. These disparities are evident from the onset of syntax, with the gap only increasing as the child becomes older.

Absolute levels of language skill

Although it is well-documented that language in Down syndrome can range from mutism to linguistic maturity, by and large, individuals with Down syndrome fail to move beyond the most rudimentary stages of syntactic development. For example, despite the fact that early vocabulary development paralleled the normal course, even the ''most accomplished'' subjects studied by Muir (1903) had acquired but a few verbs. Another study from that time described children with Down syndrome as being ''disinclined'' to use sentences (Brousseau & Brainerd, 1928). Both Thompson (1963) and Wiegel-Crump (1981) remarked upon the reliance in children with Down syndrome on short, simple sentences. Wiegel-Crump went on (1981), quantifying the productive language skills of 80 children with Down syndrome (CA 6;0 to 12;7 years; MA 2;0 to 6;11 years) using a standardized sentence scoring procedure (Lee 1974). The children with Down syndrome exhibited a *more* homogeneous pattern of syntactic usage than MA-matched nonhandicapped children, relying almost exclusively on low-level syntactic structures. Little variety of construction was observed across the entire MA range observed.

Experimental studies involving sentence comprehension, sentence repetition, and sentence completion tasks have also found that children with Down syndrome tend to cluster at very limited syntactic levels. Semmel and Dolley (1971) found that most children with Down syndrome (CA 6 to 14 years; IQ 22 to 62) could comprehend and reproduce only simple active declarative sentences. Without contextual cues, these children performed at base level on negative, passive, and negative passive sentences. Similarly, Rondal, Lambert, & Sohier (1981) reported that only three subjects out of 19 (CA 5;2 to 12;7 years; IQ 40 to 49) could successfully imitate a five-word active declarative sentence; when the declarative was negative, still five words in length, only one subject could repeat it correctly. The responses produced were echolalic and would surely be considered "deviant" if produced spontaneously. Experience in our own lab, however, indicates that these are much the same responses as produced by very young nonhandicapped children (24 to 30 months CA) when asked to repeat sentences well beyond their level of proficiency (Fowler, 1980; see also Lenneberg et al., 1964).

Generally limited language levels were also reported by Evans (1977), who was completely unsuccessful in his attempt to administer the Berko morphological cloze task (*Here is a wug, now there are two* _____) to a sample of 101 individuals with Down syndrome (CA 8.3 to 31.1 years; MA 2.5 to 7.8 years). Ninety-six of the subjects scored 6 or fewer correct responses to the 30 items in the nonsense word condition; 61 could not supply a plural for the word *wug*. In regard to his spontaneous language measures, Evans noted that "because of limited speech development no subject reached the ceiling in either the Sentence Structure Test or the Linguistic Features Count" (p. 113). In that analysis, more than a third of the utterances produced were one word long, and the ten longest utterances in each subject's corpus averaged only 5.2 words.

Finally, it should be noted that even studies ostensibly reporting a range of language skill in individuals with Down syndrome may be masking a more homogeneous pattern. In the population studied by Lenneberg et al. (1964), for example, 32 of the 35 subjects (CA 5;6 to 36;6) for which he reports data fell into his two middle categories of language development ("mostly words" or "primitive phrases"). Only two of the 35 were at the "sentence" level, while one child was still at the "babbling" stage. (This observation derives from Rosenberg, 1982.) Similarly, Andrews and Andrews (1977) report "tremendous variability" in the spontaneous speech of 39 children with Down syndrome (CA 5;8 to 17;9; IQ 31 to 60). A closer look at their data reveals that the variability stems from usage factors such as verbosity (number of utterances produced); on structural measures such as MLU, children were highly consistent in obtaining low scores.

From these various studies, the generalization seems to emerge that Down syndrome may exert considerable influence on the ultimate language level an individual will attain. Although a celebrated few will reach the language level of a 5-year-old and will have limited skills in reading and writing (Seagoe, 1965), the child with Down syndrome is not apt to move beyond the level of simple phrase structure grammar found in nonhandicapped children younger than 3 years.

Lexical versus syntactic development

There is considerable, if indirect, evidence that lexical knowledge in children with Down syndrome is spared relative to structural knowledge. In studies of lexical knowledge, whether the task is to produce, recognize, or identify vocabulary items, children with Down syndrome perform at the same level, or only slightly behind, MA-matched controls, retarded and not (Bartel, Bryen, & Keehn, 1973; Blount, 1968; Lyle, 1960; Ryan, 1975; Spreen, 1965). On the other hand, when grammatical or syntactic indices are taken, children with Down syndrome standardly perform on a lower level than their MA peers (Castellan-Paour & Paour, 1971 [cited in Gibson, 1978]; Lyle, 1960; Ryan, 1975; Spreen, 1965). Most convincing are several studies in which grammatical and lexical measures have been made on the same subjects, demonstrating a greater delay for grammatical than for lexical forms, relative to MA. This disparity is maintained whether the task involves production or comprehension of structures and appears to increase with chronological and mental age (Bless, Swift & Rosen, 1985; Hartley, 1982; Lyle, 1960; Rogers, 5; Ryan, 1975). Two studies reviewed in the paragraphs that follow illustrate the nt.

Evans (1977) provided evidence for such a lexical – structural split in a factor-analytic study using a wide range of measures including verbal and nonverbal intelligence, CA, several structural and fluency measures derived from spontaneous speech samples, and performance on the subtests of the ITPA (McCarthy & Kirk, 1961). In Evans's data there was a consistent pattern of clustering of measures according to three largely distinct factors. Significantly, there was a sharp dichotomy between the General Verbal Ability factor and the Structure of Speech factor. Stanford – Binet Mental Age was the highest loading on the Verbal factor but was insignificant on the Structural factor; CA, in contrast, loaded moderately but significantly on the Structural factor, but not on the Verbal factor. Those measures loading on the Structural factor included sentence length, complexity, ratio of nouns to verbs and other parts of speech, and a task of grammatical morphology. These were largely independent from the general Verbal measures including vocabulary, general intelligence tests, and most of the ITPA measures. Those measures tapping fluency of speech correlated only among themselves and nonsignificantly with the other two factors.

Hartley (1982) also found that difficulties in syntax surpassed those in the lexicon and went on to show that this disparity was more extreme in children with Down syndrome than in a mixed group of retarded children. Her conclusion was based on patterns of performance on The Token Test for Children (DiSimoni, 1978), which she administered to children with Down syndrome (mean CA 11;0 years), to retarded children of other etiologies (mean CA 10;7 years) and to nonhandicapped children (mean CA 4;7 years). The three groups were matched on receptive vocabulary score: mean MA on the Peabody Picture Vocabulary Test (PPVT) was 4;2 years for each group. The Token Test, which requires the subject to manipulate wooden objects of varying shapes and colors, incorporates conditions that allow the experimenter to manipulate memory demands directly as in (1) versus (2) below, as well as syntactic requirements, such as (2) versus (3). In this analysis, Hartley further divided the tasks standardly labeled syntactic into those she considered to be primarily syntactic and those she thought were lexically encoded or "spatial." This contrast is illustrated in (3) versus (4).

(1) *Give me the red circle*
(2) *Pick up the big red circle and the small green square*
(3) *Before picking up the yellow circle, touch the red square*
(4) *Put the white circle in front of the blue square*

Both groups of retarded children were significantly less successful on all parts of the test than nonhandicapped children matched for MA. Children with Down syndrome, in turn, performed less well than other non-Down syndrome children of similar age and IQ. Only on the spatial items was there no difference between the Down syndrome and the non-Down syndrome children; this was in direct contrast to the significant difference found between groups of retarded children on the sentences stressing syntactic skill. Although Hartley hypothesized that children with Down syndrome process "simultaneous" but not "sequential" information, her results can also be handled by invoking a lexical–syntactic split that holds up even when the lexical items under study are highly relational spatial terms.

Communicative skill versus structural development

A more recent body of developmentally informed research has examined the development of language structure, for instance, as indexed by MLU, within the context of more general communication skills. This literature has focused on Stage I of syntactic development, at which point children are just beginning to form two-word combinations. The general finding is that children with Down syndrome exhibit communicative skills at a level at least equivalent to, and often more advanced than, communicative behavior of nonhandicapped children also at Stage I (Coggins, Carpenter, & Owings, 1983; Coggins & Stoel-Gammon, 1982; Leifer & Lewis, 1984; Owens & MacDonald, 1982; Scherer & Owings, 1984). Beeghly and Cicchetti (1985) found not only that the communicative skills of children with Down syndrome were more mature than those of MLU-matched controls, but went on to show that they were equivalent to those of MA-matched controls whose MLU well exceeded that of the group with Down syndrome. Related findings are also reported by Weiss, Beeghly, and Cicchetti (1985) in regard to symbolic play, often thought to rest on the same cognitive basis as language behavior. On indices of symbolic play, the performance of children with Down syndrome is on a par with their general cognitive development and is generally more advanced than would be predicted on the basis of language level alone (Stage I) (see also Beeghly, Weiss-Perry, & Cicchetti, Chapter 10, this volume). Other studies of older individuals with Down syndrome also suggest that functional communicative skills may exceed verbal abilities, although these studies have not been as well controlled (Leuder, Fraser, & Jeeves, 1981; Nisbet, Zanella, & Miller, 1984; Price-Williams & Sabsay, 1979). In interpreting these results, one must be careful to keep in mind that a relative advantage on measures of communicative skill such as turn-taking or very early gestural skill need not imply that children with Down syndrome would have any real advantage in acquiring a structured sign language over spoken language. Although there is an advantage for gestural over spoken communication at the earliest stages of development in all children, this advantage appears to drop out for both nonhandicapped children and children with Down syndrome before the onset of syntax (Abrahamsen et al., 1985; Petitto, 1985).

The emergence of language as a function of "prelinguistic" abilities

The discussion thus far has been restricted to children who have already acquired at least rudimentary syntactic skill, consistent with the focus on language structure. This section discusses research that looks at the emergence of words and phrases within the context of other developmental achievements. Although Lenneberg et al. (1964) reported that the onset of first words and first sentences in children with Down syndrome intercalated nicely with major developmental milestones of walking and running, other studies conducted at that time suggest that children with Down syndrome show an inferiority in verbal skill relative to more general developmental measures, even at an early age (Dameron, 1963; Share et al., 1964). A few recent studies have made a more careful exploration of the relationship between the onset of first words and phrases, and measures of cognitive development hypothesized to underlie language skill, to yield a rather complicated story (Greenwald & Leonard, 1979; Mahoney et al., 1981; Beeghly, Weiss-Perry, & Cicchetti, Chapter 10, this volume; and Mervis, Chapter 8, this volume).

Greenwald and Leonard (1979) focused on the prelinguistic stage, comparing performance on a sensorimotor task with measures of communicative behavior in situations designed to induce either an imperative or a declarative response. Children with Down syndrome and normally developing children were selected as consistently functioning either at Stage IV or V on three scales of the Uzgiris and Hunt (1975) Ordinal Scales of Psychological Development. At Stage IV, the children with Down syndrome ranged in chronological age from 10 to 19 months (mean IQ of 52); these children were compared to nonhandicapped children between 7 and 9 months of age (mean IQ 110). At this emphatically prelinguistic level, no group differences emerged in communication measures: both groups were equally adept at using "imperative" gestures, and neither group displayed any evidence of making "declarative" gestures. More advanced levels of communicative behavior were found at Stage V in both groups and the imperative task continued to yield nonsignificant group differences. By this stage, however, a significant advantage was apparent in the declarative task: The nonhandicapped children (CA 9 to 13 months; mean IQ 125) relied upon more advanced declarative gestures than the group with Down syndrome (CA 16 to 26 months; mean IQ 68). The major source of this advantage was a greater tendency on the part of the nonhandicapped children to express themselves verbally; whereas the group with Down syndrome relied almost totally on nonverbal gestures, vocalization frequently replaced or accompanied gesture in the nonhandicapped group.

Also included in this study was a separate subgroup of older preschoolers with Down syndrome (CA 31 to 54 months; mean IQ 62). Although these children were also functioning at Stage V on the sensorimotor scale, they obtained more advanced communication scores and were more apt to use a verbal response than either of the younger groups. The authors suggest this shows some independence between the cognitive and linguistic tasks, perhaps facilitated by the massive linguistic intervention provided for these children. Although it seems that the Stage V level of sensorimotor development may be associated with a wide range of communicative skill, even within groups of children with Down syndrome, some of the variability may arise from grouping as a single category both verbal and nonverbal communication skills (see Beeghly & Cicchetti, 1985, and Beeghly, Weiss-Perry, Cicchetti, Chapter 10, this volume, for a cleaner separation of these skills in Stage I children). Greenwald and Leonard's findings that declarative, but not imperative, gestures are delayed in the infant with Down syndrome are of particular interest in light of research on referential looking in the prelinguistic infant with Down syndrome. Miller (1987) reviews several studies, most notably Jones (1977, 1980), in which children with Down syndrome (MA 8 to 22 months) exhibited significant deficits in referential looking behavior relative to general developmental level. Jones (1980), however, did not find that the children with Down syndrome vocalized significantly less than the MA-matched nonhandicapped children. Further disentanglement of what prelinguistic behaviors do and do not correlate with later linguistic patterns will surely aid our theoretical understanding of what elements constitute precursors to language learning.

Mahoney et al. (1981) provides further support that linguistic abilities lag behind sensorimotor functioning in very young children with Down syndrome. They matched children with Down syndrome (CA 24 to 38 months) and nonhandicapped children (CA 12 to 19 months) on the Bayley Mental Developmental Scale (Bayley, 1969), such that each group approximated a developmental age of 17 months (Down syndrome 13 to 23 months, mean = 16.8; nonhandicapped 12 to 23 months; mean = 17.1). Although the children with Down syndrome scored comparably or higher than the nonhandicapped children on five of the six subscales of the Uzgiris-Hunt scales of general sensorimotor development, the nonhandicapped group had a substantial advantage on the Vocal Imitation subscale and on both receptive and expressive measures of the Receptive and Expressive Early Language Test (Bzoch & League, 1970).

Finally, in a longitudinal study bridging the gap between prelanguage and language, Mervis (Chapter 8, this volume; see also Cardoso-Martins, Mervis, & Mervis, 1985) examined the ongoing relationship between cognitive development and linguistic development. Consistent with the findings of Lenneberg et al. (1964), she reports that the emergence of referential language, in both comprehension and production, is in keeping with developmental expectations. In children with Down syndrome, referential comprehension was first demonstrated at a mean MA of 14.5 months (Bayley) in children with Down syndrome, compared to a mean MA of 13.8 months in nonhandicapped children. Similarly, the onset of referential production occurred at a mean MA of 18.9 months in the group with Down syndrome compared to a mean MA of 19.5 months in the nonhandicapped group. These results were supported by a separate analysis that showed children with Down syndrome and nonhandicapped children to be comparable in their stages of sensori-motor development at the onset of referential communication.

On the other hand, Mervis reports vocabulary size is less well associated with sensorimotor measures. When groups were matched on sensorimotor development at four distinct points (all within Stages V and VI), vocabulary size was consistently smaller in the children with Down syndrome; the greatest difference in vocabulary size was apparent at the final point upon complete attainment of Stage VI. Although Mervis did not find differences in vocabulary size when she equated groups on interpolated MA levels (Bayley, 1969), she stresses that such differences were apparent in a larger-scale study conducted by Strominger, Winkler, and Cohen (1984). In that study, 36-month-old children with Down syndrome showed large deficits in vocabulary size relative to their mental age. Although they had a mean mental age of 20.6 months on the Bayley scales, their vocabulary size (mean 18.5 words; range 0 to 85) was closer to that of a normally developing child of 18 months (mean vocabulary 22 words) than to the average 21-month-old. By 21 months, the non-handicapped child has typically undergone a vocabulary explosion and has an average vocabulary of 118 words. Mervis concludes that "these results suggest that a major reason for the large differences in size of vocabulary between children with Down syndrome and non-handicapped children is that the vocabulary spurt for the child with Down syndrome does not begin at the mental age that would be expected, based on the findings concerning non-handicapped children" (p. 43). Given the close relationship between the vocabulary spurt and the onset of syntax in the non-handicapped child (Gleitman & Wanner, 1982; Lenneberg, 1967), this particular delay may presage directly the structural deficits discussed above.

Internal structure as a function of language stage

Considerable evidence has just been provided indicating that children with Down syndrome experience specific difficulties in acquiring language structures; most children advance little beyond the level attained by the normally developing 2-year-old. Further evidence seems to indicate that the bottleneck for acquiring language structure lies apart from acquisition of lexical items, and apart from general communicative and sensorimotor skills that, if necessary to acquiring language, in this population appear to be insufficient. Toward understanding the source of the difficulty of acquiring language, research focusing on the internal structure of language is reviewed here. The question is one of differential delay: When children with Down syndrome are matched with children without Down syndrome on a global measure of language structure, are there structures that are significantly more or less developed than the normal course would lead us to expect? An answer to this question should provide insight into the nature of the linguistic obstacles encountered by the child with Down syndrome. A clearer understanding of those areas of language most tied to lexical development, and those most affected in a structural delay, should provide insight into the issue of the homogeneity of developing syntax across all groups of children in the process of acquiring language.

This question of differential delay was addressed in a study by Fowler, Gelman, & Gleitman (1980), focusing on the possible dissociation between utterance length and syntactic complexity, syntax versus morphology, open class versus closed class. The subjects in that study were four adolescents with Down syndrome, attending a stimulating parochial day school. The four were selected for homogeneity of age (CA 10;9 to 13;0 years), intelligence level (Stanford–Binet IQ 46 to 56; MA 6 to 7 years), and language level (all were in Stage III, using the criteria established by Brown, 1973). This language level (MLU 2.75 to 3.25; mean 2.98) was representative of adolescent children with Down syndrome at that school and appears to be in keeping with other studies of adolescents with Down syndrome (e.g., Mein, 1961; Ryan, 1975; Semmel & Dolley, 1971). As controls, nonhandicapped youngsters were sought who had MLUs as close to 3.0 as possible. The four controls selected were between the ages of 30 and 32 months, consistent with established norms (Bloom, 1970; Brown, 1973; Miller, 1980). The young age was surprising because the adolescents appeared, at least impressionistically, to be communicating well beyond a 3-year-old level. The resulting disparity in age (CA 12 vs. 2-½ years; MA 6 vs. 3 years) made dissociation all the more likely in the various analyses employed. Half-hour spontaneous speech samples were collected under naturalistic play conditions with the experimenter at the school or day care. Internal analyses were performed on the transcript to tap the different aspects of linguistic skill hypothesized as being dissociable from the length measure used as the basis of comparison.

Performance on each of these measures was within the expectations derived from the normal literature relevant to that stage, and was confirmed on the basis of measures made on the nonhandicapped control group. The two groups did not differ at all on the types of syntactic constructions produced (or not produced); on the obligatory encoding of thematic relations (Bloom); or in the overall percentage of grammatical morphemes supplied in obligatory context. Surprisingly, where differences did occur, it was usually the child with Down syndrome who lagged behind the nonhandicapped child, despite attested higher verbal MA: They supplied early grammatical morphemes and grammatical objects less consistently, and produced less complex noun phrases. Despite relative advanced receptive vocabulary scores, in actual usage, the children with Down syndrome relied more heavily on pronouns than nouns. In those few cases where the children with Down syndrome maintained an advantage, there are important disclaimers. For instance, although they had a more extensive repertoire of closed class vocabulary (modals, pronouns, etc.), they were unable to use these same forms appropriately and consistently to serve syntactic–grammatical functions. Similarly, although they produced complex sentences of appropriate length and word order, these sentences were not supported by appropriate grammatical markers.

The children with Down syndrome in this study appeared to be at a linguistically stable, if restricted, point of development, with no syntactic or grammatical measure deviating from that stage one way or the other. Where differences occur, they relate to consistency of usage and a more enhanced vocabulary that extends even across the closed class domain. Overall, the combination of the syntactic measures employed indicate a simple phrase structure grammar. The level observed could not be reduced to semantic generalizations, perhaps (see Slobin, 1980, for a discussion of the normal course), but clearly precedes, across the board, the dramatic changes required to build the complex syntax with its associated verbal auxiliary system, sentential embedding, and movement rules.

There are, by now, many studies reiterating and extending the two main findings of Fowler et al. (1980): (1) that children with Down syndrome tend to cluster at linguistically limited, but coherent, stages of development; and (2) when appropriate matching procedures are employed, internal analyses by and large fail to distinguish the language structures employed by children with Down syndrome from those produced by other groups of children at that language stage. This seems to hold true not only at Stage III, but at earlier stages of development as well; some deviations are noted at higher language levels. The consistency of language levels within Down syndrome has resulted in a number of studies focusing on a few language stages, thus yielding a more detailed picture of language development than currently available for other, more mixed, groups.

Stages III to V

Fowler's results are consistent with those of Ryan (1975, 1977), who compared three groups of children (Down syndrome, retarded but without Down syndrome, nonhandicapped) matched on MLU (range) and found no difference in regard to the internal structure evident in spontaneous speech. At a slightly higher MLU level, Layton and Sharifi (1979) focused on verb types used by school-age children with Down syndrome (CA 7;4 to 12;2 years; MLU 3.5 to 5.5). Although the children with Down syndrome used the same types of verbs as nonhandicapped children matched on MLU, they differed in proportions of usage. A conceptual explanation was invoked to account for a much lower use in the Down syndrome group of "process" verbs involving a change of state, as in *John cut the paper*. Rondal (1978a) found no differences between children with Down syndrome and language-matched controls on syntactic complexity as assessed by Lee's (1974) Developmental Sentence Scoring procedure. Like Wiegel-Crump (1981), however, he reports that at the higher MLU levels, advanced constructions fail to develop in the child with Down syndrome at a level commensurate with normal expectations.

Studies of comprehension skill as a function of general language stage suggest that structural language deficits cut across comprehension and production equivalently. Bridges and Smith (1984) compared the performance of children with Down syndrome (CA 4;4 to 17;1) with that of nonhandicapped children (CA 1;11 to 4;4), when asked to act out active and passive semantically biased and neutral sentences. Rather than rely on MA, they used a general standardized comprehension measure (Reynell, 1969) as their criterion for selecting normal controls. There were six groups of matched pairs ranging in Verbal Comprehension Age (VCA) from 2;6 to 5;0 years. In this study, groups did not differ significantly in overall percentage correct response. The pattern of errors was comparable across groups; the groups were affected equivalently by manipulations of the semantic plausibility of the sentences presented. The children with Down syndrome, however, were 6 to 12 months behind the nonretarded children (as measured by VCA) in acquiring syntactic comprehension strategies.

Fowler (1984) also used an object manipulation procedure to examine the syntactic comprehension strategies and skills of schoolchildren with Down syndrome (CA 6;9 to 16;8). Again, they were matched to normally developing children (CA 2;3 to 3;2) on the basis of MLU (low MLU 3.15 to 3.55; high MLU 4.0 to 4.65). The children with Down syndrome had significantly higher MA scores, as assessed by the PPVT-R (Dunn & Dunn, 1981). In this study, there were no differences between groups in mean performance overall, or in their performance in the semantically reversible condition. The effect of syntactic type (actives, passives, datives and three relative clause types) was constant across groups. However, there was a significant interaction between group and effect of semantic plausibility, suggesting that the children with Down syndrome may depend more heavily on semantic inferencing skills. The children with Down syndrome performed better in the plausible conditions, and worse in the implausible conditions, than did the nonhandicapped control subjects. The apparent contradiction between Fowler (1984) and Bridges and Smith (1984) is likely a function of the matching procedure. The VCA measure employed by Bridges and Smith incorporates lexical as well as syntactic knowledge. Consistent with the lexical–syntactic split discussed earlier, it appears to have overestimated syntactic knowledge in the Down syndrome group, but to have been a fair measure of semantic inferencing skill. On the other hand, the measure selected by Fowler (MLU) turns out to be an appropriate index of syntactic comprehension knowledge, but underestimates lexical (and semantic inferencing) knowledge. The differences between groups in Fowler (1984) relevant to plausibility factors appear to be a function of large differences in vocabulary level. (See Dewart, 1978, for comparable results with a group of retarded children without Down syndrome).

Stages I to III

The virtue of comparing language structure of children with Down syndrome and without Down syndrome as a function of general language level has recently been demonstrated in several studies of mildly to moderately retarded children with Down syndrome functioning at Brown's (1973) Stage I. At this early stage, marked by the onset of two-word utterances, the focus has been on determining the "relational" or "thematic" meanings encoded in two-word combinations (Buium, Rynders, & Turnure, 1974; Coggins, 1979; Dooley, 1977; Fowler, 1984). Although these studies vary in the semantic coding systems employed, they are in full agreement that children with Down syndrome choose to encode much the same thematic relations as nonhandicapped children at the same language stage. Coggins (1979), for example, classified all two-word utterances of four children with Down syndrome (aged 3;10 to 6;2) to find that they showed as much diversity as nonhandicapped children studied in Bloom, Lightbown, and Hood (1975) and Schlesinger (1971). Approximately 70% of their utterances fell into the same nine "semantic categories" most frequently encoded by nonhandicapped at Stage I. Paralleling normal development, Coggins observed a shift from Early Stage I to Late Stage I in the tendency of the children with Down syndrome to rely increasingly on locative and stative categories. Coggins also noted that the children with Down syndrome, like nonhandicapped children at this stage, failed to make conditional or hypothetical statements, refer to past or future events, or use grammatical morphemes productively. However, within this same language stage, Harris (1983) reports that there is an effect of chronological age (CA 2;6–6;9 years) on language structure. The younger children with Down syndrome were indistinguishable from MLU-matched nonhandicapped children, but the older children employed somewhat different means to expand their utterances.

A common feature of the nonhandicapped speaker at Stage I is the spontaneous imitation of adult utterances. Coggins and Morrison (1981) found that, like nonhandicapped children studied by Bloom, Hood, and Lightbown (1974), children with Down syndrome vary considerably in the amount of spontaneous imitations produced. Of primary interest to these researchers was the finding that children with Down syndrome were selective in their choice of structures to imitate: like nonhandicapped children, they chose to imitate words that did not occur frequently in their spontaneous productions. (See Shipley, Smith, & Gleitman, 1969, for the normal case). Coggins and Morrison suggested that this selective imitation points to a strategic attempt to resolve differences between the child's productions and the adult input.

Rondal (1980) found spontaneous imitations produced by children with Down syndrome to be comparable in both number and complexity to those produced by nonhandicapped children, not only at Stage I (MLU 1.0–1.5 and 1.75–2.25) but at a somewhat higher MLU level as well (MLU 2.5–3.0). Language level was a significant factor in both groups: In children with Down syndrome as in nonhandicapped children, the absolute number of imitations decreased and the length and complexity of imitations increased as language level improved. In both groups, there was a tendency to imitate the end of a maternal utterance, which Rondal suggests shows a "perceptual centration" on the final part of adult utterances (see Slobin, 1973, for the normal case). Indeed, of a wide number of measures taken, the only difference distinguishing the children with Down syndrome from nonhandicapped children was a greater tendency to imitate modifiers from the mother's speech.

Two studies have been conducted, looking at the internal structure of language as it develops over time, starting at Stage I. Dooley (1977) conducted a year-long observational study of two children with Down syndrome (IQ 51 and 44; starting CA 3;10 and 5;2); both children were in Brown's (1973) language Stage I throughout the study. Over the year, one child made approximately one month's progress (MLU 1.48 to 1.75) relative to nonhandicapped children studied by Brown (1973); the other child actually declined somewhat in MLU (1.84 to 1.73). Except for failing to change significantly over the period, the children were similar to Stage I nonhandicapped children on internal measures (semantic relations, grammatical morphemes, utterance diversity, and size of lexicon). The only difference of note was a greater tendency on the part of the children with Down syndrome to rely more heavily on routinized expressions and proforms *(it, they, here, there, do)*, which is in keeping with the findings presented in earlier sections. Dooley stresses that this tendency also varies in the normal population.

Fowler (1984) reports on a child with Down syndrome, Rebecca (IQ 57; CA 4;3 to 7;5), who was observed on a monthly basis over a 3-year period (CA 4;3 to 6;11 years); Rebecca's language moved from Stage I to Stage III/IV over this time period. Despite a slow start in Stage I, Rebecca grew consistently from MLU 1.4 to 3.5 in a normally rapid period of time (13 months). This was followed by an extended plateau (10 months) at the 3.5 threshold. Near the close of the study, Rebecca was veering into Stage V (MLU = 4.0), but with considerable fluctuation. On internal analyses (semantic relations, grammatical morphology, negative and interrogative constructions), Rebecca's language was indistinguishable from the norm between the stages of I and III, but for a slight advance in semantic relations relative to MLU. When she reached the 3.5 threshold, progress on these internal measures halted and interesting overgeneralizations were observed in the verbal auxiliary system and wh-interrogation. Although modest further progress has been made in her syntactic development, this development appears to have diverged from the normal course in both rate and character.

Explanatory accounts of the specific language deficit in children with Down syndrome

On the basis of the research presented, it is quite clear that the course and limits on language learning in children with Down syndrome cannot be explained as a simple function of general cognitive development, as assessed either by MA, or by more sophisticated measures of communicative skill or sensorimotor development (see also Cromer, 1974, 1976). Several explanatory accounts have been put forth in an attempt to explain why there is a large discrepancy between measured MA and the final language attainment of individuals with Down syndrome; and why learning appears to stop at the point that it does. Although none of these accounts has been unequivocally ruled out, and several may play a role, they are presented here as possible directions for future research.

A commonly invoked explanation for deficits in heterogeneous retarded children above and beyond those predicted by general cognitive factors is that they are less motivated than nonhandicapped MA peers in performing the task at hand (Zigler, 1969). However, motivation fails to account for normal language learning: Whereas it is presumably extremely crucial for all individuals to have a rudimentary communication system for basic needs, the elaboration of such a system to incorporate complex linguistic syntactic forms (e.g., *can I have a cookie* vs. *cookie!*) lacks motivational explanation in all cases. And yet, it is just this elaboration that is lacking in the child with Down syndrome. Note, too, that the child with Down syndrome studied today is not the depressed institutionalized child of yesterday about whom motivational accounts were hypothesized. Today's subjects often live at home in family settings or adult workshops (e.g., Evans 1977); they receive special attention from very early ages at home and in the schools. Nonetheless, these individuals continue to perform in language well below MA expectations. Perhaps most telling concerning the role of motivation in acquiring syntax are two explicit studies of the effects of institutionalization on language in children with Down syndrome. Although McNutt and Leri (1979) found that institutionalization dampened progress across many areas of development, including vocabulary and verbosity, both they and Wiegel-Crump (1981) report no differences between institutionalized and home-reared children with Down syndrome on a wide range of syntactic measures.

A second account put forth to account for the extreme linguistic deficits in children with Down syndrome refers specifically to the language environment. Given the discrepancy between the child's age/size and linguistic capacities, it is possible that the speech directed to him or her is inappropriate. That is, whatever advantage is derived from the tendency to speak to young children in short, simple sentences (comprehensibility, perhaps), may be denied the retarded child at similar stages in the acquisition sequence. (For discussion of the facilitative effects of motherese in normal language learning, see Fernald & Simon, 1984; Furrow, Nelson, & Benedict, 1979; Gleitman, Newport, & Gleitman, 1984; and Newport, Gleitman, & Gleitman, 1977). A number of studies have addressed this issue and rendered this hypothesis implausible; mothers interact with their children with Down syndrome in much the same way as they interact with their nonhandicapped children at comparable language levels. Most compelling is the finding that MLU is a much better predictor than MA or CA of the characteristics of a mother's speech to her child. (See Peterson & Sherrod, 1982; Rondal, 1978b; and Rosenberg, 1982, for comprehensive reviews of the relevant literature.) Even where differences in mother's style of interaction do emerge, it has not been possible to assign a specific result to that difference. Mervis (Chapter 8, this volume) reports that although mothers make fewer adjustments to accommodate to the early lexical categories of their children with Down syndrome, such differences seem to have no direct effect on the categories formed and maintained by their children.

Miller (1987) agrees with these results but suggests that a lack of maternal responsiveness at the prelinguistic level may be responsible for a delay in language. In a review of the literature, he reports that mothers are less responsive to infants with Down syndrome (and vice versa); that mothers of infants with Down syndrome tend to talk while their child is vocalizing rather than to engage in turn-talking behavior; and that mothers are more directive, intrusive, and controlling while interacting with children with Down syndrome than are mothers interacting with nonhandicapped children of comparable mental age (see also Beeghly, Weiss, & Cicchetti, 1984; Hanzlik & Stevenson, 1986). The results of intervention studies seeking to mitigate these differences look promising; however, thus far, they lack controls.

Furthermore, it is not clear how one should go about "matching" prelinguistic groups as a function of language level; we know in any case that early sensorimotor and communication measures are poor indices of how far along the child has progressed toward acquiring verbal skill.

A third proposal to account for the specific language deficit suggests that the neurological structures underlying language are particularly impaired in children with Down syndrome. Although there is overwhelming evidence of anatomical, physiological, and neurochemical abnormalities in the brains of children with Down syndrome (e.g., Ross et al., 1984), such differences have not yet been specifically related to differences in language function. Two attempts have, however, been made to relate language differences to the lack of a dominant language hemisphere as assessed by dichotic listening tasks.

Looking for the biological underpinnings of a specific language impairment in individuals with Down syndrome, Zekulin-Hartley (1981) administered a dichotic listening task to children with Down syndrome, to a heterogeneous group of retarded children matched to the Down syndrome group on IQ and CA, and to nonhandicapped controls matched to the retarded groups on MA. Whereas both groups of children without Down syndrome showed the expected right-ear advantage in processing linguistic serially presented auditory stimuli (digits and common object labels), children with Down syndrome showed a significant left-ear advantage. Hartley (1985) has gone on to relate ear advantage directly to differences in syntactic processing on the Type–Token Test (DiSimoni, 1978).

Sommers and Starkey (1977) used the dichotic listening paradigm to look at differences within the syndrome, comparing two groups of children representing the extremes in language functioning. All subjects, selected from a day school population of 150 children, met a minimum criterion of being able to point correctly to each of the dichotic words and foils used in the test; all had normal hearing and were predominately right-handed. The high-language group ($n = 15$, CA 7;0 to 19;0 years, mean IQ 46, mean MA 64 months) was functioning at a language age of 5;3, as assessed by the Carrow (1973) Test for Auditory Comprehension of Language. These children had a mean MLU of 7.5 words; used both simple and complex grammatical structures; and produced appropriate and intelligible verbal responses to stimulus materials. In contrast, the low-performance group ($n = 14$, CA 7;1 to 17;8, mean IQ 39, mean MA 51 months) was functioning at a language level of 3;7 years; had a mean MLU of 2.5; and spoke in three- and four-word sentences at the base phrase structure level. Their speech was telegraphic, intelligibility was poor, and verbal perseveration and inappropriate responses were common. Despite the clear separation between groups in linguistic skill, and despite the great care taken to use a sensitive and reliable measure, the ear advantage in both groups was essentially zero. This contrasted with nonhandicapped controls (3;0 to 5;5 years CA, mean MA 5;1) who showed the expected significant right-ear advantage. Although dichotic listening tasks are fraught with methodological pitfalls (Bryden, 1982), the lack of a right-ear advantage is at least suggestive of a seriously impaired language area (though see Elliott, Weeks, & Elliott 1987). Converging evidence from other biological indices is crucial to exploring this hypothesis further.

The fourth explanation for the extreme discrepancy between language achievement and cognitive level derives from Lenneberg's (1967) critical period hypothesis discussed earlier in the chapter. As noted there, this hypothesis fails on many points. Nonetheless, a maturational account contains a great deal of merit. All longitudinal studies spanning the preschool years report that maximal language growth occurs before the age of 7 years in children with Down syndrome. For example, Share (1975) reports on the developmental progress, using Gesell norms, of 76 children with Down syndrome followed from birth; at the time of the report, these children ranged from 7 to 18 years CA. In this study most language development occurred between CA 4 and 6 years, during which time the child with Down syndrome typically moved from the developmental level of 15 months MA to 2½ or 3 years MA. This report fits with data presented in Lenneberg et al. (1964) and is corroborated in the detailed longitudinal case study reported in Fowler (1984; see also Fowler, 1988). Indirect support is provided by several cross-sectional studies in which the gap between syntactic and lexical knowledge widens with growth in CA (see Miller, 1987, for a review). A revised version of the critical period hypothesis would suggest that specialized language learning abilities are no longer available after the age of 7 years, consistent with reports from normal language development (Newport, 1982).

Finally, one might wish to account for these same facts as a function not of chronological age but of linguistic stage. If, indeed, impaired brain function sets a limit on the level of language that can be accommodated, it may well be that language skill is acquired in a timely fashion (roughly) consistent with general maturational development, but beyond the limiting language level, growth will cease or differ from the normal course (see Fowler, 1984). The considerable evidence speaking to a ceiling on language skill supports this hypothesis, but from the data presented, it is not possible to distinguish the effects of chronological age from those of language stage. (See Fowler, 1988, for a discussion of these last two hypotheses and for a more extended set of longitudinal data bearing on this issue.)

Overview

In sum, the measures and procedures that have been used to study language in Down syndrome vary in many ways. But taken together, they seem to suggest a coherent picture. Individuals with Down syndrome tend to form a well-organized human subset with regard to the prognosis for language development: They are a diminished case of the normal within the language domain and represent a particularly well-studied and straightforward case of the delay–deficit observed in retarded language generally.

1. By virtue of studying a biologically well-defined subgroup, some insight has been gained into the course and prognosis of language development under one con-

dition of retardation. Individuals with Down syndrome appear to be more consistent in terms of the degree of language delay than are more diffuse groups of retarded individuals. Language consistently develops more slowly in children with Down syndrome than do other aspects of motor or cognitive development; this lag is evident in infancy and grows wider as the children with Down syndrome become older.

2. Working from a developmental model of normal language acquisition, and finding comparable matches in terms of language stage, it becomes possible to determine what the child with Down syndrome is or is not capable of in absolute terms, rather than relative to some arbitrary MA measure. Some children with Down syndrome do acquire substantial linguistic competence, to the level of a normally developing 5-year-old. Although IQ is not totally unrelated to linguistic success, it has not yet proven possible to predict, on nonlinguistic grounds, how to distinguish the few children who will acquire syntax from the great majority whose language will level off at an early age without acquiring the complexity of syntax or morphology.

3. Global studies of language have suggested that MA overestimates structural linguistic knowledge in individuals with Down syndrome, reflecting a split between lexical and syntactic knowledge. This question has been addressed systematically, experimentally manipulating the demands on the child to tap one or the other aspect of language skill. Converging evidence from both comprehension and production strongly supports the conclusion that the language deficit in Down syndrome is most pronounced in the grammatic–syntactic components with a relative sparing within the lexical domain (also within nonverbal communication). On the other hand, within the structural components of language, it appears that the deficit is consistent across syntax and morphology and across comprehension and production (see also Beeghly, Weiss-Perry, & Cicchetti, Chapter 10, this volume).

4. Research on children with Down syndrome serves to reinforce the view that language in retarded individuals is qualitatively similar to the language of younger nonhandicapped children, particularly in Stages I through III. This holds up across a wide number of detailed internal analyses in which groups are matched for developmental level within the domain of interest (here, language), reflecting a general trend toward domain-specific research (e.g., Keil, 1981). Also in keeping with this trend, the language measures taken are not presented as a single summary index: Rather, the internal measures employed in research on children with Down syndrome (thematic relations, morphological usage, etc.) are treated as coherent rule-governed systems that are potentially separable from other language measures. Although work on other well-defined domains to contrast with syntactic growth is progressing, much more research needs to be done in this direction.

5. Although no data are available for other subgroups of retarded individuals, a small data base is accruing concerning the course of language learning over time in individuals with Down syndrome, based on longitudinal and systematic cross-sectional research. On the basis of this preliminary research, it appears that language learning does not proceed at a constant pace from birth to puberty. Rather, a great deal of language learning appears to take place by 7 years of age (CA); for brief periods it

may proceed at a near normal pace. In regard to internal analyses of the language systems acquired, conclusions derived from cross-sectional research appear to hold up across the entire developmental sequence, whether defined in terms of CA, MA, or language level, with a widening of the semantic–syntactic gap as CA increases.

Much work remains in order to understand why children with Down syndrome stop where they do in the language acquisition sequence, to determine why some children do in fact make better progress in language, to explain differences in consistency and usage that emerge on detailed internal analyses, and to explore more fully the possibility of different learning mechanisms leading to similar results. However, it should be apparent that research on Down syndrome, by taking a stance that is at once developmental, domain-specific, and biological has greatly enhanced our general understanding of the effects of retardation on language development.

References

Abrahamsen, A., Cavallo, M., & McLuer, J. A. (1985). Is the sign advantage a robust phenomenon? From gesture to language in two modalities. *Merrill-Palmer Quarterly.*

Andrews, R. J., & Andrews, J. G. (1977). A study of the spontaneous oral language of Down's syndrome children. *Exceptional Child, 24,* 86–94.

Bartel, N., Bryen, D., & Keehn, S. (1973). Language comprehension in the mentally retarded child. *Exceptional Child, 39,* 375–382.

Bayley, N. (1969). *Bayley Scales of Infant Development: Birth to two years.* New York: Psychological Corporation.

Beeghly, M., & Cicchetti, D. (1985). Development of functional communication during Stage I of syntactic development by children with Down syndrome. Presented at the Tenth Annual Boston University Conference on Language Development, October.

Beeghly, M., Hanrahan, A., Weiss, B., & Cicchetti, D. (1985). Development of communicative competence in children with Down syndrome and nonhandicapped children. Presented at the biennial meeting of the Society for Research in Child Development, Toronto, April.

Beeghly, M., Weiss, B., & Cicchetti, D. (1984). Structure and style of free play behavior in Down syndrome and non-handicapped children. Paper presented at the International Conference on Infant Studies, New York, April.

Bellugi, U. (in press). Studies of children with Williams syndrome. In H. Tager-Flusberg, (Ed.), *Constraints on Language Acquisition: Studies of Atypical Children.* Hillsdale, NJ: Erlbaum.

Berko, J. (1958). The child's learning of English morphology. *Word, 14,* 150–177.

Best, C. T., Hoffman, H., & Glanville, B. B. (1982). Development of infant ear asymmetries for speech and music. *Perception & Psychophysics, 31,* 75–85.

Bilovsky, D., & Share, J. (1965). The ITPA and Down's Syndrome: An exploratory study. *American Journal of Mental Deficiency, 70,* 78–82.

Bless, D., Swift, E., & Rosen, M. (1985). Communication profiles of children with Down syndrome. Waisman Center on Mental Retardation and Human Development. University of Wisconsin, Madison.

Bloom, L. (1970). *Language development: Form and function in emerging grammars.* Cambridge, MA: MIT Press.

Bloom, L., Hood, L., & Lightbown, P. (1974). Imitation in language development: If, when and why. *Cognitive Psychology, 6,* 380–420.

Bloom, L., & Lahey, M. (1978). *Language development and language disorders.* New York: Wiley.

Bloom, L., Lightbown, P., & Hood, L. (1975). Structure and variation in child language. *Monograph of the Society for Research in Child Development, 40*(2).

Blount, W. R. (1968). Language and the more severely retarded: A review. *American Journal of Mental Deficiency, 73,* 21 – 29.

Bowerman, M. (1982). Reorganizational processes in lexical and syntactic development. In E. Wanner & L. Gleitman (Eds.), *Language acquisition: State of the art.* Cambridge: Cambridge University Press.

Bridges, A., & Smith, J. (1984). Syntactic comprehension in Down's syndrome children. *British Journal of Psychology, 75,* 187–196.

Brousseau, K., & Brainerd, M. G. (1928). *Mongolism: A study of the psychical and mental characteristics of mongoloid imbeciles.* Baltimore: Williams & Williams.

Brown, R. (1973). *A first language.* Cambridge, MA: Harvard University Press.

Bryden, M. P. (1982). *Laterality: Functional asymmetry in the intact brain.* New York: Academic Press.

Buium, N., Rynders, J., & Turnure, J. (1974). Early maternal linguistic environment of normal and Down's syndrome language-learning children. *American Journal of Mental Deficiency, 79,* 52–58.

Burr, D. B., & Rohr, A. (1978). Patterns of psycholinguistic development in the severely retarded: a hypothesis. *Social Biology, 25,* 15–22.

Bzoch, K. R., & League, R. (1970). *The Receptive–Expressive Emergent Language Scale for the measurement of language skills in infancy.* Gainesville, FL: The Tree of Life Press.

Cardoso-Martins, C., Mervis, C. B., & Mervis, C. A. (1985). Early vocabulary acquisition by children with Down syndrome. *American Journal of Mental Deficiency, 90,* 177–184.

Carrow, M. (1968). The development of auditory comprehension of language structure in children. *Journal of Speech and Hearing Disorders, 33,* 99–111.

Carrow, E. (1973). *Test for Auditory Comprehension of Language* (5th ed.). Austin, TX: Learning Concepts.

Castellan-Paour, M., & Paour, J. (1971). Attempted syntactic structure reeducation in the adolescent mongol. *Rev. Neuropsychiatr. Infant Hyg. Ment. Enfance, 19,* 449–461. [Cited in Gibson, 1978].

Coggins, T. E. (1979). Relational meaning encoded in the two-word utterances of Stage 1 Down's Syndrome children. *Journal of Speech and Hearing Research, 22,* 166–178.

Coggins, T. E., Carpenter, R. L., & Owings, N. O. (1983). Examining early intentional communication in Down's syndrome and nonretarded children. *British Journal of Disorders of Communication, 18,* 98–106.

Coggins, T. E., & Morrison, J. A. (1981). Spontaneous imitations of Down's syndrome children: A lexical analysis. *Journal of Speech and Hearing Research, 46,* 303–308.

Coggins, T. E., & Stoel-Gammon, C. (1982). Clarification strategies used by four Down's syndrome children for maintaining normal conversational interaction. *Education and Training of the Mentally Retarded, 17,* 65–67.

Cornwell, A. (1974). Development of language, abstraction, and numerical concept formation in Down's syndrome children. *American Journal of Mental Deficiency, 79,* 179–190.

Cromer, R. F. (1974). Receptive language in the mentally retarded. In R. L. Schiefelbusch & L. L. Lloyd, *Language perspectives: Acquisition, retardation and intervention.* Baltimore: University Park Press.

Cromer, R. F. (1976). The cognitive hypothesis. In D. M. Morehead & A. E. Morehead, (Eds.), *Normal and deficient child language.* Baltimore: University Park Press.

Dameron, L. (1963). Development of intelligence of infants with Mongolism. *Child Development, 34,* 733–738.

Dennis, M., & Whitaker, H. A. (1977). Hemispheric equipotentiality and language acquisition. In S. J. Segalowitz & F. A. Gruber (Eds.), *Language development and neurological theory.* New York: Academic Press.

Dewart, M. H. (1978). Language comprehension processes of mentally retarded children. *American Journal of Mental Deficiency, 84,* 177–83.

DiSimoni, F. (1978). *The Token Test for Children.* Allen, TX: DLM Teaching Resources.

Dooley, J. (1977). Language acquisition and Down's syndrome: A study of early semantics and syntax. Unpublished doctoral dissertation, Harvard University.

Duchan, J. F., & Erikson, J. G. (1976). Normal and retarded children's understanding of semantic relations in different verbal contexts. *Journal of Speech and Hearing Research, 19,* 767–776.

Dunn, L., & Dunn, L. (1981). *Peabody Picture Vocabulary Text-Revised.* Circle Pines, MN: American Guidance Service.

Elliott, D., Weeks, D., & Elliott, C. (1987). Cerebral specialization in individuals with Down syndrome. *American Journal of Mental Deficiency, 92,* 263–271.

Evans, D. (1973). Some language abilities of severely mentally handicapped persons with special reference to Down's syndrome. Unpublished doctoral dissertation, Exeter University, England.

Evans, D. (1977). The development of language abilities in mongols: A correlational study. *Journal of Mental Deficiency Research, 21,* 103–117.

Evans, D., & Hampson, M. (1968). The language of mongols. *British Journal of Disorders of Communication, 3,* 171–181.

Fernald, A. & Simon, T. (1984). Expanded intonation contours in mothers' speech to newborns. *Developmental Psychology, 20.*

Fodor, J. A. (1983). *The modularity of language.* Cambridge, MA: MIT Press.

Fowler, A. (1980). Effects of mental retardation on the acquisition of language. Unpublished masters' thesis, University of Pennsylvania.

Fowler, A. (1984). Language acquisition in Down's syndrome children: Production and comprehension. Unpublished doctoral dissertation, University of Pennsylvania. In *Dissertation Abstracts International, 46* (1-B), 324, (1985).

Fowler, A. (1988). Determinants of rate of language growth in children with Down syndrome. In L. Nadel (Ed.), *The psychobiology of Down syndrome.* Cambridge, MA: MIT Press.

Fowler, A., Gelman, R., & Gleitman, L. (1980). A comparison of normal and retardate language equated on MLU. Presented at the Fifth Annual Boston University Conference on Child Language Development, October.

Furrow, D., Nelson, K., & Benedict, H. (1979). Mothers' speech to children and syntactic development: Some simple relationships. *Journal of Child Language, 6,* 432–442.

Gelman, R., & Cohen, M. (1988). Qualitative differences in the way Down syndrome and normal children solve a novel counting problem. In L. Nadel (Ed.), *The psychobiology of Down syndrome.* Cambridge, MA: MIT Press.

Gibson, D. (1966). Early development staging as a prophecy index in Down's syndrome. *American Journal of Mental Deficiency, 70,* 825–828.

Gibson, D. (1978). *Down's syndrome: The psychology of mongolism.* London: Cambridge University Press.

Gleitman, L., Newport, E., & Gleitman, H. (1984). The current status of the Motherese hypothesis. *Journal of Child Language, 11,* 43–79.

Gleitman, L. R., & Wanner, E. (1982). Language acquisition: The state of the art. In E. Wanner & L. R. Gleitman (Eds.), *Language acquisition. The state of the art.* Cambridge: Cambridge University Press.

Greenwald, C. A., & Leonard, L. B. (1979). Communicative and sensorimotor development of Down's syndrome children. *American Journal of Mental Deficiency, 84,* 296–303.

Hanzlik, J., & Stevenson, M. (1986). Interaction of mothers with their infants who are mentally retarded, retarded with cerebral palsy or non-retarded. *American Journal of Mental Deficiency, 90,* 513–520.

Harris, J. (1983). What does mean length of utterance mean? Evidence from a comparative study of normal and Down's syndrome children. *British Journal of Disorders of Communication, 18,* 153–169.

Hartley, X. Y. (1982). Receptive language processing of Down's Syndrome children. *Journal of Mental Deficiency Research, 26,* 263–269.

Hartley, X. Y. (1985). Receptive language processing and ear advantage of Down's syndrome children. *Journal of Mental Deficiency Research, 26,* 263–269.

Hyams, N. (1986). *Language acquisition and the theory of parameters.* Dordrecht, Holland: D. Reidel.

Johnson, J. & Newport, E. (1989). Critical period effects in second language learning: The influence of maturational state on the acquisition of English as a second language. *Cognitive Psychology, 21,* 60–99.

Johnson, R. C., & Abelson, R. B. (1969). Intellectual, behavioral and physical characteristics associated with trisomy, translocation and mosaic types of Down's syndrome. *American Journal of Mental Deficiency, 73,* 852–855.

Jones, O.H.M. (1977). Mother–child communication with prelinguistic Down's syndrome and normal infants. In H. R. Schaffer & J. Dunn (Eds.), *The first year of life: Psychological and medical implications of early experience.* New York: Wiley.

Jones, O.H.M. (1980). Prelinguistic communication skills in Down's syndrome and normal infants. In T. M. Fields, S. Goldberg, D. Stern, & A. M. Sostek (Eds.), *High risk infants and children: Adult and peer interactions.* New York: Academic Press.

Karmiloff-Smith, A. (1979). Language as a formal problem space for children. Paper presented at Beyond Description in Child Language. Nijmegen: Max Planck Gesellschaft.

Keil, F. (1981). Constraints on knowledge and cognitive development. *Psychological Review, 88,* 197–227.

Krashen, S. (1975). The critical period for language acquisition and its possible causes. *Annals of the New York Academy of Sciences, 263,* 211–224.

Layton, T. L., & Sharifi, H. (1979). Meaning and structure of Down's syndrome and non-retarded children's spontaneous speech. *American Journal of Mental Deficiency, 83,* 439–445.

Lee, L. (1974). *Developmental Sentence Analysis.* Evanston, IL: Northwestern University Press.

Leifer, J., & Lewis, M. (1984). Acquisition of conversational response skills by young Down syndrome and non-retarded children. *American Journal of Mental Deficiency, 88,* 610–618.

Lenneberg, E. H. (1967). *Biological Foundations of Language.* New York: Wiley.

Lenneberg, E. H., Nichols, I. A., & Rosenberger, E. F. (1964). Primitive stages of language development in mongolism. Research Publications, *Association for Research in Nervous and Mental Disease, 42,* 119–147.

Leuder, I., Fraser, W. I., & Jeeves, M. A. (1981). Social familiarity and communication in Down syndrome. *Journal of Mental Deficiency Research, 5,* 133–142.

Lyle, J. G. (1960). The effect of an institution upon the verbal development of imbecile children. II. Speech and language. *Journal of Mental Deficiency Research, 4,* 1–13.

Mahoney, G., Glover, A., & Finger, I. (1981). Relationship between language and sensorimotor development of Down syndrome and nonretarded children. *American Journal of Mental Deficiency, 86,* 21–27.

Marcell, M., & Armstrong, V. (1982). Auditory and visual sequential memory of Down syndrome and nonretarded children. *American Journal of Mental Deficiency, 87,* 86–95.

McCarthy, J. (1965). Patterns of psycholinguistic development of mongoloid and non-mongoloid severely retarded children. Unpublished doctoral dissertation, Urbana: University of Illinois Press.

McCarthy, J., & Kirk, S. (1961). *The Illinois Test of Psycholinguistic Abilities.* Urbana: University of Illinois Press.

McNutt, J. C., & Leri, S. M., (1979). Language differences between institutionalized and noninstitutionalized retarded children. *American Journal of Mental Deficiency, 83,* 339–345.

Mein, R. (1961). A study of the oral vocabularies of severely subnormal patients. *Journal of Mental Deficiency Research, 5,* 52–62.

Miller, J. F. (1980). *Assessing language production in children: Experimental procedures.* Baltimore: University Park Press.

Miller, J. F. (1987). Language and communication characteristics of children with Down syndrome. In S. Pueschel, C. Tinghey, J. Rynders, A. Crocker, & C. Crutcher (Eds.), *New Perspectives on Down Syndrome* (pp. 233–262). Baltimore: Brookes Publishing.

Molfese, D. L. (1977). Infant cerebral asymmetry. In S. J. Segalowitz & F. A. Gruber (Eds.), *Language development and neurological theory.* New York: Academic Press.

Muir, J. (1903). An analysis of twenty-six cases of mongolism. *Archives of Pediatrics, 20,* 161.

Newport, E. L. (1982). Task specificity in language learning? Evidence from speech perception and American Sign Language. In E. Wanner & L. R. Gleitman (Eds.), *Language acquisition: The state of the art*. Cambridge: Cambridge University Press.

Newport, E. L., Gleitman, H., & Gleitman, L. (1977). Mother I'd rather do it myself: Some effects and non-effects of maternal speech style. In C. E. Snow & C. A. Ferguson (Eds.), *Talking to children: Language input and acquisition*. Cambridge: Cambridge University Press.

Newport, E. L., & Supalla, T. C. (1980). The structuring of language: Clues from the acquisition of signed and spoken language. In U. Bellugi & M. Studdert-Kennedy (Eds.), *Signed and spoken language: Biological constraints on linguistic form*. Dahlem Konferenzem. Weinheim: Verlag Chemie.

Nisbet, J., Zanella, K., & Miller, J. (1984). An analysis of conversations among handicapped students and a nonhandicapped peer. *Exceptional Children, 51,* 156–162.

Owens, R. E., & MacDonald, J. D. (1982). Communicative uses of the early speech of nondelayed and Down syndrome children. *American Journal of Mental Deficiency, 86,* 503–510.

Paul, R., Cohen, D. J., Breg, W. R., Waxton, M., & Herman, S. (1984). Fragile X Syndrome: Its relationship to speech and language disorders. *Journal of Speech and Hearing Disorders, 49,* 328–332.

Peterson, G., & Sherrod, K. (1982). Relationship of maternal language to language development and language delay of children. *American Journal of Mental Deficiency, 86,* 391–398.

Petitto, L. (1985). Are signed languages acquired earlier than spoken languages? Presented at the biennial meeting of the Society for Research in Child Development, Toronto.

Price-Williams, D., & Sabsay, S. (1979). Communicative competence among severely retarded persons. *Semiotica, 26*(1/2), 35–63.

Reynell, J. (1969). *Reynell Developmental Language Scales. Experimental edition*. Windsor, Berks: National Foundation for Developmental Research.

Rogers, M. G. (1975). A study of language skills in severely subnormal children. *Child Care Health and Development, 1,* 113–126.

Rondal, J. A. (1975). Développement du langage et retard mental: Un revue critique de la litterature en langue anglaise. *Année Psychologique, 75,* 513–547.

Rondal, J. A. (1978a). Developmental sentence scoring procedure and the delay–difference question in language development of Down's syndrome children. *Mental Retardation, 16,* 169–171.

Rondal, J. A. (1978b). Maternal speech to normal and Down's syndrome children matched for mean length of utterance. In C. E. Meyers (Ed.), *Quality of life in severely and profoundly mentally retarded people: Research foundations for improvement*. Washington, D.C.: American Association on Mental Deficiency, Monograph 3, 193–265.

Rondal, J. A. (1980). Verbal imitation by Down Syndrome and nonretarded children. *American Journal of Mental Deficiency, 85,* 318–321.

Rondal, J. A., Lambert, J. L., & Sohier, C. (1981). Elicited verbal imitation in Down's syndrome and other mentally retarded children: A replication and extension of Berry. *Language and Speech, 24,* 245–254.

Rosenberg, S. (1982). The language of the mentally retarded: Development, processes and intervention. In S. Rosenberg (Ed.), *Handbook of applied psycholinguistics*. Hillsdale, NJ: Erlbaum.

Ross, M. H., Galaburda, A. M., & Kemper, T. L. (1984). Down's syndrome: Is there a decreased population of neurons? *Neurology, 34,* 909–916.

Ryan, J. (1975). Mental subnormality and language development. In E. Lenneberg & E. Lenneberg (Eds.), *Foundations of language development* (Vol. 2). New York: Academic Press.

Ryan, J. (1977). The silence of stupidity. In J. Morton & J. C. Marshall (Eds.), *Psycholinguistics: Developmental and pathological*. Ithaca, NY: Cornell University Press.

St. James-Roberts, I. (1981). A reinterpretation of hemispherectomy data without functional plasticity of the brain. *Brain and Language, 13,* 31–53.

Scarborough, H. S., Rescorla, L., Tager-Flusberg, H., Fowler, A., & Sudhalter, V. (unpublished ms.) Evaluations of language impairments associated with Down syndrome, Fragile X syndrome, autism, and early language delay: Utility of the Index of Productive Syntax.

Scherer, N. J., & Owings, N. O. (1984). Learning to be contingent: Retarded children's responses to their mothers' requests. *Language and Speech, 27,* 255–267.

Schlesinger, I. M., (1971). The production of utterances and language acquisition. In D. I. Slobin, (Ed.), *The ontogenesis of grammar: A theoretical symposium.* New York: Academic Press.

Seagoe, M. V. (1965). Verbal development in a mongoloid. *Exceptional Children, 31,* 269–73.

Semmel, M. I., & Dolley, D. G. (1971). Comprehension and imitation of sentences by Down's syndrome children as a function of transformational complexity. *American Journal of Mental Deficiency, 75,* 739–745.

Share, J. B. (1975). Developmental progress in Down's Syndrome. In R. Koch & F. F. de la Cruz (Eds.), *Down's syndrome (mongolism): Research, prevention and management.* New York: Brunner/Mazel.

Share, J., Koch, R., Webb, A., & Graliker, B. (1964). The longitudinal development of infants and young children with Down's syndrome (mongolism). *American Journal of Mental Deficiency, 68,* 685.

Shipley, E., Smith, C., & Gleitman, L. (1969). A study in thte acquisition of language: Free responses to commands. *Language, 45,* 322–342.

Slobin, D. I. (1973). Cognitive prerequisites for the development of grammar. In C. Ferguson & D. Slobin (Eds.), *Studies of child language development.* New York: Holt, Rinehart & Winston, 175–208.

Slobin, D. I. (1980). The repeated path between transparency and opacity in language. In U. Bellugi & M. Studdert-Kennedy (Eds.), *Signed and spoken language: Biological constraints on linguistic form.* Dahlem Konferenzem. Weinheim: Verlag Chemie GmbH, 229–243.

Sommers, R. K., & Starkey, K. L. (1977). Dichotic verbal processing in Down syndrome children having qualitatively different speech and language skills. *American Journal of Mental Deficiency, 82,* 44–53.

Spreen, O. (1965). Language functions in mental retardation: A review. I. Language development, types of retardation and intelligence level. *American Journal of Mental Deficiency, 69,* 482–494.

Strominger, A. Z., Winkler, M. R., & Cohen, L. T. (1984). Speech and language evaluation. In S. M. Pueschel (Ed.), *The young child with Down syndrome* (pp. 253–261). New York: Human Sciences Press.

Tager-Flusberg, H., Calkins, S., Nolin, T., Baumberger, T., Anderson, M., & Chadwick-Dias, A. (submitted). A longitudinal study of language acquisition in autistic and Down syndrome children.

Thompson, M. M. (1963). Psychological characteristics relevant to the education of the pre-school mongoloid child. *Mental Retardation, 1,* 148–151.

Uzgiris, I., & Hunt, J. McV. (1975). Assessment in infancy: Ordinal scales of psychological development. Urbana: University of Illinois Press.

Weiss, B., Beeghly, M., & Cicchetti, D. (1985). Development of symbolic play in children with Down syndrome and nonhandicapped children. Presented at the biennial meeting of the Society for Research in Child Development, Toronto, April.

Wiegel-Crump, C. A. (1981), The development of grammar in Down's syndrome children between the MA's of 2–0 and 6–11 years. *Education and Training of the Mentally Retarded, 6,* 24–60.

Wing, L. (1975). A study of language impairment in severely retarded children. In N. O'Connor (Ed.), *Language, cognitive deficits and retardation.* London: Butterworth.

Wisniewski, K. E., Miezejeski, C. M., & Hill, A. L. (1988). Neurological and psychological status of individuals with Down syndrome. In L. Nadel (Ed.), *The Psychobiology of Down syndrome.* Cambridge, MA: MIT Press.

Zeaman, D., & House, B. (1962). Mongoloid MA is proportional to log CA. *Child Development, 33,* 481–488.

Zekulin-Hartley, X. Y. (1981). Hemispheric asymmetry in Down's syndrome children. *Canadian Journal of Behavioral Science, 13,* 210–217.

Zigler, E. (1969). Developmental versus difference theories of mental retardation and the problem of motivation. *American Journal of Mental Deficiency, 73,* 536–556.

10 Beyond sensorimotor functioning: early communicative and play development of children with Down syndrome

Marjorie Beeghly, Bedonna Weiss-Perry,
and Dante Cicchetti

Introduction

Although there is no doubt that the rate of language development in children with Down syndrome is delayed in relation to their chronological age, results from a plethora of studies suggest that the sequence and structure of their early language development is largely similar to that observed in normally developing children (see Fowler, Chapter 9, this volume; Miller, in press; for recent reviews). An examination of different domains within language (phonology, syntax, semantics, pragmatics) and relationships of language with cognition and social development also reveals more similarities than differences (Beeghly & Cicchetti, 1985, 1986; Beeghly, Hanrahan, Weiss, & Cicchetti, 1985; Cunningham, Glenn, Wilkinson, & Sloper, 1985; Fowler, Chapter 9, this volume; Mervis, Chapter 8, this volume; Rondal, 1988). On the basis of these studies, most investigators conclude that there is not compelling evidence for a strong "difference" or "deficit" model of language development for these children, just as for mentally retarded children in general.

Nonetheless, important differences in the language development of children with Down syndrome also have been documented that are crucial to comprehend if we are to understand the process of development in these children. Perhaps the most striking difference is the dramatic delay in expressive language development of children with Down syndrome, relative to that observed in other retarded and nonretarded groups (see Chapter 9 by Fowler and Chapter 8 by Mervis, this volume, for reviews). Despite similarities in structure and sequence for most aspects of language, results of many studies document that individuals with Down syndrome

Research presented in this chapter was supported by a grant from the John D. and Catherine T. MacArthur Foundation to authors Cicchetti and Beeghly, and by grants from the March of Dimes (12-127) and the Spencer Foundation to author Cicchetti. We thank the mothers and children for their enthusiastic and loyal participation in this study. We also are grateful to the many research assistants who helped us with data collection or data reduction during the tenure of this longitudinal project. In particular, thanks are extended to Cindy Carter and Michelle Gersten for their special efforts in data collection at an early stage of this project. Moreover, we wish to acknowledge Drs. Alan Crocker and Siegfried Pueschel for their help and advice.

show increasing linguistic deficits with advancing chronological age (Gibson, 1978; Miller, in press). Indeed, some individuals do not progress beyond early stages of syntactic development (see Fowler, Chapter 9, this volume; but see Rondal, 1988, for exceptions). Moreover, expressive language skills appear to lag behind these children's nonverbal cognitive abilities (Cunningham et al., 1985; Mundy, Sigman, Kasari, & Yirmiya, 1988) and, in fact, to constitute the area of "most delay" for these children (Evans & Hampson, 1969; Share, 1975).

Because communicative abilities are thought to be a significant predictor of later competence and social adjustment (Miller, in press; Rondal, 1988; Spiker, Chapter 13, this volume), it is important to understand the nature of early symbolic development in children with Down syndrome more fully so that interventions can be better timed and guided. Indeed, many current early intervention programs for children with Down syndrome focus primarily on language development (see Spiker, Chapter 13, this volume). Despite much progress in the field of early language development, very little is known about the consequences of these children's linguistic deficits for other domains of symbolic and nonsymbolic development. Are these children's linguistic deficits part of a broader symbolic deficit that can be observed in other aspects of symbolic development, such as verbal and nonverbal communicative skills or symbolic play? Or is the expressive language delay observed in children with Down syndrome limited to structural and semantic aspects of productive language (the parameters that have been most often studied – cf. Rondal, 1988)? Answers to these questions will affect the strategies and long-term goals of early intervention programs for children with Down syndrome. Moreover, such questions are relevant to current topics of concern in the field of developmental psycholinguistics in general – namely, the controversy surrounding the modularity hypothesis in language development (see Bates, O'Connell, & Shore, 1987, for a review).

The purpose of this chapter

In this chapter, we review our own research and that of other investigators concerning the nature and course of early symbolic development in children with Down syndrome. Three basic areas are discussed from a developmental perspective.

First, we describe longitudinal changes in aspects of children's productive language development (including syntactic, lexical, and pragmatic development) over the course of 1 year. Of particular interest are the pragmatic skills of these children – that is, the way in which language is used during social interaction. In view of the dramatic delay of these children's syntactic development, do lexical and pragmatic skills develop in tandem with syntactic skills, or are they more closely tied to their chronological age and level of cognitive development?

Second, we examine the development of a nonlinguistic form of representational development – symbolic play – as well as object and social play in general. Relationships of play to aspects of cognitive, social, and affective development and to certain child and environmental factors also are reviewed.

Third, associations and dissociations among aspects of language and play development are considered in light of the current controversy surrounding the modularity and cognitive hypotheses of language acquisition (see Bates, Bretherton, & Snyder, 1988, for a review). In addition, children's representations of self and other in language and play also are examined from a developmental perspective.

By examining this body of research within the context of normal symbolic development, we intend to illuminate not only the nature and course of representational development in children with Down syndrome but also, more generally, our understanding of normal symbolic development (Cicchetti, 1984; Sroufe & Rutter, 1984).

An organizational approach to the study of communicative development

Our thinking and research involving children with Down syndrome have been guided by a developmental approach known as the ''organizational perspective,'' a theoretical position akin to the organismic-developmental approach proposed by Werner and Kaplan (1963) and the emergent ''developmental psychopathology'' approach proposed by Cicchetti (1984) and others. According to the organizational perspective, development is conceived as a dynamic series of qualitative reorganizations among and within behavioral and biological systems that take place by means of increasing differentiation and hierarchical organization (see also Cicchetti & Schneider-Rosen, 1986; Sameroff, 1983; Weiss, 1969). The character of these reorganizations is determined by variables at different levels of analysis – genetic, neurobiological, behavioral, psychological, ecological–environmental, historical, social, and so on – which are in dynamic transaction with one another throughout ontogeny. In other words, human development is viewed in terms of a hierarchical organization of transacting, interrelated systems.

In the field of developmental psychology, general behavioral systems such as cognition, affect, language, and social processes have been targeted for study by investigators attempting to adopt an organizational approach (Cicchetti, 1984). Of special concern is the organization of these behavioral systems in normal development as well as the lack of organization or different patterns of organization in abnormal development (Cicchetti & Schneider-Rosen, 1984, 1986; Gollin, 1984). According to these developmentalists, hierarchical integration occurs both within and between each of these systems (e.g., Bischof, 1975; Cicchetti & Serafica, 1981). Advances and lags in one behavioral system with respect to the others is important to study because the capacities of one behavioral system may be associated with the development or exercise of capacities for another system.

Within the domain of language development, for example, certain concurrent and preverbal social and cognitive capacities (such as those associated with object exploration, mastery motivation, joint attention and turn-taking in dyadic interaction) have been associated with the development of certain syntactic, lexical, and pragmatic abilities (Bates, Bretherton, Beeghly-Smith, & McNew, 1982; Bruner, 1983;

Golinkoff, 1983). Moreover, the absence of some of these same factors in language delayed populations has been related to later deficits in symbolic domains (Snyder, 1985).

Down syndrome and the organizational approach

Taking an organizational approach to the study of language development in children with Down syndrome can contribute meaningfully to our understanding of normal developmental processes, as well as to our understanding of Down syndrome. In normally developing children, for instance, development often proceeds so rapidly that the simultaneous emergence of behaviors or competencies in various domains may be coincidental rather than indicative of true structural or functional interrelations. In abnormal or delayed populations, such as individuals with Down syndrome, true developmental convergences and discontinuities may be more readily observed. Although children with Down syndrome develop at a delayed pace, they are quite heterogeneous in functioning, ranging from near-normal to severely retarded. Their delayed but heterogeneous development allows for a more precise examination of developmental sequences in different domains and interrelationships among behavioral systems at a particular point in ontogenesis (Cicchetti & Beeghly, Chapter 2, this volume; Cicchetti & Pogge-Hesse, 1982).

For example, studies attempting to document cognitive and social influences in the language development of children with Down syndrome have provided results that both affirm and challenge extant views of early symbolic development (Cardoso-Martins, 1984; Cardoso-Martins & Mervis, 1985; Dunst, Chapter 6, this volume). In one study, interrelations between lexical development and preverbal cognitive abilities have been observed in children with Down syndrome which mirror those reported for normally developing children (Cardoso-Martins, 1984; Cardoso-Martins & Mervis, 1985). Specifically, their first referential words (both in comprehension and production) occur in conjunction with Piaget's sensorimotor Stages 5 and 6 (for object permanence and means–ends) and general development (as measured by the Bayley Scales of Mental Development) as was observed for nonhandicapped children (see Mervis, Chapter 8, this volume, for a review). At the same time, these investigators also reported differences between the Down syndrome and nonhandicapped groups that question and broaden current thinking about language development. For example, differences in the *rate* of early lexical development were found for children with Down syndrome, relative to that seen in normal children, even when level of cognitive development was controlled. Taken together, these findings force us to refine and expand our working models of early lexical development (see also Chapter 4 by Berger and Chapter 8 by Mervis, this volume).

The Boston Down Syndrome Project

Purpose

The broad purpose of the Boston Down Syndrome Project was to examine the developmental course of children with Down syndrome as they make the transition from sensorimotor to representational functioning. Prior research on the first 2 years of life has documented that the development of infants with Down syndrome is markedly coherent and lawfully organized. Despite delays in timing and certain atypical features, such as passivity and low levels of arousal (Cicchetti & Sroufe, 1978; Lincoln, Courchesne, Kilman, & Galambos, 1985; Thompson, Cicchetti, Lamb, & Malkin, 1985), children with Down syndrome undergo developmental patterns and sequences that are highly similar to those of normal children. Evidence for this similarity has been demonstrated in a number of different behavioral systems: Piagetian stages and sequences of sensorimotor development (Cardoso-Martins & Mervis, 1985; Cicchetti & Mans-Wagener, 1987; Dunst, Chapter 6, this volume); organization of the attachment system (Cicchetti & Serafica, 1981); interrelations between affective and cognitive aspects of development (Cicchetti & Sroufe, 1976, 1978); emergence of visual self-recognition (Mans, Cicchetti, & Sroufe, 1978); self–other differentiation (Beeghly, Weiss, & Cicchetti, 1986; Cicchetti, Beeghly, Carlson, & Toth, in press); and negativism (Spiker, 1979).

While the majority of studies taking a developmental approach have focused on the sensorimotor period, far less research has been conducted on the transition from sensorimotor to representational functioning in children with Down syndrome. Does the development of these children continue to mirror that of normal children as they begin to acquire language? In light of their marked delays in expressive language development, the nature of this transition and interrelations among verbal and nonverbal as well as symbolic and nonsymbolic domains of symbol development are crucial to study in this population.

Description of the sample

All studies described in the next sections were based on the following sample of children. Groups sizes varied from study to study due to the specific purposes of each investigation and to logistic difficulties in matching children with Down syndrome to nonhandicapped children. Characteristics of the subsamples used in each study are described in detail later in the chapter.

Down syndrome sample. Forty-one children with Down syndrome (24 boys, 17 girls) and their mothers participated in our longitudinal studies of early symbolic development. All children were Caucasian and from middle-class homes; none had any obvious uncorrected sensory or motor handicaps. All children had the Trisomy 21 form of Down syndrome as confirmed by chromosomal analyses, with three having a mosaic variant. Names of the families with children with Down syndrome were obtained through listings provided by a genetic birth defects clinic at a metropolitan hospital and through inquiries made at local schools and intervention agencies. At the first observation, children with Down syndrome ranged in age from 20 to 76 months. Most children were participants in ongoing intervention programs, which is representative of the greater population of children with Down syndrome in the Boston metropolitan area.

Nonhandicapped control sample. In addition, 50 nonhandicapped children and their mothers also participated in the studies and served as controls for the children (and dyads) with Down syndrome. Children were matched for sex and demographics, and (in separate groups) for linguistic ability, developmental age, and/or chronological age, depending on the purpose of the particular study in question. Nonhandicapped children ranged in chronological age from 1 to 4 years at the time of the first observation. Families with nonhandicapped children were recruited in part through recommendations from mothers in the Down syndrome sample and in part via newspaper advertisements.

Methods of procedure

Children and their mothers participated in three laboratory visits, each spaced 6 months apart. During these sessions, subjects engaged in a variety of experimental tasks, interactive situations, and cognitive testing. All procedures took place in a large laboratory playroom and were videotaped from behind one-way mirrors. In addition, mothers were interviewed about characteristics of their children's language, communicative, and play development, and about demographic characteristics.

Data presented are based on detailed transcripts of language and interactive behavior observed during mother–child free play and during a structured mother–child picture book session. In addition, interactive behavior also was coded directly from the videotaped records. Contexts, as well as specific measures derived from these sources, are described below.

Early language development: syntax, vocabulary, pragmatics

The first set of studies (Beeghly, 1988; Beeghly & Cicchetti, 1986, 1987) was concerned with documenting the nature and course of early language development for children with Down syndrome over the course of 1 year. A range of language measures was included, tapping syntactic, lexical, pragmatic, and general productive aspects of communicative development.

Syntactic and lexical development

Although much progress has been made in our understanding of early syntactic and lexical development in children with Down syndrome (see Chapter 9 by Fowler and Chapter 8 by Mervis, this volume), our knowledge has been limited because much of this research has been based on small, cross-sectional samples. In our laboratory, we attempted to overcome these difficulties by assessing longitudinal changes in the early language of a relatively large group of children with Down syndrome over a 1-year period.

Method. In this first study, the entire sample of 41 children with Down syndrome (24 boys, 17 girls) participated. At the initial visit, children ranged in level of language development from prelinguistic to early multiword speech. Children were classified according to Brown's (1973) descriptive stages of language development. Four children were prelinguistic (*M* chronological age [CA] = 24 months, range = 20–30 months); 7 children were at the single-word stage (*M* CA = 40 months; range = 24–66 months); 19 children were beginning to combine words (early Stage 1; *M* CA = 44 months, range = 26–74 months); 8 children were in late Stage 1 (*M* = 68 months, range = 60–82 months); and 3 were in Stage 2 (*M* CA = 68 months, range = 61–76 months).

The following linguistic measures were analyzed: utterance frequency; proportion of lexicalized utterances; communicative gestures; proportion of unintelligible utterances; mean length of utterance in morphemes (MLU; Brown, 1973), including upper bound, the average of the five highest utterances (MLU-5), and MLU distribution; developmental sentence analysis (Lee, 1974); and vocabulary content and diversity.

Results. Perhaps the most striking finding was the marked expressive language delay of these children, in contrast to that observed in normally developing children, corroborating research from other studies. At the initial observation, no children with Down syndrome, not even the oldest who were approaching 6 years of age, had progressed beyond the very earliest language stages. Moreover, an examination of the longitudinal data confirmed the dramatic language delay of these children. Very minimal or no progress in language development was made over the course of the year for the majority of children with Down syndrome. Thus, 46% remained at the same syntactic level for the entire year, whereas 37% progressed one substage or stage. Only 17% of the sample progressed two language stages.

For purposes of comparison, note that most normally developing children pass through these early language stages at a relatively rapid rate. Most begin to acquire first words between the ages of 10 and 14 months. Between 18 and 24 months, most children begin to combine words, and by 24 to 28 months, the majority of children begin to acquire grammar (see Bates, O'Connell, & Shore, 1987).

Individual differences. Although MLU was correlated moderately with CA, individual differences in age among children at each level of language development were marked, indicating that heterogeneity in language development is characteristic of children with Down syndrome (see also Crawley & Spiker, 1983; Rynders, Spiker, & Horrobin, 1978). This fact is important to keep in mind when attempting to generalize about the course of language development for these children.

It is interesting that children with higher mental ages (MA) tended to progress more rapidly than children with lower mental ages, and that developmental progress was not necessarily correlated with initial chronological age. Although there was marked variation between sexes, girls tended to progress more rapidly than boys (e.g., 29% of girls but only 8% of boys progressed two stages over the year).

MLU and syntactic development. Despite their delayed syntactic development and the heterogeneity of CA at any given language level, an analysis of MLU distribution, upper bound, MLU-5, and Lee's developmental sentence analysis indicated that the structure and course of their syntactic development was otherwise similar to that observed in nonhandicapped children of comparable MLUs. These findings confirm claims by other investigators (Fowler, Chapter 9, this volume; Rondal, 1988) that MLU is a useful summary measure of syntactic complexity at early stages of syntactic development for children with Down syndrome as well as for normally developing children.

Stage-related changes in language production. Longitudinal changes in children's average scores for utterance frequency, proportion of lexicalized utterances, MLU characteristics, and observed productive vocabulary (number of different words produced during 40 minutes of social interaction) are presented in Table 10.1. Notable increases in productive language, vocabulary diversity, and the lexicalization of utterances were associated with increases in syntactic complexity, especially between early and late Stage 1. These findings support those of McCune-Nicolich and Bruskin (1982) who noted an increase in the fluency of symbol production (both verbal and nonverbal) from early to late Stage 1 for nonhandicapped children. These findings also support the theory that an increase in memory capacity (''chunking'') associated with brain development occurs around this time (see Bates et al., 1987, for a review of this research).

Increases in speech intelligibility also were noted with increasing MLU. Unexpectedly, children with Down syndrome did not differ significantly from the younger MLU-matched normally developing children on measures of intelligibility in this sample (see Miller, in press, for a discussion about the problems of speech intelligibility for research with children with Down syndrome).

Lexical development. Vocabulary development was delayed less than syntactic development in these children, especially as children's syntactic abilities increased. Vocabulary diversity also appeared to be associated with children's age and cognitive maturity, once children progressed beyond early Stage 1. The vocabulary of children with Down syndrome tended to be less diversified than that observed in nonhandicapped children matched to children with Down syndrome for receptive vocabulary on the Peabody Picture Vocabulary Test (PPVT) (Dunn & Dunn, 1981). Nonetheless, older children with Down syndrome tended to have larger productive vocabularies than younger MA- and MLU-matched children at any given language stage. A bar graph comparing the vocabulary production of children with Down syndrome and nonhandicapped children in early and late Stage 1 is presented in Figure 10.1. In this figure, nonhandicapped children were matched to the children with Down syndrome for sex, demographics, and, in three groups, for CA, MA, and MLU. Subject characteristics of these groups are presented in the following section.

An examination of the content of children's early productive vocabularies revealed no striking group differences for the children with Down syndrome and the nonhandicapped children. Individual differences for both groups were pronounced.

Table 10.1. *Longitudinal changes in the expressive language of children with Down syndrome (Selected language measures presented as group means)*

| Child group | Vocalizations | | MLU (in morphemes) | | | Vocabulary |
	# utterances	% speech	MLU	MLU5	Upper bound	# Different words produced
Prelinguistic (at visit 1) (N = 4; M CA = 24 mo)						
Visit 1	41	0	—	—	—	—
Visit 2	31	0–26	0–1.0	—	—	0–1
Visit 3	54	0–46	0–1.2	—	—	0–8
One-word stage (at Visit 1) (N = 7; M CA = 40 mo)						
Visit 1	93	28	1.00	1.00	1	9
Visit 2	102	59	1.09	2.08	3	13
Visit 3	109	49	1.29	2.64	4	23
Early Stage 1 (at Visit 1) (N = 19; M CA = 44 mo)						
Visit 1	133	51	1.18	2.14	3	24
Visit 2	164	68	1.29	2.51	3	36
Visit 3	136	73	1.35	2.84	4	38
Late Stage 1 (at Visit 1) (N = 8; M CA = 68 mo)						
Visit 1	235	80	1.68	4.65	6	81
Visit 2	232	91	1.98	5.43	6	99
Visit 3	185	91	2.49	6.10	7	119
Stage 2 (at Visit 1) (N = 3; M CA = 68 mo)						
Visit 1	216	87	2.16	6.20	8	105
Visit 2	178	94	2.48	7.20	8	129
Visit 3	193	97	3.01	7.60	8	142

Note: Visits were spaced six months apart. Children were placed into groups according to their level of linguistic performance at the first visit (Brown, 1973). MLU was calculated according to Brown's specifications. MLU5 refers to the average of the 5 longest utterances; upper bound refers to the longest observed utterance. Utterances included both lexicalized and nonlexicalized utterances; % speech refers to the porportion of utterances which were lexicalized. Number of different words produced during two interactive contexts (40 min).

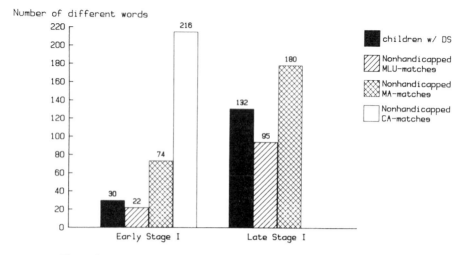

Figure 10.1. Vocabulary production in early and late Stage 1

Note that these children's linguistic corpora were based on child utterances produced during a laboratory session and do not necessarily reflect children's completed productive vocabularies. In this study, children's *relative* linguistic performance on a group level was of interest.

Summary. Children with Down syndrome showed dramatic delays in syntactic development relative to nonhandicapped children which were robust over the course
of a 1-year period. Importantly, individual differences in MA and gender were
associated with language progress in these children.

In contrast, lexical development appeared to be somewhat less delayed than syntactic development for children with Down syndrome and was associated with CA
and MA. These results point to the role of experience and cognitive maturity in
vocabulary acquisition. Because children with Down syndrome are significantly
older and more cognitively advanced than nonhandicapped children at equivalent
levels of syntactic development, it is not surprising that they would tend to have
productive vocabularies in line with their cognitive attainments.

The role of social experience and cognitive maturity for other aspects of language
– the "social" aspects of language such as pragmatics – are addressed next. It was
hypothesized that children with Down syndrome would be advanced in these skills
relative to their syntactic abilities, in light of their documented propensities for
social interaction (Mundy et al., 1988; Serafica, Chapter 11, this volume).

Pragmatics and communicative skills

Mirroring trends in the field of social development, language researchers have moved
away from a study of single utterances and have devoted increased attention to the

dyad-in-context as the unit of analysis during the past decade (Greenberg, 1983). More and more, investigators have devoted time and effort to documenting aspects of children's *pragmatic* development. This shift undoubtedly reflects the current Zeitgeist, but it also indicates a prevalent belief among developmentalists and interventionists that communicative functioning is a significant predictor of later social competence and adaptive functioning (Greenberg, 1983; Schiefelbusch & Pickar, 1984; Spiker, Chapter 13, this volume), as well as later cognitive attainments such as literacy (Galda & Pellegrini, 1985).

Because children with Down syndrome typically are less impaired cognitively than linguistically, and because of their reported strengths in social domains, we hypothesized that children with Down syndrome would be more communicatively competent during social interaction than would nonhandicapped children at a similar level of syntactic development. In addition, we predicted that their pragmatic skills would not differ from those of MA-matched counterparts and would be in line with their cognitive attainments. The thesis that linguistic and pragmatic abilities can emerge asynchronously is supported by research with different atypical populations of children (see Rosenberg, 1982, for a review). For example, the pragmatic skills of autistic children appear to lag behind their syntactic skills (see Schopler & Mesibov, 1985; Sigman & Mundy, 1987; Tager-Flusberg, 1981), whereas the reverse appears to be true for children with Down syndrome.

Support for this hypothesis has been provided by several studies of communicative competence in individuals with Down syndrome. For example, several investigators (Coggins, Carpenter, & Owings, 1984; Coggins & Stoel-Gammon, 1982; Leifer & Lewis, 1984; Owings & MacDonald, 1982; Scherer & Owings, 1984) have reported that children with Down syndrome in Stage 1 of syntactic development (Brown, 1973) exhibit communicative skills that are as, or more, advanced than that of MLU-matched nonhandicapped children. Coggins and Stoel-Gammon (1982), for instance, found that 5- to 7-year-old children with Down syndrome were able to respond appropriately to requests for clarification, as evidenced by repetitions or revisions of their utterances.

Similar findings have been reported for older children, teenagers, and adults with Down syndrome. For example, some researchers (Leuder, Fraser, & Jeeves, 1981; Price-Williams & Sabsay, 1979) have documented that adults with Down syndrome appear to be more advanced communicatively, relative to their linguistic abilities, when nonlinguistic aspects of communication (e.g., gestures, body movements) are also taken into account. Other researchers (Nisbet, Zanella, & Miller, 1984) report that teenage subjects with Down syndrome showed more advanced communicative skills during peer interactions when observed in social contexts demanding higher levels of communicative competence.

Discrepant findings also exist in the literature (see Miller, in press). These divergent results may be due, at least in part, to a variety of methodological problems that plague this field, including the wide variation in measures of ''discourse'' employed in different studies and the use of MLU as a matching device for older children and adults. Several investigators stress that MLU may not be an adequate summary measure of individuals' syntactic complexity beyond early stages of syntactic development (Fowler, Chapter 9, this volume; Rondal, 1988).

Context differences (e.g., adult vs. peer partners) among studies also may help explain inconsistent reports of communicative competence in children with Down syndrome. It is well documented that adults tend to do more "conversational housekeeping" than peers when interacting with young language-learning children. Children with Down syndrome may exhibit less mature communicative behavior in more unstructured contexts with peers than in more structured situations with adults. In support of this, Sinson and Wetherick (1982) reported that children with Down syndrome who were mainstreamed in school with normal peers failed to observe some of the conventional "rules" of conversation with peers (i.e., they failed to maintain mutual gaze and did not respond verbally to peers' initiations). Perhaps as a consequence, these children were rejected by their peers and became socially isolated. The "communicative incompetence" of these children may have stemmed, in part, from difficulties in the timing and appropriate use of eye contact, which, in turn, may reflect underlying problems in information processing, arousal modulation, and visual attention (Cicchetti & Pogge-Hesse, 1982; Kopp, Krakow, & Johnson, 1983; Krakow & Kopp, 1982; Wagner, Ganiban, & Cicchetti, Chapter 5, this volume; see Berger, Chapter 4, this volume for a discussion of these problems for infants with Down syndrome). These difficulties may have been more pronounced under less structured circumstances.

In our laboratory, we extended this body of research by examining the communicative skills of children with Down syndrome and nonhandicapped children at two levels of syntactic development – early and late Stage 1. Stage 1 is an important stage of syntactic development to study because it marks children's transition from one-word to multiword speech (see Bretherton, McNew, Snyder, & Bates, 1983; Shore, Bates, Bretherton, Beeghly, & O'Connell, in press; Shore, O'Connell, & Bates, 1984). This linguistic transition has been associated with similar transitions in object play (McCune-Nicolich & Bruskin, 1982) and with other cognitive attainments in normally developing children such as memory capacity (see Bates et al., 1987). Documenting similarities and differences in developmental sequences for the communicative development of both Down syndrome and nonhandicapped groups during this transition is thus important for both theoretical and practical reasons.

Subjects. Twenty-eight children with Down syndrome (17 boys, 11 girls) and 35 nonhandicapped children participated in this study, along with their mothers. Data from one of the three longitudinal visits are reported here. Children with Down syndrome and their MLU-matched counterparts were selected for inclusion if they fell into either early or late Stage 1 of syntactic development. Children with MLUs between 1.01 and 1.49 were classified into the early Stage 1 group, whereas those with MLUs between 1.50 and 1.99 were classified into the late Stage 1 group. Down syndrome children were then individually matched to normal children for sex, demographics, and MLU.

There were large differences in both CA and MA for the children with Down syndrome and their MLU-matched controls. Thus, the average CA of the children with Down syndrome in early Stage 1 was 50 months (range = 31–69 months), whereas the average CA of the normal chilren in early Stage 1 was 19 months (range = 18–22 months). Similarly, in late Stage 1, the average CAs of the children with Down syndrome and the normal children were 75 months (range = 50–93 months) and 24 months (range = 23–27 months), respectively.

Children also were individually matched to a second set of normal children for mental age–equivalent scores (MA). Pairs were matched either on the Bayley Mental Scales (Bayley, 1969) or on the revised PPVT, depending on their level of functioning. Children were matched within one month of MA.

The average MA of the children with Down syndrome and their language controls in early stage one was 27 months and 21 months, respectively, while the mean MA of those children with Down syndrome and their controls in late Stage 1 was 44 months and 28 months, respectively. Note that the mental ages of the children with Down syndrome were significantly higher than those of their linguistically matched controls. Note, too, that mental age increased significantly for both groups between early and late Stage 1.

Method. Measures of communicative skills were derived from detailed transcripts of mother–child interaction in two situations varying in task demands for conversation maintenance – a structured picture book reading task and a 30-minute semi-structured free play situation. During the book situation, mothers and children were told to look through a picture book together and to talk about the photographs of people in different situations (e.g., children at a birthday party, children struggling over an object, a child at the doctor's office). During the free play situation, mothers and children were led into a laboratory playroom furnished with a box of standard, age-appropriate toys and several beanbag chairs. The free play situation was divided into three 10-minute segments (A-B-A). During the first and third "A" segments, mothers were asked to sit on a beanbag chair and to refrain from initiating or directing play or interaction with their child. If the child initiated play or conversation, the mothers were free to respond but not to seek to maintain the interaction. During the middle "B" segment, mothers were instructed to get down and interact "as they normally would" at home. Thus, for two-thirds of the play session, the initiation and maintenance of conversation was left up to the child.

In addition to measures of utterance form, intelligibility, productivity, syntactic complexity, and vocabulary diversity (described above), the following measures of pragmatic development were included. First, at the level of the utterance, the diversity and content of speech acts, or "functional communication," were scored. A mutually exclusive and exhaustive coding system tapping the major communicative functions of early language (adapted from Dore, 1974, 1979) was used, including such speech act summary categories as requests for action; requests for information; attentionals; statements (including internal reports of self and other); object labels and object descriptions; conversational devices (turn markers); imitations; repetitions; and so on. In addition, at the level of the dyad, a measure of "conver-

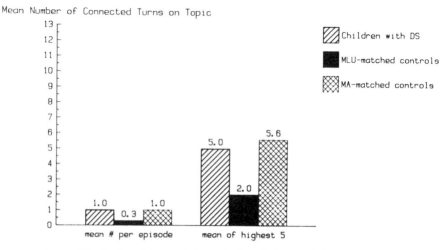

Figure 10.2. Topic maintenance during early Stage 1 of syntactic development: (MLU 1.01–1.49)

sational relevance'' [or mean length of episode (MLE), Brown, 1980] was included which tapped the semantic and pragmatic as well as the syntactic relevance of children's utterances to the caregivers' preceding utterances. In addition, an assessment of topic maintenance (average number of connected child turns that were on topic) and several measures of turn-taking skills (initiations, responses) were analyzed.

Results. Results in both interactive contexts were similar, so data was collapsed across contexts for the purposes of this chapter.

Speech acts. As expected, children with Down syndrome produced a greater diversity of speech acts than did MLU-matched normal children, but did not differ from their MA-matched counterparts in this regard. Children with Down syndrome also differed from their MLU-matched controls (but not their MA matches) in the content of their speech acts, exhibiting proportionally more responses, descriptions, and statements but proportionally fewer conversational devices and nonlexical turn fillers (both considered less mature categories). There was one notable exception: Children with Down syndrome made fewer requests than did their MA-matched controls, but did not differ in this regard from their MLU-matched controls (see also Mundy et al., 1988, and Smith & Tetzchner, 1986, for comparable results for nonlinguistic ''request'' measures).

Turn-taking and discourse skills. Similar findings were obtained for measures of communicative skills at the level of the dyad. Children with Down syndrome engaged in significantly longer sequences of on-topic turns and longer conversationally relevant turns, and were better able to make appropriate responses to adult

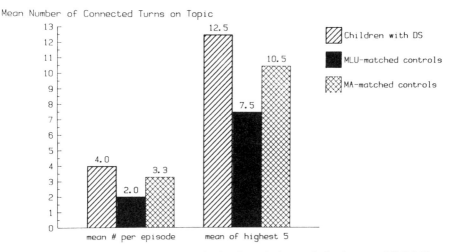

Figure 10.3. Topic maintenance during late Stage 1 of syntactic development: (MLU 1.50–1.99)

demands than their younger, linguistically matched counterparts. Again, children with Down syndrome did not differ from their MA-matched counterparts with respect to these dyadic measures.

Stage-related changes in pragmatic skills. Both children with Down syndrome and nonhandicapped children in late Stage 1 had significantly more mature communicative behavior than children in early Stage 1. Compared to children in early Stage 1, children in late Stage 1 produced proportionally more lexicalized utterances, a larger vocabulary, a greater diversity of speech acts, longer chains of connected, conversationally relevant turns, and longer sequences of on-topic turns. Compared to children in early Stage 1, children in late Stage 1 also differed in the content of their speech acts, evidencing more requests, statements, and descriptions, and fewer turn fillers and conversational devices. Thus, although children with Down syndrome differed significantly from younger MLU-matched controls on a variety of pragmatic measures at a given language stage, the sequence of their development from early to late Stage 1 bore remarkable similarities to those observed for nonhandicapped children.

Figures 10.2 and 10.3 portray stage-related changes in topic maintenance for each group of children. Both the average number of on-topic turns per episode and the average of the longest five bouts are depicted.

Summary and discussion. These data reflect an asynchrony or dissociation between syntactic and pragmatic development for children with Down syndrome that was not observed for nonhandicapped children. Although the communicative skills and mental ages of all children advanced significantly as MLU increased from early to late Stage 1, the children with Down syndrome had more mature communicative skills than their MLU matches at each substage.

When one considers the significant differences in children's MAs and CAs in the two groups, these results seem less surprising. More notable is the fact that the communicative performance of the children with Down syndrome did not differ from that of the MA-matched controls, who were significantly older than the MLU controls and who had significantly longer MLUs and more elaborated vocabularies than the children with Down syndrome. Taken together, these data highlight the significant role of both cognitive development and experience in the acquisition of social–communicative skills.

One important difference observed between the children with Down syndrome and their MA-matched counterparts was for the speech act category ''requests'': Children with Down syndrome produced fewer requests than did their MA-matched controls. Similar findings have been reported in other studies for nonverbal initiating behavior of infants and children with Down syndrome (Jones, 1980; Mundy et al., 1988; Smith & Tetzchner, 1986). For example, as in our studies of verbal communicative competence, Mundy and his colleagues examined the *nonverbal* communicative competence of children with Down syndrome and found that these children exhibited strengths and weaknesses in nonverbal communicative skills. A specific strength, relative to MA-matched normal children, was in their nonverbal social interactive skills. In contrast, a marked problem area was in their nonverbal requests for objects and requests for assistance with objects. Importantly, nonverbal requests were correlated significantly with expressive language. Moreover, Mundy and his associates demonstrated that this pattern was unique to children with Down syndrome, since MA-matched, retarded children without Down syndrome did not display this pattern.

Similarly, Smith and Tetzchner (1986) reported in their longitudinal sample of 13 children with Down syndrome that a measure of nonverbal requesting (as opposed to a measure of nonverbal indicating) taken at 24 months of age was significantly associated with children's expressive language skills at 36 months, even when variance due to differences in developmental level was removed statistically. Viewed concomitantly, these studies suggest that the linguistic deficit observed in children with Down syndrome is associated with, among other things, a deficit in verbal and nonverbal requesting behavior. Thus, while children with Down syndrome were relatively proficient at certain pragmatic abilities such as topic maintenance and basic turn-taking skills, they showed deficiencies in certain communicative abilities within the domain of pragmatics.

Symbolic play development

In this section, we examine the development of another nonlinguistic aspect of representation – symbolic play – from a developmental perspective. Do children with Down syndrome follow the same sequences of play development as nonhandicapped children? Are similar strengths and weaknesses observed for different aspects of symbolic play as were observed for communicative development? To explore this idea, we examine both structural (action complexity, object substitution) and social (independent agency, social roles) aspects of symbolic play.

Background. During the past ten to fifteen years, investigators adopting a developmental perspective have demonstrated that the course and content of symbolic play development in children with Down syndrome is markedly similar to that observed in normal children. Thus, investigators now have compelling evidence that the sequence of early play development in children with Down syndrome mirrors that of normal children (Beeghly, Weiss-Perry, & Cicchetti, 1989; Hill & McCune-Nicolich, 1981; Quinn & Rubin, 1984; Weiss, Beeghly, & Cicchetti, 1985). Although emerging at a delayed pace, the symbolic play of children with Down syndrome progresses through the same developmental sequences of decentration, decontextualization, and integration in object and social play that characterize the play development of nonhandicapped children in early childhood (see Bretherton, 1984, for a recent review).

In addition, investigators of play development in abnormally developing populations have replicated studies in the play literature documenting a significant association between symbolic play and level of cognitive development (e.g., Beeghly et al., 1989; Hill & McCune-Nicolich, 1981; Motti, Cicchetti, & Sroufe, 1983; Riguet, Taylor, Benaroya, & Klein, 1981; Weiss et al., 1985). In a study of handicapped children of varying etiology and degree of handicap, Wing, Gould, Yeates, and Brierly (1977) reported that no child with a mental age under 20 months engaged in symbolic play. It is interesting that these investigators also found that, among the organically retarded subgroups they studied, children with Down syndrome exhibited the most fluent and flexible symbolic play. Moreover, relations of play with cognition, affect, and social development also have been observed for both children with Down syndrome and cognitively matched nonhandicapped children (Beeghly et al., 1989; Motti et al., 1983). These studies are discussed in greater detail in the sections that follow. Taken in tandem, research findings suggest that the nonverbal symbolic play of children with Down syndrome is coherent, lawfully organized, and similar in developmental course to that observed in nonhandicapped children.

For the past several years, longitudinal changes in the structure, content, and style of play in children with Down syndrome have been studied intensively in our laboratory (Beeghly, 1988; Beeghly et al., 1989; Weiss et al., 1985). In the following sections, we describe three such play studies. The first involves structural dimensions of object and social play development, while the second explores interrelations among play, cognitive development, affect, and social behavior. Finally, we describe the development of four different aspects of symbolic play in children with Down syndrome and nonhandicapped children.

Subjects. The sample comprised 35 children with Down syndrome and 41 nonhandicapped children. Children were divided by age into two subsamples that were studied separately. In the younger cohort, 15 children with Down syndrome (*M* CA = 41 months; range = 27–56 months) were matched individually to 15 nonretarded children (*M* CA = 22 months, range = 17–24 months) for sex, demographics, and for mental age–equivalent scores (MA) derived from the Bayley Mental Scale. The average MA for both groups was 23 months. Eight boys and seven girls were represented in each group. In addition, these children with Down syndrome also were individually matched to a second set of nonhandicapped children for sex, demographics, and CA.

In the second (older) cohort, 20 children with Down syndrome (*M* CA = 74 months, range = 68–93 months) were matched individually to twenty normal children for sex, demographics, and MA (*M* MA = 48 months, range = 34–61 months). MA was based on age-equivalent scores from the Wechsler Scales for Preschool and Primary Children (WPPSI) or the revised PPVT, depending on their level of functioning.

Method. All play measures in the studies that follow were derived from a 30-minute mother-child free play session (''A–B–A'') described in the language section above. Descriptions of specific measures used in each study are provided below.

Structural dimensions of object and social play

In this study (Beeghly et al., 1989), we examined age-related changes in the proportion of time children engaged in different categories of object and social play. The purpose was to determine whether similar developmental sequences of play could be observed in children with Down syndrome as have been reported for nonhandicapped children.

In nonhandicapped children, age-graded changes in play behavior have been observed during the first year of life and are thought to form the foundation for true symbolic play, which emerges sometime during the second year of life. Until around 8 or 9 months, play is characterized primarily by visual–tactile object exploration and manipulation. Near the end of the first year, infants start to manipulate objects in relational, combinatorial ways. At the start of the second year of life, infants start to use objects in functionally appropriate ways. During the second year, actual symbolic use of objects emerges and becomes elaborate (Belsky & Most, 1981; Nicolich, 1977; Piaget, 1962; Ungerer, Zelazo, Kearsley, & O'Leary, 1981).

Measures. Play measures used in this study were adapted from those used by Belsky and Most (1981). Eight mutually exclusive summary categories were included in the analyses. Five more were concerned with object play: simple object manipulation–exploration; relational object manipulation; functional (conventional) object play; self-related (autosymbolic) pretend play; and decontextualized symbolic play. Three additional categories included structured social play involving turn-taking, simple attending to mother, and no play (disengagement). Play categories were coded in 15-second intervals from videotapes.

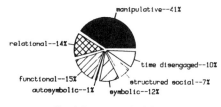

Children with DS

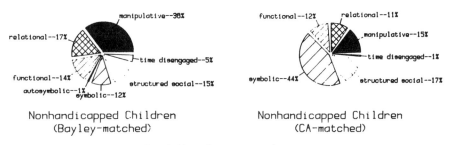

Nonhandicapped Children
(Bayley-matched)

Nonhandicapped Children
(CA-matched)

Figure 10.4. Categories of object play: younger cohort

Results. Results from this study indicated that similar mental age-related changes in the distribution of categories of object and social play occurred both for children with Down syndrome and for cognitively comparable nonhandicapped children in both cohorts. As children increased in level of cognitive development, the time engaged in simple object manipulation decreased significantly, whereas the reverse trend was observed for time engaged in decontextualized symbolic play and in structured social interaction.

However, despite significant increases in more mature forms of play, both children with Down syndrome and MA-matched controls in the younger cohort spent the greatest proportion of time engaged in simple object manipulation. Relational, functional, and symbolic play categories occurred next in frequency for both groups. Least frequent were the no play, attends, and autosymbolic categories. Pie charts of these play categories for the children with Down syndrome, their MA-matched controls, and their CA-matched controls are given in Figure 10.4.

In contrast, both children with Down syndrome and nonhandicapped children in the older cohort spent a significantly greater amount of time engaged in decontextualized symbolic play than did children in the younger cohort (see Figure 10.5). Children with Down syndrome in both cohorts did not differ significantly from their MA-matched controls on any object play category. The one exception was that children with Down syndrome in the younger cohort spent a significantly greater amount of time engaged in simple manipulative play than did their MA counterparts. In contrast, children with Down syndrome in both cohorts engaged in fewer structured turn-taking games with their mothers than did their controls.

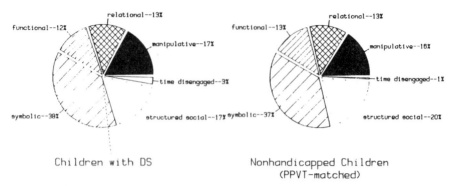

Children with DS   Nonhandicapped Children
                              (PPVT-matched)

Figure 10.5. Categories of object play: older cohort (0% autosymbolic in both groups)

As expected, the CA-matched controls engaged in significantly more symbolic play and structured social interaction than either the younger children with Down syndrome or their MA-matched controls. Taken together, these results corroborate the age-related trends reported for normally developing children in the play literature (Belsky & Most, 1981).

Play, affect, and cognition

Although emerging cognitive abilities may underlie the structure of children's play, as just seen, the *force* behind play is often affective in nature (Cicchetti & Hesse, 1983; Cicchetti & Pogge-Hesse, 1982; Piaget, 1962, 1981; Piaget & Inhelder, 1969). In the following study, interrelations between affective–motivational and social dimensions of play were examined for children with Down syndrome and nonhandicapped children.

In the play literature, cognitive–affective relations have been observed within the domain of object play that have been interpreted to be indicative of "mastery motivation" (Jennings, Harmon, Gaiter, & Yarrow, 1979) or "play style" (Fein & Apfel, 1979). In these studies, children's enthusiasm and persistence in object play have been found to be correlated significantly with the complexity and maturity of object play and with children's level of cognitive development.

Interrelations among cognitive and affective dimensions of object play also have been observed in a longitudinal sample of 31 children with Down syndrome (Motti et al., 1983). Like other investigators of symbolic play, Motti and her colleagues found that symbolic play behavior in children with Down syndrome was qualitatively similar to that reported for normally developing children (Nicolich, 1977). Yet, individual differences were seen in the symbolic play of the children with Down syndrome that were related to their level of cognitive development and to the degree of their affective engagement in play. Children with more mature levels of play not only had higher levels of cognitive development but also exhibited more positive affect and were more enthusiastic during play and explored toys more thoroughly.

These investigators also found that both symbolic play maturity and affective play behavior at 3 to 5 years were correlated significantly with indices of cognitive and affective development assessed during the first and second years of these children's lives. That is, affect ratings of these children at 10 months and scores from the Bayley Mental Scales at 24 months both predicted children's symbolic play maturity at 3 to 5 years. In addition, significant relations between cognitive and affective behavior were observed in this sample throughout infancy, and level of cognitive development at 16 months was predicted by affective ratings made at several earlier developmental points during the first year (Cicchetti & Sroufe, 1976, 1978). These results point to the coherence of cognitive and affective development throughout the first five years of life for children with Down syndrome.

Method. The findings of Motti and her collaborators were partially replicated in our own play studies (Beeghly et al., 1989). In addition to the assessments of object play just described, dimensions of affective–motivational play style were independently rated from videotapes of mother–child free play. These 5-point scales were adapted from scales used by Motti and colleagues and tapped dimensions of children's object exploration (active vs. passive), children's positive affect, and children's affective engagement in play. In addition, aspects of mother–child interactive behavior (e.g., dyadic harmony, initiating behavior, contingent responsivity) also were rated from the videotapes (see Beeghly et al., 1989, for further details of these coding systems). Within-group and between-group analyses were performed for both the younger and older cohorts of children.

Results. Results of correlational analyses revealed that affective–motivational play style (enthusiasm, persistence, positive affect) was correlated significantly with level of cognitive development and with symbolic play behavior in both the younger and the older cohorts of children with Down syndrome and in the cognitively matched nonhandicapped children. Similarly, results of group comparisons indicated that no differences existed between the children with Down syndrome and their MA-matches on these affective ratings, but that children with Down syndrome exhibited significantly less affect, enthusiasm, and active object exploration than did their CA-matched counterparts.

Dimensions of social play (structured turn-taking games) and social interaction (child responsiveness, initiating behavior, dyadic harmony) also were correlated significantly with both level of play maturity and cognitive development. It is notable that these relations were found even though, as a group, children with Down syndrome engaged in significantly less social play and were rated as being less responsive and less initiating than their cognitively matched controls during social interaction (see Beeghly et al., 1989). Similar characteristics have been reported in other studies of children with Down syndrome (Jones, 1980; MacTurk, Hunter, McCarthy, Vietze, & McQuiston, 1985).

Summary. These results suggest that the affective, cognitive, and social aspects of symbolic functioning are organized similarly in children with Down syndrome and in nonhandicapped children of comparable cognitive development, despite areas of weakness in certain aspects of social interactive behavior of children with Down syndrome. Such results attest to the coherence of symbolic development for children with Down syndrome.

Symbolic play development

In this third study of play development in our laboratory (Weiss et al., 1985), children's symbolic play was examined in greater detail. Although it has been well documented that children with Down syndrome progress through sequences of symbolic play similar to those found in normal children, the developmental scale used most often in these studies (Nicolich, 1977) has ceiling limitations when used with older preoperational children with Down syndrome. Several other developmental scales generated by investigators probing separate aspects of symbolic play maturity (e.g., agent use, role representation, object representation, scheme complexity) have been used and partially validated in normally developing populations of children (see Bretherton, 1984, and Rubin, Fein, & Vandenberg, 1983, for reviews). However, these different sequences of symbolic play have yet to be investigated concurrently in the same study. Moreover, the development of these components of symbolic play has not been studied in children with Down syndrome.

The purpose of this present study was to extend and integrate the findings of previous play research by examining the development of these different aspects of symbolic play conjointly in a cross-sectional sample of children with Down syndrome and two control groups of nonhandicapped children. To achieve this end, a coding system was devised combining four different scales of symbolic play that have been used separately in the play literature. Comparisons of children with Down syndrome's relative strengths and weaknesses on different dimensions of play, including both structural dimensions (such as scheme complexity, and decontextualization of object use [e.g., object substitutions]), and more socially relevant aspects of play (such as independent agency and social role representations), were of particular interest. These dimensions were considered to be roughly analogous to structural and social aspects of early communicative development (e.g., MLU, pragmatics).

Method. Children's play was coded from transcripts of mother–child free play behavior. Each bout of symbolic play was then scored for level of symbolic maturity on four different play scales that were derived from empirical data reported in the literature. The first scale focused on the increasing complexity and integration of action schemes, ranging from single schemes to scheme combinations of hierarchically integrated, multischemed play. Two scales were concerned with role representation. One was concerned with social roles depicted in play with small figures (replica play) and the other involved play with human partners (sociodramatic play). Both of these scales ranged from self-related pretend play to the integration of roles of several actors. The fourth scale measured children's tendency to use objects in a decontextualized fashion (object substitution). This fourth scale ranged from the use of objects in a prototypical manner (i.e., using a cup as a cup), to simple object substitutions, and, finally, to gestural miming and verbal ideation. For purposes of comparison, we also included a fifth play scale, Nicolich's (1977) play scheme.

Two scores were derived for each play scale: the highest level of spontaneous symbolic play observed at least twice, and the average level of play, as indexed by the weighted mean of the summed spontaneous play scores. In addition, the density (number of connected symbolic play schemes per play bout) and the complexity (number of different connected symbolic schemes per play bout) were assessed.

Results. As in the first play study, the play behavior of the children with Down syndrome were compared to their MA- and CA-matched counterparts. Correlations of play behavior with MA, CA, and MLU were also assessed within each child group. Age-related differences in symbolic play behavior between the younger and older cohorts were also examined.

Younger cohort. When compared to the play of their CA-matched controls, the children with Down syndrome's play was significantly less complex, dense, and mature on each of the play scales. In contrast, children with Down syndrome did *not* differ significantly from their cognitively comparable controls on any aspect of symbolic play assessed.

Older cohort. Slightly different findings were obtained for the older sample of children. As with the younger children with Down syndrome, the older children with Down syndrome were not significantly different from their cognitively comparable matches on the highest level of play observed for the action complexity, agent use, or role enactment play scales. Nor did they differ from their controls on most measures of play density and complexity. The one exception was for the total number of symbolic schemes produced. Children with Down syndrome had significantly more schemes overall than did their nonretarded controls, though the groups did not differ in the total number of *different* schemes produced. Another difference was that the older children with Down syndrome were significantly *less* advanced than their MA-matched counterparts on all play scales in terms of their *average* (but not highest) scores, and on the object substitution scale for all scores (average and highest).

In addition, correlations between play variables and indices of child development (MA, CA, MLU) also were examined within child groups. For each group of children in both cohorts, symbolic play variables were correlated significantly with both MA and MLU, but less strongly with CA.

Somewhat different patterns of correlations were seen in the older cohort. As in the younger cohort, both the children with Down syndrome and their MA-matched controls had more significant correlations of play with MA than with CA (7 vs. 2 and 9 vs. 6, respectively, out of 16). However, different patterns were observed with respect to MLU. The MA-comparable controls in the older cohort had 11 out of 16 play variables correlated significantly with MLU, whereas the children with

Down syndrome had only 4 out of 16. These differences possibly may be explained by the fact that the MLUs of the older children with Down syndrome were much more restricted in range than those of the nonhandicapped children. These results attest to the increasing dissociation of syntactic development and other forms of symbolic development (play, communicative skills) with age for children with Down syndrome.

Age-related changes in symbolic play. Age-related changes in play also were tested by comparing the younger and older subsamples of children within each child group. Results indicated that all children in the older cohort had significantly higher means on all play variables than did the younger children.

Summary and discussion. Results suggest that children with Down syndrome continue to develop similarly (although at a slower pace) to nonhandicapped children with respect to symbolic play during the preoperational period. In the main, children with Down syndrome did not differ significantly from their MA-matched counterparts on most symbolic play measures. Moreover, similar patterns of correlations were observed among play, language, and cognitive variables for both the children with Down syndrome and their nonretarded controls.

As was found for communicative measures, children with Down syndrome also had strengths and weaknesses among different aspects of symbolic play. A particular strength was in the more socially related aspects of symbolic play that involved independent agency and social role representations. An area of deficit emerged for older children with Down syndrome that involved the ability to use objects in a decontextualized fashion (object substitution scale). One explanation for this deficit may be their alleged difficulty with abstractions (Gibson, 1978). An alternative explanation for these differences might be the expressive language differences observed between children with Down syndrome and their MA-matched controls. Recall that the higher levels of the object substitution scale required verbal transformations or verbal ideation. In support of this, MLU was correlated highly with the object use scale for both groups of children. On the other hand, the relative linguistic deficits of the children with Down syndrome did not preclude them from engaging in long, connected bouts of play that were as complex and hierarchically integrated as that of their controls.

In addition, older children with Down syndrome produced more symbolic schemes than their controls overall (yet their play did not differ in complexity) and had lower average scores for all play scales. This finding suggests that these children were more perseverative in play, repeating schemes more often than did their controls (a finding also noted by Kopp, Krakow, & Vaughn, 1983, and Riguet et al., 1981). Perhaps these differences reflect their slower information processing abilities (Lincoln et al., 1985). Because the highest levels of their play did not differ from that of their controls, however, these play differences did not interfere greatly with their ultimate play achievements.

In sum, the findings of these three studies attest to the coherence of play development in preoperational children with Down syndrome. Despite certain differences, the Down syndrome and MA-matched groups showed equivalent performances on most measures of play and displayed similar correlational patterns among cognitive, linguistic, and play measures. These results confirm and extend prior research documenting the relationship between symbolic play and cognitive development, and among play and affective–motivational, cognitive, and social development during early childhood.

Associations and dissociations between language and play development

The purpose of the third set of studies was to examine whether similar correspondences between early linguistic and play development that have been reported previously for normally developing children could be observed for children with Down syndrome (McCune-Nicolich & Bruskin, 1982). The theoretical rationale for these studies stems from the current debate between proponents of the modularity hypothesis of language development, who claim that language develops separately and independently from other emerging systems of development, and investigators proposing that aspects of language and other symbolic skills may be interrelated and may have common roots in nonlinguistic domains such as cognition (see Bates et al., 1988, for a review).

Piaget (1962) and other classical developmental theorists such as Werner and Kaplan (1963) have stressed that language and symbolic play are two aspects of the same emergent representational capacity – the "semiotic function." Based on this hypothesis, one might expect language and other forms of symbolic development to correspond closely in development (see Werner & Kaplan, 1963). Language and play *do* share similar features and functions. In symbolic play, for example, children used objects, sounds, and gestures to symbolize other aspects and events, as is the case with early language (McCune-Nicolich & Bruskin, 1982; Shore et al., in press). Language and play also serve similar functions in early life. For example, children use both to transform and "play with" early representations of familiar events and social understanding; children also use both in a communication fashion to share objects and object transformations (see Bretherton, 1984).

Although most studies largely have discredited a strong version of this "cognitive" hypothesis, partial support for a more limited "neo-Piagetian" version has in fact been generated for both normally developing and language delayed children (see Bates, Bretherton, & Snyder, 1988 for a review). For example, McCune-Nicolich and Bruskin (1982) provided longitudinal evidence for close correspondences in certain language and symbolic play abilities at particular periods in early development: first words and the appearance of single symbolic play schemes; early word combinations and combinatorial play; and the emergence of grammar and planned symbolic play. Other investigators have found relationships among specific aspects of sensorimotor development (imitation, tool use) and early language development at specific points in time (see Bates & Snyder, 1987). Likewise, certain cognitive and linguistic skills have been associated with the development of nonlinguistic symbolic skills such as communicative gestures and symbolic play (Bates, Benigni, Bretherton, Camaioni, & Volterra, 1979; McCune-Nicolich & Bruskin, 1982; Piaget, 1962). Significant associations between more general aspects of language development and symbolic play maturity also have been reported (Fein, 1979; Largo & Howard, 1979).

A stronger case for these associations could be made with supporting evidence from children with delayed language or cognitive development, such as children with Down syndrome. Some limited support exists from studies of language-delayed children of varying etiology. For example, Sigman and Ungerer (1984) reported significant correlations between receptive language and symbolic play maturity, as well as between receptive language and imitation skills, in mentally retarded children, autistic children, and normal children of equivalent mental age. In our play studies (described earlier), both MLU and MA were correlated strongly with indices of symbolic play maturity for children with Down syndrome as well as for non-handicapped children. In addition, both Smith and Tetzchner (1986) and Mundy and his colleagues (1988) found that nonverbal communicative skills predicted expressive language development in their sample of children with Down syndrome.

Structural parallels between language and play

In this first study, we investigated whether we could observe similar parallels between early language and symbolic play development as were reported for normally developing children by McCune-Nicolich and Bruskin (1982), Shore et al., (in press), and others.

Method. All 41 subjects with Down syndrome from our sample participated. Children's expressive language abilities were assessed as described in the studies on early language development in this chapter. Children ranged in language ability from prelinguistic to multiword speech. Children's symbolic play was assessed from videotapes of mother–child free play using Nicolich's (1977) symbolic play coding scheme. This system is based on Piagetian theory (Piaget, 1962) and has five developmental levels: presymbolic; autosymbolic (self-related pretend); single scheme decontextualized pretend play; multischemed symbolic play; and planned symbolic play. This coding system was employed so we could compare our results with those reported for normally developing children by McCune-Nicolich and Bruskin (1982).

Results. The following play–language correspondences were observed, which are consistent with prior findings reported in the literature. First, no prelinguistic children engaged in symbolic play at any of the longitudinal visits. Second, children in the one-word stage of language development produced only single symbolic schemes during play. For most of these children, symbolic play rarely was observed. Third, all children in early and late Stage 1 of syntactic development (initial word combinations) were observed to combine symbolic schemes in play. However, children in early Stage 1 varied in how frequently and consistently they combined schemes in play. Fourth, a marked increase in productivity for both language and symbolic play was observed for children in late Stage 1 and beyond. Most of these children were observed to engage in planned, hierarchically organized symbolic play consisting of long episodes of connected symbolic schemes. One child, for instance, produced a 10-minute-long "camping trip" using small toy figures. This episode consisted of many logically ordered, connected bouts of play (e.g., packing the car, traveling, stopping for lunch, traveling, stopping for a snack, traveling, stopping for a swim, traveling, getting into an accident, and getting transported to the hospital by a superhero doll). Although this level of play was not common among the children with Down syndrome, the child's MLU was only 1.83 at the time of the play observation.

It is important to note that these correspondences are based on children's spontaneous play and language, as were those reported by McCune-Nicolich and Bruskin. As such, our data do not necessarily reflect these children's true competencies. A different pattern might have emerged had we tried to elicit symbolic play through modeling techniques, since children often show somewhat higher levels of play under those conditions (Fenson, 1984).

Associations and dissociations between play and language during Stage 1

Based on the results of our studies, which suggest that certain aspects of symbolic play and language development are closely associated at specific times in ontogeny for children with Down syndrome, one might expect that the level of symbolic play exhibited by children with Down syndrome would not differ significantly from that observed in MLU-equivalent nonhandicapped children. We hypothesized that this would *not* be the case, because of the findings reported in the studies on the structural dimensions of object and social play and on symbolic play development described earlier in this chapter. In those studies, the symbolic play abilities of children with Down syndrome did not differ from those observed in cognitively comparable normal children, who had significantly longer MLUs than the children with Down syndrome. However, not all aspects of symbolic play were advanced equally for children with Down syndrome. Recall that children with Down syndrome had significantly *lower* play scores for one form of symbolic play–object substitution. Transforming objects into other objects or using objects in decontextualized ways occurred less frequently for children with Down syndrome than for their MA-matched controls.

In the present study, we compared children with Down syndrome's symbolic play scores on the four play scales described in the symbolic play development studies to those of MLU-matched nonhandicapped children. Based on the results from our studies on pragmatics, communication, and symbolic development, we expected that children with Down syndrome would be significantly more advanced in the more social types of symbolic play (independent agency, role representations), rel-

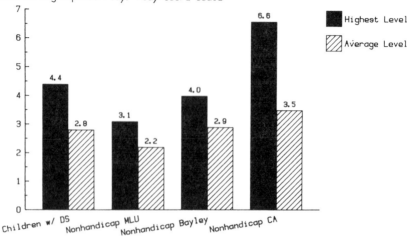

Figure 10.6. Symbolic play performance of children during early Stage 1: agent use during replica play

ative to their MLU-matched controls, but would not differ from these controls in object substitution.

Method. In this study, we used the sample of 28 children with Down syndrome who were in Stage 1 described in the language section of this chapter. Each child with Down syndrome was matched to two control children: one for MLU and one for MA. In addition, unlike the former language study, we included a third control group (matched to the children with Down syndrome for sex and CA).

Results. As expected, the symbolic play of children with Down syndrome was significantly more advanced than that observed in their MLU-matched controls (but not their MA matches) for the action complexity, replica use, and social role play scales. These results mirror the results for pragmatic development reported in our studies on pragmatics and communicative skills and attest to the role of social experience and cognitive development in the acquisition of two kinds of symbolic abilities: communicative skills and socially oriented symbolic play.

In contrast, on the object substitution scale, children with Down syndrome performed at a significantly *less* mature level than their MA-matched (but not MLU-matched) counterparts. Thus, transforming objects and using objects in decontextualized ways appear to be especially difficult for children with Down syndrome. This type of symbolic play has been associated with an ''analytical'' style (as opposed to a holistic style) of language learning in normally developing children (Bates et al., 1988). Bates and her colleagues reported that an analytical style of language learning predicted children's later acquisition of grammar in their longitudinal study.

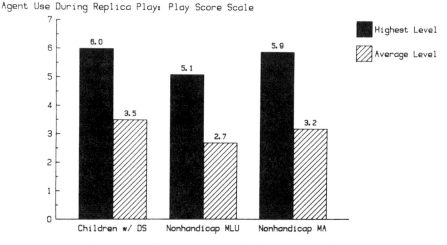

Figure 10.7. Symbolic play performance of children during late Stage 1: agent use during replica play

Stage-related changes in symbolic play. Stage-related changes in children's play behavior also were observed. Children in late Stage 1 engaged in more mature symbolic play as measured by all four scales than did children in early Stage 1. These results are similar to those reported for lexical and communicative skills in an earlier section of this chapter.

Figures 10.6 and 10.7 display group and stage differences in children's symbolic play performance on the replica use scale, which assessed the emergence of independent agency and role relations during play with small figures.

Early linguistic and nonlinguistic representations of self and other

During the second and third years of life, children become increasingly aware of themselves as agents and recipients of action (Kagan, 1982). During this time, self–other differences also become more and more salient. The use of language and play to represent early conceptions of self and other is an age-appropriate manifestation of these developmental trends (Bretherton, 1984; Wolf, Rygh, & Altschuler, 1984). For example, children begin to use their own names and personal pronouns and describe their own activities more frequently (Kagan, 1982). In addition, children start to label the emotional states, intentions, and volitions of both themselves and other persons. At first, children tend to speak primarily about self and other in the here and now; however, with increasing cognitive development, they begin to use self-related language in more decontextualized ways (i.e., they discuss nonpresent or hypothetical actions and states).

As seen in the studies on symbolic play development, children also represent their early conceptions of self and other during symbolic play. Young children first play at being themselves and later project their own behavior onto other recipients such as dolls or toys. By the end of the third year, children are able to engage in sociodramatic play involving role-taking and to represent the behavior of several interacting replicas in an integrated fashion (see Watson & Fisher, 1977). As in other forms of symbolic development, these age-related changes in children's representations of self and other reflect a process of decentration, decontextualization, and integration (Fenson, 1984).

The purpose of this study was to examine early linguistic and nonlinguistic representations of self and other by children with Down syndrome during Stage 1 of syntactic development. As in other forms of symbolic development, replication of developmental trends in self-other representation found for normally developing children in delayed or deviant populations can offer important insight into current developmental theories such as self–other differentiation. Of particular interest was the effect of extreme expressive language delays on children's early representations of self and other in language and play.

Method. In this study, we used the sample described in the play and language section. Measures of language and symbolic play were derived from detailed transcripts of mother–child interaction. The following measures of self-related language were included: proportion of statements describing self and other's actions; proportion of statements describing self and other's internal states; number of different internal state labels; number of different personal pronouns; and decontextualized use of internal state language (e.g., in questions, negations, nonpresent contexts). Children's ability to use an internal state word for both self and other also was scored.

Symbolic play was coded using the two scales described in the symbolic play section which measured developmental trends in children's representations of self and other in play (role representation scales). These scales ranged from predominantly self-related pretending to increasingly decentered and hierarchically integrated play depicting the interaction and roles of several different social actors.

We hypothesized that children's representations of self and other in both language and play would be related to children's level of cognitive development based on prior research in normally developing populations (Bretherton & Beeghly, 1982).

Results. Results indicated that children with Down syndrome showed similar but delayed sequences of self-related language and play development compared to that observed for nonhandicapped children. In both language and play, children first represented themselves symbolically, and with increasing age and cognitive maturity, children's language and play became more decentered, decontextualized, and integrated. Only the most cognitively mature children used language and play to represent self and other in hypothetical or nonpresent situations.

As reported in the study on the relation between play and language, children with Down syndrome were significantly more mature in symbolic play than their MLU-matched controls (but not their MA-matched controls). In contrast to these findings, and unexpectedly, the children with Down syndrome were significantly less advanced than their MA controls (but not their MLU controls) on most *linguistic* measures of self–other representation. However, both linguistic and nonlinguistic variables were significantly correlated with MA for children with Down syndrome. Interestingly, children with Down syndrome produced significantly more utterances about others' actions and internal states than they did about their own actions and states, a pattern not seen in the nonhandicapped children.

In sum, findings from these three studies provide support for a "neo-Piagetian" or "local homologies" model of early language development, rather than a strong version of Piaget's "semiotic hypothesis." Language, play, and cognitive development shared specific but limited proportions of variance in our Down syndrome sample. Important.y, the overall pattern of interrelations reveal that for children with Down syndrome, symbolic development is multimodal and polyphasic in nature (Gollin, 1984).

Overview and general discussion

We began our research program by asking two broad questions that are crucial for a more complete understanding of the expressive language deficit of children with Down syndrome and for the nature and course of symbolic development more generally. Are the language deficits of children with Down syndrome part of a broader symbolic deficit that can be observed in other aspects of representational functioning, such as communicative skills or symbolic play? Or are their expressive language delays limited to more structural aspects of language? Our results have shed some preliminary light on these issues, although clearly much more work remains to be done. An overview of our findings to date is provided.

Expressive language development

Like other investigators (e.g., see Chapter 9 by Fowler and Chapter 8 by Mervis, this volume), we found dramatic delays in the expressive language development of children with Down syndrome, which persisted over the course of our study. The majority of children in our sample showed little or no linguistic progress over the year. Although there were wide variations in MA in this sample, children with Down syndrome all clustered in very early levels of language development.

Compared to MLU-matched nonhandicapped children, children with Down syndrome had significantly higher MAs and CAs. These discrepancies grew larger as children grew older. Nonetheless, MLU proved to be a good summary measure of syntactic development for children at this early level of syntactic development (see also Fowler, Chapter 9, this volume).

What can account for these inordinate delays in language? The answer is likely to be multivariate and multidimensional, involving a consideration of both child and environmental characteristics that are unique to individuals with Down syndrome. For example, an increased incidence of hearing and visual deficits, otitis media, structural anomalies in the speech apparatus, and motor control problems (all of which are associated with Down syndrome) may affect children's ability to comprehend and produce language (see Miller, in press). Moreover, certain neuro-physiological and cognitive deficits such as slowed information processing, problems in visual attention, difficulties in verbal coding and decoding, memory deficits, as well as problems in arousal modulation, visual–proprioceptive feedback, dampened affect, and pronounced passivity are characteristic of children with Down syndrome and may well interfere with children's language acquisition (Cicchetti & Beeghly, Chapter 2, this volume; Cicchetti & Pogge-Hesse, 1982; Ganiban et al., Chapter 3, this volume; Kopp et al., 1983; Loveland, 1987; Thompson et al., 1985; Wagner et al., Chapter 5, this volume).

In turn, these unique characteristics may affect the quality of social interaction that children with Down syndrome experience, since social interaction patterns are reciprocal in nature (Bell & Harper, 1977). For example, it is well documented that children with Down syndrome engage in less initiating, parental referencing, and joint attention during object play and social interaction, which may interfere with the establishment of turn-taking and reciprocity (Berger, Chapter 4, this volume; Sorce, Emde, & Frank, 1982). These qualities may make it more difficult for adults to read, mark, and reward these children's behavior (Berger, Chapter 4, this volume), which may contribute to a less than optimal linguistic environment for these children.

In addition, these characteristics of children with Down syndrome, along with their delayed developmental progress, may influence parents' beliefs and expectations for their children, which in turn could affect the type of input such children receive. Although the structural aspects of caregiver speech to children with Down syndrome (e.g., syntactic complexity) appear to be similar to that addressed to normally developing children at equivalent levels of language maturity (Buckhalt, Rutherford, & Goldberg, 1978; Buium, Rynders, & Turnure, 1974), other *functional* features of caregiver input to children with Down syndrome may be less than optimal for facilitating early language development. For example, Cardoso-Martins and her colleagues (Cardoso-Martins, 1984; see also Mervis, Chapter 8, this volume, for a review) have demonstrated that mothers of language-learning children with Down syndrome are more likely to be directive and less likely to tailor their utterances to their children in a semantically contingent way. This style of interaction is not unique to caregivers of children with Down syndrome but, rather, is characteristic of interactions with language-delayed individuals in general (Cross, Nienhuys, & Kirkman, 1985).

Lexical and pragmatic development

Lexical development was somewhat less delayed than syntactic development, especially for older, more cognitively mature children with Down syndrome. Moreover, the content of the productive vocabularies of children with Down syndrome did not differ markedly from that observed in their nonhandicapped controls.

In contrast, the area of least delay within the language domain was in pragmatics and conversation skills. Compared to MLU-matched controls, children with Down syndrome had consistently higher scores on most measures of pragmatic development, including the diversity of speech acts produced, conversational relevance (MLE) (Brown, 1980), topic maintenance, and turn-taking skills. Although we observed a dissociation between MLU and pragmatic skills for children with Down syndrome that was not observed for nonhandicapped children, age-related increases in pragmatic skills were found for all groups of children. These increases were especially marked as children made the transition from early to late Stage 1 of syntactic development.

One notable exception to the superior conversational skills of children with Down syndrome was observed. Children with Down syndrome produced proportionally fewer requests than did MA-matched controls. This finding is consistent with those reported by both Mundy and colleagues (1988) and Smith and Tetzchner (1986) for nonverbal requesting behavior by children with Down syndrome. This deficit may be related to other factors that may interfere with children's tendency to take the initiative (e.g., passivity, low levels of arousal, etc.)

Symbolic play development

Parallel strengths and weaknesses were seen in the symbolic play development of children with Down syndrome as were observed for pragmatic development. Though delayed in the pace of their development, children with Down syndrome exhibited similar sequences of play development as have been observed in normally developing children. Moreover, for the most part, children with Down syndrome did not differ significantly from their MA-matched controls in the relative proportion of time they engaged in various types of object play nor in the complexity of their symbolic play.

Three notable exceptions to this pattern were observed. Relative to their MA-matched controls, younger children with Down syndrome tended, first, to spend more time engaged in simple manipulative object play and, second, to repeat symbolic schemes in a perseverative fashion. Both of these behavior patterns are consistent with behaviors reported by Kopp and her colleagues (1983), Loveland (1987), and Vietze and his colleague (1983) in their studies of children with Down syndrome. Third, children with Down syndrome engaged in fewer object transformations and object substitutions during symbolic play than did their MA-matched controls. This deficit was related to these children's syntactic abilities. Interestingly, Bates and her colleagues (Bates et al., 1987, 1988) reported that children who engaged in frequent object substitutions during symbolic play were more likely to have adopted an ''analytical'' (versus a ''holistic'') approach to language acquisition. This style predicted more advanced grammatical development in her longitudinal study of normal children.

Results from both the language and play assessments have methodological as well as theoretical implications. Thus, the asynchronies or dissociations among specific aspects of both language and play behavior (e.g., MLU and pragmatics; de-contextualized symbolic play [object substitutions]; and social-oriented symbolic play) observed for children with Down syndrome suggest that neither language nor play is fruitfully conceptualized as a unitary construct. Rather, both are multidimensional in nature. Moreover, weaknesses observed for children with Down syndrome within a particular area of relative strength such as pragmatics or symbolic play suggest that caution should be taken when attempting to generalize about more specific symbolic domains.

The role of affect and social behavior

More qualitative aspects of play, such as affective play engagement and exploration, did not differentiate children with Down syndrome from their MA-matched controls and were correlated with both symbolic play and level of cognitive maturity. In contrast, more systematic differences were observed for a variety of social behaviors for children with Down syndrome. As others have reported (Jones, 1980), these children were rated as being less initiating and less directing than MA-matched nonhandicapped children. These findings mirror reports of depressed rates of requesting behavior in children with Down syndrome, discussed in an earlier section.

Despite their deficits and differences in aspects of linguistic and social behavior, and the delayed pace of their development, children with Down syndrome displayed similar patterns of correlations among indices of cognitive development, symbolic play maturity, affective play style, and specific aspects of social behavior as were seen for nonhandicapped children.

These results suggest that the early symbolic behavior of children with Down syndrome is organized in much the same way as in nonhandicapped children and attest to the coherence of play development for children with Down syndrome. Play proved to be an excellent context in which to study the social, emotional, cognitive, and linguistic aspects of representational development.

Implications for assessment. If these results can be replicated systematically, our findings have implications for the developmental evaluation of children with Down syndrome. Adult–child play situations may prove to be useful alternatives and/or additions to standardized testing for evaluating the cognitive–motivational competence of children with Down syndrome (see Cicchetti & Wagner, in press). During play, for instance, examiners can avoid problems associated with evaluations of developmentally delayed children in more demanding testing contexts (e.g., increased passivity, avoidance, learned helplessness; Zigler & Balla, 1982).

In conclusion, our research provides descriptive evidence consistent with a ''neo-Piagetian'' or ''local homologies'' model of early symbol language development (Bates et al., 1988). Specific parallels among aspects of symbolic play and language were observed at limited points in development for children with Down syndrome. These results are corroborated by similar findings in the play literature. Despite relative strengths and weaknesses among types of symbolic play and language for children with Down syndrome, measures of play and language were correlated significantly with MA and MLU in all groups of children. In addition, similar stage-related changes in children's symbolic play abilities also were observed. These results attest to the coherence of early symbolic development in children with Down syndrome and suggest that, despite their extreme linguistic deficits, their symbolic capacities are relatively intact during this age period.

The implications of these findings for children's later adaptation and social–communicative competence remain unclear. Studies of the long-term sequelae of individual differences in early symbolic skills are lacking (Rondal, 1988). In our laboratory, we plan to remedy this by following up our Down syndrome sample into middle childhood. Educators and other professionals directing intervention and other support programs for older children and adults with Down syndrome and their families are in dire need of this type of information.

References

Bates, E., Benigni, L., Bretherton, I., Camaioni, L., & Volterra, V. (1979). *The emergence of symbols.* New York: Academic Press.

Bates, E., Bretherton, I., Beeghly-Smith, M., & McNew, S. (1982). Social bases of language development: A reassessment. In H. Reese & L. Lipsitt (Eds.), *Advances in child development and behavior* (Vol. 16). New York: Academic Press.

Bates, E., Bretherton, I., & Snyder, L. (1988). *From first words to grammar.* New York: Cambridge University Press.

Bates, E., O'Connell, B., & Shore, C. (1987). Language and communication in infancy. In J. Osofsky (Ed.), *Handbook of Infant Development.* New York: Wiley.

Bates, E., & Snyder, L. (1987). The cognitive hypothesis in language development. In I. Uzgiris & J. McV. Hunt (Eds.), *Research with scales of psychological development in infancy.* Urbana: University of Illinois Press.

Bayley, N. (1969). *Bayley Scales of Infant Development.* New York: Psychological Corporation.

Beeghly, M. (1988). *Associations and dissociations in language and symbolic play of children with Down syndrome.* Symposium presented at the International Conference on Infant Studies, Washington, DC.

Beeghly, M., & Cicchetti, D. (1985). *Development of functional communication during Stage 1 of syntactic development by children with Down syndrome.* Presented at the 10th Annual Boston University Conference on Language Development, Boston, October.

Beeghly, M., & Cicchetti, D. (1986). *Early language development of children with Down syndrome: A longitudinal study.* Presented at the 11th Annual Boston University Conference on Language Development, Boston, October.

Beeghly, M., & Cicchetti, D. (1987). An organizational approach to symbolic development in children with Down syndrome. In D. Cicchetti & M. Beeghly (Eds.), *Atypical symbolic development.* San Francisco: Jossey-Bass.

Beeghly, M., Hanrahan, A., Weiss, B., & Cicchetti, D. (1985). *Development of communicative competence in children with Down syndrome.* Presented at the biennial meetings of the Society for Research in Child Development, Toronto, April.

Beeghly, M., Weiss, B., and Cicchetti, D. (1986). *Early linguistic and nonlinguistic representations of self and other by children with Down syndrome.* Presented at the International Conference on Infant Studies, Los Angeles, April.

Beeghly, M., Weiss-Perry, B., & Cicchetti, D. (1989). Structural and affective dimensions of free play behavior in children with Down syndrome. *International Journal of Behavioral Development, 12,* 257–277.

Bell, R. Q., & Harper, L. V. (1977). *Child effects on adults*. Hillsdale, NJ: Erlbaum.

Belsky, J., & Most, R. (1981). From exploration to play: A cross-sectional study of infant free play behavior. *Developmental Psychology, 17*, 630–639.

Bischof, N. (1975). A systems approach toward the functional connections of attachment and fear. *Child Development, 46*, 801–817.

Bretherton, I. (Ed.). (1984). *Symbolic play*. New York: Academic Press.

Bretherton, I., & Beeghly, M. (1982). Talking about internal states: The acquisition of an explicit theory of mind. *Developmental Psychology, 18*, 906–921.

Bretherton, I., McNew, S., Snyder, L. & Bates, E. (1983). Individual differences at 20 months: Analytic and holistic strategies. *Journal of Child Language, 10*, 293–320.

Brown, R. (1973). *A first language*. Cambridge, MA: Harvard University Press.

Brown, R. (1980). The maintenance of conversation. In D. Olson (Ed.), *Social foundations of language and thought*. New York: Oxford University Press.

Bruner, J. (1983). The acquisition of pragmatic commitments. In R. Golinkoff (Ed.), *The transition from prelinguistic to linguistic communication*. Hillsdale, NJ: Erlbaum.

Buckhalt, T. A., Rutherford, R. B., & Goldberg, K. E. (1978). Verbal and nonverbal interactions of mothers and their Down syndrome and nonretarded infants. *American Journal of Mental Deficiency, 72*, 337–343.

Buium, N., Rynders, J. & Turnure, J. (1974). Early maternal linguistic environment of normal and Down's syndrome language-learning children. *American Journal of Mental Deficiency, 79*, 52–58.

Cardoso-Martins, C. (1984). *Early vocabulary acquisition by Down syndrome children: The roles of cognitive development and maternal language input*. Unpublished doctoral dissertation. University of Illinois, Urbana-Champaign.

Cardoso-Martins, C., & Mervis, C. B. (1985). Maternal speech to prelinguistic Down syndrome children. *American Journal of Mental Deficiency, 89*, 451–458.

Cardoso-Martins, C., Mervis, C. B., and Mervis, C. A. (1985). Early vocabulary acquisition by children with Down syndrome. *American Journal of Mental Deficiency, 90*, 177–184.

Cicchetti, D. (1984). The emergence of developmental psychopathology. *Child Development, 55*, 1–7.

Cicchetti, D., Beeghly, M., & Carlson, V. (in press). The development of the self in atypical populations: An organizational perspective. In D. Cicchetti & M. Beeghly (Eds.), *The self in transition: Infancy to childhood*. Chicago: University of Chicago Press.

Cicchetti, D., & Hesse, P. (1983). Affect and intellect: Piaget's contributions to the study of infant emotional development. In R. Plutchik & H. Kellerman (Eds.), *Emotion: Theory and research* (Vol. 2). New York: Academic Press.

Cicchetti, D., & Mans-Wagener, L. (1987). Stages, sequences, and structures in the organization of cognitive development in Down syndrome infants. In I. Uzgiris & J. McV. Hunt (Eds.), *Research with scales of psychological development in infancy*. Urbana: University of Illinois Press.

Cicchetti, D., & Pogge-Hesse, P. (1982). Possible contributions of the study of organic mentally retarded children to developmental theory. In E. Zigler & D. Balla (Eds.), *Mental retardation: The developmental–difference controversy*. Hillsdale, NJ: Erlbaum.

Cicchetti, D., & Schneider-Rosen, K. (1984). Theoretical and empirical considerations in the investigation of the relationship between affect and cognition in atypical populations of infants: Contributions to the formulation of an integrative theory of development. In C. Izard, J. Kagan, & R. Zajonc (Eds.), *Emotions, cognition, and behavior*. New York: Cambridge University Press.

Cicchetti, D., & Schneider-Rosen, K. (1986). An organizational approach to childhood depression. In M. Rutter, C. Izard, & P. Read (Eds.), *Depression in young people: Clinical and developmental perspectives*. New York: Guilford.

Cicchetti, D., & Serafica, F. (1981). The interplay among behavioral systems: Illustrations from the study of attachment, affiliation, and wariness in young Down syndrome children. *Developmental Psychology, 17*, 36–49.

Cicchetti, D., & Sroufe, L. A. (1976). The relationship between affective and cognitive development in Down's syndrome infants. *Child Development, 47*, 920–929.

Cicchetti, D., & Sroufe, L. A. (1978). An organizational view of affect: Illustration from the study of Down's syndrome infants. In M. Lewis & L. Rosenblum (Eds.), *The development of affect.* New York: Plenum.

Cicchetti, D., & Wagner, S. (in press). Alternative assessment strategies for the evaluation of infants and toddlers: An organizational perspective. In S. Meisels & J. Shonkoff (Eds.), *Handbook of early intervention.* New York: Cambridge University Press.

Coggins, T. E., Carpenter, R., & Owings, N. (1984). Examining early intentional communication in Down syndrome and nonretarded children. *British Journal of Disorders of Communication, 18,* 98–106.

Coggins, T. E., & Stoel-Gammon, L. (1982). Clarification strategies used by four Down syndrome children for maintaining normal conversational interaction. *Education and Training of the Mentally Retarded, 17,* 65–67.

Crawley, S., & Spiker, D. (1983). Mother–child interactions and mental development in two-year-olds with Down syndrome. *Child Development, 54,* 1312–1323.

Cross, T., Nienhuys, T., & Kirkman, M. (1985). Parent–child interaction with receptively disabled children: Some determinants of maternal speech style. In K. Nelson (Ed.), *Children's language* (Vol. 5). Hillsdale, NJ: Erlbaum.

Cunningham, C., Glenn, S., Wilkinson, P., & Sloper, P. (1985). Mental ability, symbolic play, and expressive language of young children with Down syndrome. *Journal of Child Psychology and Psychiatry, 26,* 255–265.

Dore, J. (1974). A pragmatic description of early language development. *Journal of Psycholinguistic Research, 3,* 343–350.

Dore, J. (1979). Children's illocutionary acts. In R. Freedle (Ed.), *Discourse processes: Advances in research and theory.* Norwood, NJ: Ablex.

Dunn, L. M., & Dunn, L. (1981). *The Peabody Picture Vocabulary Test – revised.* Circle Pines, MN: American Guidance Service.

Evans, D., & Hampson, M. (1969). The language of mongols. *British Journal of Disorders of Communication, 3,* 171–181.

Fein, G. (1979). Echoes from the nursery: Piaget, Vygotsky, and the relationship between language and play. *New Directions for Child Development, 6,* 1–14.

Fein, G. & Apfel, N. (1979). The development of play: Style, structure, and situation. *Genetic Psychology Monographs, 99,* 231–250.

Fenson, L. (1984). Developmental trends for action and speech in pretend play. In I. Bretherton (Ed.), *Symbolic play.* New York: Academic Press.

Galda, L., & Pellegrini, A. (1985). *Play, language, and stories: The development of children's literate behaviors.* Norwood, NJ: Ablex.

Gibson, D. (1978). *Down's syndrome: The psychology of mongolism.* London: Cambridge University Press.

Golinkoff, R. (1983). *The transition from prelinguistic to linguistic communication.* Hillsdale, NJ: Erlbaum.

Gollin, E. (1984). *Malformations of development.* New York: Academic.

Greenberg, M. (1983). Pragmatics and social interaction: The unrealized nexus. In L. Feagans, R. Golinkoff, & C. Garvey (Eds.), *The origins and growth of communication.* Norwood, NJ: Ablex.

Hill, P., & McCune-Nicolich, L. (1981). Pretend play and patterns of cognition in Down's syndrome infants. *Child Development, 23,* 43–60.

Jennings, K., Harmon, R., Gaiter, J., & Yarrow. L. (1979). Exploratory play as an index of mastery motivation: Relationships to persistence, cognitive functioning, and environmental measures. *Developmental Psychology, 15,* 386–394.

Jones, O. H. M. (1980). Prelinguistic communication skills in Down's syndrome and normal infants. In T. Field (Ed.), *High risk infants and children.* New York: Academic Press.

Kagan, J. (1982). *The second year: Growth of self awareness.* Cambridge, MA: Harvard University Press.

Kopp, C., Krakow, J., & Johnson, K. (1983). Strategy production by young children with Down syndrome. *American Journal of Mental Deficiency, 88,* 164–169.

Kopp, C. B., Krakow, J., & Vaughn, V. (1983). Patterns of self-control in young handicapped children. *Minnesota Symposia on Child Psychology* (Vol. 16). Hillsdale, NJ: Erlbaum.

Krakow, J., & Kopp, C. (1982). Sustained attention in young children with Down syndrome. *Topics in Early Childhood Special Education, 2,* 32–42.

Largo, J., & Howard, J. (1979). Developmental progression in play behavior of children between nine and thirty months, II. *Developmental Medicine and Child Neurology, 21,* 492–503.

Lee, L. (1974). *Developmental Sentence Analysis.* Evanston, IL: Northwestern University Press.

Leifer, J., & Lewis, M. (1984). Acquisition of conversational response skills by young Down syndrome and nonretarded young children. *American Journal of Mental Deficiency, 88,* 610–618.

Leuder, I., Fraser, W., & Jeeves, M. (1981). Social familiarity and communication in Down syndrome. *Journal of Mental Deficiency Research, 25,* 133–142.

Lincoln, A., Courchesne, E., Kilman, B., & Galambos, R. (1985). Neurophysiological correlates of information processing by children with Down syndrome. *American Journal of Mental Deficiency, 89,* 403–414.

Loveland, K. (1987). Behavior of young children with Down syndrome before the mirror: Exploration. *Child Development, 58,* 768–778.

MacTurk, R., Hunter, R., McCarthy, M., Vietze, P., & McQuiston, S. (1985). Social mastery motivation in Down syndrome and nondelayed infants. *Topics in Early Childhood Special Education, 4,* 93–109.

Mans, L., Cicchetti, D., & Sroufe, L. A. (1978). Mirror reactions of Down's syndrome infants and toddlers: Cognitive underpinnings of self-recognition. *Child Development, 49,* 1247–1250.

McCune-Nicolich, L., & Bruskin, C. (1982). Combinatorial competency in symbolic play and language. In D. Pepler & K. Rubin (Eds.), *The play of children.* New York: Karger.

Miller, J. F. (in press). Language and communication characteristics of children with Down syndrome. In A. Crocker, S. Pueschel, J. Rynders, & C. Tinghey (Eds.), *Down syndrome: State of the art.* Baltimore, MD: Brooks.

Motti, F., Cicchetti, D., & Sroufe, L. A. (1983). From infant affect expression to symbolic play: The coherence of development in Down syndrome children. *Child Development, 54,* 1168–1175.

Mundy, P., Sigman, M., Kasari, C., & Yirmiya, N. (1988). Nonverbal communication skills in Down syndrome children. *Child Development, 59,* 235–249.

Nicolich, L. (1977). Beyond sensorimotor intelligence: Assessment of symbolic maturity through analysis of pretend play. *Merrill-Palmer Quarterly, 23,* 89–99.

Nisbet, J., Zanella, K., & Miller, J. (1984). An analysis of conversations among handicapped students and a non-handicapped peer. *Exceptional Children, 51,* 156–162.

Owings, R., & MacDonald, J. (1982). Communicative uses of the early speech of nondelayed and Down syndrome children. *American Journal of Mental Deficiency, 86,* 503–510.

Piaget, J. (1962). *Play, dreams, and imitation in childhood.* New York: Norton.

Piaget, J. (1981). *Intelligence and affectivity: Their relationship during child development.* Palo Alto, CA: Annual Reviews.

Piaget, J., & Inhelder, B. (1969). *The psychology of the child.* (H. Weaver, Trans.) London: Routledge & Kegan Paul.

Price-Williams, D., & Sabsay, S. (1979). Communicative competence among severely retarded persons. *Semiotica, 26*(1/2), 35–63.

Quinn, J., & Rubin, K. (1984). The play of handicapped children. In T. Yawkey & A. Pellegrini (Eds.), *Child's Play: Developmental and Applied.* Hillsdale, NJ: Erlbaum.

Riguet, C., Taylor, N., Benaroya, S., & Klein, L. (1981). Symbolic play in autistic, Downs, and normal children of equivalent mental age. *Journal of Autism and Developmental Disorders, 11,* 439–448.

Rondal, J. (1988). Language development in Down's syndrome: A lifespan perspective. *International Journal of Behavioral Development, 11,* 21–36.

Rosenberg, S. (1982). The language of the mentally retarded: Developmental processes and intervention. In S. Rosenberg (Ed.), *Handbook of applied psycholinguistics*. Hillsdale, NJ: Erlbaum.

Rubin, K., Fein, G., & Vandenberg, B. (1983). Play. In P. Mussen (Ed.), *Handbook of child psychology*, Vol. 4: *Socialization*. New York: Wiley.

Rynders, J., Spiker, D., & Horrobin, M. (1978). Underestimating the educability of Down's syndrome children: Examination of methodological problems in recent literature. *American Journal of Mental Deficiency, 82*, 440–448.

Sameroff, A. (1983). Developmental systems: Contexts and evolution. In P. Mussen, *Handbook of child psychology* (4th ed.), Vol. 1: *Infancy* (pp. 237–294). New York: Wiley.

Scherer, N., & Owings, N. (1984). Learning to be contingent: Retarded children's responses to their mothers. *Language and Speech, 27*, 255–267.

Schiefelbusch, R., & Pickar, J. (1984). *The acquisition of communicative competence*. Baltimore: University Park Press.

Schopler, E., & Mesibov, G. (1985). *Communication problems in autism*. New York: Plenum.

Share, J. (1975). Developmental progress in Down syndrome. In R. Koch & F. de la Cruz (Eds.), *Down's syndrome (mongolism): Research, prevention, & practice*. New York: Brunner/Mazel.

Shore, C., Bates, E., Bretherton, I., Beeghly, M., and O'Connell, B. (in press). Vocal and gestural symbols: Similarities and differences from 13 to 28 months. In V. Volterra & C. Erting (Eds.), *From gesture to language in hearing and deaf children*. New York: Springer-Verlag.

Shore, C., O'Connell, B., & Bates, E. (1984). First sentences in language and play. *Developmental Psychology, 20*, 872–880.

Sigman, M., & Mundy, P. (1987). Symbolic processes in young autistic children. In D. Cicchetti & M. Beeghly (Eds.), *Symbolic development in atypical children*. San Francisco: Jossey-Bass.

Sigman, M., & Ungerer, J. (1984). Cognitive and language skills in autistic, mentally retarded, and normal children. *Developmental Psychology, 20*, 293–302.

Sinson, J., & Wetherick, N. (1982). Mutual gaze in preschool Down's and normal children. *Journal of Mental Deficiency Research, 26*, 123–129.

Smith, L., & Tetzchner, S. (1986). Communicative, sensorimotor, and language skills of young children with Down syndrome. *American Journal of Mental Deficiency, 91*, 57–66.

Snyder, L. (1985). Communicative competence in children with delayed language development. In R. Schiefelbusch & J. Pickar (Eds.), *Communicative competence*. Baltimore: University Park Press.

Sorce, J., Emde, R., & Frank, M. (1982). Maternal referencing in normal and Down syndrome infants: A longitudinal analysis. In R. Emde & R. Harmon (Eds.), *The development of attachment and affiliative systems*. New York: Plenum.

Spiker, D. (1979). *A descriptive study of mother–child teaching interaction with high- and low-functioning Down syndrome preschoolers*. Unpublished doctoral dissertation, University of Minnesota.

Sroufe, L. A., & Rutter, M. (1984). The domain of developmental psychopathology. *Child Development, 55*, 17–29.

Tager-Flusberg, H. (1981). On the nature of linguistic functioning in early infantile autism. *Journal of Autism and Developmental Disorders, 11*, 45–56.

Thompson, R., Cicchetti, D., Lamb, M., & Malkin, C. (1985). The emotional responses of Down syndrome and normal infants in the Strange Situation: The organization of affective behavior in infants. *Developmental Psychology, 21*, 828–841.

Ungerer, J., Zelazo, P., Kearsley, R., & O'Leary, K. (1981). Developmental changes in the representation of objects in symbolic play from 18 to 34 months of age. *Child Development, 52*, 186–195.

Vietze, P., McCarthy, M., McQuiston, S., MacTurk, R., & Yarrow, L. (1983). Attention and exploratory behavior in infants with Down syndrome. In T. Field & A. Sostek (Eds.), *Infants born at risk: Perceptual and physical processes* (pp. 251–268). New York: Grune & Stratton.

Watson, M., & Fischer, K. (1977). A developmental sequence of agent use in late infancy. *Child Development, 48*, 828–836.

Weiss, P. (1969). *Principles of development*. New York: Hafner.

Weiss, B., Beeghly, M., & Cicchetti, D. (1985). *Symbolic play development in children with Down syndrome and nonhandicapped children.* Presented at the biennial meetings of the Society for Research in Child Development, Toronto, April.

Werner, H., & Kaplan B. (1963). *Symbol formation.* New York: Wiley.

Wing, L., Gould, J., Yeates, S. & Brierly, L. (1977). Symbolic play in severely mentally retarded and in autistic children. *Journal of Child Psychology and Psychiatry, 18,* 167–178.

Wolf, D., Rygh, J., & Altschuler, J. (1984). Agency and experience: Representations of people in early play narratives. In I. Bretherton (Ed.), *Symbolic play.* New York: Academic Press.

Zigler, E., & Balla, D. (1982). *Mental retardation: The developmental–difference controversy.* Hillsdale, NJ: Erlbaum.

11   Peer relations of children with Down syndrome

Felicisima C. Serafica

The significance of peer relations for psychological development and mental health was recognized years ago by some eminent theorists. Piaget (1932) assigned a critical role to peer relations in his theory of cognitive development. According to him, peer interaction exposes the child to diverse viewpoints, including some that differ from those held by his or her parents. The cognitive conflict induced by such exposure facilitates transition from one level of cognitive development to the next. Furthermore, within the more egalitarian context of the peer system, it is easier for the child to examine, analyze, and reflect on the nature and bases of social rules. It is such critical analysis and reflection, Piaget hypothesized, that brings about the realization that social intercourse and order are based on reciprocal exchanges between people.

Relations with peers were also deemed essential for optimal personality development and psychological adjustment by personality theorists. Adler (1930) asserted that the greatest personal growth occurs in an environment where positive interpersonal relations enhance a child's intrinsic social feelings and make him or her comfortable. Children who feel that they are part of a group will empathize and cooperate with others, thereby contributing to the well-being of the group; those who feel left out may perceive themselves as inferior and engage in maladaptive behavior in order to prove their own worth. To Sullivan (1953), peer relations permitted the developing child to define his or her sense of self and to learn modes of relating required for successful adult relations. More specifically, Sullivan considered friendships important because, unlike the parent-child relationship, they tend to be egalitarian and therefore more conducive to the emergence of mutuality and intimacy in a relationship.

Since the above theoretical propositions about the significance of peer relations were formulated, scientific evidence has accumulated. Research has shown that 4- to 7-year-old children's conservation of liquid, number, graphic space, and length is facilitated by social interaction (Murray, 1972; Perret-Clermont, 1980). Similarly, development of moral judgment has been found to be significantly related to such varied indices of peer relations as participation in clubs and special activity

369

groups, popularity among peers, and service in leadership roles (Harris, Mussen, & Rutherford, 1976; Keasey, 1971; Kohlberg, 1958). More specifically, positive justice has been reported to be significantly related to socially constructive behavior in the classroom, sociometric ratings of popularity, and parent ratings of social skills and adjustment (Enright & Sutterfield, 1980; Kurdek, 1980). The positive contributions of peer relations to the development of communicative competence and play have also been noted (Guralnick, 1981). Moreover, it has been shown that a child's personal–social effectiveness is related to his or her interactions and sociability with peers (Baumrind, 1972; Becker, 1977; Bronson, 1975; Rubenstein & Howes, 1976).

The role of peers in socialization is well documented. Through their reactions, peers can strengthen, maintain, decrease, or in some cases virtually extinguish a child's social behaviors (Charlesworth & Hartup, 1967; Patterson, Littman, & Bricker, 1967; Wahler, 1967). Peers also serve as models for a variety of behaviors that are acquired through observational learning, including achievement (McArthur & Eisen, 1976); altruism (Hartup & Coates, 1976); compliance or resistance to deviation (Wolf, 1973; Wolf & Cheyne, 1972); delay of gratification (Stumphauzer, 1972); and moral judgment (Bandura & McDonald, 1963; Dorr & Fey, 1974). It is, however, in regard to the attitudes and behaviors dealing with aggression, gender role, and sexuality that peers as socialization agents often exert the greatest influence. The modulation of aggression is learned primarily within the context of peer interactions, initially in rough-and-tumble play and later in the physical and verbal aggressive behaviors that mark the interactions of children in the playground and elsewhere (Hartup, 1974, 1980; Patterson & Cobb, 1971). Studies have consistently demonstrated that acquisition, maintenance, or extinction of behaviors that are appropriate or inappropriate with a child's gender are under the control of peer behaviors (Fagot, 1977a & 1977b; Kobasigawa, 1968; Wolf, 1973, 1975). Last, research indicates that the most profound influences on adolescent sexuality come from dating partners and peers (Spanier, 1976).

In addition to functioning as socialization agents, peers can also be effective tutors and "therapists." Children tutored by their peers have been found to show significant improvement in both reading and mathematics, as measured by mastery of tutorial content and standardized tests, particularly when the tutor is somewhat older than the tutee (Allen, 1976; East, 1976). The potential that peers have for alleviating the miseries of another child was dramatically illustrated in the study by Freud and Dann (1951) of children separated from their parents during World War II. Since their pioneering work, others have shown that social withdrawal can be modified through symbolic peer modeling (O'Connor, 1969) or social initiations made by a trained peer confederate (Strain & Fox, 1981).

Finally, a link between peer relations during childhood and mental health status in adolescence and adulthood has been demonstrated by major predictive studies (Cowen, Pederson, Babigian, Izzo, & Trost, 1973; Roff, 1961, 1963; Roff, Sells, & Golden, 1972). These studies consistently showed that negative peer ratings or poor peer relations during middle childhood predict mental health client status in adulthood, particularly as related to adult neuroses, psychoses, or disturbances in sexual behavior and adjustment.

In sum, both theory and research indicate that the company and interactions of peers are essential for optimal psychological development and mental health. What happens, then, if opportunities for constructive engagement are less readily available? This may be the case for certain groups such as developmentally delayed children, including those with Down syndrome. The aims of this chapter are: (1) to review critically the available research on peer relations in children with Down syndrome; (2) to discuss the relevant conceptual and methodological issues; and (3) to suggest directions for future research.

To provide a background for the review of the peer relations of children with Down syndrome, the research literature on development of peer interaction during infancy and early childhood in normal and developmentally delayed without Down syndrome populations will be selectively reviewed. This brief review will be limited to age trends in peer interaction for both groups. In addition, the effects on peer interaction of mainstreaming children without Down syndrome will also be discussed. For a more extensive coverage of research on peer relations of normal and developmentally delayed children, the interested reader is referred to Guralnick (1986), Hartup (1983), and Mueller and Vandell (1979).

Peer interactions of children

The origins of peer interaction may be seen in the emergence of social responsiveness and social behaviors directed toward peers. The latter evolve from a single socially directed behavior (SDB) to a combination of behaviors usually involving different modalities (coordinated SDB) and eventually to a pattern interchange consisting of two or more interactions (Mueller & Vandell, 1979). With increasing age, there are quantitative and qualitative changes in peer interaction.

Infancy and toddlerhood

Social responsiveness to peers is manifest as early as the first year of life. This fact was established by a brief flurry of descriptive studies carried out in the 1930s. Several decades later, it was confirmed by Eckerman, Whatley, and Kutz (1975). The onset of an interest in peers has been observed as early as the second month of life (Bridges, 1933). The amount of interest steadily increases over time such that by 24 months, when mother or familiar adult and a peer are both present, play with the adult will have markedly declined whereas play with the peer will have significantly increased (Eckerman et al., 1975; Lewis, Young, Brooks, & Michalson, 1975; Rubenstein & Howes, 1976). Moreover, there is a qualitative difference between a toddler's interactions with his or her mother and that with a peer. More proximal behaviors are manifested toward the mother whereas distal behaviors dominate interaction with a peer (Lewis et al., 1975).

With increasing age, there is also an increase in the number of peer-directed behaviors as well as in the frequency that each behavior is exhibited. Visual regard, observed in infants as young as 2 months, is the earliest form of social behavior directed to a peer (Bridges, 1933; Vincze, 1971). At 3 to 4 months, infants have been noted to touch a peer who happens to be near by (Shirley, 1933; Vincze, 1971). Social smiles directed toward a peer have been manifested by 6-month-old infants (Bridges, 1933; Buhler, 1933; Maudry & Nekula, 1939; Vincze, 1971). From this point on, interest in a peer is expressed in more active ways. With the development of locomotor skills at 7 to 8 months, infants begin to approach, follow, and reach for peers (Bridges, 1933; Durfee & Lee, 1973). Having established contact, infants initially may "explore" their peers by patting or banging (Bridges, 1933), but they rapidly progress to behaviors that observers consider social. From 9 to 12 months, infants "offer" objects to familiar peers and "take" from them (Vincze, 1971). Within this age period, infants start playing games such as peek-a-boo with each other (Bridges, 1933; Maudry & Nekula, 1939; Vincze, 1971). Infant imitation of a peer has been reported as early as 10 months (Bridges, 1983), although its occurrence was not noted until 13 to 14 months of age by Eckerman et al. (1975). Displays of positive affect also increase with age. Bridges (1933) found that smiling and affectional gestures had become more prominent by 15 months of age while Mueller and Rich (1976) noted that smiles and laughs increased between 13 and 15 months. Ross and Goldman (1976) also found an increase in the incidence of positive affect between 12 and 24 months.

Besides a broadening of the social repertoire, there is an increase in the frequency of peer interaction. Jacobson (1981), who observed pairs of home-reared infants engaged in free play in a laboratory setting of 10, 12, and 14½ months of age, reported that the rate per minute of peer-directed behavior increased linearly from 2.0 at 10 months to 3.8 at 14½ months.

Not surprisingly, the increment in amount of social interaction is accompanied by an increase in negative exchanges. Fights over toys, hitting, hair pulling, and biting occur more frequently during the second year (Eckerman et al., 1975; Mueller & Vandell, 1979). It has been reported that disagreements constituted 45% of playroom peer encounters of toddlers observed in the second year of life (Bronson, 1975). However, positive social behaviors still predominate (Rubenstein & Howes, 1976).

In addition to quantitative changes, there are also qualitative changes in peer interaction during infancy and the toddler years. The complexity of coordinated or combined social behavior increases over time, particularly between 12 and 23 months of age (Mueller & Brenner, 1977; Mueller & Rich, 1976). Also, interchanges or social interactions containing two or more elicitations increase in length and occur more often (Mueller & Brenner, 1977). In addition, the organizational characteristics of peer exchanges change. Three qualitatively different stages in the ontogeny of early peer relations have been identified by Mueller and Lucas (1975). Stage 1, observed among 1-year-olds, is characterized by object-centered contacts. At this stage, children typically do not interact; instead they act unilaterally on a common object. Stage 2 is distinguished by simple and complex interchanges that more closely approximate social interactions. Toddlers seek and receive "contingencies" from one another. Stage 3, apparent by the end of the second year, is defined by the emergence of complementary interchanges. Social interactions at this stage reflect more organized role relations, reciprocity, and complementarity. Furthermore, positive social exchanges are accompanied by smiling, laughter, or other appropriate expressions of positive affect (Mueller & Brenner, 1977; Mueller & Rich, 1976).

Early childhood

During the preschool years, the trend toward an increase with age in the amount of social interaction continues (Beaver, 1932; Parten, 1932; Washburn & Hilgard, 1934; Wright, 1967). By the age of 4 or 5 years, children in a free play situation show much more interest in their peers than they do in toys (Scholtz & Ellis, 1975). Five-year-olds interact more frequently with their peers than do 3-year-olds (Lougee, Grueneich, & Hartup, 1977).

Changes also occur in the frequency of specific peer-oriented behaviors. As children grow older, they talk more frequently and use more words in conversation with peers (Blurton Jones, 1972; Garvey & BenDebba, 1974; Mueller, 1972; Smith & Connolly, 1972). They seek attention and praise from their peers with greater frequency (Hattwick & Sanders, 1938; Martin, 1964). Some specific techniques for initiating and maintaining social interaction can be identified in the behavioral repertoire of 3-year-olds. Garvey (1974) described one such technique, a ritualized pattern of turns that constituted what she terms "rounds." In this type of dyadic interaction, one partner makes a verbal or nonverbal contribution that elicits a response from the other partner, whose content may be the same or complementary to the content of the first child's behavior. In either case, one turn is contingent upon another.

More importantly, peer interaction becomes more positive with increasing age. A study by Walters, Pearce, and Dahms (1957) of children aged 2 to 5 years showed that at all age levels, the children were more affectionate (i.e., exhibited to another person warm regard, friendliness, sympathy, or helpfulness) than aggressive (i.e., attacked or threatened to attack another person) in their response to others, and more frequently employed affection than aggression in initiating contact. This study also revealed an increase with age in the relative dominance of verbal over physical expressions of affection. At age 2 the difference between verbal and physical indices of affection was not statistically significant. By ages 3, 4, and 5, the children were more verbally than physically affectionate.

In addition to initiating positive behaviors, preschoolers exhibit significantly more positive responses to the overtures of their peers (Manwell & Mangert, 1934). Blurton-Jones (1972) observed that older preschoolers engaged in more talks and play with their peers. Also, they manifested more positive affective behaviors such as smiling and laughing. In addition, older children provided positive reinforcement to their peers at a significantly higher rate. Charlesworth and Hartup (1967) reported that positive attention and approval, affection and personal acceptance, submission, and tangible objects were dispensed with significantly greater frequency by 4-year-olds than by 3-year-olds.

Early studies of young children's peer relations reported that as positive behaviors increase, so do competition and rivalry (Greenberg, 1932; Leuba, 1933). However, subsequent studies do not consistently indicate a positive linear increase in negative behaviors. Depending upon the ages studied, subsequent studies have shown either a decline or a curvilinear trend. Smith and Connolly (1972) observed that in a sample of 40 children ranging in age from 2 years, 9 months to 4 years, 9 months, the older children manifested less staring, crying, sucking, pointing, and submissive-flight behavior; instead they engaged in more conversation and social play with peers. On the other hand, several studies (Blurton-Jones, 1972; Hartup, 1974; Walters et al., 1957) found that total frequencies of aggressive peer interactions increase between the ages of 2 and 4 years, then decline.

The issue, however, may actually be more complex than simply the rise and fall of negative behaviors in peer interaction. Although most studies show that such behaviors ultimately decrease as children grow older, there is also evidence that with increasing age, the negative interactions that do occur may be more intense and of longer episodic duration. In addition, the modes of aggression change, becoming increasingly verbal (Hartup, 1974). An early study (Green, 1933) of group play and quarreling among young children showed that quarrels increased from age 2 to 3 years, then decreased steadily. It also revealed, however, that among the age-groups studied 4-year-olds were the most retaliatory while 2-year-olds reacted most passively to a quarrel initiated by a peer. Similarly, Dawes (1934) demonstrated that although older preschoolers engaged in fewer quarrels than younger ones, their quarrels lasted longer.

Other qualitative changes have been observed in dyadic peer interactions during the preschool years. Young children use more material objects when initiating social contact, whereas older ones rely more on verbal means (Beaver, 1932). With increasing age, there is a greater tendency for a child to adapt his or her responses to those of a partner. A study of preschool dyads by Garvey and BenDebba (1974) showed that with increasing age, a child engaged in verbal communication with another child is more likely to adapt the number of utterances he or she makes to the number of utterances made by his or her partner. In social problem solving, older children collaborate more (Cooper, 1980). Among kindergarten children, the ratio of positive social initiations is significantly related to the positive initiations received (Kohn, 1966). Finally, the more reinforcements a child gives to others, the more he or she receives in return (Charlesworth & Hartup, 1967).

Sex differences in peer interaction become more obvious during the preschool years. Walters et al., (1957) found that at all ages represented in their sample, boys consistently initiated significantly more affectional contacts with boys than with girls. In contrast, only the 2-year-old and 5-year-old girls initiated significantly more affectional contacts with girls than with boys; at ages 3 and 4 years, girls initiated affectional contacts with boys about as often as they did with girls. Green's

(1933) data are more perplexing. When mean frequencies of occurrence are considered, boys appear to start more quarrels and retaliate more than girls do, yet they also behave passively more often. However, when percentages of quarrels are considered, the girls are found to start slightly more quarrels and are more retaliatory. Also, girls are slightly more inclined to use verbal arguments in quarrels, whereas boys are more inclined to use physical force, a difference that might be related to sex differences in language development or socialization, or both. More recent studies have yielded more evidence for sex differences. Interaction among boys, compared to girls, is more likely to be boisterous, include rough-and-tumble play, and to be more competitive (DiPietro, 1981; Lever, 1976). Perhaps because of these emerging sex differences in play behavior, as well as the sex-role stereotypes common during the preschool years, a cleavage between the sexes emerges during the preschool years. Same-sex interactions are more common than mixed-sex ones, and each type of pairing acquires its own distinguishing characteristics (Hartup, 1983).

To summarize, interest in peers appears as early as the first year of life. Although this social responsiveness is initially manifested as visual regard, it rapidly becomes expressed in many other ways. During the first 2 years of life, the infant's social repertoire broadens to include a wide range of peer-directed behaviors. In addition, these behaviors increase in complexity. Further development occurs during the early childhood years. The amount of social interaction increases substantially. More mature, socially desirable behaviors are substituted for the earlier simpler and less socially desirable ones (e.g., verbal request in lieu of grabbing). The nature of social interaction becomes generally more positive. Mutual adaptation increasingly characterizes interchanges between peers.

These developments do not take place in a vacuum. They are influenced by personal characteristics, setting conditions, amount of peer group experience and the relationships a child has with parents and siblings. For a more detailed presentation of research on these influential variables, the reader is referred to Hartup (1983).

Peer interactions of developmentally delayed children

Children with developmental delays may be especially vulnerable to difficulties in relating to their peers. The slow development of motor, perceptual, cognitive, language, and communicative skills that underlie social competence may hinder them from initiating interactions with their peers. If they do make social bids, they may be unable to maintain the exchange and the other child will look elsewhere for other more rewarding peer interactions. In addition to having limited cognitive and other abilities, developmentally delayed children may lack the exposure to peers so necessary for the development of social skills. Their encounters with agemates may be limited because, as indicated earlier, their agemates may lose interest in interacting with them, or their apprehensive parents may curtail opportunities to interact freely with peers. Thus, their encounters with agemates are most likely confined to children with similar handicaps who are themselves experiencing social difficulties. In general, developmentally delayed children have limited access to agemates who can serve as appropriate models and provide constructive feedback.

Social interaction

Although educators, clinicians, and researchers are agreed that children with developmental delays are at risk for a developmental lag or even disturbances in peer relations, few investigations into the peer relations of this group have been conducted. In an observational study of developmentally delayed 4- and 5-year-olds, Field (1980) found that they engaged in fewer social interactions than a group of 3- to 4-year-old normal children with matching developmental levels. Similarly, Crawley and Chan (1982) reported that mild and moderately delayed children observed in an outdoor playground setting did not engage in peer interactions of any form, even as recipients of a single initiation, in over 90% of the intervals observed. Consistent results were also reported by Mindes (1982) for a group of mildly delayed 5-year-olds enrolled in noncategorical special education preschool classes. Deviations from developmental norms were also noted by Guralnick and Weinhouse (1984) in their short-term longitudinal study of 52 mild and moderately delayed children with a mean chronological age of 54.4 months. Observations were made at the beginning and end of the schoolyear, during free play periods in the specialized community programs attended by the children. Sequential interactive measures of individual episodes of social exchanges occurring between children, ratings of social participation, and constructiveness of play were coded. In contrast to prior research findings on nonhandicapped children of a similar age range, only about 20% of the sample were able to turn simple two-unit initiation response encounters into longer social exchanges. The dominant forms of social participation were still solitary and parallel play. Associative and cooperative play occurred infrequently, far less than would be expected on the basis of the children's developmental levels.

Overall, developmentally delayed children as a group show social skills deficits. Nonetheless, there are also within-group differences. Field (1984) has reported differences in the play behaviors of handicapped children with and without close friends. Having a close friend was operationally defined as playing with a particular peer 66% or more of the time sample. The two groups did not differ significantly in chronological age, developmental age, developmental quotient, type of developmental delay, or height, although the children with friends were found to be more extraverted on the Buck affect scale than those who had no friends. Inside the classroom, the group with close friends were generally more assertive in initiating, leading, and terminating play interactions than the other group. They were also more verbal and emotionally expressive. Children without friends spent more time wandering around, watching the teachers and the other children, than did the children who had friends. Outside the classroom, no significant group differences emerged, not surprising because except for vocalizing and taking toys, behaviors that were differentially affected by setting were different from those differentiating the groups from one another.

Developmental changes

In addition to describing the social behaviors of developmentally delayed children, investigators have also assessed developmental changes. Crawley and Chan (1982) noted that with increasing chronological age, involvement in unoccupied and on-looker activities decreased while participation in solitary or parallel play increased. Also, within the mildly delayed group, the older children engaged in peer interactions far more than the younger ones. The social participation patterns, however, were highly similar in both age-groups, suggesting that they were operating largely within the same developmental level, differing only in response rate. This slow pace of developmental change was also noted by Guralnick and Weinhouse (1984) in the study cited in the preceding section. Their cross-sectional analysis (across ages 3 to 5½ years) did not reveal any developmental changes for a wide range of peer-related measures. According to Guralnick (1984), this highly atypical pattern suggests that most developmentally delayed children enrolled in specialized settings reach an asymptotic level of interacting with their peers during the early preschool period and remain there until they enter their elementary school years.

Interactions in mainstreamed environments

Several investigators concerned about the developmental lag in cognitively delayed children's peer relations have proposed educational mainstreaming as a more facilitative setting. They (Guralnick, 1978) contend that such children when placed with the more socially active normal children will also emit social behaviors with greater frequency. Furthermore, developmentally delayed children will imitate the appropriate social behaviors of the normal youngsters who would serve as models. In addition, a classroom containing normally developing children would provide a richer and more varied language environment, thereby facilitating the development of linguistic and communications skills that are an integral part of social competence (Guralnick, 1984).

However, studies of handicapped children in mainstreamed settings show that the availability of normally developing playmates has no substantial effect on the social and play interactions of developmentally delayed youngsters (Field, Roseman, DeStefano, & Koewler, 1981). At most, the evidence suggests that mainstreaming reduces the level of inappropriate play of severely delayed children (Guralnick, 1981) and increases the frequency of certain specific but isolated behaviors for children with and without developmental delay during the mainstreamed condition (Field et al., 1981).

Guralnick (1984) has suggested that the minimal effects of mainstreaming imply that although mildly delayed children appear to be well integrated in that they do not receive numerous or extensive negative interactions and are the beneficiaries of rather impressive communicative adjustments by their nonhandicapped classmates, the integration may be superficial. There may be a greater social cleavage between children with and without cognitive delay that emerges during the most elaborate forms of social play and extensive, complex verbal exchanges. Moreover, when nonhandicapped children interact with the handicapped, they adjust downward their own social, play, and verbal behaviors. When integrated close friendships are formed, they are likely to be between handicapped and nonhandicapped children who hold similar status in their respective groups (Field, 1984). Thus, it appears that "like seeks out like." Children prefer to interact with those who have approximately the same developmental levels. Through such behavior, children are underscoring equality as the hallmark of peer relations.

Peer relations of children with Down syndrome

The growth of research on normal and developmentally delayed children's peer relations leads one to expect a parallel increase in studies on this topic involving children with Down syndrome. However, this is not the case. Although researchers have become increasingly interested in the psychological development of children with Down syndrome, they have been attracted primarily to the study of cognition, language, or learning. The minority who investigated socio-emotional development usually focused on attachment, emotion, or temperament. Studies of peer relations are few. The state of the art in research on peer relations of this clinical population is dramatically illustrated by the fact that the major books on Down syndrome published between 1976 and 1986 (De la Cruz & Gerald, 1981; Gibson, 1978; Pueschel, 1984) do not directly address this topic. In these volumes, peer relations are rarely differentiated from relations with adults. Moreover, discussions about inter-personal relations are embedded in sections on personality or socialization.

In order to understand the apparent lack of interest in the peer relations of children with Down syndrome, it seems necessary to review the conception of Down syndrome that guided early studies of this clinical population. Down (1866, 1867) identified four distinguishing personality characteristics of this group: mimicry, humor, amiability, and obstinacy. This constellation of attributes were also noted by other clinicians (e.g, Fennel, 1904). In time, Down's conception of the group eventually named after him was expanded to include such qualities as cheerful, good-tempered, and submissive to authority (Barr, 1904; Brushfield, 1924; Sherlock & Donkin, 1911). Thus emerged a positive social image that became a stereotype of the Down syndrome individual. This social stereotype strongly influenced the thinking of investigators. The first 100 years of research on social aspects of Down syndrome largely consisted of attempts to validate the social stereotype or to test hypotheses predicated on it. Only within the last few decades have researchers become interested in the study of the peer relations of children with Down syndrome. This shift in emphasis is probably the result of several factors. First, the results of empirical studies eroded belief in the social stereotype. Second, the conceptualization of personality characteristics as generalized, stable, enduring traits lost favor among personality theorists. Last, but not least, among developmental psychologists there was a revival of interest in the study of peer relations. These simultaneous developments within the fields of mental retardation, personality theory, and developmental psychology brought about a paradigm shift (Kuhn, 1970) in the study of Down syndrome, resulting in the few studies on peer interaction and social play of children with Down syndrome that will be reviewed following a discussion of their sociability as inferred from the earlier research.

Sociability: myth or reality?

Early clinical descriptions of individuals with Down syndrome imbued them with a high degree of social responsiveness and potential for socialization, at least compared to others who also exhibited developmental delay (Down, 1866, 1867; Fennel, 1904). Those descriptions generated four hypotheses: (1) Retarded individuals with Down syndrome are more sociable than those without Down syndrome; (2) sociability is a universal characteristic of individuals with Down syndrome; (3) sociability is inherent in the population with Down syndrome; and (4) retarded individuals with Down syndrome are more amenable to socialization than those without Down syndrome. The first three hypotheses are directly relevant to the study of peer relations, so the empirical evidence bearing on them will be examined. The last hypothesis, dealing with the extent to which individuals with Down syndrome can acquire self-help and other skills required for successful adaptation to society, is less directly relevant and will not be discussed.

The hypothesis that individuals with Down syndrome are more sociable than developmentally delayed individuals without Down syndrome guided much of the early research, yet not until the second half of the 20th century was it tested in a study that included a control group. Blacketer-Simmonds (1953) compared the behavior checklist ratings received by individuals with and without Down syndrome who had similar intellectual and physical status, prior to and following institutionalization. Among the behavior items were: friendly, sociable, mimics, solitary, and docile. Pre-institutionalization, intake nurses rated a significantly higher percent of the group with Down syndrome as solitary and a significantly lower percent as docile than they rated the group without Down syndrome. Following institutionalization, 20% of the group with Down syndrome were described as sociable in comparison to 23.6% of the controls. Also, 16.6% of the group with Down syndrome were rated as solitary and poor mixers while only 15% of the control group received the same rating. Among the individuals with Down syndrome, 31.6% were rated as docile. In addition, 10% were rated as mimics while only 7% of the control group were rated thus. The results do not provide strong support for the hypothesis that individuals with Down syndrome are more sociable than developmentally delayed individuals without Down syndrome, prior to or following institutionalization.

The Blacketer-Simmonds (1953) study is noteworthy because for its time it included a control group, attempted to equate intellectual and physical status, obtained pre- and post-institutionalization ratings, employed an objective measure, took precautions so that the experimental and control subjects could not be separately identified by observers, and analyzed the data using chi-square. Nonetheless, the study had some conceptual and methodological limitations. Conceptually, it did not attempt to separate behavioral indices of sociability from other behaviors such as restlessness. Methodologically, it did not specify the age ranges for the two samples, nor did it indicate the number of males and females in each group. Furthermore, it did not control for the health and psychiatric status of the subjects and the reasons for institutionalization. Test–retest reliability was not provided, nor was there an attempt to obtain interrater reliability.

Another study comparing the social characteristics of institutionalized individuals with and without Down syndrome, but limited to females, was conducted by Domino, Goldschmid, and Kaplan (1964). The 21 subjects with Down syndrome had a mean chronological age (CA) of 11.25 years and a mean IQ of 30. They were institutionalized at a mean CA of 6.75 years and had been there for 4.50 years at the time of the study. The 35 subjects without Down syndrome had a mean CA of 10.42 years, and a mean IQ of 35. They were institutionalized at a mean CA of 7.33 years and had been there for a mean of 2.92 years at the time of the study. The subjects were rated by professional and ward personnel on the Sonoma Checklist, an objective checklist devised for the study. To control for observer bias, staff ratings were used to generate a staff acceptance index and a familiarity score was defined by each staff observer for each subject. Descriptive social adjectives such as friendly, sociable, and open correlated significantly and positively with a diagnosis of Down syndrome. The investigators interpreted these results as support for the social stereotype with Down syndrome and also claimed that observer bias had been effectively managed. Domino et al. speculated that the favorable social stereotype might be evidenced only in contrast with the subjects without Down syndrome who also manifested a significantly greater number of central nervous anomalies, such as irritability, shortened attention, and drive disorder. Gibson (1978) suggests an alternative interpretation, that is, that the traditional social stereotype might be specific to females with Down syndrome who may receive different and superior care compared to males with Down syndrome in the same institutions. Furthermore, the greater length of hospitalization for the sample with Down syndrome might have contributed to greater stability and homogeneity of their behavioral characteristics.

In order to determine whether the results obtained for females also apply to males, and to investigate whether a positive social image of the institutionalized individual with Down syndrome is merely a phenomenon reflecting the expectations of a well-indoctrinated staff, Domino and his colleagues (1965) asked 210 college students to rate 21 pairs of retarded individuals with and without Down syndrome. This time, 56 of the 210 items on the Sonoma Checklist were found to differentiate significantly between the two groups. The individuals with Down syndrome were rated significantly more often as cooperative and pleasing though also shy, show-off, unfriendly, and hostile. The individuals without Down syndrome were significantly more likely to be rated as outgoing but also as withdrawn, unsociable, and rude. Domino (1965) interpreted these results as a confirmation of the classical social stereotype. An alternative interpretation is that the data yielded only partial support.

The favorable social image of institutionalized individuals with Down syndrome might reflect a bias induced by institutional policies and practices, but a study of community-reared individuals with Down syndrome might reveal a more accurate portrayal. Blessing (1959) asked teachers of 83 children with Down syndrome living at home and attending special classes in their communities to complete a questionnaire including 11 favorable and 19 unfavorable behavior traits. For the children with Down syndrome, the favorable traits mentioned most frequently were: amenable, good nature, gay, happy, cheerful, independent, and, to a lesser extent, obedient or docile. The problems reported most frequently for the group were: short attention span, poor communication, stubborn, attention seeker, and tires easily. Blessing concluded that type and quality of social responsiveness in Down syndrome varies widely. The results also suggest that children with Down syndrome may have a lower physical fatigue threshold that lessens their self-control so they cannot sustain socially appropriate behaviors. Further, their poor communication skills may make it difficult for them to engage in the more complex social behaviors expected of children in community settings.

Evidence that communication disorder or speech lag is common among children with Down syndrome has also been reported by other investigators (Moore, Thuline, & Capes, 1968; Spreen, 1965). It has been suggested that the communication deficit retards social development, particularly as age increases (Spreen, 1965). This was found to be the case by Johnson and Abelson (1969) in their study comparing 2,606 individuals who had Down syndrome with a mean CA of 21 years and an IQ of 28.6 with developmentally delayed controls whose mean of CA and IQ were 24.45 years and 32, respectively. The most striking deficiency was in the social aspects of communication, with the children who had Down syndrome being notably inferior compared to the controls.

Overall, the hypothesis that individuals with Down syndrome are more sociable than their counterparts without Down syndrome has not received strong support from studies of both institutionalized and community-reared samples. At most, they yield only partial support. The findings have usually been mixed, indicating that although in some ways individuals with Down syndrome seem more sociable than the controls, in other ways they appeared less so. As a result of these studies, refinements of the social stereotype were introduced. It was suggested that the group with Down syndrome may appear more sociable only when compared to a retarded group that did not have Down syndrome but had significantly more neurological problems. Another modification limited the social stereotype to females with Down syndrome who might receive more favorable treatment than their male peers, at least in institutions.

Earlier, it was assumed that sociability was a universal characteristic of individuals with Down syndrome. Subsequent observations, however, revealed exceptions that on closer examination seemed to be systematically linked to age. Observers of infants with Down syndrome and very young children noted minimal social alertness and responsiveness. Brousseau and Brainerd (1928) reported that these age groups showed little or no social expression and offered no response to a social initiative except a tendency to grimace. Similarly, Tredgold (1947) described an infant with Down syndrome as socially inert and lethargic. Along the same lines,

Siegert and Scharling observed in 1910 (see Oster, 1953) that at 2 to 3 years of age, children with Down syndrome alternate between "torpor and erithism."

During the early and middle childhood years, children with Down syndrome appear to be quite sociable. They have been described as affectionate, amiable, good-natured, and extroverted (Engler, 1949; Rollin, 1946; Wallin, 1949). There is, however, a different image that begins to emerge during these years and becomes more prominent with increasing age. Wallin (1949) hypothesized that a positive personality is primarily characteristic of children with Down syndrome, although some are shy, reticent, apathetic, and negativistic. Other investigators have also reported that sociability seems more characteristic of younger than of older individuals with Down syndrome (Benda, 1956, 1960; Oster, 1953; Tredgold, 1947). A relationship between social behavior and age in the population with Down syndrome was observed by Francis (1970), too. She found that social contact was significantly but negatively correlated with CA for low-grade institutionalized individuals with Down syndrome. Although a greater proportion of the group with Down syndrome was mobile and hence able to approach and initiate social contact with other patients as well as nurses, social contact decreased rather than increased with age.

Following a review of the relevant personality research, Gibson (1978) concluded that allowing for the methodological limitations of these early studies, there is a compelling impression of characteristic developmental changes. In his view, the placid sensorially insufficient infant becomes an emotionally intact, outgoing child who turns subsequently into a sullen, stubborn adolescent and finally faces premature aging as well as marked behavioral deterioration in early adulthood. He cautions, though, that this life-span view may not hold true always, perhaps not even for the majority of individuals with Down syndrome.

Several explanations have been advanced for the observed age changes in sociability. Oster (1953) attributed them to an early and progressive leveling of intellectual development, combined possibly with restrictive care practices. Benda (1956) initially posited an explanation that emphasized the role of situational conditions. Later, he assigned greater importance to a stubbornness originating from a discrepancy in the development of the nervous system in this clinical population (Benda, 1960). Stubbornness continues to be a popular explanation for age changes in sociability, although its origins are now attributed to factors other than those proposed earlier (Gibson, 1978).

Sociability in the population with Down syndrome varies not only with age but also with sex. According to Gibson, the traditional positive image of the individual with Down syndrome is probably more true for the young female. Sex differences have been attributed to variations in institutional and home-care practices as a function of the sex of the child, as well as to early mortality rates that are sex and IQ selective. However, more direct studies of sex differences in sociability and its antecedents among individuals with Down syndrome are needed.

Another early assumption about the population with Down syndrome was that its highly touted sociability was inherent. Sociability was viewed as having little to do with other organismic characteristics such as physical status, temperament, or intelligence. Nor was it attributed to caretaking environment or socioeconomic status. Direct investigations into the relationship between sociability and intelligence, temperament, or physical status of individuals with Down syndrome have yet to be carried out. Studies of their social maturity as measured by the Vineland Social Maturity Scale suggest that intellectual and communication deficits may place limits on the manifestations of sociability possible for them. Other studies indicate that although children with Down syndrome may approach other individuals with high frequency, vigor, and direction, they are less adept at the more complex social skills. Gibson (1978) has proposed that the positive social stereotype can be reinterpreted as social-behavioral manifestations of extroversion and imitation. He has also speculated that environment and socioeconomic status may contribute to the positive social image. According to him, within the largely regimented sparse environment of the institution, the young child with Down syndrome, because of his or her relatively uncomplicated neurophysiological and emotional status, may be able to compete more vigorously for the attention of the staff with developmentally delayed children without Down syndrome who have similar IQ. Also, Gibson adds, the social origins of the child with Down syndrome are often superior to those of the general population of retarded. Insofar as the child with Down syndrome is often a manifestation of the late childbearing age, he or she tends to have older siblings as agents of socialization, and/or parents who left school later and married later. In contrast, educable retarded children of unspecified etiology originate disproportionately from the lower socioeconomic stratum (Gibson & Butler, 1954). Thus, the child with Down syndrome may arrive in the institution or school seeming more socially adept than the intellectually similar child without Down syndrome, and is subsequently reinforced by the staff for his or her apparent social skills. Finally, in the population with Down syndrome, a variety of somatic factors including fatigability, heart problems, and neurophysiological disturbances may contribute to the observed decline in sociability with increasing age.

In sum, evidence for the hypothesis that individuals with Down syndrome are more sociable than individuals whose developmental delays are attributable to other causes is mixed. Although there is some empirical support for the hypothesis, these results come from studies that have serious methodological flaws. Furthermore, they are based largely on ratings rather than direct observation, so they might be more appropriately considered a measure of the social attractiveness rather than the sociability of the Down syndrome population. The evidence is more conclusive with respect to the universality, or lack thereof, of sociability in this clinical group. Studies have consistently shown age-related changes in sociability. There is also some evidence suggesting sex differences. Finally, there is no evidence as yet bearing on the inherentness of sociability in individuals with Down syndrome, but the results of studies on intelligence and social maturity suggest that intelligence, temperament, and somatic factors may affect sociability and that behavioral manifestations of sociability may also be influenced by caretaking environment and socioeconomic status.

Social interaction

Several investigations of peer interaction among children with Down syndrome, or comparing them with other developmentally delayed or normally developing populations, have been conducted in recent years. These studies differ from the earlier ones in several ways. They have focused exclusively on children or adolescents. They have examined specific peer-related behaviors. Finally, they have employed direct observations of peer interaction instead of asking raters to identify and/or rate social characteristics of individuals with Down syndrome.

The hypothesis that children with Down syndrome are more sociable than developmentally delayed children with a different etiology has received only partial support from more recent research. Schlottman and Anderson (1975) compared the interactions within a dyadic free play situation of 12 children with Down syndrome and 12 developmentally delayed children who did not exhibit Down syndrome with same or opposite sex peers belonging to their own clinical group. Males and females were equally represented in the experimental and contrast group. The mean CA, Stanford–Binet Form L–M MA and IQ were, respectively, 10–3, 3–0, and 34 for the children with Down syndrome and 9–11, 3–1, and 35 for those without. Consistent with the traditional social image, boys with Down syndrome smiled significantly more often than boys without Down syndrome, but only in same-sex dyads. They also exhibited significantly more positive social vocalization (laughing and singing) than boys without Down syndrome, again only in the same-sex condition. Conversely, they engaged significantly less in solitary toy play than did the contrast boys while with a same-sex peer. On the other hand, contrary to the social stereotype, the children with Down syndrome obtained significantly higher scores for negative verbal behavior than did the children without Down syndrome. Across sex, children with Down syndrome were more likely to express verbally their dislike or displeasure directed toward another child. In addition, girls with Down syndrome had significantly higher reject scores than girls without Down syndrome. They tended to physically reject contact or another child's attempt to play with them by pushing, walking away, or turning away from the other child.

The results of the Schlottman and Anderson (1975) study indicate that children with Down syndrome are not generally more sociable than developmentally delayed children without Down syndrome. They also cast doubt on the hypothesized universality of sociability for the group with Down syndrome. Sex differences in sociability were found. Furthermore, even the boys with Down syndrome, who seemed more sociable than the boys who did not exhibit the condition, appeared thus only in the same-sex condition. The investigators hypothesized that the observed variability in the behavior of boys with Down syndrome, as a function of the dyadic partner's sex, might have been an artifact of cottage placement. Whereas all the girls in the study lived in the same cottage, only 10 of the 12 boys with Down syndrome shared living quarters. Allowing for the possibility, the results still suggest that sociability in this group may vary as a function of familiarity with the other person, a challenge to the hypothesis that for this population, sociability is inherent rather than the outcome of organism–environment interaction.

Interaction in mainstreamed environments

The social interaction between Down syndrome and normally developing children has been the subject of several investigations. Proponents of integrated educational environments (Guralnick, 1980) argue that it provides a more stimulating, normalizing educational setting for a handicapped child than does a classroom attended only by developmentally delayed children. Supposedly, both handicapped and nonhandicapped children stand to gain from their mutual association. For handicapped children, an integrated classroom offers opportunities to observe, interact with, and imitate normally developing and, presumably, more socially competent peers. The extent to which the expected benefits are realized, however, depends on the quantity and quality of actual interaction between handicapped and nonhandicapped children. As noted earlier for developmentally delayed children without Down syndrome, integrated environments do not also always result in increased interaction between normal children and those with Down syndrome.

An exploratory study by Sinson and Wetherick (1981) showed that preschool children with Down syndrome who, to the casual observer and even to the playground staff, appeared to be socially accepted and little different from other children in normal playgroups actually engaged in no verbal interaction with normal peers and spent relatively little time in constructive behavior. Instead, they spent more of their time in inappropriate or nonconstructive behaviors, including aggressive and attention-seeking behaviors. When they interacted socially, it was with adults. Furthermore, they established eye contact with adults but, unlike their normal counterparts, had little or no eye contact with any of the other children. This behavior was in contrast to their behavior in a nursery school limited to handicapped children. In that context, they showed a pattern of eye contact similar to that exhibited by normal children. They also engaged in constructive and imaginative play.

Similar results were reported by Rogers-Warren (1980) from a study of the social interactions and play behavior of four children who were normal (ages 4½–5 years) and four (ages 5–6½ years) with Down syndrome. Both sexes were equally represented in each group. These children attended in integrated (40% nonhandicapped) early interaction program designed primarily for handicapped children. In this setting, children with Down syndrome interacted more with handicapped peers while normal children interacted more with nonhandicapped peers. This finding was consistent across the two settings of classroom free play period and outdoor playground. There was, however, considerable variability among subjects. On the average, handicapped subjects chose handicapped playmates about one and one-half times as frequently as they chose nonhandicapped playmates. Nonhandicapped children selected nonhandicapped playmates twice as often as they selected handicapped peers. Because the ratio of handicapped to nonhandicapped children in the class favored the selection of handicapped playmates, it appears that nonhandicapped children actively sought nonhandicapped playmates. The differences between handicapped and nonhandicapped children's playmate preferences were statistically significant for the playground, but not the classroom setting. In sum, despite the best efforts of adults to promote interaction between children with Down syndrome and their normal counterparts, children seem to seek out other members of their respective groups as playmates. In order to account for these phenomena, researchers have examined the possible influences of several variables on peer interaction of children with Down syndrome.

Correlates of peer interaction

It has been hypothesized that mutual gaze is a precursor to verbal and play interactions (Argyle & Cook, 1976). Sinson and Wetherick (1981) observed that children with Down syndrome established eye contact with other handicapped children in a nursery school for mentally handicapped children only, but did not do so with nonhandicapped children in a normal playgroup. They also noted that when the children with Down syndrome were first introduced into the playgroups, nonhandicapped children repeatedly attempted to establish mutual eye gaze with them, with no success. The normal children then became increasingly uneasy and over time ceased to make overtures. Observations of three children with Down syndrome who remained in the normal playgroups for 2 years showed that the normal children eventually ceased their attempts to establish mutual gaze and the children with Down syndrome became social isolates, interacting with no one except the adult helpers.

The tendency of normal children to withdraw from children with Down syndrome was further demonstrated in a subsequent study by Sinson and Wetherick (1982). Four 3-year-olds, two boys and two girls, who knew one another well but had no previous encounters with Down syndrome, were allowed to play for 10 minutes, then introduced to a 3-year-old child with Down syndrome who remained in the group for 15 minutes. Following a 10-minute distractor task, the children were introduced to a normal child of the same age and sex as the child with Down syndrome. This normal child left after 15 minutes. The group then had a snack period before being introduced to a baby with Down syndrome aged 22–24 months but of the same sex as the previous visitors. This sequence was repeated over 8 weeks with two alternating groups of normal children. Sex of the visiting child was alternated. The introduction of the child with Down syndrome, whether 3-year-old or infant, male or female, was followed by a period of intense scrutiny by all the normal children, lasting up to 20 seconds. The normal children then retreated away from the child with Down syndrome to the farthest part of the room, where they positioned themselves and played. If directed by an adult to engage in cooperative play with the child with Down syndrome, they did so but mutual gaze did not occur. Apart from these adult-instigated interactions, the child with Down syndrome was ignored by the normal children, who played cooperatively with each other for the remainder of the 15-minute period. In contrast, the normal though unfamiliar children who were introduced in the same way were absorbed into the group immediately. Sinson and Wetherick (1982) concluded that the convention of mutual gaze may govern relatively casual interactions between children who are not familiar with each other. Because the children with Down syndrome in their study used the gym equipment and read or did simple number work that the normal 3-year-olds did, Sinson and Wetherick (1982) speculated that the normal children's indifference to the child with Down syndrome was not due to academic inferiority, special physical weakness, or lack of social adjustment on the part of the latter. It appears, they said, that 3-year-old normal children are able at a glance to identify as "different" unfamiliar children with Down syndrome, without ever having encountered the syndrome previously.

The possibility that the playmate choices of children with and without Down syndrome may be linked to their level of play has also been examined. Before discussing this possible linkage, the meager data thus far on play behaviors and social participation of children with Down syndrome will be reviewed to provide a background. Schlottman and Anderson (1975) reported that children with Down syndrome obtained higher scores on social object manipulation than did developmentally delayed children without Down syndrome. They were significantly more likely to manually manipulate or inspect a toy or other object in the room in cooperation with another child, or to assist in transporting or moving objects. They also engaged in significantly more social play, that is, actually playing with one or more toys while orienting toward, or in response to, the other child, such as throwing a ball or rolling a truck toward another child. Thus, children with Down syndrome seem more advanced in their play when compared with other developmentally delayed children without Down syndrome who are matched closely in CA and MA. Nonetheless, they may differ significantly from normal children.

Rogers-Warren's (1980) study of preschool children with Down syndrome and their normal peers enrolled in an integrated program showed that the most and least frequented areas on the playground were similar for both groups. In the classroom, the most preferred and least preferred areas were also the same for both groups. Beyond these shared preferences, children with Down syndrome spent their time in more structured areas of the classroom (art table and table work), whereas normal children preferred more creative, nonstructured play areas. Distributions of time spent in no-play, solitary play, parallel play, and cooperative play were generally similar for both groups. In both playground and classroom setting, however, children with Down syndrome engaged in more solitary than parallel play, whereas the normal children were involved in more parallel than solitary play. Furthermore, the two groups differed significantly in the amount of solitary play in the playground but not in the classroom, where teachers probably encouraged them to interact. Both groups exhibited similar rates of cooperative play on the playground (approximately 6%) and in the classroom (approximately 3%–4%). In general, parallel play exceeded cooperative play for all combinations of handicapped and nonhandicapped playmates, suggesting that type of play was not strongly influenced by type of peer. Very little cooperative play was observed even among the normal children, a finding that is not surprising in view of their age and developmental status and the way in which cooperative behavior was operationally defined (i.e., mutual give-and-take in pursuit of a common goal). Finally, interaction between children with Down syndrome and normal children occurred in all activities in the classroom and on the playground, although children preferred playmates from their own group. Because potential playmates from both groups were available in all play areas, as shown by the activity preference data, Warren (1980) concluded that interaction with play-mates of similar skill levels was a matter of choice and not of simple availability.

It has also been hypothesized that the language difficulties of children with Down syndrome might preclude them from being sought as playmates by normal and other handicapped children. According to Coggins, Carpenter, & Owings (1983), studies have shown that developmentally delayed children accomplish similar linguistic achievements within the same developmental stages as children developing nor-mally. Furthermore, their own study of communicative intentions encoded by a group of normally developing preschool children and a group of children with Down syndrome matched for cognitive level and linguistic abilities revealed no significant group differences with respect to their use of various intentional communicative behaviors directed toward their mothers. Young children with Down syndrome at a two-word stage of linguistic development may be as flexible and diverse in their use of language during social interactions as are children who do not have developmen-tal delay. However, differences in rate of acquisition or frequency of use have been reported (Lackner, 1976; Naremore & Dever, 1975). Furthermore, young devel-opmentally delayed children may use language during communicative interactions with peers differently from normally developing children. Finally, they may be unable to take advantage of the "press for development" (Guralnick & Paul-Brown, 1980, 445) generated by the variation and complexity that remain, after adjustments to the development level of retarded peers, in normal children's communications with them.

At least one study suggests, however, that children with Down syndrome respond positively to the "press for development" (Guralnick & Paul-Brown, 1980, 445). A study of the verbal interactions over a 9-week period that preschool (ages 3½–4 years) and school (ages 6–7 years) children with Down syndrome had with their nonretarded peers in an unstructured normal playground setting found that over time the children with Down syndrome used language more frequently to initiate inter-actions with their retarded peers (Knox, 1983). They also showed a marked increase in responding to verbal directions over the 9-week observation period. These find-ings suggest that as time went on the nonretarded children became more able to adapt their language to ensure communication with the child who exhibited Down syndrome or that the latter became more able to comprehend the former's language, or both. However, these changes varied as a function of age. Schoolchildren with Down syndrome showed a higher percentage of time spent in interaction and cor-respondingly greater increases in frequency of language use in interaction than did the preschool children. Also, although both age groups showed decreases in fre-quencies of nonverbal imitation and responding to nonverbal directions from peers, the difference was more marked for the schoolchildren. Finally, although as a group the children with Down syndrome demonstrated increased language use, there were marked individual differences, suggesting aptitude–treatment interaction effects. These findings suggest that mutual language adaptation can take place between children with Down syndrome and nonretarded children. Furthermore, this seems to co-occur with increased social interaction between the two groups. On the other hand, the increases were quite small (the data were not submitted to statistical tests of significance). Besides, measures of social behavior other than number of inter-actions were not used, so more detailed information is needed to clarify relation-ships between peer relations and language skills of children with Down syndrome.

Summing up, no conclusive statements about the correlates of peer relations in children with Down syndrome can be made based on the findings of the studies reviewed. Although these studies suggest that group differences in mutual gaze behavior, level of social play, and communication skills might affect the amount of interaction between children with Down syndrome and their normally developing peers, any conclusions drawn would be premature.

Conceptual and methodological issues

At a conceptual level, it has to be said that progress in the study of peer relations in children with Down syndrome was considerably slowed down by the earlier focus on sociability. Quite apart from the inaccuracy of early assumptions about the so-ciability of the population with Down syndrome, the lack of clear conceptual and operational definitions for this construct limited the extent to which the findings from various studies could be interpreted as valid indicators. Furthermore, there was very little attempt to relate the diverse behavior indices in order to demonstrate that all of them were measures of the same construct. In addition, sociability was rarely differentiated from other constructs such as compliance, conformity, or adaptability to socialization. Hence, even after decades of research, a coherent de-scription of sociability in the population with Down syndrome still eludes us. So-ciability can be a heuristic construct, but only if it is clearly defined, conceptually and operationally.

Another conceptual issue that must be raised concerns the usefulness of the the-oretical bases. Very much in keeping with the Zeitgeist at that time, research on sociability was strongly influenced by two fields of psychology – personality theory and individual differences. The former provided the conceptualization of the prob-lem, while the latter furnished the methodological strategy. The influences of de-velopmental psychology and social psychology are not readily apparent. Hence, questions concerning developmental change or social acceptance did not receive a great deal of attention. On the other hand, contemporary research on the peer rela-tions of this clinical population is more closely aligned with developmental psy-chology. Nonetheless, this research seems largely atheoretical. Nor is there any attempt to integrate the findings as a preliminary step toward theory building. Un-derstandably, the research has a pronounced pragmatic orientation. Its significance, if any, is applied rather than theoretical. In general, the research could be improved if it were more closely linked to relevant theories.

In terms of methodology, many of the studies are flawed. Sampling problems are common. The sample sizes of many early studies on sociability were too small. The later studies had larger sample sizes but there were other problems, chiefly, the representativeness of the sample and heterogeneity. Obviously, it is difficult to obtain a random sample of individuals with Down syndrome. The samples of the early studies were frequently drawn from institutions, which limits the generalizability of their findings. In addition, the samples were often heterogeneous as to chronological age, sex, social class, rearing environment, karyotype, IQ, mental age, language abilities, and medical–neurological complications, yet the influence of these variables was rarely examined, or at least adjusted for, in the data analyses. Finally, appropriate control or comparison groups were often lacking. Contemporary studies of peer relations have more homogeneous samples and appropriate controls or comparison groups, but the sample sizes continue to be quite small. This limits both the number of variables that can be examined and the types of statistical analysis possible in a single study. The sample size problem is going to be difficult to solve simply because the population of individuals with Down syndrome is small, and trying to find an adequate sample size matched for CA, MA, and all the other relevant variables presents a challenge. The proposed Down syndrome registry should help, but there are limits to how far and how long subject recruitment should extend. This practical problem heightens the importance of replication in research on Down syndrome. Replication can take place either sequentially, as it is usually done, or simultaneously with a network of investigations in different facilities working on the same problem and employing identical methods.

The early research relied heavily on the Vineland Social Maturity Scale, objective personality tests, survey questionnaires and rating scales, some with weak psychometric properties. Also, the studies did not always control for respondent or rater differences in familiarity with the subjects or other possible sources of bias. The shift to direct observation methodology in contemporary research on peer relations is a change for the better, provided that adequate interrater reliabilities are obtained, which has not always been the case.

Directions for future research

Research on peer relations of individuals with Down syndrome has barely begun. The basic questions have yet to be asked. These can be grouped together into the following.

1. Questions dealing with development require attention. For this clinical population, when is the onset of interest in and responsiveness to peers? What is the nature of the developmental sequence for different peer-directed social behaviors? What age-related changes occur in their frequency and complexity? Similarly, what quantitative and qualitative changes characterize the amount of peer interaction,

patterns of interaction and interchange, ratio of positive to negative interactions, or social participation through play? Finally, what factors facilitate development of peer relations? What are the relative influences of opportunities for peer group experience, placement in integrated environments, and the like? Previous research suggests that the rate of development would be slower in Down syndrome, but more information is needed about differential rates of development for different developmental variables. Prior research with developmentally delayed children who do not have Down syndrome has shown that the developmental level achieved in peer relations is not commensurate with progress in other domains such as cognition. If this is found to be true for children with Down syndrome, it has to be accounted for through explanatory research.

2. The effects of various setting conditions on peer interaction of children with Down syndrome also have yet to be studied. At a given age, does the quantity and quality of these children's interaction vary as a function of the situation or context, the partner's characteristics, the presence or absence of adults, the types of toys, materials, or tasks? Past research with both normal and developmentally delayed populations has demonstrated these effects and some studies involving children with Down syndrome suggest that at least context (classroom vs. playground) and partner characteristics (normal vs. developmentally delayed, familiar vs. unfamiliar) exert influences. Similarly, the effect of a physical fatigue threshold (Blessing, 1959) on their peer interaction remains an intriguing question.

3. Individual differences in sociability and peer relations still constitute a worthwhile area of investigation. Sex differences are revealed by some early studies, but because their methodologies were flawed, further research is needed to clarify this issue. On the basis of previous research, it can also be hypothesized that individual differences associated with such personal characteristics as temperament, IQ, communicative competence, and medical–neurological complications are likely to characterize sociability and peer relations in this population.

4. The social acceptance of individuals with Down syndrome remains a fascinating question. As noted earlier, the population with Down syndrome seems to be socially attractive, at least to adults and in contrast to other developmentally delayed individuals. It would be interesting, therefore, to determine whether they are similarly perceived by their peers. Although some studies reviewed earlier in this chapter suggested that they are not sought out as playmates, these studies were not designed as studies of peer acceptance, nor did they involve comparisons of children with and without Down syndrome as target playmates.

5. Friendships, social networks, and peer group relations of individuals with Down syndrome, particularly older children, adolescents, and adults, also need to be explored. Increased opportunities to be with both developmentally delayed and normal peers in schools and in the community have enhanced the possibilities for individuals with Down syndrome to establish friendships, form social networks, and become part of a group. These aspects of their peer relations have never been studied.

6. Linkages between relational systems, that is, parent–child, sibling, and peer

relations of the population with Down syndrome, also have yet to be investigated. Similarities and differences between these systems as well as their influences on one another require investigation.

7. The relative contributions of peer relations to development and mental health of children with Down syndrome also need to be examined. Do the relationships between peer relations, development, and psychological adjustment that have been found in the normally developing population also hold true for this clinical population? Who are their peer referent groups and do these groups play as important a role as socialization agents?

In time, intervention studies may also need to be done. But until we have more basic information about the development of peer relations in this population, it seems premature to institute social skills training and other forms of intervention on a large scale. It is also important to keep in mind that studies have consistently shown that despite our best efforts to integrate children, ultimately, for both delayed and normally developing children, playmate preferences seem to be based on compatibility of developmental status or equality between partners. A return to segregation is not being advocated here. Rather, it is suggested that we reconsider the objectives of integration. Interactions between normally developing children and children with Down syndrome are desirable for the purpose of instilling greater awareness, understanding, and empathy, as well as forming positive attitudes in the former that will ensure peer acceptance for the latter. Also, to the extent that integration facilitates development and social adaptation of Down syndrome children, then it is useful. However, we need to be careful lest unrealistic expectations on our part are conveyed, which could damage the self-concept and self-esteem of the children with Down syndrome.

Finally, it is suggested that investigators of peer relations in the population with Down syndrome adopt an organizational view of development and a life-span perspective. The organizational view (Cicchetti & Beeghly, Chapter 2, this volume; Cicchetti & Sroufe, 1978; Sroufe & Waters, 1976) suggests that in this population, perhaps more so than in some other groups, behavior is strongly influenced by physiological factors, somatic state, and neuropsychological status. Furthermore, development in one domain such as peer relations remains closely linked to similar processes in other domains such as cognition and language. Moreover, contemporary research on social relations (Hartup, 1983) now indicates that peer relations are related to other interpersonal relationships such as those between siblings or between parent and child. Hence, a broader, organizational view of development is required for a proper understanding of systemic relationships at different levels of analysis. A life-span perspective (Baltes & Goulet, 1970) is also important because of the observed deterioration with increasing age in the social relations of this population. Although the results of previous studies must be treated with caution because of their conceptual and methodological limitations, the reports of increased serious medical complications, neurological problems, and even accelerated aging in the individual with Down syndrome make the possibility of a decline, at least in sociability, a viable hypothesis. Thus, we need to conceptualize processes over a long range even though we may focus for the moment on a single age-period, such as early childhood. An organizational view of development combined with a life-span focus would result in a more comprehensive understanding about peer relations of individuals with Down syndrome.

References

Adler, A. (1930). *The education of children*. New York: Greenberg.

Allen, V. L. (1976). *Children as teachers: Theory and research on tutoring*. New York: Academic Press.

Argyle, M., & Cook, M. (1976). *Gaze and mutual gaze*. Cambridge: Cambridge University Press.

Baltes, P. B., & Goulet, L. R. (1970). Status and issues of a life-span developmental psychology. In L. R. Goulet & P. B. Baltes (Eds.), *Life-span developmental psychology; Research and theory* (pp. 4–21). New York: Academic Press.

Bandura, A., & McDonald, F. J. (1963). The influence of social reinforcement and the behavior of models in shaping children's moral judgment. *Journal of Abnormal Social Psychology, 67,* 274–281.

Barr, M. W. (1904). *Mental defectives: Their history, treatment, and training*. Philadelphia: Philip Blakiston's Son.

Baumrind, D. (1972). Socialization and instrumental competence in young children. In W. W. Hartup (Ed.), *The young child: Reviews of research* (Vol. 2, pp. 202–244). Washington, DC: National Association for the Education of Young Children.

Beaver, A. P. (1932). *The initiation of social contacts by preschool children: A study of technique in recording social behavior*. New York: Teachers College.

Becker, J.M.T. (1977). A learning analysis of the development of peer-oriented behavior in nine-month-old infants. *Developmental Psychology, 13,* 481–491.

Benda, C. E. (1956). Mongolism: A comprehensive review. *Archives of Pediatrics, 73,* 391–407.

Benda, C. E. (1960). *The child with mongolism*. New York: Grune & Stratton.

Blacketer-Simmonds, D. A. (1953). An investigation into the supposed differences existing between mongols and other mentally defective subjects with regard to certain psychological traits. *Journal of Mental Science, 99,* 702–719.

Blessing, K. R. (1959). The middle range mongoloid in trainable classes. *American Journal of Mental Deficiency, 63,* 812–821.

Blurton-Jones, N. (1972). Categories of child–child interaction. In N. Blurton-Jones (Ed.), *Ethological studies of child behavior* (pp. 97–128). New York: Cambridge University Press.

Bridges, K.M.B. (1933). A study of social development in early infancy. *Child Development, 4,* 36–49.

Bronson, W. C. (1975). Developments in behavior with agemates during the second year of life. In M. Lewis & L. A. Rosenblum (Eds.), *Friendship and peer relations* (pp. 131–152). New York: Wiley.

Brousseau, K., & Brainerd, M. G. (1928). *Mongolism: A study of the physical and mental characteristics of mongoloid imbeciles*. Baltimore: Williams & Wilkins.

Brushfield, T. (1924). Mongolism. *British Journal of Children's Diseases, 21,* 240.

Buhler, C. (1933). The social behavior of children. In C. Murchison (Ed.), *Handbook of child psychology*. Worcester, MA: Clark University Press.

Charlesworth, R., & Hartup, W. W. (1967). Positive social reinforcement in the nursery school peer group. *Child Development, 38,* 993–1002.

Cicchetti, D., & Sroufe, L. A. (1978). An organizational view of affect: Illustration from the study of Down's syndrome infants. In M. Lewis & L. A. Rosenblum (Eds.), *The development of affect* (pp. 309–350). New York: Plenum.

Coggins, T. E., Carpenter, R. L., & Owings, N. O. (1983). Examining early international communications in Down syndrome and non-retarded children. *British Journal of Disorders of Communication, 18,* 98–106.

Cooper, C. R. (1980). Development of collaborative problem solving among preschool children. *Developmental Psychology, 16,* 433–441.

Cowen, E. L., Pederson, A., Babigian, M., Izzo, L. D., & Trost, M. A. (1973). Long-term follow-up of early detected vulnerable children. *Journal of Consulting and Clinical Psychology, 41,* 438–446.

Crawley, S. B., & Chan, K. S. (1982). Developmental changes in the free play behavior of mildly and moderately retarded preschool-aged children. *Education and Training of the Mentally Retarded, 17,* 234–239.

Dawes, H. C. (1934). Analysis of two hundred quarrels of preschool children. *Child Development, 5,* 139–157.

De la Cruz, F., & Gerald, P. S. (Eds.). (1981). *Trisomy 21 (Down Syndrome).* Baltimore, MD: University Park Press.

DiPietro, J. A. (1981). Rough and tumble play: A function of gender. *Developmental Psychology, 17,* 50–58.

Domino, G. (1965). Personality traits in institutionalized mongoloids. *American Journal of Mental Deficiency, 69,* 568–570.

Domino, G., Goldschmid, M., & Kaplan, M. (1964). Personality traits of institutionalized mongoloid girls. *American Journal of Mental Deficiency, 68,* 498–502.

Dorr, D., & Fey, S. (1974). Relative power of symbolic adult and peer models in the modification of children's moral choice behavior. *Journal of Personality and Social Psychology, 29,* 335–341.

Down, J.L.N. (1866). Observations on ethnic classification of idiots. *Clinical Lectures and Reports, London Hospital, 3,* 259.

Down, J.L.N. (1867). Observations on an ethnic classification of idiots. *Mental Science, 13,* 121–128.

Durfee, J. T., & Lee, L. C. (1973). Infant–infant interaction in a daycare setting. Paper presented at the meeting of the American Psychological Association, Montreal, August.

East, B. A. (1976). Cross-age tutoring in the elementary school. *Graduate Research in Education and Related Disciplines, 8,* 88–111.

Eckerman, C. O., Whatley, J., & Kutz, S. (1975). Growth of social play with peers during the second year of life. *Developmental Psychology, 11,* 42–49.

Engler, M.(1949). *Mongolism.* Bristol: John Wright & Sons.

Enright, R. D., & Sutterfield, S. J. (1980). An ecological validation of social cognitive development. *Child Development, 51,* 156–161.

Fagot, B. I, (1977a). Consequences of moderate cross-gender behavior in preschool children. *Child Development, 48,* 902–907.

Fagot, B. I. (1977b). Variations in density: Effect on task and social behaviors of preschool children. *Developmental Psychology, 13,* 166–167.

Fennel, C. H. (1904). Mongolian imbecility. *Journal of Mental Science, 50,* 32.

Field, T. M. (1980). Self, teacher, toy, and peer-directed behaviors of handicapped preschool children. In T. M. Field, S. Goldberg, D. Stern, & A. M. Sostek (Eds.), *High-risk infants and children: Adult and peer interactions* (pp. 313–326). New York: Academic Press.

Field, T. (1984). Play behaviors of handicapped children who have friends. In T. Field, J. L. Roopnarine, & M. Segal (Eds.), *Friendships in normal and handicapped children* (pp. 153–162). Norwood, NJ: Ablex.

Field, T., Roseman, S., DeStefano, L., & Koewler, J. H. III (1981). Play behaviors of handicapped preschool children in the presence and absence of nonhandicapped peers. *Journal of Applied Developmental Psychology, 2,* 49–58.

Francis, S. H. (1970). Behavior of low-grade institutionalized mongoloids: Changes with age. *American Journal of Mental Deficiency, 75,* 92–101.

Freud, A., & Dann, S. (1951). An experiment in group upbringing. In R. S. Eisler, A. Freud, H. Hartmann, & E. Kris (Eds.). *The psychoanalytic study of the child* (Vol. 6). New York: International Universities Press.

Garvey, C. (1974). Some properties of social play. *Merrill-Palmer Quarterly, 20,* 163–180.

Garvey, C., & BenDebba, M. (1974). Effects of age, sex, and partner on children's dyadic speech. *Child Development, 45,* 1159–1162.

Gibson, D. (1978). *Down's syndrome: The psychology of mongolism.* London: Cambridge University Press.

Gibson, D., & Butler, A. J. (1954). Culture as a possible contributor to feeble-mindedness. *American Journal of Mental Deficiency, 58,* 490–495.

Green, E. H. (1933). Group play and quarreling among preschool children. *Child Development, 4,* 302–307.

Greenberg, P. J. (1932). Competition in children: An experimental study. *American Journal of Psychology, 44,* 221–248.

Guralnick, M. J. (1978). *Early intervention and the integration of handicapped and nonhandicapped children.* Baltimore: University Park Press.

Guralnick, M. J. (1980). Social interactions among preschool children. *Exceptional Children, 46,* 248–253.

Guralnick, M. J. (1981). The social behavior of preschool children at different developmental levels. Effects of group composition. *Journal of Experimental Child Psychology, 31,* 115–130.

Guralnick, M. J. (1984). The peer interactions of young developmentally delayed children in specialized and integrated settings. In T. Field, J. L. Roopnarine, & M. S. Segal (Eds.), *Friendship in normal and handicapped children* (pp. 139–152). Norwood, NJ: Ablex.

Guralnick, M. J. (1986). The peer relations of young handicapped and nonhandicapped children. In P. S. Strain, M. J. Guralnick, & H. M. Walker (Eds.), *Children's social behavior: Development, assessment, and modification.* New York: Academic Press.

Guralnick, M. J., & Paul-Brown, D. (1980). Functional and discourse analyses of nonhandicapped preschool children's speech to handicapped children. *American Journal of Mental Deficiency, 84,* 444–454.

Guralnick, M. J., & Weinhouse, E. M. (1984). Peer-related social interactions of developmentally delayed young children: Their development and characteristics. *Developmental Psychology, 20,* 815–827.

Harris, S., Mussen, P., & Rutherford, E. (1976). Some cognitive, behavioral, and personality correlates of maturity of moral judgment. *Journal of Genetic Psychology, 128,* 123–135.

Hartup, W. W. (1974). Aggression in childhood: Developmental perspectives. *American Psychologist, 29,* 336–341.

Hartup, W. W. (1980). Two social worlds: Family relations and peer relations. In M. Rutter (Ed.), *Scientific foundations of developmental psychiatry.* London: Heinemann.

Hartup, W. W. (1983). Peer relations. In P. H. Mussen (Ed.), *Handbook of child psychology,* Vol. 4: *Socialization, personality, and social development* (pp. 104–196). New York: Wiley.

Hartup, W. W., & Coates, B. (1976). Imitation of a peer as a function of reinforcement from the peer group and rewardingness of the model. *Child Development, 38,* 1003–1016.

Hattwick, L. A., & Sanders, M. K. (1938). Age differences in behavior at the nursery school. *Child Psychology, 9,* 27–47.

Jacobson, J. L. (1981). The role of inanimate objects in early peer interaction. *Child Development, 52,* 618–626.

Johnson, R. C., & Abelson, R. B. (1969). The behavioral competence of mongoloid and non-mongoloid retardates. *American Journal of Mental Deficiency, 73,* 856–857.

Keasey, C. B. (1971). Social participation as a factor in the moral development of preadolescents. *Developmental Psychology, 5,* 216–220.

Knox, M. (1983). Changes in the frequency of language use by Down's syndrome children interacting with non-retarded peers. *Education and Training of the Mentally Retarded, 18,* 185–190.

Kobasigawa, A. (1968). Inhibitory and disinhibitory effects of models on sex-inappropriate behavior in children. *Psychologia, 11,* 86–96.

Kohlberg, L. (1958). *The development of moral thinking and choice in the years ten to sixteen.* Unpublished doctoral dissertation, University of Chicago.

Kohn, M. (1966). The child as a determinant of his peers' approach to him. *Journal of Genetic Psychology, 109,* 165–174.

Kuhn, T. S. (1970). *The structure of scientific revolutions* (2nd ed.). Chicago: University of Chicago Press.

Kurdek, L. A. (1980). Developmental relations among children's perspective taking, moral judgment, and parent-rated behaviors. *Merrill-Palmer Quarterly, 26,* 103–122.

Lackner, J. (1976). A developmental study of language behavior in retarded children. In D. Morehead & A. Morehead (Eds.), *Normal and deficient child language.* Baltimore: University Park Press.

Leuba, C. (1933). An experimental study of rivalry in young children. *Journal of Comparative Psychology, 16,* 367–378.

Lever, J. (1976). Sex differences in the games children play. *Social Problems, 23,* 479–487.

Lewis, M., Young, G., Brooks, J., & Michalson, L. (1975). The beginning of friendship. In M. Lewis & L. A. Rosenblum (Eds.), *Friendship and peer relations* (pp. 27–66). New York: Wiley.

Lougee, M. D., Grueneich, R., & Hartup, W. W. (1977). Social interaction in same and mixed age dyads of preschool children. *Child Development, 48,* 1353–1361.

McArthur, L. Z., & Eisen, S. V. (1976). Achievements of male and female storybook characters as determinants of achievement behavior by boys and girls. *Journal of Personality and Social Psychology, 33,* 467–473.

Manwell, E. M., & Mangert, I. G. (1934). A study of the development of two- and three-year-old children with respect to play activities. *University of Iowa Studies in Child Welfare, 9,* 69–111.

Martin, W. (1964). Singularity and stability of social behavior. In C. B. Stendler (Ed.), *Readings in child behavior and development.* New York: Harcourt Brace.

Maudry, M., & Nekula, M. (1939). Social relations between children of the same age during the first two years of life. *Journal of Genetic Psychology, 54,* 193–215.

Mindes, G. (1982). Social and cognitive aspects of play in young handicapped children. *Topics in Early Childhood Education, 2,* 39–52.

Moore, B. C., Thuline, H. C., & Capes, L. V. (1968). Mongoloid and non-mongoloid retardates: A behavioral comparison. *American Journal of Mental Deficiency, 73,* 433–436.

Mueller, E. (1972). The maintenance of verbal exchanges between young children. *Child Development, 43,* 930–938.

Mueller, E., & Brenner, J. (1977). The origins of social skills and interaction among playgroup toddlers. *Child Development, 48,* 854–861.

Mueller, E., & Lucas, T. (1975). A developmental analysis of peer interaction among toddlers. In M. Lewis & L. A. Rosenblum (Eds.), *Friendship and peer relations* (pp. 223–258). New York: Wiley.

Mueller, E., & Rich, A. (1976). Clustering and socially-directed behaviors in a play-group of 1-year-old boys. *Journal of Child Psychology and Psychiatry, 17,* 315–322.

Mueller, E. C., & Vandell, D. (1979). Infant–infant interaction. In J. D. Osofsky (Ed.), *Handbook of infant development* (pp. 591–622). New York: Wiley.

Murray, F. (1972). Acquisition of conservation through social interaction. *Developmental Psychology, 6,* 1–6.

Naremore, R., & Dever, R. (1975). Language performance of educable mentally retarded and normal children at five age levels. *Journal of Speech and Hearing Research, 18,* 82–95.

O'Connor, R. (1969). Modification of social withdrawal through symbolic modeling. *Journal of Applied Behavior Analysis, 2,* 15–22.

Oster, J. (1953). *Mongolism.* Copenhagen: Danish Science Press.

Parten, M. B. (1932). Social participation among preschool children. *Journal of Abnormal and Social Psychology, 27,* 243–269.

Patterson, G. R., & Cobb, J. A. (1971). A dyadic analysis of aggressive behaviors. In J. P. Hill (Ed.), *Minnesota symposia on child psychology* (Vol. 5, pp. 72–129). Minneapolis: University of Minnesota Press.

Patterson, G. R., Littman, R. A., & Bricker, W. (1967). Assertive behavior in children: A step toward a theory of aggression. *Monographs of the Society for Research in Child Development, 32,* (5, Serial No 113).

Perret-Clermont, A. (1980). *Social interaction and cognitive development in children.* New York: Academic Press.

Piaget, J. (1932). *The moral judgment of the child.* Glencoe, IL: Free Press.

Pueschel, S. M. (1984). *The young child with Down syndrome.* New York: Human Sciences Press.

Roff, M. (1961). Childhood social interactions and young adult bad conduct. *Journal of Abnormal and Social Psychology, 63,* 333–337.

Roff, M. (1963). Childhood social interactions and young adult psychosis. *Journal of Clinical Psychology, 19,* 152–157.

Roff, M., Sells, S. B., & Golden, M. M. (1972). *Social adjustment and personality development in children.* Minneapolis: University of Minnesota Press.

Rogers-Warren, A. (1980). *Playing and learning together.* Lawrence: University of Kansas, Early Childhood Institute. (ERIC Document Reproduction Service No. ED 231 104).

Rollin, H. R. (1946). Personality in mongolism with special reference to the incidence of catatonic psychosis. *American Journal of Mental Deficiency, 51,* 219–237.

Ross, H. S., & Goldman, B. M. (1976). Establishing new social relations in infancy. In T. Alloway, L. Krames, & P. Pliner (Eds.), *Advances in communication and affect* (Vol. 3, pp. 61–78). New York: Plenum.

Rubenstein, J., & Howes, C. (1976). The effects of peers on toddler interaction with mother and toys. *Child Development, 47,* 597–605.

Schlottman, R. S., & Anderson, V. H. (1975). Social and play behaviors of institutionalized mongoloid and nonmongoloid retarded children. *Journal of Psychology, 91,* 201–206.

Scholtz, G., & Ellis, M. (1975). Repeated exposure to objects and peers in a play setting. *Journal of Experimental Child Psychology, 19,* 448–455.

Sherlock, E. B., & Donkin, H. B. (1911). *The feeble minded: A guide to study and practice.* London: Macmillan.

Shirley, M. (1933). *The first two years: A study of twenty-five babies* (Vol. 2). Minneapolis: University of Minnesota Press.

Sinson, J. C., & Wetherick, N. E. (1981). The behavior of children with Down syndrome in normal playgroups. *Journal of Mental Deficiency Research, 25,* 113–120.

Sinson, J. C., & Wetherick, N. E. (1982). Mutual gaze in preschool Down and normal children. *Journal of Mental Health Deficiency Research, 26,* 123–129.

Smith, P. K., & Connolly, K. (1972). Patterns of play and social interaction in preschool children. In N. Blurton Jones (Ed.), *Ethological studies of child behavior* (pp. 65–96). Cambridge: Cambridge University Press.

Spanier, G. B. (1976). Formal and informal sex education as determinants of premarital sexual behavior. *Archives of Sexual Behavior, 5,* 39–67.

Spreen, O. (1965). Language functions in mental retardation: A review of language development, types of retardation and intelligence. *American Journal of Mental Deficiency, 69,* 482–494.

Sroufe, L. A., & Waters, E. (1976). The ontogenesis of smiling and laughter: A perspective on the organization of development in infancy. *Psychological Review, 83,* 173–189.

Strain, P. S., & Fox, J. E. (1981). Peers as behavior change agents for withdrawn classmates. In A. E. Kazdin & B. Lahey (Eds.), *Advances in clinical child psychology.* New York: Plenum.

Stumphauzer, J. S. (1972). Increased delay of gratification in young prison inmates through imitation of high-delay peer models. *Journal of Personality and Social Psychology, 21,* 10–17.

Sullivan, H. S. (1953). *The interpersonal theory of psychiatry.* New York: Norton.

Tredgold, A. F. (1947). *A textbook of mental deficiency.* London: Bailliere, Tindall.

Vincze, M. (1971). The social contacts of infants and young children reared together. *Early Child Development and Care, 1,* 99–109.

Wahler, R. G. (1967). Child–child interactions in five field settings: Some experimental analyses. *Journal of Experimental Child Psychology, 5,* 278–293.

Wallin, J.E.W. (1949). *Children with mental and physical handicaps.* Englewood Cliffs, NJ: Prentice-Hall.

Walters, J., Pearce, D., & Dahms, L. (1957). Affectional and aggressive behavior of preschool children. *Child Development, 28,* 15–26.

Washburn, R. W., & Hilgard, J. R. (1934). A quantitative clinical method of recording the social behavior of young children. *Pediatrics Seminars, 45,* 390–405.

Wolf, T. M. (1973). Effects of live modeled sex-inappropriate play behavior in a naturalistic setting. *Developmental Psychology, 9,* 120–123.

Wolf, T. M. (1975). Response consequences to televised modeled sex-inappropriate play behavior. *Journal of Genetic Psychology, 127,* 35–44.

Wolf, T. M., & Cheyne, J. A. (1972). Persistence of effects of live behavioral, televised behavioral, and live verbal models on resistance to deviation. *Child Development, 43,* 1429–1436.

Wright, H. F. (1967). *Recording and analyzing child behavior.* New York: Harper.

12 Families of children with Down syndrome: ecological contexts and characteristics

Keith A. Crnic

Children with Down syndrome constitute a group with unique developmental characteristics as well as developmental parameters more common to the general population of mentally retarded children. The preceding chapters have documented many of these developmental characteristics through representative reviews of previous research and new data-based studies. Although it is apparent that we have learned a good deal about the developmental functioning of Down syndrome children, it is likewise also apparent that little of this research has attempted to understand these developmental processes within an ecological framework. In this regard, the study of Down syndrome children mirrors that of normal child development. In fact, Bronfenbrenner (1979), in a discussion of the ecological contexts of child-rearing, made the point succinctly when he stated, "We know much more about children than about the environments in which they live or the processes through which these environments affect the course of development" (p. 844).

The family provides the primary developmental context influencing the psychological growth, development, and well-being of children. This notion is pervasive in the literature from the earliest theoretical formulations of psychodynamic models to the overwhelming number of empirical investigations of the influence of parental attitudes, perceptions, and behavior on child development as well as the more reciprocal notions involving the child's influence on the parent. Yet these studies deal with the family context only in the narrowest sense. We have generally not studied the family as an integrated interactive system nor have we made concerted efforts to understand the various ecological contexts that affect families and thereby directly and indirectly influence child development. While such considerations are important within all families, the presence of a child with significant developmental disabilities such as Down syndrome presents a unique stressor on the family and impacts both the family system and the various ecological contexts in which the family interacts (Crnic, Friedrich, & Greenberg, 1983).

Ecological contexts include the various environmental settings in which children and families live and interact as well as the pervasive institutional and cultural factors that influence attitudes and behavior. Of particular relevance for this chapter

399

is the separation of ecological contexts into those which are intrafamilial and those which are extrafamilial. The intrafamilial context pertains to factors only within the family itself. These would involve the complex interrelationships between various familial factors that include the marital relationship, parent–child relationships, and individual parent and child characteristics within an interactive dynamic system (Belsky, 1981; 1984). Extrafamilial contexts pertain to factors outside the immediate family. These would include those diverse environmental settings in which families and their individual members interact, including workplaces, schools, neighborhoods, communities, peer groups, and social networks as well as numerous others (Bronfenbrenner, 1977). Although extrafamilial contexts can have direct influences on child development (Cochran & Brassard, 1979), the family frequently serves to moderate or filter the effect of extrafamilial contexts. The family accomplishes this through selectively exposing children to various contexts, situations, and activities that will influence their development. Thus, the ways in which extrafamilial contexts affect children are often indirect and mediated through the family context.

Presently, we know very little about the impact that a handicapped child has on the family system and the extrafamilial environmental contexts that influence it. We know even less about how, in turn, the family and extrafamilial contexts subsequently affect the development of a handicapped child. A recent review of the literature on families of mentally retarded children (Crnic, Friedrich, & Greenberg, 1983) suggests that there is frequently an adverse impact on numerous aspects of familial functioning, most likely as a result of the added stress associated with the presence of a retarded child. In these regards, *stress* refers generally to notions of anxiety around the child's abilities, skills, and appearance, and the social response by friends and the community at large; the increased caretaking burdens, potential major changes in family life-style, and worries over both minor and major, short- and long-term care provision. The presence of a handicapped child in the family, however, will not only impact the intrafamilial context but is also likely to affect extrafamilial contexts as families become involved with various service agencies, parent groups, special education school systems, and as changes occur in the social networks of the family members. How the stresses and changes within both intra- and extrafamilial contexts influence familial functioning will be a function of how well the family and its individual members cope with and subsequently adapt to the presence of a handicapped child. Adaptations to this situation are certainly not uniform across families, nor are they necessarily dysfunctional. Despite the general trend of previous research to focus on dysfunctional outcomes, it is clear that some families remain intact and functional through the adaptation process, a process that is most likely to vary depending upon the degree of stress perceived, the coping resource available to the family, and the ecological contexts that mediate those resources. It should also be noted that adaptation is not an outcome or end point. In this respect, adaptation must be considered as a life-span developmental process. It does not imply successful or unsuccessful resolution to the reality of having a handicapped child. It seems unlikely that final resolution, either successful or unsuccessful, is feasible if we accept development as a dynamic process involving change over time and across contexts. Adaptation, therefore, is an ongoing process necessitated by the occurrence of minor and major crises arising during developmental and life changes that occur in families of handicapped children.

Ecological context and normal development

To attempt to understand the complex interrelationships that exist between the child with Down syndrome and his or her family, we need to begin by examining those factors we know to be operative within the normal development literature. The study of children with some handicapping conditions falls within the spectrum of the emergent field of developmental psychopathology, and Cicchetti (1984) has eloquently stated that "we can learn more about the normal functioning of an organism by studying its pathology and, likewise, more about its pathology by studying its normal condition" (p. 1). Therefore, we need to consider how functioning within normal families in normative contexts operates to influence and be influenced by the child, with specific attention to the way in which these processes are either similar or dissimilar to like studies of children with some pathological condition.

The suggestion that ecological contexts are important to human development is not necessarily a novel one. For example, the Skeels studies of the late 1930s and early 1940s are classic examples of contextual influences on development (Skeels, 1966). Skeels showed that placing children in adoptive homes following early rearing in orphanages resulted in greatly increased IQs. However, it is only recently that Bronfenbrenner has proposed a theoretical formulation of the issues involved in an ecological model of development (1977; 1979b; Bronfenbrenner & Crouter, 1983). Basically, he has proposed that development can be best understood within a person–process–context model (Bronfenbrenner & Crouter, 1983), which purports that variations in the developmental process are best explained by an interaction of the characteristics of the person and the context in which the person is involved. Contexts include the immediate setting that contains the person (microsystem), the interrelationships between settings in which the person interacts (mesosystem), the influence of larger social structures which do not necessarily contain the person such as neighborhoods, media, governments (ecosystem), and the overarching societal and cultural value systems (macrosystems).

A brief review of studies of ecological influences on normal child development provides a relevant context for the few studies that have attempted to measure similar facets of families of children with Down syndrome or other handicaps. Within the literature of normal child development, there is an overwhelming number of studies concerning intrafamilial contexts and their impact on child development, with a particular focus on parent–child interactions. This research has been well summarized elsewhere (Maccoby & Martin, 1983), and is too voluminous to begin to be discussed here. Ample evidence, however, indicates that parents' attitudes and behavior affect children's development and conversely that children's development and behavior influence parental responding, thereby creating notions that the parent–child relationship is normally reciprocal and bidirectional. Fewer by far, however, are studies that attempt to examine the influence of extrafamilial factors on intrafamilial process.

Social class is a factor uniformly included in developmental research but not often assessed within a process model or in terms of its developmental implications over time. A series of studies by Tulkin (Tulkin, 1973a, 1973b; Tulkin & Covitz, 1975; Tulkin & Kagan, 1972), which are exemplary of a more ecological approach, found that middle-class mothers engaged in more reciprocal interactions with their infants, and had attitudes that valued meeting the child's needs and the importance of mother–child interaction. Further, middle-class mothers showed much greater correspondence between their attitudes and behavior, and long-term positive effects on child developmental outcome were found for middle-class mothers.

Recent research on specific ecological contexts has also demonstrated specific effects on families and child development. Studies of day care have traditionally focused on direct effects on the child with generally optimistic results, although a recent review of the latest studies (Belsky, 1984) suggests that the security of infant–mother attachment in infants placed in day care may be more problematic and less stable. Parental employment status has also been investigated, with differences noted between paternal and maternal employment in relation to the family and child development (Kammerman & Hayes, 1982). Fathers' occupational status has been found to influence the son's occupational choices (Mortimer, Lorence, & Kumka, 1983), and fathers' time schedules can produce greater family conflicts if they interfere with other family members' schedules (Mott, Mann, McLoughlin, & Warwick, 1965). The issue of maternal employment has grown much in importance as mothers enter the work force in greater numbers. Analyses of research studies of maternal employment (Hoffman, 1983) have produced the consistent finding that it tends to have a positive influence on daughters (they admire their mothers more, have a more positive conception of female role, and are more independent) but a negative impact on sons (they show lower academic achievement in middle-class families).

Some intriguing findings are beginning to emerge from studies of parental social networks and their effects on families and child development, which have particular relevance to families of handicapped children. Much of this research was spurred by Cochran and Brassard (1979), who suggested that parental social networks directly and indirectly impact parenting styles and child development. Subsequently, a number of studies have found that mothers with more adequate social support from spouses, friends, and families have more positive attitudes toward parenting and their child (Colletta, 1981, 1983; Crnic, Greenberg, Ragozin, Robinson, & Basham, 1983; Crnic, Greenberg, Robinson, & Ragozin, 1984; Mercer, Hackley, & Bostrom, 1983; Tietjen & Bradley, 1982). More adequate support has also been found to be related to more positive maternal behavior toward children (Crnic et al., 1983; Crnic et al., 1984; Crockenberg, in press; Wandersman & Unger, 1983; Weinraub & Wolf, 1983), and more positive child behavior during interactions with mother (Crnic, et al., 1983; Crnic et al., 1984). Further, these effects of social network support appear to have particularly positive effects under certain conditions of greater familial stress (Crnic et al., 1983; Crockenberg, 1987; Weinraub & Wolf, 1983). It is this final point that is particularly relevant to the ecological contexts of families of children with Down syndrome or other handicaps, as these children clearly precipitate greater stresses within families. Yet, regardless of the presence of stress, parents' social networks appear to be important contributors to parental psychological well-being, parenting attitudes and behavior, and child development.

The studies just described are certainly not exhaustive of those which explore contexts of families of normal children. A comprehensive review can be found in Bronfenbrenner and Crouter (1983). Nonetheless, these studies exemplify the importance of ecological context to various aspects of family functioning and child development, in particular regard to the processes that influence these as well as outcomes obtained.

Ecological contexts and mentally retarded children

In rather sharp contrast to the data available concerning intra- and extrafamilial contexts involved in normal child development, only a few studies have attempted to measure similar factors in families of retarded children and many of those that have done so are plagued with methodological problems of inadequate control groups and measures. The paucity of such studies is indeed rather surprising considering the generally accepted clinical observations of greater stress and less optimal family functioning in these groups. Nevertheless, there appears to be a growing interest in these families reflected by a number of recent studies. These studies have perhaps been stimulated by earlier work on various intrafamilial factors suggesting that specific psychological difficulties are present in family members of retarded children. There is also the question of whether families of Down syndrome children differ from families of other handicapped children or whether the presence of a child with a handicap regardless of the specific diagnosis produces a comparable effect across families. This is a particularly difficult question to address from previous research, as studies related to family context typically have mixed samples of children with Down syndrome and children with undifferentiated mental retardation, or study children with Down syndrome only in comparison to nonhandicapped peer groups.

Intrafamilial context

Studies which have attempted to assess families of retarded children have focused primarily on intrafamilial factors. In general, these studies have had a rather narrow focus, reflecting a unidimensional (primary focus on one member or one factor) and unimodal (utilizing one type of measurement) character. Further, many of these investigations have used measures of questionable psychometric status, and did not include adequate controls. Nevertheless, there are consistent indications across studies and measurement domains that the presence of a retarded child adversely impacts various aspects of family functioning.

Parental child-rearing attitudes appear to be impacted by retarded children, as

parents (primarily mothers) of retarded children have been found to be more reject-
ing, punitive, overprotective, and angry (Caldwell & Guze, 1960; Cook, 1963;
Ricci, 1970; Waisbren, 1980). Further, such attitudes appear to have significant
implications for the retarded child's development, as parental attitudes have been
found to be related to skill on performance tests (Landman, 1979) and parent involvement in home-based programming (Strom, Rees, Slaughter, & Wurster, 1981).
Less positive attitudes were related to less positive performances on tests of developmental skill acquisition and to less parental involvement in home-based programming. Parents of retarded children have also been found to show more personality
and emotional problems than parents of normal children, including problems with
impulse control and aggressive feelings (Erickson, 1968, 1969; Miller & Keirn,
1978), greater depressive and dysphoric affect, less sense of parental competence
and enjoyment (Cummings, Bayley, & Rie, 1966), and general greater "malaise"
(Tew & Lawrence, 1975).

Studies of the marital relationship in families with a retarded child present a
somewhat less clear picture of effect. Farber's (1959) early landmark work with
families of severely retarded children found that marital integration decreased with
the presence of a severely retarded child, although outcome was more related to the
perceived marital integration before the child's birth. He also found a significant
effect for sex of child, as retarded male children had a more significant negative
impact on marital integration. Two more recent studies, both using the Locke Wallace Marital Adjustment Inventory, have produced directly conflicting results. Friedrich
and Friedrich (1981) found that parents of handicapped children report significantly
less marital satisfaction than parents of nonhandicapped children, while Waisbren
(1980) found no differences between 60 well-matched couples, half of whom were
parents of developmentally delayed infants. These differences may be attributed to
sampling effects, as the Waisbren (1980) sample children averaged 13 months of
age while the Friedrich and Friedrich (1981) sample children averaged over 9 years
of age. Marital satisfaction may indeed decrease over time in families of retarded
children; as the children grow older, the extent of the handicap becomes more clearly
predictable, and the effects of stress accumulate, thus helping to create more frequent and intense marital conflicts.

The retarded child's apparent negative impact on parents' attitudes, emotional
functioning, and marriage has been most frequently explained with a stress-reaction
hypothesis (Erickson, 1969; Miller & Keirn, 1978). This hypothesis suggests that
the detrimental functioning observed in these families is a reaction to the stress that
is precipitated by the presence of the retarded child. Yet only recently have studies
actually attempted to measure the stresses in these families. The development of the
Questionnaire on Resources and Stress (QRS) (Holyroyd, 1974) has provided the
most frequently used measure, and studies have indicated that the QRS relates well
to interview ratings of stress (Holroyd, Brown, Wikler, & Simons, 1975), successfully differentiates families both within and between groups of handicapped and
nonhandicapped children (Friedrich & Friedrich, 1981; Holroyd & McArthur, 1976),
and shows a significant positive relationship to severity of child's handicap (Beck-

man, 1983; Holroyd & Guthrie, 1979). A recent revision of the QRS (Friedrich, Greenberg, & Crnic, 1983) has reduced the length of the instrument (from 285 to 52 items) and provided a more manageable and reliable form. The data acquired from the QRS measures indicate, in sum, that the notion of a stress-reaction hypothesis has some validity; although there remains a need for prospective longitudinal studies to detail such relationships. Such studies should begin at the time the child is identified as handicapped and follow these families over extended periods of time.

Studies of intrafamilial factors have not focused solely on parents; siblings have also been a focus of some concern, with interesting results. Sibling relationships have been found to be problematic, with the normal sibling (especially female siblings) encouraged to function as surrogate parent (Farber, 1960), and feel less free to express negative feelings toward the retarded sibling (Miller, 1974). Pfouts (1976) reported that normal siblings feel ambivalent toward their retarded sibling, while the retarded sibling was noted to be hostile toward the nonretarded sibling on projective testing. A number of studies indicate that beyond relationship difficulties, normal siblings are adversely affected by the presence of a retarded sibling, depending somewhat upon the demographic characteristics of family social class and age and sex of the normal sibling. Normal siblings have been found to show greater anxiety, more conflict with parents, and lower sociability (Farber, 1960, 1963; Fowle, 1964), although the degree of effect is somewhat less when parental reaction and ability to cope are more positive, the family's socioeconomic status (SES) is higher, and the normal sibling is older (Grossman, 1972). Detrimental effects are most apparent on female siblings (Farber, 1959, 1960), a finding also clearly demonstrated in a study of siblings of 174 Down syndrome children (Gath, 1973). She found that parents and teachers rated siblings of Down syndrome children as having significantly more behavior problems ($p < .05$) than siblings of normal children. When female siblings alone were considered, the significance rose to $p < .001$, indicating that nearly the entire group difference could be accounted for by the increase in deviant behavior of female siblings.

Another area that bears on intrafamilial factors is parent–child interactions. This research has been discussed in Chapter 4 of this volume and need not be repeated here. Nonetheless, the research would appear to indicate that parent–child interactions with Down syndrome and other retarded children are significantly different from those with nonretarded children, particularly in terms of the use of greater control and directiveness, less responsiveness, less positive affect, and less reciprocity.

The studies just reviewed have focused on individual aspects of familial functioning without attempting to view the family as a more complex integrated system. Yet this would appear to remain the greatest need in the area. One group of investigators has begun such a research program and these studies deserve more specific attention as they detail more fully the family system as a context for development of retarded children, and also include a sizable population of Down syndrome children. Nihira and his colleagues (Nihira, Meyers, & Mink, 1980; Nihira, Mink, &

Meyers, 1981; Mink, Nihira, & Meyers, 1983) have explored the complex interrelationships between home environment, family adjustment, and parent and child
characteristics in families of 268 mildly and moderately retarded children approximately half of which were Down syndrome. A beginning taxonomy of family lifestyles has resulted (Mink et al., 1983).

In the first study (Nihira et al., 1980), family adjustment and functioning were
related not only to the severity of the child's retardation and degree of maladaptive
behavior, but to family demographic characteristics, the psychosocial climate of the
family (cohesion, expressiveness, harmony), specific parental behavior, marital dis-
harmony, and conflicts unrelated to the retarded child (e.g., life stress events).
Further, the parents' perceived impact of the child on the family was negatively
related to the child's adaptive competency, whereas the child's adaptive competency was positively related to the parents' ability to cope. These relationships clearly
suggest the interactional and reciprocal nature of the family–retarded child system.
The child's behavior and competency affects the parents' responsivity and ability to
cope, which in turn again affects the child's behavior and competency. Subsequently, Nihira et al. (1981) showed that family harmony, quality of parenting,
family cohesiveness, and emotional support for learning were positively related to
the retarded child's school adjustment.

In attempting to determine a descriptive taxonomy of families of retarded children, Mink et al. (1983) utilized a cluster analysis of their family measures, which
included the Home Observation for Measurement of the Environment, the Family
Environment Scale, and their Home Quality Rating Scale. The sample consisted of
115 families of trainable mentally retarded children, 48% of which had Down syndrome. Analyses showed that families tended to cluster into 5 types: (1) cohesive,
harmonious families ($N = 35$); (2) control-oriented, somewhat nonharmonious families ($N = 34$); (3) low disclosure, nonharmonious families ($N = 7$); (4) child-oriented,
expressive families ($N = 27$); and (5) disadvantaged, low morale families ($N = 12$).
Families with a Down syndrome child constituted 65% of the cohesive, harmonious
families and nearly 45% of the child-oriented, expressive families. In contrast, the
Down syndrome families comprised only 33% of the disadvantaged low morale
group and 38% of the control-oriented, somewhat nonharmonious families. Mink
et al. speculated that Down syndrome children may have a positive effect on the
climate of the home, although such an interpretation is highly speculative at this
time.

In total, this brief review of intrafamilial contexts in families of retarded children
suggests two major conclusions. First, ample evidence suggests that various aspects
of familial functioning are adversely impacted by the presence of a retarded child;
and second, adverse impacts and less optimal family functioning are not necessary
outcomes. Clearly, there is great variation within families of retarded children,
which is well documented by the Mink et al. (1983) taxonomy study. This leads to
the question as to what factors may account for these variations in response. There
are indications that certain parental characteristics, such as attributions and belief
systems, may be important (Affleck, Allen, McGrade, & McQueeney, 1983), as

well as child characteristics (severity of retardation, Down syndrome versus non-Down syndrome-retarded children), and degree of perceived stress. It is also likely that extrafamilial ecological contexts play a significant role in the coping process related to family functional outcomes to explain adaptational variations.

Extrafamilial contexts

As noted previously, few studies have addressed the extrafamilial contexts and their influence on family systems or individual family members. Yet several studies do provide some insights into such relationships. Studies of psychosocial variables have indicated that family social mobility is reduced and SES declined in families who kept their retarded children at home (Farber, 1960, 1968, 1970), mothers of retarded children were less likely to work full-time, and parents went out less as child care was more difficult to arrange (Watson & Midlarsky, 1979).

Other data suggest that religious beliefs and involvement in community church groups has a positive impact on parents and families with retarded children in general (Zuk, 1959; Zuk, Miller, Bartram, & Kling, 1961), and Down syndrome children in particular (Vadasy, Fewell, Meyer, Schell, & Greenberg, 1984). There are also indications that societal and cultural factors influence family functioning, particularly in regard to acceptance of normalization practices (Ferrara, 1979) and dealing with the stigma of the handicap (Goffman, 1963). The Nihira et al. (1981) study clearly demonstrated the efficacy of mesosystem models by finding important relationships between family and school contexts for Down syndrome and other retarded children, and Mink et al. (1983) contributed extrafamilial context data into the family clusters described by including parental work status, community involvement, and life stress events associated with the five identified clusters discussed earlier.

Perhaps reflecting the trend in the normal child development literature, the extrafamilial context that has received the greatest attention is parental social networks and support systems. In a cross-sectional survey of 330 families of retarded children, Suelzle and Keenan (1981) found that parents of younger retarded children utilized more support networks, whereas parents of older children had less support, were more isolated, and perceived a greater need for expanded services. Parents of retarded children reported less social support than parents of nonhandicapped children (Friedrich & Friedrich, 1981), although parental support in families of retarded children is positively related to coping and measures of parental well-being (Friedrich, 1979; Vadasy et al., 1984). In a study of 24 mothers of children with Down syndrome, Spiker (1982) found that participating in a parent support group was noted as the most beneficial aspect of parent involvement in an early intervention program, with mothers reporting that the shared emotional support was the most important facet of the group. Early intervention programs are a frequent extrafamilial context for families of children with Down syndrome, but the impact that such programs have on families and parents are complex and not always uniformly positive (see Spiker, Chapter 13, this volume). Although few, the studies related to extrafamilial context would appear to indicate that such contexts are important determinants of family status.

Together, the research on intrafamilial and extrafamilial ecological contexts of families of mentally retarded children suggests that the functioning of the family system and its subsequent effects on the child are dependent upon the degree of stress perceived by the family members, specific parent and child characteristics, the coping resources that are available to the family, and the ecological contexts that mediate these resources. This model has been detailed elsewhere (Crnic, Friedrich, & Greenberg, 1983), and data are only now beginning to accumulate detailing the processes of stress, coping, and family ecologies and their relationship to family adaptation and the development of retarded children.

It is important to emphasize the relationship between family functioning and children's development, especially for those children who have some atypical status. Specifically, understanding the family context of these children will assist in furthering the understanding of such children's development from an organizational perspective (Cicchetti & Pogge-Hesse, 1982). While intraorganismic variables associated with Down syndrome certainly influence the course and the organization of the child's development, this development also occurs within context, that context being primarily defined by the family. Therefore, development and its organization in atypical populations, (and Down syndrome in particular), will be a function of the complex interactions between intraorganismic state and the environmental context provided as a function of that state.

The complex interactions between an atypical or high-risk child and the subsequent environmental contexts that affect developmental process and outcome are descriptive of a *transactional model* (Sameroff & Chandler, 1975). In essence, the notion of transactional explanations of developmental outcome have gained in popularity as research has indicated that biomedical status or intraorganismic variables alone (e.g., the continuum of reproductive casualty, Passaminick & Knoblock, 1961) does not well account for the range of developmental outcomes seen with high-risk and atypical populations (Sameroff & Chandler, 1975). In fact, the majority of developmental research with high-risk and atypical children indicates that environmental context factors appear to explain outcomes better than does birth or biomedical status alone (Crnic & Greenberg, 1987; Greenberg & Crnic, 1988; Field, 1980; Sameroff & Seifer, 1983; Werner & Smith, 1982).

The transactional model of development suggests that given a risk or atypical status (biomedical or environmental), the outcome for any particular child is dependent upon the active interaction between the child and his or her caretaking environment, such that each is changing and being changed as a function of these interactions. Predominantly, studies have focused on SES factors as measures of the caretaking context, and a number of studies have included indices of parent–child interaction. Few studies, however, have attempted to investigate broadly the notion of family contexts as they relate to the behavioral and developmental outcomes of risk and atypical children. The work previously described by Nihira, Mink, and

Meyers is one exception, and clearly shows the validity and potential utility of a transactional approach to studying these families.

The transactional model does not necessarily suggest that birth or biomedical intraorganismic factors are not important to developmental organization. In fact, these factors are important as they appear to create the conditions that enhance the various environmental contexts and their influence. For example, several recent studies by Crnic and Greenberg (1987, 1988) have found that for high-risk premature infants there appear to be more relationships between family factors and maternal and child behavior and development than there are between family factors and normal mother–child pairs. Yet these groups do not appear to differ on measures of child developmental status, or on the measures of family and maternal functioning. What does differentiate the groups is the pattern of relationships found. There are many more relationships between the family and child and maternal factors for preterms than for full terms, intrafamilial psychosocial factors are more predictive of preterm outcomes than full-term outcomes, mother and high-risk child interactions are more related to family status than are the interactions of mother–normal child pairs, and extrafamilial factors (e.g., life stresses) are more related to normal child and mother factors than high-risk child and mother factors. Given the lack of differences in developmental competence between the two groups, it seems likely that the more extensive family focus in the high-risk group served as a self-righting mechanism in relation to the high-risk child's development. The notion that family contexts can serve as self-righting mechanisms for children at risk has been previously suggested by Sameroff and Seifer (1983). The differential importance of the family context between the groups suggests that it is the presence of the high-risk birth status or biomedical condition that creates the specific importance of the family context to outcome for the family and child. The process of transactional phenomena must then be understood within the context of the biomedical or risk factor itself. Within the focus of the present chapter, the Down syndrome condition can be assumed to provide the catalyst through which the family functions to influence the development of the child with Down syndrome.

As families clearly have differential responses to the presence of retarded children, it may well be that the specific diagnosis or characteristics of the handicap are critical in determining variability in response. Although studies have not specifically differentiated between families of Down syndrome and other retarded children, the study by Mink et al. (1983) is particularly suggestive in this regard. Families of children with Down syndrome constituted a greater proportion of the better functioning families, and smaller proportions of dysfunctional families. The suggestion that children with Down syndrome can have a positive effect on the climate of the home is intriguing, and needs to be more fully explored. The fact that children with Down syndrome are generally included along with non-Down syndrome retarded children in studies of family factors has generally served to obscure such differences, and studies that specifically assess the characteristics of the families of children with Down syndrome are needed to address such issues.

A pilot study

In an attempt to address a number of the issues presented above, a pilot study of families of children with Down syndrome was conducted. These data were collected in preface to a planned, larger prospective and longitudinal study of the factors that influence coping and adaptations of families of young, handicapped children.

The families

The sample consisted of 22 children with Down syndrome and their families, who were recruited through their contacts with service professionals at the Child Development and Mental Retardation Center at the University of Washington and through various special programs in the surrounding area. The children ranged in age from 23 months to 7 years, 4 months ($\chi = 4.5$ years) and all functioned within the mild to moderate range of mental retardation. Mothers ranged in age from 23 to 45 years ($\chi = 29.0$) and had completed 10 to 18 years of education ($\chi = 13.8$). The families were primarily two-parent and middle class.

The mothers of the children were contacted by telephone to explain the study protocol and the measures included. The mothers were then mailed the study questionnaires along with a stamped, preaddressed envelope in which to return the questionnaires. A total of 24 questionnaires were originally sent, and 22 were returned. This high return rate (91%) was primarily due to the willingness of many of these families to participate and to follow-up phone calls to families to encourage the return of the questionnaires.

The questionnaires

The measures included in this pilot study focused exclusively on parental and family factors with the exception of one measure related to the child's characteristics. The measures of interest included life stress and stresses associated with the handicapped child, attitudes toward parenting and child-rearing, maternal characteristics, social support networks, and the family environment.

Stress. The measures of stress included the Life Experiences Survey (LES) (Sarason, Johnson, & Siegel, 1978), a measure of general life stress that specifically focuses on negative life change, a factor frequently associated with various adverse psychological effects; and the QRS-F (Friedrich, Greenberg, & Crnic, 1983), a short form of the Questionnaire on Resources and Stress. The QRS-F provides four indices of stress related to handicapped children, including parental problems, parental pessimism, child characteristics, and physical incapacitation.

Parental attitudes. The Satisfaction with Parenting Scale (SWPS) (Crnic et al., 1983) and Cohler's Maternal Attitude Scale (MAS) (Cohler, Weiss, & Grunebaum, 1970) were completed by the mothers. The SWPS provides an index of maternal satisfaction with parenting role (such as child-care chores) and satisfaction with the child, while the MAS assesses child-rearing philosophy across three dimensions: appropriate control of aggression, encouragement of reciprocity, and acceptance of emotional complexity.

Maternal characteristics. Berger's Scale for Expressed Acceptance of Self was completed by the mothers. This is a 36-item self-concept scale in which the mother rates statements on a 5-point scale from *True of Myself* to *Not at all True of Myself* (e.g., ''I don't question my worth as a person, even if I think others do''). Mothers' general life satisfaction (GLS) was assessed with a single-item 5-point rating scale used in several previous research studies (Crnic et al., 1983). This measure provides an index of how good or bad mothers feel about their present life situation on the whole and is not solely related to parenting.

Social support networks. Mothers completed a 16-item questionnaire on social support development by Crnic et al. (1983). This measure assesses support across three ecological levels (intimate relationships, friendships, neighborhood/community involvement) and along two dimensions (availability or amount of support and satisfaction with availability or amount of support). The measure provides scores for each support index as well as a total support score.

Family environment. The Family Environment Scale (FES) (Moos, 1974) was also included in the protocol to provide a measure of perceived family style along 10 dimensions of family functioning (cohesiveness, expressiveness, conflict, independence, achievement orientation, intellectual–cultural orientation, active–recreational orientation, moral–religious emphasis, organization, and control). This measure basically describes a family's psychological orientation and functioning as a system.

Study findings

The basic questions of interest in this study involved the relationships between stress and the various factors involved in parental and family functioning, relationships between maternal self-concept and family factors, and relationships between social support indices and the family factors. Although regression equations would have been preferred as a data analytic technique, the sample size was too small to allow for confidence in such techniques. As such, partial correlations were computed controlling for mothers' age and education. Age and education were chosen as covariates as both factors were related to a number of the maternal and family variables measured.

Stress and family status. Interestingly, mothers of the Down syndrome children reported generally low life stress, and only moderate degrees of stress associated with the child. The only exception was on the parental problems index of stress

Table 12.1. *Partial correlations between life stress, child-related stresses, and indices of parental and family functioning*

	LES	QRS-F		
	Negative life stress	Parent problems	Pessimism	Child characteristics
SWPS	−.07	−.57***	−.40**	−.43**
GLS	−.49**	−.13	−.01	−.26+
MAS:				
Control of aggression	−.50**	−.32*	−.09	−.25+
Encourage reciprocity	−.18	−.12	−.05	−.18
Acceptance of complexity	−.14	−.33*	−.06	−.02
Intimate support	−.12	.03	−.01	−.20
Friendship support	−.08	.13	.18	−.11
Community support	−.17	−.15	−.12	−.30*
Total support	−.11	.07	.12	−.17
FES:				
Cohesion	−.13	.09	−.07	−.30*
Expressiveness	−.05	.12	−.08	−.11
Conflict	.05	−.15	.06	.13
Independence	−.06	.07	−.15	−.31*
Achievement	−.33*	.11	−.08	.06
Intellectual/cultural	−.24+	.12	.27+	−.08
Moral/religious	.45**	−.08	.22	.19
Organization	−.04	.28*	.37*	.19
Control	.24+	.01	.36*	.13
Maternal self-concept	−.58***	.01	−.06	−.30*

Note: $^+p<.08$; $^*p<.05$; $^{**}p<.01$; $^{***}p<.001$.

from the QRS-F, which had a relatively high mean score ($\chi = 11.3$; $SD = 4.7$; total possible score of 20).

Table 12.1 presents the partial correlations between the stress factors and the measures of parental and family functioning. Physical incapacitation was omitted as this was not a variable of concern to these families. As expected, both negative life stress and the stress associated with having a child with Down syndrome produced significant relationships with various aspects of parental and family functioning. Interestingly, the varying types of stress are differentially related to aspects of parent and family functioning. Life stress was not related to satisfaction with parenting, although the stresses associated with the child with Down syndrome were. Conversely, child-related stresses had generally little relation to maternal life satisfaction or self-concept, whereas life stress produced strong relationships to these maternal characteristics. In addition, life stress was related to a lower achievement orientation in families and a greater moral–religious orientation, whereas child stresses were related to neither of these family attributes. These findings support earlier suggestions about the need to assess stress along a number of dimensions in these families (Crnic, Friedrich, & Greenberg, 1983), as stresses other than those related to the handicapped child impact parent and family status. Measuring life stress, then, serves a control function in relation to the stress associated with the child with Down syndrome.

Differential relationships are also apparent between the QRS-F subscales and the parent and family factors, although they are somewhat less dramatic. The stress associated with child characteristics produced the greatest number of significant relationships, generally indicating that the more severe the child's impairments and the subsequent stress perceived by the mother, the less optimal were the parenting and family characteristics in general. Relationships for stresses of parent problems and pessimism were similar in nature, especially for mothers' satisfaction with parenting.

Intriguing also is the lack of significant relationships between the various stress factors and the social support measures. Only 1 of 16 possible correlations reached significance, and one has to entertain the possibility of that effect occurring by chance. Yet the lone relationship apparent – a negative correlation between the stress associated with child characteristics and perceived social support from community and neighborhood sources – certainly makes sense. The more deviant the child's characteristics and perceived parental stress over them, the less likely the family will be to engage in community or neighborhood events or feel easily accepted into them. They may also relate to the concept of perceived stigma of the handicap. Further delineation of such relationships will depend upon larger and more sophisticated investigations.

In summary, it is apparent that both intrafamilial and extrafamilial stress bear significant negative relationships to various intrafamilial characteristics of families of Down syndrome children, and perhaps to some extent extrafamilial community relationships. These findings corroborate much of the earlier work by Holroyd (Holroyd & McArthur, 1976), Friedrich and Friedrich (1981), and Mink et al. (1983) with other populations of retarded and handicapped children and further extend the implications of stress to novel measures of parenting satisfaction, general life satisfaction, mothers' self-concept, and perceived social support. Certainly, both intrafamilial and extrafamilial sources of stress are important parameters in the functional status of families with Down syndrome children and require attention in further studies.

Maternal characteristics. Two specific measures of mothers' psychological well-being were general life satisfaction and self-concept. Belsky's (1984) model of the determinants of parenting as well as the Crnic et al. (1983) model of familial adaptation, predict that parental personality characteristics are one major determinant of these processes within families, so measures of life satisfaction and self-concept

Table 12.2. *Partial correlations of maternal characteristics with indices of parental and family functioning*

	Maternal characteristics	
Parental and family factors	GLS	Self-concept
SWPS	.42**	.25$^+$
MAS:		
Control of aggression	.38*	.42**
Encourage reciprocity	.21	.34**
Acceptance of complexity	.09	−.07
Intimate support	.13	.28$^+$
Friendship support	.38*	.36*
Community support	.40**	.19
Total support	.41**	.39**
FES:		
Cohesion	.27$^+$	.38*
Expressiveness	.25$^+$	.31*
Conflict	−.15	−.14
Independence	.30*	.42**
Achievement	−.21	−.20
Intellectual/cultural	.21	.27$^+$
Moral/religious	−.16	−.20
Organization	.18	.08
Control	−.16	−.40**
GLS	—	.53***
Self-concept	.53***	—

Note: $^+ p < .08$; $* p < .05$; $** p < .01$; $*** p < .001$.

should relate to the adequacy of family functioning. Table 12.2 presents the relevant partial correlations between these maternal characteristics and the intra- and extra-familial indices of parental and family status in this Down syndrome population.

As predicted, both mothers' GLS and self-concept were significantly related to maternal parenting satisfaction and child-rearing attitudes, a number of the family environment subscales, and to the extrafamilial social support variables. Likewise, the GLS and self-concept factors showed a significant positive relationship with each other. Maternal self-concept would appear to be a more powerful predictor of parental and family status as the relationships were more frequent and generally stronger for this factor in these families of Down syndrome children. The relationships are particularly striking in regard to the FES factors, as mothers of Down syndrome children who have generally strong self-concepts perceive their families as more highly oriented to positive emotional relationships between members and much less involved in control of members. These findings are consistent with those of Mink et al.'s (1983) report of their families of Down syndrome children, and support the earlier theoretical formulations of Belsky (1984) and Crnic, Friedrich, & Greenberg (1983) suggesting that maternal personality characteristics are important determinants of parenting and family factors. Of additional interest are the relationships between maternal characteristics and the social support factors, and these will be discussed in the following section.

Social support as an extrafamilial context. As with maternal characteristics, perceived social support of mothers of Down syndrome children has been proposed as a factor relevant to competent parenting (Belsky, 1984) and as an influential ecological context and major coping resource for families of retarded children (Crnic, Friedrich, & Greenberg, 1983). The data from this small sample of families of Down syndrome children, however, provide only partial support for these notions.

As can be seen in Table 12.2, the support indices and particularly friendship, community, and total support had significant positive relationships with measures of maternal life satisfaction and self-concept. Community support was positively related to mothers' satisfaction with parenting their Down syndrome child ($r = .36$, $p < .05$), but no other significant relationships were found between any of the support variables and the SWPS and MAS factors. Similarly, none of the individual support indices were significantly related to any of the FES factors, although the total social support index was positively related to the FES factors of Cohesion ($r = .35, p < .05$) and Expressiveness ($r = .31, p < .05$).

It seems apparent that within these families of Down syndrome children, social network support has only specific direct relationships with a limited number of intrafamilial factors, such as maternal satisfaction with parenting, life satisfaction, self-concept, and, to some extent, family status, all of which nonetheless are in the predicted positive direction. It is impossible to conclude that greater social support influences such positive maternal responses, as correlational evidence allows no causal inference. Further, it has been well argued in numerous other literatures that more competent persons may enlist greater support networks, and this hypothesis must be entertained for these families as well. Nevertheless, it is plausible to propose that social support networks are indeed important determinants of parental response in families of Down syndrome children.

The failure to find specific relationships between the individual support indices and the FES factors was somewhat surprising, as data from other studies of various risk populations suggest that such relationships may well exist (Crnic et al., 1984; Friedrich, 1979; Mink et al., 1983; Suelze & Keenan, 1981). Although the failure to find direct relationships in this pilot study does not preclude the possibility that such relationships will be apparent in later, more sophisticated studies, several interpretations of the current findings are worthy of note. First, there was little variability within this sample on the FES factors, and the scores on the factors indicated that mothers perceived their families as well functioning, low in conflict and control, and not extreme in any particular interest or pursuit. This general lack of variability may have inhibited relationships that would be apparent in larger samples of families of Down syndrome children. Additionally, it may well be that the effect of social network support systems on these families is more indirect than direct, and is perhaps mediated through other variables related to the family context. For example, mothers with greater support from various social sources reported greater life satisfaction and self-concepts, and these factors in turn were significantly related to a number of the family status factors of the FES. In this way, maternal life satisfaction and self-concept may function to mediate the influence of social network support on the family system of Down syndrome children resulting in indirect influences. Future studies utilizing path analysis models can address this possibility more specifically.

Summary and conclusions

In this chapter, I have attempted to detail a theoretical rationale for studying intra- and extrafamilial ecological contexts of families of Down syndrome children as well as to provide a succinct review of the relevant studies of family ecologies of normal and handicapped children. Certainly, previous research has established the validity of this approach, and the potential explanatory power of ecological models has been clearly detailed for both normal (Belsky, 1984; Bronfenbrenner, 1977) and handicapped (Crnic, Friedrich, & Greenberg, 1983) populations.

The data from the small pilot project presented here, however, have a number of important limitations that should be kept in mind. First, the small sample size and lack of variability on some measures limit the power of the findings as well as the generalizability. It may well be that the results reported from this sample are specific to this sample only and may not apply to other families of Down syndrome children. Second, no control data with other populations of handicapped, risk, or normal children were included. This is an important consideration because without other control groups, it is impossible to know whether the data reported here are specific to Down syndrome families. However, given the nature of this project as a pilot study to provide a context for more elaborate future studies, the findings do suggest that further study may prove fruitful. A final limitation involves the lack of specific measures related to the development and behavior of the Down syndrome children themselves. This precluded the possibility of assessing the impact of the ecological context on the developmental functioning of the children – clearly an issue of great interest and importance.

These limitations notwithstanding, the data from this study are suggestive of important intra- and extrafamilial relationships within families of Down syndrome children that have not been previously explored. In many respects, these families of Down syndrome children appear to be quite positive and functional. Scores on the measures of life stress, parenting satisfaction, general life satisfaction, and family environment are comparable to the scores obtained in other studies of families of normal children using the same measures (e.g., Crnic & Greenberg, 1987). This corresponds with the similar report of Mink et al. (1983), who likewise found greater proportions of Down syndrome families in the more positive and functional clusters of families of handicapped children. The generally functional quality of these families suggests that the intrafamilial context of Down syndrome families is distinctly different from families of other non-Down syndrome retarded children who appear to exhibit greater dysfunction (Crnic, Friedrich, & Greenberg, 1983), and families of children who are not retarded but are at-risk for various developmental problems (Crnic & Greenberg, 1984; Mink, Nihira, & Meyers, 1983).

Why families of Down syndrome children are distinct from other families of handicapped children is an empirical question, yet several interpretations are plausible beyond Mink et al.'s (1983) suggestion that these children have a positive impact on families. First, Down syndrome children can be identified at birth, which provides the benefit of developmental and familial intervention from early infancy, and these families begin the adaptational process earlier than families whose handicapped children are not identified until late infancy or preschool years. Spiker (Chapter 13, this volume) has well detailed how these early intervention programs influence parents and families. Second, the major developmental parameters of the syndrome are well known, as is the etiology, which reduces the impact of issues such as long-term predictability of developmental course, parental expectations for development, and parental feelings of guilt. These are issues that clinicians frequently face with families of retarded or developmentally delayed children, as the lack of knowledge and predictability create additive stresses within families of these children. Also, as Down syndrome children share the unique constellation of physical characteristics and developmental difficulties, these families have a readily identifiable peer group and are often involved in support groups of other families with Down syndrome children from early infancy (again, see Spiker, Chapter 13, this volume).

Despite the apparently distinct ecologies of Down syndrome families, the data from this study suggest that they experience added stresses associated with the presence of the child that do adversely impact parental and family functioning. This suggests that Mink et al.'s (1984) conclusion that these children have a positive impact on the family may not be entirely correct. Further, stress, various parental characteristics, and extrafamilial social contexts are differentially related to positive or negative aspects of familial functioning through either direct or indirect paths. The differential nature of these relationships is important, as it underlines the need to examine a multiplicity of factors that can potentially influence these families in various ways. The stress relationships to family factors demonstrate this most clearly, as life stress that is generally unrelated to the Down syndrome child impacts the intra- and extrafamilial context in ways quite distinct from those affected by the stresses associated with the child. It was also apparent that within families of Down syndrome children, social support from friends and community was more relevant to maternal and family status than was support from a spouse. This finding is clearly different from other studies of handicapped children (Friedrich, 1979) and normal and at-risk children (Crnic et al., 1983) that emphasize the role of the marital relationship and spouse as a source of major support for parenting and the parent–child relationship. Perhaps intimate support sources are less influential than either friendships or community sources once children reach later preschool years, because families increase their external involvements as children grow older and increase the family's social networks through their own peer and school involvements (Crnic et al., 1984). It may also be that spouses become less influential in populations of Down syndrome children as the child grows older and the family has had an extended period to adapt. Once the family unit becomes organized and mobilized in regard to the presence of the Down syndrome child, the more extrafamilial sources of friendships and community relationships take on greater significance. Obviously, we need to attend further to such possibilities in future work. Yet such relationships strongly suggest transactional processes operating within the family context of children with Down syndrome that are likely to influence the developmental process.

It is also important to stress the potential indirect pathways of influence that may operate within families of Down syndrome children. The earlier suggestion that friendships and community support networks may indirectly impact family status as mediated through their impact on maternal characteristics (and perhaps paternal and child characteristics as well) is but one example of such possibilities. The absence of specific direct effects of extrafamilial factors, then, does not obviate the fact that they may yet be influential within the family context, and our future research designs with families of Down syndrome children must allow for such possibilities. Identifying the indirect pathways of influence of these ecological factors is likely to be a difficult and complex task, yet one necessary to understand the transaction of context and person.

In sum, it does appear that the adaptation of families of Down syndrome children and their subsequent functioning along a number of dimensions is related to the perceived stress involved with and external to the Down syndrome child, which is subsequently moderated by various coping resources available to the family from both intrafamilial and extrafamilial sources (e.g., mothers' well-being, beliefs, social supports). These findings, however, only begin to illuminate the issues raised at the beginning of this chapter. A good deal more research is needed to broaden our understanding of and confidence in the relationships found in this study. Within the context of this chapter, the issues raised and the rather meager data presented are meant to be a catalyst and perhaps a stimulus to further and more sophisticated research.

There are still numerous questions to be asked and the direction of future research in this area to be decided. If, indeed, additional and more sophisticated research substantiates that families of Down syndrome children are unique compared to families of handicapped or other risk populations, we must try to answer why these families differ and what factors might account for such differences. Are these differences stable across age levels of the Down syndrome children, being present at birth and continuing through childhood and adolescence? Do these differences have implications for the long-term developmental and behavioral outcomes for Down syndrome children? Do these differences impact service resource allocation and families' use of available resources, and do these resources in turn promote continued more positive adaptational patterns? What are the factors that might account for individual variation in developmental process within groups of families of Down syndrome children, and are these the same factors responsible for between group differences in Down syndrome and families of other handicapped children? These complex questions will require similarly complex and comprehensive research strategies to answer. Studies directed at explicating these processes must, however, have a clearly developmental focus if the research is to add to our understanding.

Clearly, more comprehensive data on the ecologies of families of Down syndrome children is needed, and can be accomplished by research designs such as that employed by Mink et al. (1984). Combined cross-sectional and longitudinal designs should also be informative in delineating the potential effects of age and development on the family context of Down syndrome children. The strategy that should prove most effective, however, will be one employing a prospective, longitudinal and cross-sectional design following families of Down syndrome children from identification of the syndrome through adolescence or further. The addition of other handicap controls and normal controls should allow the multitude of issues mentioned above to be addressed. Such a design has its own limitations, to be sure (it's very expensive, and family attrition is a problem), but the effort may well prove worth the trouble. The continued need for longitudinal studies is great, and their value will be immeasurable in understanding the process of development.

Regardless of design methodology, future studies must be multidimensional in measurement. The children and families must be assessed in context, which will require attention to ecological variables across the spectrum of settings likely to influence them. We should consider just what the ecologies of these families are and what they encompass. These ecologies may include special school settings, service agencies, specific support groups, nonspecific friendships or acquaintances with other families with handicapped children and families without handicapped children, sibling social networks, contacts within extended families, day-care settings, community and neighborhood involvements, and aspects of these families' status within society in general. If we are to develop a comprehensive model of child development and family functioning, one that applies to Down syndrome, other handicaps, and nonhandicapped groups as well, then we must attend to issues of the child within the family system and the family within the greater social system. Acquiring such knowledge will be to the benefit of all children and families regardless of developmental status.

References

Affleck, G., McGrade, B., Allen, D., & McQueeney, M. (1983). Maternal and child characteristics associated with the mothers' perceptions of their high risk/developmentally delayed infants. *Journal of Genetic Psychology, 142,* 171–180.

Beckman, P. J. (1983). The influence of selected child characteristics on stress in families of handicapped infants. *American Journal of Mental Deficiency, 88,* 150–156.

Belsky, J. (1981). Early human experience: A family perspective. *Developmental Psychology, 17,* 3–23.

Belsky, J. (1984). The determinants of parenting: A process model. *Child Development, 55,* 83–96.

Bronfenbrenner, U. (1977). Toward an experimental ecology of human development. *American Psychologist, 32,* 513–531.

Bronfenbrenner, U. (1979). Context of child-rearing. *American Psychologist, 34,* 844–850.

Bronfenbrenner, U., & Crouter, A. C. (1983). The evolution of environmental models in developmental research. In W. Kessen (Ed.), *History, theories and methods.* Vol. 1 of P. H. Mussen (Ed.), *Handbook of child psychology* (4th ed.), New York: Wiley.

Caldwell, B. M., & Guze, S. B. (1960). A study of the adjustment of parents and siblings of institutionalized and non-institutionalized retarded children. *American Journal of Mental Deficiency, 64,* 845–861.

Cicchetti, D. (1984). The emergence of developmental psychopathology. *Child Development, 55,* 1–7.

Cicchetti, D. & Pogge-Hesse, P. (1982). Possible contributions of the study of organically retarded persons to developmental theory. In E. Zigler & D. Balla (Eds.), *Mental retardation: The developmental–difference controversy.* Hillsdale, NJ: Erlbaum.

Cochran, M. M., & Brassard, J. A. (1979). Child development and personal social networks. *Child Development, 50,* 601–616.

Cohler, C., Weiss, J., & Grunebaum, H. (1970). Child care attitudes and emotional disturbance among mothers of young children. *Genetic Psychology Monographs, 82,* 3–47.

Colletta, N. (1981). Social support and the risk of maternal rejection by adolescent mothers. *Journal of Psychology, 109,* 191–197.

Colletta, N. (1983). At risk for depression: A study of young mothers. *Journal of Genetic Psychology, 142,* 301–310.

Cook, J. J. (1963). Dimensional analysis of child-rearing attitudes of parents of handicapped children. *American Journal of Mental Deficiency, 68,* 354–361.

Crnic, K. A., Friedrich, W. N., & Greenberg, M. T. (1983). Adaptation of families with mentally retarded children: A model of stress, coping, and family ecology. *American Journal of Mental Deficiency, 88,* 125–138.

Crnic, K. A., & Greenberg, M. T. (1987). Transactional relationships between family style, risk status, and mother–child interactions in two year olds. *Journal of Pediatric Psychology, 12*(3), 343–362.

Crnic, K. A., Greenberg, M. T., Ragozin, A. S., Robinson, N. M., & Basham, R. (1983). Effects of stress and social support on mothers and premature and full-term infants. *Child Development, 54,* 209–217.

Crnic, K. A., Greenberg, M. T., Robinson, N. M., & Ragozin, A. S. (1984). Maternal stress and social support: Effects on the mother–infant relationship from birth to eighteen months. *American Journal of Orthopsychiatry, 54,* 224–235.

Crockenberg, S. B. (1987). Support for adolescent mothers during the postnatal period: Theory and research. In Z. Boukydis (Ed.), *Research on support for parents and infants in the postnatal period.* Norwood, NJ: Ablex.

Cummings, S., Bayley, H., & Rie, H. (1966). Effects of the child's deficiency on the mother: A study of mothers of mentally retarded, chronically ill and neurotic children. *American Journal of Orthopsychiatry, 36,* 595–608.

Erickson, M. T. (1968). MMPI comparisons between parents of young emotionally disturbed and organically retarded children. *Journal of Consulting and Clinical Psychology, 32,* 701–706.

Erickson, M. T. (1969). MMPI profiles of parents of young retarded children. *American Journal of Mental Deficiency, 73,* 728–732.

Farber, B. (1959). Effects of a severely mentally retarded child on family integration. *Monographs of the Society for Research in Child Development, 24* (Whole No. 71).

Farber, B. (1960). Family organization and crisis: Maintenance of integration in families with a severely retarded child. *Monographs of the Society for Research in Child Development, 25,* 1–95.

Farber, B. (1963). Interaction with retarded siblings and life goals of children. *Marriage and Family Living, 25,* 96–98.

Farber, B. (1968). *Mental retardation: Its social context and social consequences.* Boston: Houghton Mifflin.

Farber, B. (1970). Notes on sociological knowledge about families with mentally retarded children. In M. Schreiber (Ed.), *Social work and mental retardation.* New York: John Day.

Ferrara, D. M. (1979). Attitudes of parents of mentally retarded children toward normalization activities. *American Journal of Mental Deficiency, 84,* 145–151.

Field, T. (1980). Interaction of high risk infants: Quantitative and qualitative differences. In D. Sawin, R. Hawking, L. Walker, & J. Penticuff (Eds.), *Exceptional infant,* Vol. 4: Psychosocial risks in infant–environment transactions. New York: Brunner/Mazel.

Fowle, C. M. (1968). The effect of a severely mentally retarded child on his family. *American Journal of Mental Deficiency, 73,* 468–473.

Friedrich, W. N. (1979). Predictors of the coping behavior of mothers of handicapped children. *Journal of Consulting and Clinical Psychology, 47,* 1140–1141.

Friedrich, W. N., & Friedrich, W. L. (1981). Comparison of psychosocial assets of parents with a handicapped child and their normal controls. *American Journal of Mental Deficiency, 85,* 551–553.

Friedrich, W. N., Greenberg, M. T., & Crnic, K. A. (1983). A short form of the Questionnaire on Resources and Stress. *American Journal of Mental Deficiency, 88,* 41–48.

Gath, A. (1973). The school-age siblings of mongol children. *British Journal of Psychiatry, 123,* 161–167.

Goffman, E. (1963). *Stigma.* Englewood Cliffs, NJ: Prentice-Hall.

Greenberg, M. T., & Crnic, K. A. (1988). Longitudinal predictors of developmental status and social interaction in premature and full term infants at age two. *Child Development, 59,* 554–570.

Grossman, F. K. (1972). *Brothers and sisters of retarded children: An exploratory study.* Syracuse, NY: Syracuse University Press.

Hoffman, L. W. (1983). Work, family, and the socialization of the child. In R. D. Parke (Ed.), *Review of child development research,* Vol. 7: *The family.* Chicago: University of Chicago Press.

Holroyd, J. (1974). The Questionnaire on Resources and Stress: An instrument to measure family response to a handicapped family member. *Journal of Community Psychology, 2,* 92–94.

Holroyd, J., Brown, N., Wikler, L., & Simons, H. (1975). Stress in families of institutionalized and noninstitutionalized autistic children. *Journal of Community Psychology, 3,* 26–31.

Holroyd, J., & Guthrie, D. (1979). Stress in families with neuromuscular disease. *Journal of Clinical Psychology, 35,* 734–739.

Holroyd, J., & McArthur, D. (1976). Mental retardation and stress on the parents: A contrast between Down's syndrome and childhood autism. *American Journal of Mental Deficiency, 80,* 431–436.

Kammerman, S. B., & Hayes, C. D. (Eds.). (1982). *Families that work.* Washington, DC: National Academy Press.

Landman, S. H. (1979) A study of the relationship between parental overprotectiveness and the achievement of selected life skills among mildly retarded adolescents. *Dissertation Abstracts International.*

Maccoby, E. E., & Martin, J. A. (1983) Socialization in the context of the family: Parent–child interaction. In E. M. Hetherington (Ed.), *Socialization, personality, and social development,* Vol. 4 of P. H. Mussen (Ed.), *Handbook of child psychology* (4th ed.). New York: Wiley.

Mercer, R. T., Hackley, K. C., & Bostrom, A. (1983) Social support of teenage mothers. *Birth Defects: Original Articles Series.*

Miller, S. G. (1974). An exploratory study of sibling relationships in families with retarded children. *Dissertation Abstracts International, 35,* 2994B–2995B. (University Microfilms No. 74-26, 606).

Miller, W. H., & Keirn, W. C. (1978). Personality measurement in parents of retarded and emotionally disturbed children: A replication. *Journal of Clinical Psychology, 34,* 686–690.

Mink, I. T., Nihira, K., & Meyers, C. E. (1983). Taxonomy of family lifestyles: I. Homes with TMR children. *American Journal of Mental Deficiency, 87,* 484–497.

Mink, I. T., Meyers, C. E., & Nihira, K. (in press). A taxonomy of family lifestyles: II. Homes with slow learning children. *American Journal of Mental Deficiency*.

Moos, R. H. (1974) *Preliminary Manual for the Family Environment Scale*. Palo Alto, CA: Consulting Psychologists Press.

Mortimer, J. T., Lorence, J., & Kumka, D. (1983). Work and family linkages in the transition to adulthood: A panel study of highly educated men. *Western Sociological Review*.

Mott, P. E., Mann, F. C., McLoughlin, Q., & Warwick, D. P. (1965) *Shift work: The social, psychological, and physical consequences*. Ann Arbor: University of Michigan Press.

Nihira, K., Meyers, C. E., & Mink, I. T. (1980). Home environment, family adjustment, and the development of mentally retarded children. *Applied Research in Mental Retardation, 1*, 5–24.

Nihira, K., Mink, I. T. & Meyers, C. E. (1981). Relationship between home environment and school adjustment of TMR children. *American Journal of Mental Deficiency, 86*, 8–15.

Passaminick, B., & Knobloch, H. (1961). Epidemiologic studies on the complications of pregnancy and the birth process. In G. Gaplan (Ed.), *Prevention of mental disorders in children*. New York: Basic.

Pfouts, J. H. (1976) The sibling relationship: a forgotten dimension. *Social Work, 21*, 200–204.

Ricci, C. S. (1970) Analysis of child-rearing attitudes of mothers of mentally retarded, emotionally disturbed, and normal children. *American Journal of Mental Deficiency, 74*, 756–761.

Sameroff, A., & Chandler, M. (1975). Reproductive risk and the continuum of caretaking casualty. In F. D. Horowitz, M. Hetherington, S. Scarr-Salapatek, & G. Siegel (Eds.), *Review of Child Development Research* (Vol. 4). Chicago: University of Chicago Press.

Sameroff, A., & Seifer, R. (1983). Familial risk and child competence. *Child Development, 54*, 1254–1268.

Sarason, I. G., Johnson, J. H., & Siegel, J. M. (1978). Assessing the impact of life changes: Development of the Life Experiences Survey. *Journal of Consulting and Clinical Psychology, 45*, 932–946.

Skeels, H. M. (1966). Adult status of children with contrasting early life experiences: A follow-up study. *Monographs of the Society for Research in Child Development, 31* (Serial No. 77).

Spiker, D. (1982). Parent involvement in early intervention activities with their children with Down syndrome. *Education and Training of the Mentally Retarded, 17*, 24–29.

Strom, R., Rees, R., Slaughter, H., & Wurster, S. (1981). Childrearing expectations of families with atypical children. *American Journal of Orthopsychiatry, 51*, 285–296.

Suelzle, M., & Keenan, V. (1981). Changes in family support networks over the life cycle of mentally retarded persons. *American Journal of Orthopsychiatry, 51*, 285–296.

Tew, B. J., & Laurence, K. M. (1975). Some sources of stress found in mothers of spina bifida children. *British Journal of Preventive and Social Medicine, 29*, 27–30.

Tietjen, A. M., & Bradley, C. F. (1982). *Social networks, social support and transition to parenthood*. Unpublished paper. University of British Columbia, Vancouver, Division of Family Studies.

Tulkin, S. R. (1973a). Social class differences in infants' reactions to mother's and stranger's voices. *Developmental Psychology, 8*(1), 137.

Tulkin, S. R. (1973b). Social class differences in attachment behaviors of ten-month-old infants. *Child Development, 44*(1), 171–174.

Tulkin, S. R., & Covitz, F. E. (1975). *Mother–infant interaction and intellectual functioning at age six*. Paper presented at the meeting of the Society for Research in Child Development, Denver, April.

Tulkin, S. R., & Kagan, J. (1972). Mother–child interaction in the first year of life. *Child Development, 43*, 31–41.

Vadasy, P. F., Fewell, R. R., Meyer, D. J., Schell, G., & Greenberg, M. T. (1984). Involved parents: Characteristics and resources of fathers and mothers of young handicapped children. *Journal of the Division of Early Childhood, 8*, 13–25.

Waisbren, S. E. (1980). Parents' reactions after the birth of a developmentally disabled child. *American Journal of Mental Deficiency, 84*, 345–351.

Wandersman, L. P., & Unger, D. G. (1983). *Interaction of infant difficulty and social support in adolescent mothers*. Paper presented at the biennial meeting of the Society for Research in Child Development, Detroit, April.

Watson, R. L., & Midlarsky, E. (1979). Reactions of mothers with mentally retarded children: A social perspective. *Psychological Reports, 45,* 309–310.

Weinraub, M., & Wolf, B. M. (1983). Effects of stress and social supports on mother–child interactions in single- and two-parent families. *Child Development, 54,* 1294–1311.

Werner, E. E., & Smith, R. S. (1982). *Vulnerable but invincible: A longitudinal study of resilient children and youth.* New York: McGraw-Hill.

Zuk, G. H. (1959). Religious factors and the role of guilt in parental acceptance of the retarded child. *American Journal of Mental Deficiency, 64,* 139–147.

Zuk, G. H., Miller, R. L., Bartram, J. B., & Kling, F. (1961). Maternal acceptance of retarded children: A questionnaire study of attitudes and religious background. *Child Development, 32,* 525–540.

13 Early intervention from a developmental perspective

Donna Spiker

Introduction

Strictly speaking, the notion of a developmental perspective in the field of mental retardation applies to the developmental–difference controversy associated with Zigler (Zigler & Balla, 1982). Its major emphasis is on understanding the development of nonorganically impaired individuals with mental retardation. Cicchetti & Pogge-Hesse (1982) have adopted a more "liberal" developmental perspective to explicate the early development of infants and preschoolers with Down syndrome. Rather than summarize their excellent reviews of the issues in this area, this chapter will draw upon their work to provide the definitional framework for approaching the topic of intervention strategies for individuals with Down syndrome from a developmental perspective.

After a summary of some of the definitional issues, a brief history of early intervention programs will be presented. This history will show that social, political, and child development research factors influenced the emergence and proliferation of early intervention programs for infants and preschoolers with Down syndrome. A review of early intervention programs for infants and preschoolers with Down syndrome will follow and will include discussion of basic developmental research findings on Down syndrome that have influenced the design of these programs (or might be considered more seriously in the future). The links between the goals of early intervention programs and the goals for the later development of children with Down syndrome are summarized in the conclusion.

For purposes of this chapter, a developmental perspective toward intervention refers to an approach toward programming decisions based on developmental theory and research. Every intervention program must adopt a set of working assumptions to make decisions about the "who, what, why, when, where, and how" of the program's objectives and its strategies to accomplish them. The historical review that follows will show that a developmental approach toward intervention with chil-

Special thanks go to Daniel Harris and Cindy Duenas for excellent word processing of drafts on this chapter. This chapter is dedicated to Chris Hebein.

424

dren with Down syndrome is a relatively new phenomenon. A developmental approach suggests that the objectives of intervention should focus on promoting optimal functioning in basic areas of development (e.g., cognition, language, social–emotional development, motor development, etc.). Attention should be paid to the timing and the context (social and physical) of activities. This is based on the assumption that development proceeds in an orderly sequence of stages that is supported by the appropriate match between the developing child and characteristics of the social and physical environment. This is what is meant by the concept of "readiness."

Also involved in the concept of "readiness" is the assumption that there are significant relationships between different areas of development. Such interrelationships will affect decisions about program objectives and activities. For example, an infant with Down syndrome with significant gross motor delays may be limiting its ability for continued growth in other areas of development because of its reduced locomotor ability (see Gustafson, 1984). Similarly, an understanding of the links between the emergence of a mature object concept and certain prelinguistic skills should help inform decisions about the types and sequence of program activities.

Cicchetti & Pogge-Hesse (1982) have suggested that the early development of infants with Down syndrome should be approached from an organizational perspective. This means examining the developmental *process*. It involves providing a description of the developmental sequencing of stages, their hierarchical organization and consolidation, explanations for stage transitions and for organization across developmental domains. While such a broad perspective presents many challenges for basic research on Down syndrome, it presents even more significant challenges for those interested in designing early intervention programs.

A brief history of early intervention

A history of early intervention programs for infants and young children with Down syndrome requires describing social and political events surrounding the development of early intervention programs in general. The idea of early education of young children outside the family existed in the United States in the form of nursery schools for normally developing children early in this century. However, the enormous proliferation of programs began in the 1960s (Clarke-Stewart & Fein, 1983).

The War on Poverty gave birth to the Head Start movement, which sought to improve the development of socially disadvantaged preschoolers. More specifically, it sought to provide them with early structured experiences aimed at improving their long-range school achievement (Zigler & Valentine, 1979). This ambitious movement was an outgrowth of several prior historical developments. Socially and politically, the 1960s represented a period of important change in this country's attitudes toward the poor, blacks, and the handicapped. The civil rights movement, the trauma of the Vietnam war, the birth of the community mental health and its resultant trend toward deinstitutionalization, all contributed to an increase in social programs (including early intervention programs). This movement was based on optimism about improving the lot of less privileged and less competent members of the society.

In terms of programs for infants and young children, it is fair to conclude that the emergence of these programs was influenced by the enormous increase in basic research on infants and young children. New infant research methodologies (e.g., Fantz, 1963) and an interest in early cognitive development (spurred by the introduction of Piaget's ideas brought to the United States by Flavell, 1963) served to promote the view that infants and young children were competent creatures capable of benefiting from properly structured early experiences (Caldwell, 1970). Thus, increased knowledge about infants coupled with a spirit of optimism about intervening to produce change, contributed to the beginning of the early intervention movement as we know it today.

It may be argued that the development of programs for young handicapped children was influenced by the Head Start movement, but it also was influenced by several other unique factors. Although many parents rejected the advice of physicians who recommended that they place their newborn with Down syndrome in an institution as soon as possible, before the 1960s there was little hope or optimism about the wisdom of such a decision. Only anecdotal reports about the possibility of favorable developmental growth in persons with Down syndrome reared at home were available (see Hunt, 1967, for an inspiring book by a young man with Down syndrome raised at home by his parents). With a decline in early institutionalization came an increasing interest and need for early programs for families who were deciding to raise their baby with Down syndrome at home. These families were confronted with dire predictions of very low levels of intellectual and behavioral functioning based on accounts of persons with Down syndrome reared in institutions (e.g., Johnson & Abelson, 1969).

Two of the first well-documented research and early intervention programs for infants with Down syndrome in the United States were carried out at the University of Washington (Hayden & Haring, 1976) and the University of Minnesota (Rynders & Horrobin, 1975). Both programs were comprehensive in their approach toward the total development of the children, with a special emphasis on early language stimulation, as this was seen as the most significant deficiency in these children. These programs began with home-visiting components aimed at teaching parents about ways to stimulate the baby's development, and moved to center-based formats as the children reached preschool age. Periodic developmental assessments and monitoring of major developmental milestones indicated that both programs were effective in enhancing the rate of development in the participants. As these and other early intervention programs continued to proliferate, researchers and educators began to take a closer look at the assumptions, objectives, and strategies underlying their programs.

The introduction of Public Law 94–142 in 1975, guaranteeing the right of all handicapped children to a free and appropriate education, served to reinforce further the acceptance of education and intervention with handicapped children (Public Law 94–142, 1976). It also signaled a growing trend of parents' involvement in the process of education and advocacy for their children (Bricker & Casuso, 1979), since a major factor in the passage of this important piece of legislation was the grassroots movement of parents. Interestingly, this latter development corresponds to a time in child development research when there was a growing interest in a general systems model of development (see review by Sameroff, 1983), a surge of research attention about parent–infant interaction and attachment (Ainsworth, 1979), and an expanded interest in how the family context (e.g., its life stresses, social networks, marital interactions, and harmony) relates to child development (Bronfenbrenner, 1979). These latter trends required us to expand our developmental perspective about intervention strategies. Theorists now discuss the individual development of the child as well as the development of the family in which the child is reared. Our view now includes consideration of the effects of normal transitions and stresses on families (McCubbin & Figley, 1983) and the special considerations involved in a family's adjustment and coping with a handicapped child (Arnold, 1978). The research review to follow considers the implications of a developmental perspective toward intervention from the point of view of the individual child and from its family context.

Early intervention programs for children with Down syndrome

History and the need for a developmental perspective

Before the emergence of early intervention programs for infants and young children with Down syndrome, there was a body of literature indicating that home-reared children were functioning significantly better than were children reared in institutions (e.g., Carr, 1970; Francis, 1971).

Based on results of some of the earliest programs, Rynders, Spiker, & Horrobin (1978) challenged the notion that children with Down syndrome are uneducable. There is now a substantial body of research to indicate that early intervention programs with infants and young children with Down syndrome can lead to improved developmental functioning (Aronson & Fallstrom, 1977; Bidder, Bryant, & Gray, 1975; Clunies-Ross, 1979; Connolly, Morgan, Russell, & Richardson, 1980; Connolly & Russell, 1976; Cullen, Cronk, Pueschel, Schnell, & Reed, 1981; Hanson, 1981; Hayden & Haring, 1976; Ludlow & Allen, 1979; Oelwein, Fewell, & Pruess, 1985; Rynders & Horrobin, 1975; Salzberg & Villani, 1983; Seitz & Terdal, 1972; Simeonsson, Cooper, & Scheiner, 1982). Several recent reviews summarize the effects of early intervention programs on infants with Down syndrome (Gibson & Fields, 1984; Hanson, 1981) and on these and other biologically impaired infants (Simeonsson, Cooper, & Scheiner, 1982) and will not be repeated here. The latter authors concluded that early intervention has been shown to be effective, although much of the support for it has lacked the rigorous statistical methodology that would provide the most convincing evidence for program effectiveness. This methodological skepticism about the significance of studies that have indicated that infants with Down syndrome who have participated in early intervention programs show in-

creases in developmental functioning and earlier attainment of developmental milestones is thoroughly explored by Gibson and Fields (1984). These authors carefully
review the published literature on 11 major early intervention programs for infants
with Down syndrome. They raise the following concerns (which will be elaborated
on in the paragraphs that follow: (1) lack of well-matched control groups; (2) use
of small, self-selected samples; (3) lack of long-term follow-up to establish dura-
bility of early developmental gains; (4) vague and/or inconsistent reporting of results; (5) "atheoretical-pragmatic approach" toward program design, especially the
lack of attention paid to biological–psychological relationships affecting development in children with Down syndrome. They conclude that the "clearest benefit"
of early intervention programs has been the "assistance, comfort, and remotiva-
tion" they provide for parents during the early years of their baby's life.

Gibson and Fields (1984) are especially skeptical about the long-range significance of early increases in rate of development for infants with Down syndrome.
Just as several studies have shown that there is notable variation in later tested
intelligence among children with Down syndrome (e.g., Clements, Bates & Hafer,
1976; Connolly, 1978), Clunies-Ross (1979) reported that there is considerable individual variation in the developmental progress of infants with Down syndrome
who participate in early programs; some infants make considerably more progress
than others. Aronson & Fallstrom (1977) reported that the gains made by many
infants with Down syndrome in early intervention programs are not maintained
unless there are carefully designed follow-through educational programs to continue
to support those gains. (This finding reminds us of the questionable impact on later
school achievement of a short-term early educational program for socially disadvantaged preschoolers in Head Start [Zigler & Valentine, 1979]).

Other reports also provide data on individual differences and program efficacy.
Cullen, Cronk, Pueschel, Schnell, & Reed (1981) found the Down syndrome infants with better muscle tone and mild or no cardiac problems achieved selected
developmental milestones earlier while in early intervention programs than did their
counterparts with these problems. Similarly, Mahoney & Snow (1983) reported that
the progress made by preschoolers with Down syndrome in a language-training
program was directly related to their cognitive and sensorimotor status before entering the training program. Such results suggest that variations in infants' biological–
developmental functioning and/or parents' responsiveness to those variations affect
program effectiveness. Gibson and Fields (1984) go even further to suggest that
most evaluation studies have failed to distinguish between developmental gains due
to the program curriculum and gains due to typical growth sustained by the care
from motivated parents. (Parent involvement is discussed in a later section.)

Instead of reaching pessimistic conclusions about their results, Mahoney and Snow
(1983) argue that their results suggest the need to train the youngsters on specific
pre-verbal communication or sensorimotor skills thought to be prerequisites for benefiting from a verbal training program. This insightful paper is a good example of
the developmental perspective that requires a closer look at the interrelationships
among different areas of development. By noting ways in which deficits in one area

of development may be hindering the acquisition of skills in another area, interventionists may make beneficial adjustments in program objectives and activities. Instead of assuming that a failure to advance the infant's development is a sign of an inherent deficiency in the infant, this developmental perspective advocates a closer look at the developmental prerequisites for a particular skill and seeks to identify the appropriate activities and context for promoting the prerequisites.

Program Objectives and Strategies

The idea that there are interrelationships among different areas of early development and that some skills are prerequisites or co-emergent skills for development in another area is a relatively new idea in basic developmental research. In particular, there is growing interest in the relationships between early cognitive, language, affective, and play development in normally developing children (Rubin, Fein, & Vandenberg, 1983). For example, Smolak (1982) reported that a minimum of Stage 5 object permanence skill was necessary before the onset of language production. McCune-Nicolich (1981) has shown that the early stages of symbolic play are related to early linguistic abilities. And Sroufe and Wunsch (1972) outlined a sequence of early affective behaviors following an orderly developmental sequence in normal infants that are closely linked to overall cognitive development.

Studies of this sort have led researchers studying Down syndrome to examine in close detail the process of early development in infants and young children with Down syndrome. For example, both Dunst & Rheingrover (1983) and Cicchetti and Mans-Wagener (1987) studied the performance of infants with Down syndrome on the Uzgiris–Hunt Ordinal Scales of Development. Both found a structure and sequence in the sensorimotor performance of these infants that was similar to that reported for normally developing infants, but there was more variability in the performance of the infants with Down syndrome. In a similar study, Casby and Ruder (1983) compared normal and mentally retarded young children matched on mean length of utterance (MLU) on stages of symbolic play. They found that the ability to use one object to represent another was a strong correlate of early language development. Cunningham, Glenn, Wilkinson, and Sloper (1985) studied the performance of 73 children with Down Syndrome on the Lowe and Costello Symbolic Play Test, the Bayley Scales or Stanford–Binet, and the Reynell Developmental Language Scales. They found that by age 2 years there was a significant lag in expressive language relative to other skills, that level of play maturity was significantly related to mental age, and that differences between performance on mental age tests and language tests widened with increasing age. Other studies of prelinguistic vocalizations, gaze, and pointing gestures of infants with Down syndrome have shown both similarities and differences in comparison to normally developing infants (Beeghley, Weiss-Perry, & Cicchetti, Chapter 10, this volume). Finally, studies of affective development add an additional dimension by showing that the emergence of affective responses is also closely linked to cognitive development in infants with Down syndrome (Cicchetti & Sroufe, 1976).

The empirical efforts to describe these early behaviors in infants with Down syndrome offer important data for developers of early intervention programs. *First,* they suggest that deficits in one area may hinder development in another area. *Second,* these data provide clues about underlying functional skills and deficits of infants with Down syndrome that are not identified very well by global developmental tests. Assessment of infants on early sequences of sensorimotor, prelinguistic and affective development and play behaviors might be used in planning program activities to facilitate emerging skills. *Third,* such research suggests links and possible prerequisites or co-emerging skills in one developmental area to support the emergence and acquisition of skills in another area. Early interventionists may be making a futile attempt to promote the development of skills that *cannot* emerge until other prerequisite skills are attained. Moreover, it might be possible to facilitate development in one area by attending to behaviors in another area. For example, because it is known that early cognitive and affective development are interrelated (Cicchetti & Sroufe, 1976), how might cognitive development be enhanced by exclusive selection of program activities that elicit a high degree of interest and positive affective involvement of the infant? Anecdotal suggestions by early interventionists that activities should be fun and interesting for the infant show the conventional wisdom implicit in this suggestion. The use of play to promote cognitive and linguistic skills has also been suggested (McCune-Nicolich & Carroll, 1981). In addition to promoting the developmental skills of infants, a focus on play interactions with parents can enhance the quality of the parent–infant relationship, a worthy goal for early intervention programs. McConkey and Martin (1983) report on such a program with Down syndrome infants.

In relation to the area of play development, Esenther (1984) describes an early intervention program based on improving the motor and sensory skills of infants with Down syndrome. Conceptually, the curriculum is based on the assumption that the quality of fine motor movements, their self-controlled stability and coordination, serves to promote meaningful exploration and improved attention. Coordination of touch and vision has been shown to be less coordinated in Down syndrome infants in comparison to normal MA-matched infants (Lewis & Bryant, 1982). Furthermore, fine motor coordination in preschoolers with Down syndrome has been shown to be impaired (Hogg & Moss, 1983). The hope of Esenther's intervention model is to promote basic primitive motor skills in support of more advanced exploratory behavior. Research with preschoolers with Down syndrome on problem solving using a manipulative toy known as the "Lock-Box" (both with and without the mother present) has shown the presence of deficits in organized exploration and perseverance in problem solving that may be the logical outgrowth of earlier fine motor difficulties (Berry & Gunn, 1984; Berry, Gunn & Andrews, 1984).

One of the most consistently reported suggestions about strategies for working with infants with Down syndrome in early intervention programs is that these infants need an instructional environment that is highly structured and individualized (Hanson, 1977, 1981; Keogh & Kopp, 1978; Rynders, Behlin, & Horrobin, 1979; Simeonsson & Wiegerink, 1974; Tawney, 1974). The search for specific educational techniques uniquely suited for promoting the learning of young children with Down syndrome has not been demonstrated. For example, Rynders, Behlin, and Horrobin (1979) found that preschoolers with Down syndrome had difficulty with both augmented verbal and manual guidance support for learning tasks. Although research indicates that children with Down syndrome may have more trouble in processing incoming information that is auditory rather than visual (Hartley, 1982; Marcell & Armstrong, 1982), it is clear from recent research that these infants have significant difficulties with both types of information processing. For example, Miranda and Fantz (1973) reported impaired visual attention abilities in infants with Down syndrome on a laboratory habituation task. Gunn, Berry, and Andrews (1982) reported that infants with Down syndrome show delays in visual exploration of the environment in a ϳlay situation with their mothers as early as 6 months of age, suggesting delays in the functional deployment of visual exploration. (See also Serafica and Cicchetti, 1976.)

A developmental perspective helps us recognize that the early visual and auditory information-processing difficulties of infants and young children with Down syndrome interfere with learning and acquisition of basic developmental skills. As more is learned about early information processing, the challenge for early interventionists is how to use these data to find techniques to remediate such information processing deficiencies and/or to minimize their negative impact on contemporary and future development.

When the first early intervention programs for infants and young children with Down syndrome were being developed, basic research on the information-processing abilities of infants was just beginning. Since there was no precedent for considering the notion that children with Down syndrome might be understood from a developmental perspective (as we had with normal children), early program developers were left with two options. They could approach the task of promoting the learning of these children as they would approach this task with normal children. Or they could adopt the hypothesis that these children had special learning characteristics requiring unique and novel approaches because the learning mechanisms were qualitatively different. In either case, they were embarking on uncharted ground: They would try to teach qualitatively different children using traditional methods and current knowledge about normal development, or they would have to be extremely creative to generate new methods for promoting learning in qualitatively different types of children.

It is probably fair to conclude that the early program developers approached this task by assuming an optimism that was based on these strategies: (1) observe and note the similarities and differences between learning in children with Down syndrome and normal children; and (2), specify and implement the conditions that promote normal development, while paying close attention to understanding the ways in which this approach was failing (if it was failing). Since the major goal of the earliest early intervention programs with infants and children with Down syndrome was promoting their intellectual development, and there was a growing awareness of the important relationships between intellectual and language development, it is not surprising that these programs became concerned with promoting development in these two areas.

The heightened concern with deficiences in auditory information processing in infancy is related to concerns that this deficiency signals the beginning of the difficulties that children with Down syndrome have with language acquisition (Rynders, 1982). Most early intervention programs have been interested in promoting language development in children with Down syndrome (e.g., Rynders & Horrobin, 1975). This occurred because it is recognized that communicative abilities are a significant predictor of long-range adjustment and competence and because the development of language and intellectual abilities is so intricately interwoven. Thus, the choice of language stimulation as a major target of intervention efforts has been motivated by its significant contribution to the long range developmental outcomes for children with Down syndrome. Here again it has been shown that infants with Down syndrome have particular difficulties with early language skills. By the time infant tests begin to include a significant number of items tapping receptive and expressive language skills, infants with Down syndrome begin to show significant declines in Developmental Quotient (DQ) (Share, 1975). They have also been shown to have notable problems with verbal imitation (Mahoney, Glover, & Finger, 1981; Rondal, 1980).

Studies have suggested that when children with Down syndrome are already using speech and are matched on mean length of utterance (MLU) with normally developing younger peers, they show similar patterns of linguistic development and usage (Beeghly, Weiss-Perry, & Cicchetti, Chapter 10, this volume; Rondal, 1978; Wiegel-Crump, 1981). There are, however, notable differences in pragmatics when mental age–matched normal and Down syndrome children are compared (Cardoso-Martins and Mervis, 1985; Harris, 1983; Leifer and Lewis, 1984). Furthermore, there is evidence that prelinguistic development and functional use of language in infants with Down syndrome is different from matched normally developing peers. For example, Berger and Cunningham (1981) have shown that infants with Down syndrome show delays in the onset of eye contact behavior and in the establishment of high levels of it (see Berger, Chapter 4, this volume). These researchers also found deficiencies in the functional uses of eye contact to explore the environment while maintaining intermittent social contact with the mother in interactive situations. They suggest that there are normal changes from relatively long to relatively short durations of eye contact that are delayed in infants with Down syndrome, suggestive of immaturities in inhibitory mechanisms and the development of the peripheral vision system. Longer gazes may also be an indication of slower information processing, suggesting that the timing and discriminative uses of eye contact may be different for infants with Down syndrome. This is an important area in need of further study.

The role of such differences in the development of social interactive behaviors has implications for the role of nonlinguistic factors in later difficulties in social interactions with peers. For example, it has been reported that preschoolers with Down syndrome who are mainstreamed in an educational program with normal peers are discriminated by their peers, tend to become isolated socially from them, and fail to observe some of the conventional rules of conversational interactions. That is, they fail to observe the normal conventions of mutual gaze in social interactions (Sinson & Wetherick, 1981) and they tend to violate the expected conventions of responding verbally to the initiations of peers (Knox, 1983). These findings about young children parallel the findings from studies of adults with Down syndrome that indicate that these adults have difficulty with the social conventional rules of the functional uses of language for conversation. Leudar, Fraser, and Jeeves (1981) have reported that adults with Down syndrome frequently broke the rules of conversation by not responding to questions and tended to restrict their comments to the current ongoing activity.

Because of interest in early language deficits in children with Down syndrome, insights gained from basic developmental research on language acquisition are influencing recent developments in early intervention programs (Schiefelbusch & Bricker, 1981). Our understanding of the process by which infants come to acquire an intention to communicate (Harding, 1982) has influenced the changes seen in philosophies of early language-training programs for young children with Down syndrome. Owens and MacDonald (1982) described a recent language training program for young children with Down syndrome that is based on a view of language as social-communicative behavior. They underscore the need to evaluate and train for functional speech. Clark and Seifer (1983) described a program for infants with Down syndrome that focuses on the mother–infant communicative interactions. They found that many of the infants showed social responses that were less frequent, less intense, and more developmentally delayed than seen in their normally developing peers. Their mothers tended to compensate with more frequent and intensive forms of social interaction. An intervention model that evaluates the mother's sensitivity on a hierarchy of social behavior is used in this program to promote a better match between the interactive styles of mothers and infants. Weistuch and Lewis (1985) describe a similar program based on the goal of improving mother–infant language interactions.

These latter types of intervention program models have been influenced by recent developmental research findings on the role of mother–infant interactions on infant development and on the differences in interaction patterns for normally developing and retarded or delayed infants. Brooks-Gunn and Lewis (1984) found that maternal responsiveness in interaction with their 3- to 36-month-old children with Down syndrome increased proportionately to their infants' behavior as the infants became more mature mentally. Crawley & Spiker (1983) found significant individual differences in the behavioral interactive styles of mothers with their 2-year-olds with Down syndrome as well as in the behaviors of children. Furthermore, specific features of maternal style were significantly positively correlated with child developmental level (indexed by the Bayley Scales of Infant Development). While causal statements could not be made from this study about the direction of effects in maternal and child characteristics, the patterns of relationship between maternal and child interactive behavior and developmental outcomes were similar to those found with normally developing counterparts (e.g., Clarke-Stewart, 1973). In two recent reviews of early intervention programs and mother–child interactions with handicapped infants and young children (Kysela & Marfo, 1983; Marfo, 1984) it is suggested that mothers of at-risk and handicapped infants need help from early programs to enhance their interaction skills, but that there are important individual differences in these needs.

Three major points about early intervention programs are highlighted by the above discussion. *First*, there is a growing endorsement of the notion that early intervention programs should focus on mother–infant interaction patterns in ways that are informed by research on interaction patterns and their relationship to infant development (Kysela & Marfo, 1983). Although the role of parents in stimulating their infant's development was acknowledged and utilized in the earliest programs (e.g., Hayden & Haring, 1976; Rynders & Horrobin, 1975), Keogh and Kopp (1978) concluded that most early intervention programs up until that time involved a strategy of nonspecific stimulation utilizing the parents as mediators. A subtle but significant shift of focus has occurred recently: Earlier programs sought to help the parent to stimulate the infant, whereas current programs seek to promote an optimal quality in the interaction patterns between parents and infants. Exclusive emphasis on infant behavior and characteristics is being replaced by increased attention to the parent–infant dyad as a unit, with attention to qualities such as mutuality, synchrony, conflict, and reciprocity (e.g., Affleck, McGrade, McQueeney, & Allen 1982; Clark & Seifer, 1983). McConachie and Mitchell (1985) have described an early intervention program that focuses on mother– and father–infant interactions. Based on recent research on pragmatics, they direct their interventions toward improving parental responsivity to the child; they are concerned that the need for parental structuring of child behavior can lead to overdirectiveness and unresponsiveness to child initiations.

A *second* point highlighted above is that individual differences are important considerations in programming objectives and strategies. The variability in the developmental functioning, interactional styles, and responsiveness to intervention of infants and children with Down syndrome is now well recognized and receiving more research attention (Cicchetti and Sroufe, 1976, 1978; Clunies-Ross, 1979; Crawley & Spiker, 1983; Hanson, 1981; LaVeck & Brehm, 1978; Mahoney & Snow, 1983; Morgan, 1979; Rynders, Spiker, & Horrobin, 1978; Simeonsson, Huntington, & Short, 1982; Spiker, 1982b). Similarly, the needs, styles and involvement of parents with regard to early intervention programs are now being conceptualized in more individualized ways than they have been in the past (e.g., MacMillan & Turnbull, 1983; Mink, Nihira, & Meyers, 1983). (This topic will be discussed in depth in the sections that follow.)

And *third*, these changes are moving the intervention field toward different and broader views of assessment. Hanson & Bellamy (1977) argued that programs for infants with Down syndrome should abandon a normed-based periodic strategy of assessment and adopt a criterion-based continuous strategy of evaluation. This suggestion is congruent with a developmental perspective and with a focus on individualized approaches toward programming. Program goals have been defined previously in terms of a nonspecific general stimulation model focusing mainly on global infant outcomes. There has been a recent shift in defining program objectives; included is a more differentiated view of infant development as well as attention to parental interactional styles and family adjustment. Such a shift requires an expansion of evaluation strategies, which is just beginning to emerge.

Infants and young children are now being evaluated for progress in specific areas of development in addition to being periodically tested for overall developmental level and monitored for attainment of key developmental milestones. Descriptive research on normal development and on Down syndrome provides numerous suggestions for alternative targets for assessment: play behavior (McCune-Nicolich & Carroll, 1981; Motti, Cicchetti, & Sroufe, 1983; Beeghly, Weiss-Perry, & Cicchetti, Chapter 10, this volume); temperament (Bridges & Cicchetti, 1982; Gunn, Berry & Andrews, 1983; Rothbart & Hanson, 1983); mother–infant attachment (Cicchetti & Serafica, 1981; Berry, Gunn, & Andrews, 1984; Serafica & Cicchetti, 1976); mother–infant interaction patterns (Berger, Chapter 4, this volume; Clark & Seifer, 1983; Crawley & Spiker, 1983); attention span (Krakow & Kopp, 1983); and sensorimotor development (Cicchetti & Mans-Wagener, 1987; Dunst & Rheingrover, 1983). In each of these areas, sequences of development or individual differences relevant to social interactional skills have been identified. Furthermore, these more differentiated descriptions of developmental progress and infant characteristics offer the more fine-grained information needed for the day-to-day program planning of teachers and parents that is not really available from global developmental assessment instruments.

The expansion of program evaluation to include assessment of parents and families as they provide the context for the development of the infant and child with Down syndrome is the most recent development in early program assessment. There is growing interest in the ways families cope with raising a young handicapped child, replacing a pathology model with a coping model (Crnic, Friedrich, & Greenberg, 1983; Gallagher, Beckman, & Cross, 1983). This will be explored further in the next section.

Parent involvement in early intervention programs

Research on parent involvement in early intervention programs with young children with Down syndrome has undergone some important changes in the last 20 years. Two bodies of literature on the subject exist. The first is research on initial family adjustment to the birth of an infant with Down syndrome. The second is the literature on the ways that parents have been participating in early intervention programs. From the very beginning, early intervention programs sought to involve parents in efforts to improve the developmental functioning of infants with Down syndrome (Hayden & Haring, 1976; Rynders & Horrobin, 1975). In the earliest programs, parents were recruited to become active in the teaching and stimulation of their infants through home-based instruction and support. It became apparent that parents of young infants were experiencing significant emotional reactions and upset related to the fact that they had given birth to a handicapped infant, and that this "crisis" required attention from intervention staff. Earlier research on parental reactions to the birth of a handicapped infant provided a psychoanalytical perspective. Parents were described as experiencing the birth of the handicapped infant as a loss of the expected normal infant (Solnit & Stark, 1961). They were described as having a mourning reaction requiring a readjustment in order to accept the "defective" infant that had actually been born (Ferholt & Solnit, 1978). Such a model proposed that there were "stages" of mourning and adjustment that had to be experienced in order to move to a state of "acceptance" of the child. It became fashionable for professionals to accept this "stage" model and "help" parents move through the stages toward the final state of "adjustment" (a model derived from the work of Kübler-Ross (1969) on the stages of dying patients who were experiencing life's greatest loss).

Although this model may have helped both professionals and parents realize that many of the emotional reactions, such as anger (often directed toward professionals or the infant) were natural responses, recent research and commentary have questioned the rigidity with which this model has been applied (Blancher, 1984). While it is now clear that parents experience an initial shock after the birth of an infant with Down syndrome (Murphy, 1982; Pueschel & Murphy, 1977; Waisbren, 1980), a broader view of parental reaction and adjustment is emerging.

Blancher (1984) questions the universal sequence of "stages" of adjustment. She has suggested that the timing, duration, and behaviors related to parental reactions to their new handicapped infant vary across parents. She points out that this stage model has been supported mainly by anecdotal evidence and there has been little research on a variety of factors that are likely to affect adjustment. Such factors include socioeconomic status, family composition, availability of support services, social networks, religion, physical appearance of the child, severity of the child's handicap, and parental access to information on mental retardation. Implicit in her point of view is an assumption that factors shown to be influential in understanding normal development and parenting will help to explicate the processes of adjustment and parenting with a child with Down syndrome.

In a review of research on family adaptation with mentally retarded children, Crnic, Friedrich, & Greenberg (1983) propose a model of adaptation that considers the perceived stress and coping resources available to families. In such a model, the concept of coping replaces an emphasis on pathology. While not denying that parents with a mentally retarded child may encounter special problems and issues in child rearing, the authors suggest that most families can make adequate adjustments and manage well in rearing their children (see Crnic, Chapter 12, this volume). In a review of parents' reports of life with a developmentally delayed child, Wishart, Bidder, and Gray (1981) found that these families were not strikingly different in their everyday lives when compared with families with same-age normally developing children.

To understand further the process of family adjustment with a child with Down syndrome, it is important to distinguish between the initial reactions and adjustments after the birth of the infant and the long-term impact of the child on the family life after the infancy period. Most research has dealt with the former. From the point of view of early intervention, several key points are worth noting. First, parents need early emotional support and accurate information (Cunningham, Aumonier, & Sloper, 1982; Ferholt & Solnit, 1978; Murphy, 1982). Second, the initial diagnosis is reported to parents by physicians and the initial information about Down syndrome given to parents is communicated to them in medical settings. This requires a closer working alliance between professionals in medical settings and early intervention programs. Parental dissatisfaction with the lack of accurate information and emotional sensitivity surrounding the initial diagnosis has been abundantly noted in anecdotal reports and research studies (e.g., Gath, 1978; Murphy, 1982), although notable progress has been documented for recent early counseling practices (Pueschel, 1985). Some of this dissatisfaction is probably a function of the parental shock and disappointment upon hearing the diagnosis. However, some of it is related to genuine deficiencies in the knowledge and attitudes of the helping professionals. For example, Kelly and Menolascino (1975) examined the knowledge and attitudes of physicians about mental retardation and found that many of them were unfamiliar with available community services for these families. Similarly, Wolraich and Siperstein (1983) found that many professionals hold very pessimistic views about the ultimate abilities of persons with mental retardation, with physicians' attitudes being significantly more pessimistic than those of psychologists and educators.

It is likely that there has been a decline in the dire negative prognoses given to parents by physicians in the last 10 to 15 years, however, as evidenced by a study by Springer and Steele (1980). These authors interviewed 37 couples with a school-age child with Down syndrome who were born since 1970. They found that parents of the more recently born children were given a more optimistic picture of the developmental potential of their children than were the parents of the earlier born children. In addition, they reported that the parents cited the emotional support and information obtained from parent groups in the community as having increasing influence on their own attitudes about their new infant, whereas physicians' input was declining in importance.

This shift away from physicians as the sole or primary source of information and counseling after the birth of an infant with Down syndrome is probably related to the growth of early intervention services. After the initial diagnosis, these services have the potential of providing parents with the ongoing support and practical help necessary for actually living with and rearing the infant on a daily basis. The need for continuing efforts to educate physicians should not be minimized or ignored, however, for two reasons. *First,* physicians will continue to be the first professional contact the family will have after the infant's birth. *Second,* many infants and children with Down syndrome will have continuing medical problems requiring not only proper medical intervention and care but sensitive parental guidance.

Another major point about initial family adjustment to the birth of an infant with

Down syndrome is that families are not homogeneous in terms of this initial period of adjustment. Gath (1977, 1978) interviewed families with an infant with Down syndrome over the first 2 years of the infant's life and found notable individual differences in the impact of the infant on the family. Some families reported increased marital stress; others reported more harmonious marriages based on both shared sorrow and happiness. It appeared that the pre-birth characteristics of the parents and marriages contributed more toward understanding the effects of the infant with Down syndrome on the family than did the actual birth of the infant. Nevertheless, Gath noted that during the first year after the birth, the couples with infants with Down syndrome experienced more unhappiness than did comparison couples who had given birth to a normal infant. These results suggest that there are unique needs of parents during the first year after the birth of an infant with Down syndrome, but significant individual variation exists in the adjustment process.

In a follow-up of these families when the children were 8 to 9 years old, Gath and Gumley (1984) found continuing problems in parental emotional adjustment and desires for guidance in providing a satisfactory caregiving environment, but without further deterioration in marital problems if they existed during the early years. Parents expressed particular needs in the areas of teaching their children communication skills and in understanding and dealing effectively with difficult behavior, results that highlight continuing developmental problems with language and social skills. These findings are also significant because these skills have been the most consistently reported predictors of adult adjustment for individuals with Down syndrome (Cunningham and Preshall, 1978; Hirst, 1983; Willer and Intagliata, 1981).

The implications for early intervention programs of these variations in initial reactions of parents are complex. Interventionists who seek to involve parents as teachers of their infants must balance their zeal to involve parents in stimulation activities with the obvious needs parents have for coping with their own emotional concerns. Gath (1978) concluded from her research that most parents "should not be treated as potential psychiatric patients or social work clients" (p. 119).

Research indicates that parent discussion groups are important sources of support and information for parents. When asked to name the most beneficial aspect of their involvement in an early intervention program with their infant with Down syndrome, the majority of a group of 24 mothers questioned by Spiker (1982a) cited participation in a parent support group. Furthermore, the mothers reported that the shared emotional support was the most important aspect of the group experience, with gains in information as a second benefit. It has been suggested that meeting with parents who are undergoing similar emotional adjustments provides a unique forum for expressing feelings, validating the "normality" of those feelings, and gaining confidence in one's ability to make a reasonable adjustment toward rearing the child (Schoenig, 1978).

Because most early intervention programs seek to involve parents in stimulation activities with their infant or preschooler, programmers must be sensitive and responsive to parental emotional adjustment. Earlier reports documented that mothers of infants and young children with Down syndrome could be taught to stimulate the infants' development (e.g., Cheseldine & McConkey, 1979; Filler, 1977). Although it is assumed that the amount and quality of parent involvement in early intervention activities with the infant is directly related to infant developmental progress, few studies have actually established this link empirically (Gibson & Fields, 1984). A study by Cullen et al., (1981) is an exception. They studied 89 young children with Down syndrome between 6 and 36 months of age, monitoring health and developmental functioning at 6-month intervals. Their results indicated that parent follow-through with stimulation activities was significantly associated with higher scores on the Vineland Social Maturity Scale and earlier achievement of selected feeding milestones. They also found, however, that infants with significantly greater developmental progress had better muscle tone and either mild or no cardiac problems. These results suggest that parent stimulation contributes to developmental growth, but that variations in infant biological vulnerability mediate the influence of parental stimulation efforts. This is an important study because it highlights the interplay between biological and environmental factors in the developmental functioning observed in children with Down syndrome (Clements et al., 1976; Connolly, 1978; Rynders et al., 1978).

The above study also raises two important questions about parent involvement in early intervention programs that are receiving increased research attention. *First,* what are the possible sources and implications of individual differences in parents' ability and willingness to follow through with guidance given by programmers? *Second,* how might individual differences in infant characteristics that may influence parent stimulation efforts be incorporated in the design of early programs? A study by Gallagher, Jens, and O'Donnell (1983) showed that handicapped infants' ability to express laughter was impaired in relation to degree of muscle tone abnormalities (hypotonicity or hypertonicity). Such limitations in affective expression may affect parent–infant interaction and may in turn be implicated in the results found by Cullen et al. (1981) just described.

Several cautionary comments should be made about the role of parent involvement in early intervention programs and about family adjustment beyond the infancy and preschool period. Although active parent involvement in early intervention programs has been generally hailed as beneficial and desirable (e.g., Bricker & Casuso, 1979), its widespread endorsement has been questioned recently. MacMillan & Turnbull (1983) have argued that the nature and extent of parent involvement should be individualized. They cite a number of factors that can affect the parent's ability or willingness for program involvement, including severity of the child's condition, and family factors such as parental age, income level, and other socioeconomic variables. In particular, some research has questioned whether the parent-as-teacher model of some programs might be inappropriate for some families.

Spiker (1982a) asked mothers of 2- to 4-year-olds with Down syndrome to rate their behavioral interactions with the children during times in which they were "working" on stimulation activities suggested to them by early intervention program staff. Mothers of the lower functioning children rated their children as less attentive and less happy during these activities than did mothers of higher functioning children. Mothers of males also rated these interactions as more difficult than did mothers of females. Especially notable were anecdotal reports that program planners did not ask parents about the difficulties they might be having in implementing program suggestions. Such a lack of explicit concern about parents' problems in carrying out program activities may lead to frustration that can undermine the parents' confidence in their parenting with the young child with Down syndrome.

Sloper, Cunningham, and Arnljotsdottir (1983) interviewed 48 parents with an infant with Down syndrome who were participating in a home stimulation program. They found that the parents valued the information they received about Down syndrome, child development, and stimulation activities. However, they expressed resentment over the record-keeping involved in the program and expressed anxiety about how they were helping the infants even when the infants were progressing well. Schell (1981) has suggested that parents of young handicapped children may experience "burn-out", a progressive loss of energy and sense of purpose associated with helping activities (Edelwich & Brodsky, 1980). Such "burn-out" may result from frustration due to the cumulative slow developmental progress of the child that does not match parental expectations. Such frustration can be exacerbated if parents perceive covert (and sometimes overt) messages from professionals that they may be inadequately involved in stimulating their child. Schilling, Gilchrist, and Schinke (1984) describe a parent discussion group model for parents of handicapped children that aims to teach them to use personal coping and social supports to deal with stress and to give up what they call idealized images of the "super parent." Such an approach is an important addition to intervention programs because it recognizes the variations among families and supports the concept of individualized parental involvement.

While most of the literature about families with handicapped children and children with Down syndrome in particular has dealt with the infancy and preschool period, a few recent studies address issues of family functioning beyond this time. It has been suggested that stress in families with handicapped children increases as the child grows older (Gallagher, Beckman, & Cross, 1983). Similarly, Kornblum and Anderson (1982) have questioned the notion that parents of handicapped children resolve their feelings associated with mourning early in the child's life and reach a final stage of "acceptance." They argue that parental grief is ongoing and periodic, exacerbated by the normal developmental transitions that highlight the child's continuing differences from the normally developing child. To make matters worse, Suelze and Keenan (1981) reported data on 330 families with children with mental retardation (including children with Down syndrome) indicating that parents of older children felt less well supported and more socially isolated than did parents of younger children. Spiker (1982a) also reported that mothers of preschoolers with Down syndrome were less involved in parent support groups than they had been when the children were infants. The author suggested that the parent groups did not appear to be evolving to meet the changing needs of the parents.

These studies indicate that our knowledge base for understanding the long-term developmental needs of families with children with Down syndrome is seriously limited. The current family systems models are a step on the right direction because they attempt to describe child development in the context of a continuously evolving family system in which stresses, supports, and resources are viewed as reciprocal influences on the child's development.

In one of the few applications of a family systems approach to families with children with mental retardation, researchers at UCLA are examining family styles in families with school-age trainably mentally retarded (TMR) children, many of whom have Down syndrome. Mink et al., (1983) examined family styles in 115 families of school-age children (average age of 12½ years) in TMR classes (mean IQ = 41.5, range = 12 − 70), with 48% of the sample having Down syndrome. They categorized families into five types: cohesive, harmonious; control-oriented, somewhat unharmonious; low-disclosure, unharmonious; child-oriented, expressive; and disadvantaged, with low morale. A very high percentage of the families with a child with Down syndrome were categorized as cohesive, harmonious. These families were low on life stress and were characterized as ''caring'' homes with parents who encouraged their children to develop their potential. In a related study, these researchers found that certain home characteristics were positively associated with the children's school adjustment. The characteristics included harmony and quality of parenting, availability of educational and cognitive stimulation in the home, emotional support for learning in the home, and cohesiveness of family members (Nihira, Mink, & Meyers, 1981). Note that these variables are the same ones associated with school achievement in normally developing children.

Summary of review of early intervention programs

This review of early intervention programs highlights several important considerations. *First,* as we begin to learn more about infants and young children with Down syndrome, we are struck with the individual variation in the development of this population. Both biological and environmental factors and their interactions appear to be implicated in these individual differences.

Second, our initial assumptions about family characteristics and adjustments to rearing such a child at home and about the use of early intervention services have not adequately considered the individual variations that exist. In particular, we are only just beginning to be serious about the individualized family characteristics that both affect and are affected by early program participation. This can lead to a broader perspective about the goals and activities being promoted by early intervention programs. A focus on infant cognitive and language development can be expanded to include curriculum aimed at promoting stimulating and mutually gratifying parent–infant interactions. Such a perspective would place infant cognitive and language development in a context that includes social and affective development as a more integrated whole, which, by the way, is how parents of normal infants experience their infants.

Third, one is struck by the fact that our understanding of normal development continues to help us in our understanding of these children and their families, despite the differences in the children that emerge from comparative studies. In particular, the organizational perspective that suggests that there is a logical structure to the relationships across developmental domains has helped to elucidate the complexities of the delays and possible deficits in the development of children with Down syndrome. For example, if arousal–attentional deficits serve to reduce infant exploration and interest in social interaction, which in turn serve to retard developmental progress, how might early interventionists design activities and promote parent involvement that recognizes these linkages in ways that will promote early development?

And *fourth,* the targets of early intervention programs have been soundly based on our evolving understanding of the ways in which early development provides the groundwork for the later development of competencies and behaviors associated with childhood and adult adjustment. This chapter ends with a brief comment on the latter topic.

Future directions for intervention with older children

Although this chapter has not focused on the interactions between parents and children (see Spiker, 1982b; and Berger, Chapter 4, this volume), it is apparent that a better understanding of parental behavior with their children with Down syndrome is essential for understanding the long-range development and adjustment of these children. The later educational goals for these children follow the goals of infant–preschool programs in that they aim to promote cognitive, linguistic, and social skills, by encouraging parents to do the best that they can do. Family and educational support of the development of intellectual and linguistic skills, of behavioral and social–emotional adjustment, and of the attainment of maximal adult independence are the ultimate goals. As we seek to improve early intervention programs for infants with Down syndrome and their families, it is imperative that we keep an eye toward the long-range goals of these enterprises. Data with older children and adults suggest that well-developed communicative abilities and social skills (such as role-taking skills, lack of behavior problems) are critical to the attainment of adult functioning and independence (Cunningham & Preshall, 1978; Hirst, 1983; Willer & Intagliata, 1981). Furthermore, we have more success in designing programs to promote significant gains in these areas than in intellectual and language areas with older children, adolescents, and adults.

Our challenge in the early intervention field is twofold. We must continue to examine questions about the relationship between the early development of competencies that appear to be precursors to later competencies. And we must continue to question the validity of these links, especially in light of major developmental shifts after the infancy period, so that we discover the best ways to support the optimal development of children with Down syndrome. We owe that much to these children and to their parents.

References

Affleck, G., McGrade, B. J., McQueeney, M., & Allen, D. (1982). Relationship-focussed early intervention in developmental disabilities. *Exceptional Children, 49,* 259–261.

Ainsworth, M.D.S. (1979). Infant–mother attachment. *American Psychologist, 34,* 932–937.

Arnold, L. E. (Ed.). (1978). *Helping parents help their children.* New York: Brunner/Mazel.

Aronson, M., & Fallstrom, K. (1977). Immediate and long-term effects developmental training in children with Down's syndrome. *Developmental Medicine and Child Neurology, 19,* 489–494.

Berger, J., & Cunningham, C. C. (1981). The development of eye contact between mothers and normal versus Down's syndrome infants. *Developmental Psychology, 17,* 678–689.

Berry, P., & Gunn, P. (1984). Maternal Influence on the task behavior of young Down's syndrome Children. *Journal of Mental Deficiency Research, 28,* 269–274.

Berry, P., Gunn, P., & Andrews, R. J. (1984). The behaviour of Down's syndrome children using the "Lock Box": A research note. *Journal of Child Psychology and Psychiatry, 25,* 125–131.

Bidder, R. T., Bryant, G., & Gray, O. P. (1975). Benefits of Down's syndrome children through training their mothers. *Archives of Diseases of Children, 50,* 383–386.

Blancher, J. (1984). Sequential stages of parental adjustment to the birth of a child with handicaps: Fact or artifact? *Mental Retardation, 22,* 55–68.

Bricker, D., & Casuso, V. (1979). Family involvement: A critical component of early intervention. *Exceptional Children, 46,* 108–116.

Bridges, F. A., & Cicchetti, D. (1982). Mothers' ratings of the temperament characteristics of Down syndrome infants. *Developmental Psychology, 18,* 238–244.

Bronfenbrenner, U. (1979). *The ecology of human development.* Cambridge, MA: Harvard University Press.

Brooks-Gunn, J., & Lewis, M. (1984). Maternal responsivity in interactions with handicapped infants. *Child Development, 55,* 782–793.

Caldwell, B. M. (1970). The rationale for early intervention. *Exceptional Children, 36,* 717–726.

Cardoso-Martins, C., & Mervis, C. B. (1985). Maternal speech to prelinguistic children with Down syndrome. *American Journal of Mental Deficiency, 89,* 451–458.

Carr, J. (1970). Mental and motor development in young mongol children. *Journal of Mental Deficiency Research, 14,* 205–220.

Casby, M. W., & Ruder, K. F. (1983). Symbolic play and early language development in normal and mentally retarded children. *Journal of Speech and Hearing Research, 26,* 404–411.

Cheseldine, S., & McConkey, R. (1979). Parental speech to young Down's syndrome children: An intervention study. *American Journal of Mental Deficiency, 83,* 612–620.

Cicchetti, D., & Mans-Wagener, L. (1987). Stages, sequences and structures in the organization of development in infants with Down syndrome. In I. Uzgiris & J. McV. Hunt (Eds.), *Research with scales of psychological development.* Champaign: University of Illinois Press.

Cicchetti, D., & Pogge-Hesse, P. (1982). Possible contributions of the study of organically retarded persons to developmental theory. In E. Zigler & D. Balla (Eds.), *Mental retardation: The developmental–difference controversy.* Hillsdale, NJ: Erlbaum.

Cicchetti, D., & Serafica, F. C. (1981). Interplay among behavioral systems: Illustrations from the study of attachment, affiliation, and wariness in young children with Down's syndrome. *Developmental Psychology, 17* 36–49.

Cicchetti, D., & Sroufe, L. A. (1976). The relationship between affective and cognitive development in Down's syndrome infants. *Child Development, 47,* 920–929.

Cicchetti, D., & Sroufe, L. A. (1978). An organizational view of affect: Illustrations from the study of Down's syndrome infants. In M. Lewis & L. A. Rosenblum (Eds.), *The development of affect*. New York: Plenum.

Clark, G. N., & Seifer, R. (1983). Facilitating mother–infant communication: A treatment model for high-risk and developmentally-delayed infants. *Infant Mental Health Journal, 4*, 67–81.

Clarke-Stewart, K. A. (1973). Interactions between mothers and their young children: Characteristics and consequences. *Monographs of the Society for Research in Child Development, 38*, (6–7, Serial No. 153).

Clarke-Stewart, K. A., & Fein, G. G. (1983). Early childhood programs. In P. H. Mussen (Ed.), *Handbook of child psychology*, Volume 2: *Infancy and developmental psychobiology*. New York: Wiley.

Clements, P. R., Bates, M. V., & Hafer, M. (1976). Variability within Down's syndrome (trisomy-21): Empirically observed sex difference in IQs. *Mental Retardation, 14*, 30–31.

Clunies-Ross, G. G. (1979). Accelerating the development of Down's syndrome infants and young children. *Journal of Special Education, 13*, 169–177.

Connolly, B., Morgan, S., Russell, F. F., & Richardson, B. (1980). Early intervention with Down's syndrome children. *Physical Therapy, 60*, 1405–1408.

Connolly, B., & Russell, F. (1976). Interdisciplinary early intervention program. *Physical Therapy, 56*, 155–158.

Connolly, J. A. (1978). Intelligence levels of young Down's syndrome children. *American Journal of Mental Deficiency, 83*, 193–196.

Crawley, S. B., & Spiker, D. (1983). Mother–child interactions involving two-year-olds with Down syndrome: A look at individual differences. *Child Development, 54*, 1312–1323.

Crnic, K. A., Friedrich, W. N., & Greenberg, M. T. (1983). Adaptation of families with mentally retarded children: A model of stress, coping, and family ecology. *American Journal of Mental Deficiency, 88*, 125–138.

Cullen, S. M, Cronk, C. E., Pueschel, S. M., Schnell, R. R., & Reed, R. B. (1981). Social development and feeding milestones of young Down syndrome children. *American Journal of Mental Deficiency, 85*, 410–415.

Cunningham, C. C., Aumonier, M. E., & Sloper, P. (1982). Health visitor support for families with Down's syndrome infants. *Child: Care, Health, and Development, 8*, 1–19.

Cunningham, C. C., Glenn, S. M., Wilkinson, P., & Sloper, P. (1985). Mental ability, symbolic play, and receptive and expressive language of young children with Down's syndrome. *Journal of Child Psychology and Psychiatry, 26*, 255–265.

Cunningham, T., & Preshall, D. (1978). Relationship between dimensions of adaptive behavior and sheltered workshop productivity. *American Journal of Mental Deficiency, 82*, 386–393.

Dunst, C. J., & Rheingrover, R. M. (1983). Structural characteristics of sensorimotor development among Down's syndrome infants. *Journal of Mental Deficiency Research, 27*, 11–22.

Edelwich, J., & Brodsky, A. (1980). *Burn-out: Stages of disillusionment in the helping professions*. New York: Human Sciences Press.

Esenther, S. E. (1984). Developmental coaching of the Down syndrome infant. *American Journal of Occupational Therapy, 38*, 440–445.

Fantz, R. L. (1963). Pattern vision in newborn infants. *Science, 140*, 296–297.

Ferholt, J. B., & Solnit, A. J. (1978). Counselling parents of mentally retarded children. In L. E. Arnold (Ed.), *Helping parents help their children*. New York: Brunner/Mazel.

Filler, J. W., Jr. (1977). Modifying maternal teaching styles: Effects of task arrangement on the match-to-sample performance of retarded preschool-age children. *American Journal of Mental Deficiency, 80*, 602–612.

Flavell, J. H. (1963). *The developmental psychology of Jean Piaget*. New York: Van Nostrand Reinhold.

Francis, S. H. (1971). The effects of own-home and institution-rearing on the behavioural development of normal and mongol children. *Journal of Child Psychology and Psychiatry, 12*, 173–190.

Gallagher, J. J., Beckman, P., & Cross, A. H. (1983). Families of handicapped children: Sources of stress and its amelioration. *Exceptional Children, 50*, 10–19.

Gallagher, R. J., Jens, K. G., & O'Donnell, K. J. (1983). The effect of physical status on the affective expression of handicapped infants. *Infant Behavior and Development, 6,* 73–77.

Gath, A. (1977). The impact of an abnormal child upon the parents. *British Journal of Psychiatry, 130,* 405–410.

Gath, A. (1978). *Down's syndrome and the family: The early years.* New York: Academic Press.

Gath, A., & Gumley, D. (1984). Down's syndrome and the family: Follow-up of children first seen in infancy. *Developmental Medicine and Child Neurology, 26,* 500–508.

Gibson, D., & Fields, D. L. (1984). Early infant stimulation programs for children with Down syndrome: a review of effectiveness. *Advances in Developmental and Behavioral Pediatrics, 5,* 331–371.

Gunn, P., Berry, P., & Andrews, R. J. (1982). Looking behavior of Down syndrome infants. *American Journal of Mental Deficiency, 87,* 344–347.

Gunn, P., Berry, P., & Andrews, R. J. (1983). The temperament of Down's syndrome toddlers: A research note. *Journal of Child Psychology and Psychiatry, 24,* 601–605.

Gustafson, G. (1984). Effects of the ability to locomote on infants' social and exploratory behaviors: An experimental study. *Developmental Psychology, 20,* 397–405.

Hanson, M. J. (1977). *Teaching your Down's syndrome infant: A guide for parents.* Baltimore: University Park Press.

Hanson, M. J. (1981). Down's syndrome children: Characteristics and intervention research. In M. Lewis & L. A. Rosenblum (Eds.), *The uncommon child.* New York: Plenum.

Hanson, M. J., & Bellamy, G. T. (1977). Continuous measurement of progress in infant intervention programs. *Education and Training of the Mentally Retarded, 12,* 52–58.

Harding, C. G. (1982). Development of the intention to communicate. *Human Development, 25,* 140–151.

Harris, J. (1983). What does mean length of utterance mean? Evidence from a comparative study of normal and Down's syndrome children. *British Journal of Disorders of Communication, 18,* 153–169.

Hartley, X. Y. (1982). Receptive language processing of Down's syndrome children. *Journal of Mental Deficiency Research, 26,* 263–269.

Hayden, A. H., & Haring, N. G. (1976). Early intervention for high risk infants and young children: Programs for Down's syndrome children. In T. D. Tjossem (Ed.), *Intervention strategies for high risk infants and young children.* Baltimore: University Park Press.

Hirst, M. A. (1983). Young people with disabilities: What happens after 16? *Child: Care, Health, and Development, 9,* 273–284.

Hogg, J., & Moss, S. C. (1983). Prehensile development in Down's syndrome and nonhandicapped preschool children. *British Journal of Developmental Psychology, 1,* 189–204.

Hunt, N. (1967). *The world of Nigel Hunt: The diary of a mongoloid youth.* Beaconsfield, England: Darwen Finlayson.

Johnson, R. C., & Abelson, R. B. (1969). Intellectual, behavioral, and physical characteristics associated with trisomy, translocation and mosaic types of Down's syndrome. *American Journal of Mental Deficiency, 73,* 852–855.

Kelly, N. K., & Menolascino, F. J. (1975). Physicians' awareness and attitudes toward the retarded. *Mental Retardation, 13,* 10–13.

Keogh, B. K., & Kopp, C. B. (1978). From assessment to the intervention: An elusive bridge. In F. D. Minifie & L. L. Lloyd (Eds.), *Communicative and cognitive abilities – Early behavioral assessment.* Baltimore: University Park Press.

Knox, M. (1983). Changes in the frequency of language use in Down's syndrome children interacting with nonretarded peers. *Education and Training of the Mentally Retarded, 18,* 185–190.

Kornblum, H., & Anderson, B. (1982). "Acceptance" reassessed: A point of view. *Child Psychiatry and Human Development, 12,* 171–178.

Krakow, J. B., & Kopp, C. B. (1983). The effects of developmental delay on sustained attention in young children. *Children Development, 54,* 1143–1155.

Kübler-Ross, E. (1969). *On death and dying.* New York: Macmillan.

Kysela, G. M., & Marfo, K. (1983). Mother–child interactions and early intervention programmes for handicapped infants and young children. *Educational Psychology, 3*, 201–212.

LaVeck, B., & Brehm, S. S. (1978). Individual variability among children with Down's syndrome. *Mental Retardation, 16*, 135–137.

Leifer, J. S., & Lewis, M. (1984). Acquisition of conversational response skills by young Down's syndrome and nonretarded children. *American Journal of Mental Deficiency, 88*, 610–618.

Leudar, I., Fraser, W. I., & Jeeves, M. A. (1981). Social familiarity and communication in Down syndrome. *Journal of Mental Deficiency Research, 25*, 133–142.

Lewis, V., & Bryant, P. E. (1982). Touch and vision in normal and Down's syndrome babies. *Perception, 11*, 691–701.

Ludlow, J. R., & Allen, L. M. (1979). The effect of early intervention and pre-school stimulus on the development of the Down's syndrome child. *Journal of Mental Deficiency Research, 23*, 29–44.

MacMillan, D. L., & Turnbull, A. P. (1983). Parent involvement with special education: Respecting individual preferences. *Education and Training of the Mentally Retarded, 18*, 4–9.

Mahoney, G., Glover, A., & Finger, I. (1981). Relationship between language and sensorimotor development of Down syndrome and nonretarded children. *American Journal of Mental Deficiency, 86*, 21–27.

Mahoney, G., & Snow, K. (1983). The relationship of sensorimotor functioning to children's response to early language training. *Mental Retardation, 21*, 248–254.

Marcell, M. M., & Armstrong, V. (1982). Auditory and visual sequential memory of Down syndrome and nonretarded children. *American Journal of Mental Deficiency, 87*, 86–95.

Marfo, K. (1984). Interactions between mothers and their mentally retarded children: Integration of research findings. *Journal of Applied Developmental Psychology, 5*, 45–69.

McConachie, H., & Mitchell, D. R. (1985). Parents teaching their young handicapped children. *Journal of Child Psychology and Psychiatry, 26*, 389–405.

McConkey, R., & Martin, H. (1983). Mothers' play with toys: A longitudinal study with Down's syndrome infants. *Child: Care, Health, and Development, 9*, 215–226.

McCubbin, H. I., & Figley, C. R. (1983). *Stress and the family*, Vol. 1: *Coping with normative transitions*. New York: Brunner/Mazel.

McCune-Nicolich, L. (1981). Toward symbolic functioning: Structure of early pretend games and potential parallels with language. *Child Development, 52*, 785–797.

McCune-Nicolich, L., & Carroll, S. (1981). Development of symbolic play: Implications for the language specialist. *Topics in Language Disorders, 2*(1), 1–15.

Mink, I. T., Nihira, K., & Meyers, C. E. (1983). Taxonomy of family life styles: I. Homes with TMR children. *American Journal of Mental Deficiency, 87*, 484–497.

Miranda, S. B., & Fantz, R. L. (1973). Visual preferences of Down's syndrome and normal infants. *Child Development, 44*, 555–561.

Morgan, S. B. (1979). Development and distribution of intellectual and adaptive skills in Down's syndrome children. *Mental Retardation, 17*, 247–249.

Motti, F., Cicchetti, D., & Sroufe, L. A. (1983). From infant affect expression to symbolic play: The coherence of development in Down syndrome children. *Child Development, 54*, 1168–1175.

Murphy, A. (1982). Positive and supportive counseling of parents of infants with Down syndrome. In S. M. Pueschel & J. E. Rynders (Eds.), *Down syndrome: Advances in biomedicine and the behavioral sciences*. Cambridge, MA: Ware Press.

Nihira, K., Mink, I. T., & Meyers, C. E. (1981). Relationship between home environment and school adjustment of TMR children. *American Journal of Mental Deficiency, 86*, 8–15.

Oelwein, P. L., Fewell, R. R., & Pruess, J. B. (1985). The efficacy of intervention at outreach sites of the program for children with Down syndrome and other developmental delays. *Topics in Early Childhood Special Education, 5*, 78–87.

Owens, R. E., & MacDonald, J. D. (1982). Communicative uses of the early speech of nondelayed and Down syndrome children. *American Journal of Mental Deficiency, 86*, 503–510.

Public Law 94–142 (1976). Education for All Handicapped Children of 1975. Reston, VA: The Council for Exceptional Children.

Pueschel. S. M. (1985). Changes of counseling practices at the birth of a child with Down syndrome. *Applied Research in Mental Retardation, 6,* 99–108.

Pueschel, S. M., & Murphy, A. (1977). Assessment of counselling practices at the birth of a child with Down's syndrome. *American Journal of Mental Deficiency, 81,* 325–330.

Rondal, J. (1978). Maternal speech to normal and Down's syndrome children matched for mean length of utterance. In C. E. Meyers (Ed.), *Quality of life in severely and profoundly mentally retarded people.* Washington, DC: American Association on Mental Deficiency.

Rondal, J. (1980). Verbal imitation of Down syndrome and nonretarded children. *American Journal of Mental Deficiency, 85,* 318–321.

Rothbart, M. K., & Hanson, M. J. (1983). A caregiver report comparison of temperamental characteristics of Down syndrome and normal infants. *Developmental Psychology, 19,* 766–769.

Rubin, K. H., Fein, G. G., & Vandenberg, B. (1983). Play. In P. H. Mussen (Ed.), *Handbook of child psychology,* Vol. 4: *Socialization, personality, and social development.* New York: Wiley.

Rynders, J. E. (1982). Research on promoting learning in children with Down syndrome. In S. M. Pueschel & J. E. Rynders (Eds.), *Down syndrome: Advances in biomedicine and the behavioral sciences.* Cambridge, MA: Ware Press.

Rynders, J. E., Behlin, K. L., & Horrobin, J. M. (1979). Performance characteristics of preschool Down's syndrome children receiving augmented or repetitive verbal instruction. *American Journal of Mental Deficiency, 84,* 67–73.

Rynders, J. E., & Horrobin, J. M. (1975). Project EDGE: The University of Minnesota's communication program for Down's syndrome infants. In B. Z. Friedlander, G. M. Sterritt, & G. E. Kirk (Eds.), *Exceptional infant,* Vol. 3: *Assessment and intervention.* New York: Brunner/Mazel.

Rynders, J. E., Spiker, D., & Horrobin, J. M. (1978). Underestimating the educability of Down's syndrome children: Examination of methodological problems in recent literature. *American Journal of Mental Deficiency, 82,* 440–448.

Salzberg, C. L., & Villani, T. V. (1983). Speech training by parents of Down syndrome toddlers: Generalization across settings and instructional contexts. *American Journal of Mental Deficiency, 87,* 403–413.

Sameroff, A. J. (1983). Developmental systems: Contexts and evolution. In P. H. Mussen (Ed.), *Handbook of child psychology,* Vol. 1: *History, theory and methods.* New York: Wiley.

Schell, G. C. (1981). The young handicapped child: A family perspective. *Topics in Early Childhood Special Education, 1*(31), 21–27.

Schiefelbusch, R. L., & Bricker, D. D. (Eds.) (1981). *Early language: Acquisition and intervention.* Baltimore: University Park Press.

Schilling, R. F., Gilchrist, L. D., & Schinke, S. P. (1984). Coping and social support in families of developmentally disabled children. *Family Relations: Journal of Applied Family and Child Relations, 33,* 47–54.

Schoenig, B. (1978). P.E.E.R.S.: Parents are effective early education resources. *Exceptional Parent, 8,* 8–12.

Seitz, S., & Terdal, L. (1972). A modeling approach to changing parent–child interactions. *Mental Retardation, 10,* 39–43.

Serafica, F. C., & Cicchetti, D. (1976). Down's syndrome children in the strange situation: Attachment and exploration behaviors. *Merrill-Palmer Quarterly, 22,* 137–150.

Share, J. B. (1975). Developmental progress in Down's syndrome. In R. Koch & F. F. de la Cruz (Eds.), *Down's syndrome (mongolism): Research, prevention, and management.* New York: Brunner/Mazel.

Simeonsson, R. J., Cooper, D. H., & Scheiner, A. P. (1982). A review and analysis of the effectiveness of early intervention programs. *Pediatrics, 69,* 635–641.

Simeonsson, R. J., Huntington, G. S., & Short, R. J. (1982). Individual differences and goals: An approach to the evaluation of child progress. *Topics in Early Childhood Special Education, 1*(4), 71–80.

Simeonsson, R. J., & Wiegerink, R. (1974). Early language intervention: A contingent stimulation model. *Mental Retardation, 12,* 7–11.

Sinson, J. C., & Wetherick, N. E. (1981). The behavior of children with Down's syndrome in normal playgroups. *Journal of Mental Deficiency Research, 25,* 113–120.

Sinson, J. C., & Wetherick, N. E. (1982). Mutual gaze in pre-school Down's and normal children. *Journal of Mental Deficiency Research, 26,* 123–129.

Sloper, P., Cunningham, C. C., & Arnljotsdottir, M. (1983). Parental reactions to early intervention with their Down's syndrome infants. *Child: Care, Health, & Development, 9,* 357–376.

Smolak, L. (1982). Cognitive precursors of receptive vs. expressive language. *Journal of Child Language, 9,* 13–22.

Solnit, A. J., & Stark, M. (1961). Mourning the birth of a defective child. *The Psychoanalytic Study of the Child, 16,* 523–537.

Spiker, D. (1982a). Parent involvement in early intervention activities with their children with Down's syndrome. *Education and Training of the Mentally Retarded, 17*(1), 24–29.

Spiker, D. (1982b). Early intervention for young children with Down syndrome: New directions in enhancing parent–infant synchrony. In S. M. Pueschel & J. E. Rynders (Eds.), *Down syndrome: Advances in biomedicine and the behavioral sciences.* Cambridge, MA: Ware Press.

Springer, A., & Steele, M. W. (1980). Effects of physician's early parental counseling on rearing of Down's syndrome children. *American Journal of Mental Deficiency, 85,* 1–5.

Sroufe, L. A., & Wunsch, J. (1972). The development of laughter in the first year of life. *Child Development, 43,* 1326–1344.

Suelze, M., & Keenan, V. (1981). Changes in family support networks over the life cycle of mentally retarded persons. *American Journal of Mental Deficiency, 86,* 267–274.

Tawney, J. W. (1974). Acceleration of vocal behavior in developmentally retarded children. *Education and Training of the Mentally Retarded, 9,* 22–27.

Waisbren, S. E. (1980). Parents' reactions after the birth of a developmentally disabled child. *American Journal of Mental Deficiency, 84,* 345–351.

Weistuch, L., & Lewis, M. (1985). The Language Interaction Intervention Program. *Analysis and Intervention in Developmental Disabilities, 5,* 97–106.

Wiegel-Crump, C. A. (1981). The development of grammar in Down's syndrome children between the mental ages of 2–0 and 6–11 years. *Education and Training of the Mentally Retarded, 16,* 24–30.

Willer, B., & Intagliata, J. (1981). Social–environmental factors as predictors of adjustment of deinstitutionalized mentally retarded adults. *American Journal of Mental Deficiency, 86,* 252–259.

Wishart, M. C., Bidder, R. T., & Gray, O. P. (1981). Parents' report of family life with a developmentally delayed child. *Child: Care, Health, & Development, 1,* 267–279.

Wolraich, M. L., & Siperstein, G. N. (1983). Assessing professionals' prognostic impressions of mental retardation. *Mental Retardation, 21,* 8–12.

Zigler, E., & Balla, D. (Eds.) (1982) *Mental retardation: The developmental–difference controversy.* Hillside, NJ: Erlbaum.

Zigler, E., & Valentine, J. (1979). *Project Head Start: A legacy of the War on Poverty.* New York: Free Press.

Name index

449

Swift, E., 309
Sylvester-Bradley, B., 119

Tager-Flusberg, H., 256, 257, 263, 287, 288,
    303, 339
Takashima, S., 33, 75, 79
Tawney, J. W., 430
Taylor, D. G., 51
Taylor, L., 113
Taylor, N., 345
Teller, D., 151
Terdal, L., 125, 427
Terman, L. M., 265
Tetzchner, S., 342, 344, 354, 361
Tew, B. J., 404
Thase, M., x, 34, 75
Thoa, N., 773
Thoman, E. B., 105
Thomas, A., 63, 64, 85
Thompson, J., 256
Thompson, J. R., 256
Thompson, M. M., 279, 306, 307
Thompson, R., 30, 42, 51, 84, 93, 237, 333,
    360
Thorpe, J., 64, 86
Thorpe, J. K., 41, 116, 237
Thuline, H., ix, x
Thurline, H. C., 381
Tietjen, A. M., 402
Tingey, C., x
Tomkins, S., 42
Tomlin, C., 45, 52
Toth, S., 40, 47, 56
Tredgold, A. F., 381, 382
Trevarthen, C., 39, 103, 107, 108, 112, 124,
    130
Trevarthen, N. C., 119
Tronic, E., 130
Trost, M. A., 370
Troutman, B. R., 63
Tucker, D. M., 70, 72
Tucker, L. R., 212
Tulkin, S. R., 402
Turnbull, A. P., 434, 439
Turnure, J., 132, 283, 316, 360
Turpin, R., ix
Tversky, B., 262, 276

Unger, D. G., 402
Ungerer, J., 346, 354
Uzgiris, I. C., 11, 14, 21, 43, 180, 182, 184,
    185, 186, 187, 192, 193, 194, 195, 196,
    197, 199, 200, 202, 203, 204, 205, 206,
    211, 213, 217, 218, 219, 265, 279, 294,
    311

Vadasy, P. F., 407
Valentine, J., 425, 428

Vance, S., 206
Vandell, D., 371, 372
Vandenberg, B., 52, 350, 429
Varnhagen, C., 171, 175
Varnhagen, S., 171
Vaughn, B. E., 239, 241, 243
Vaughn, V., 352
Velleman, S. L., 258
Vernon, P., 18
Vietze, P., 13, 64, 79, 81, 93, 94, 166, 167,
    168, 349, 361
Villani, T. V., 427
Vincze, M., 372
Vine, I., 104, 112
Volterra, V., 13, 21, 133, 354
Voss, D. K., 139
Vygotsky, L. S., 233

Wachs, T., 206, 211, 213, 214, 222
Wachs, T. C., 64
Wagner, S., 42, 50, 56, 63, 64, 76, 78, 81, 94,
    95, 147, 151, 152, 154, 157, 163, 174,
    340, 360, 362
Wahler, R. G., 370
Waisbren, S. E., 404, 436
Walk, R., 82
Walker, L., 72
Wall, S., 50, 233
Wallace, C., 67, 75
Wallace, I., 150, 155, 156, 170
Wallin, J. E. W., 382
Walters, J., 373, 374
Wandersman, L. P., 402
Wanner, E., 313
Wapner, S., 1
Warwick, D. P., 402
Washburn, R. W., 373
Waters, E., 43, 49, 50, 233, 392
Watson, J. S., 117, 118, 130
Watson, M., 53, 358
Watson, M. W., 185, 193, 206, 207
Watson, R. L., 407
Waxton, M., 303
Webb, A., 306
Weeks, D., 321
Weinhouse, E. M., 376, 377
Weinraub, M., 402, 403
Weinshilbaum, R., 73, 79
Weintraub, D., 109
Weisberg, P., 130
Weiss, B., 304, 310, 319, 329, 333, 345, 350
Weiss, J., 410
Weiss, M., 41
Weiss, P., 331
Weiss-Perry, B., 11, 33, 45, 46, 53, 54, 164,
    198, 237, 302, 304, 310, 311, 312, 329,
    345, 429, 432, 435
Weistuch, L., 283, 433

Subject index

accessibility, of knowledge, 247
acetylcholine, and reactivity, 72
achievement orientation, of families, 413
ACTH, 71
activation, laterality, 70
activity level, 242
adrenaline, and activation, 73
affectionate behavior, 382
affective development
  and cognitive development, 44–7, 82–5, 168
  interactionism, 46–7
  motor aspects, 71, 82, 221
  parental perception, 88, 92
  play development relationship, 348–9
  sensorimotor development role, 221
  symbolic play correlation, 84
aggression, 374
Alzheimer's disease, 75–6
analytical language style, 356, 361
anxiety, 129
approach behavior
  maternal stimulation, 130–1
  temperament, 93–4
arousal
  biology of, 69–77
  and cognition, 42–4, 68, 77–85
  developmental stages, 49–50
  and temperament, 66–8
assessment
  alternate approaches, 56
  early intervention, 434–5
  psychometric test weaknesses, 150–1
attachment, 50–1, 108–9
attention, 147–79
  assessment paradigms, in infants, 151–66
  development, 147–79
  evaluative capacity influence, 80–1
  and eye contact, in infants, 112
  group designs, assessment, 157–8

in infants and toddlers, 150–69
  methodology, 170–1
  naturalistic studies, 166–9
  parental perceptions, 94–5
attitudes, parental, 403–4, 410, 414–15
attribute words, 294
attributions, parental, 406–7
auditory deficits
  early intervention implication, 431–2
  and language delay, 306, 432
auditory evoked potentials, 163
autism, and syntactic skills, 339
autonomic nervous system, 70–1
autonomous self, 51–2
avoidance behavior, 130–1

babbling, 13, 15
"baby talk," *see* motherese
Bayley scales, 170
Berkeley Growth Studies, 17
Berko cloze task, 308
blinking, 83–4
bonding, 108–9
Boston Down Syndrome Project, 332–63
"bottom up" language processing, 165
brain maturation, 75–6
"burn-out," 440

Carey Infant Temperament Questionnaire, 85–7
Casati-Lezine scales, 206
categorization, 252–301
  in infants, 154
  longitudinal study, 264–96
  methods of study, 255–7
  in older children, 287–9
  taxonomy, 261–4
  theory, 266–72
cerebral hemispheres, 70, 320
child rearing, 216–19

463

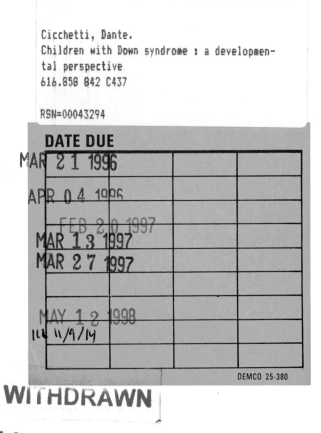